Management of Pancreatic Cancer

Management of Pancreatic Cancer

Guest Editor

Traian Dumitrascu

MDPI

Basel • Beijing • Wuhan • Barcelona • Belgrade • Novi Sad • Cluj • Manchester

Guest Editor
Traian Dumitrascu
Center of General Surgery and
Liver Transplantation
Carol Davila University of
Medicine and Pharmacy
Bucharest
Romania

Editorial Office
MDPI AG
Grossspeteranlage 5
4052 Basel, Switzerland

This is a reprint of the Special Issue, published open access by the journal *Cancers* (ISSN 2072-6694), freely accessible at: https://www.mdpi.com/journal/cancers/special_issues/N9QS9B1RXQ.

For citation purposes, cite each article independently as indicated on the article page online and as indicated below:

Lastname, A.A.; Lastname, B.B. Article Title. *Journal Name* **Year**, *Volume Number*, Page Range.

ISBN 978-3-7258-6069-2 (Hbk)
ISBN 978-3-7258-6070-8 (PDF)
https://doi.org/10.3390/books978-3-7258-6070-8

Contents

About the Editor

Traian Dumitrascu

Traian Dumitrascu is currently a senior surgeon at the Center of General Surgery and Liver Transplant of Fundeni Clinical Institute, Bucharest, Romania, and is an academic staff member at the Carol Davila University of Medicine and Pharmacy. His primary clinical and research interest is HPB surgery, particularly pancreatic cancer surgery. He has published many scientific studies and reviews in peer-reviewed journals, gaining a Hirsch index of 18 and more than 2000 citations in Google Scholar.

Preface

This reprint includes a variety of original studies and reviews addressing the diagnosis and management of pancreatic cancer, a highly lethal disease that still has poor prognosis and limited curative-intent therapeutic resources. This reprint also includes studies addressing potential predictors of pancreatic cancer development and exploring the mechanisms of carcinogenesis in pancreatic cancer. A number of studies presenting real-life data regarding the outcomes of different therapeutic options in pancreatic cancer and the potential impact of diagnosis on the quality of life of these patients are considered a valuable asset.

Traian Dumitrascu
Guest Editor

cancers

MDPI

Article

The Role of ENHO in Pancreatic Adenocarcinoma: A Bioinformatics Approach †

Osama M. Younis [1,2], Zeid K. Al-Sharif [2], Ahmad E. Saeed [2], Fares B. Qubbaj [2], Jehad A. Yasin [2], Tasnim Nour [2], Yassine Alami Idrissi [1] and Anwaar Saeed [1,*]

1 Division of Hematology & Oncology, Department of Medicine, University of Pittsburgh Medical Center (UPMC), Pittsburgh, PA 15232, USA; osamayns301@gmail.com (O.M.Y.); yalamiidr@gmail.com (Y.A.I.)
2 School of Medicine, The University of Jordan, Amman 11942, Jordan; zaidalsharif123@gmail.com (Z.K.A.-S.); fares.baha@hotmail.com (F.B.Q.); jehadamerjehadyasin@gmail.com (J.A.Y.); t.nour@ju.edu.jo (T.N.)
* Correspondence: saeeda3@upmc.edu; Tel.: +1-412-623-2091

† This article is a revised and expanded version of a paper entitled "ENHO's Protective Role in Pancreatic Adenocarcinoma", which was presented at the ESMO Gastrointestinal Cancers Congress 2024, Munich, Germany, 26–29 June 2024.

Simple Summary: Pancreatic adenocarcinoma is an aggressive cancer that has a 5-year overall survival rate of 13%. *ENHO* encodes for Adropin, a protein that is known to modulate glucose and fat metabolism. Previous studies have shown that exogenous Adropin administration to pancreatic cancer cell lines results in cancer growth. In this study, we sought to study the role of endogenous *ENHO* expression by assessing the transcriptomic landscape associated with *ENHO* expression in pancreatic adenocarcinoma. We identified that increased *ENHO* expression was associated with better overall survival. Further exploration of this discrepancy revealed that *ENHO* expression was associated with a protective immune microenvironment, protective noncoding RNA expression profile, and a microenvironment with downregulated extracellular matrix reorganization and epithelial-mesenchymal transition. We propose *ENHO* as a protective prognostic biomarker in pancreatic adenocarcinoma.

Abstract: Background: Pancreatic adenocarcinoma (PAAD) is an aggressive subtype of pancreatic cancer that is estimated to have a 5-year overall survival rate of only 13%. Most patients present with advanced disease with unpredictable outcomes. The identification of prognostic biomarkers is important to accurately stratify these patients. Methods: We investigated the molecular and survival-related role of *ENHO* in PAAD by analyzing TGCA mRNA and miRNA data. Survival analysis was conducted using TIMER2.0, "survival", and "survminer". Gene set enrichment analysis was conducted using enrichr, while miRNA-mRNA interactions were identified using "multiMiR". Immune infiltration was assessed using CIBERSORT ABS and ImmuCellAI. Results: We observed that *ENHO* was strikingly downregulated in PAAD tissues ($p = 3.68 \times 10^{-68}$), and patients with higher *ENHO* levels enjoyed significantly better overall survival (HR = 0.597; 95% CI: 0.419–0.852; $p < 0.01$). Pathway analysis showed that genes co-upregulated with *ENHO* were enriched for insulin secretion and ion channel activity, whereas those co-downregulated were related to epithelial–mesenchymal transition and extracellular matrix remodeling. Higher *ENHO* also tracked with increased $CD8^+$ T-cell infiltration and correlated positively with PDCD1 and LAG3 but negatively with B7-H3, CD70, and NT5E. Conclusions: Our results point to a protective role for *ENHO* in pancreatic adenocarcinoma.

Keywords: ENHO; pancreatic adenocarcinoma; Adropin; bioinformatics

 https://doi.org/10.3390/cancers17132139

1. Introduction

Pancreatic adenocarcinoma (PAAD) is an aggressive malignancy by all standards. It is the third leading cause of cancer-related deaths amongst males and females in 2024 in the United States [1], and some estimate it will soon become the second leading cause by 2030 [2]. PAAD is notoriously linked with a poor prognosis, highlighted by a five-year survival rate of roughly 13% [3]. This underscores the urgent need for comprehensive investigations into the genetic underpinnings of its pathogenesis and the prognostic implications.

One genetic factor of emerging interest is the energy-homeostasis-associated (*ENHO*) gene, which plays a vital role in lipid and glucose metabolism. Experimental studies indicate that *ENHO* is regulated by the nuclear Liver X Receptor (LXR), a sensor that adjusts its activity in response to lipid and glucose levels. Specifically, when high fat levels are detected, *ENHO* expression is upregulated, and its protein product, Adropin, subsequently facilitates fat storage through the modulation of hepatic lipogenic proteins and interaction with the Peroxisome Proliferator-Activated Receptor Gamma (PPAR-γ), a key mediator of adipogenesis [4]. Additionally, Adropin has shown its influence on endothelial cell function and promotes angiogenesis by stimulating Endothelial Nitric Oxide Synthase (eNOS) expression via the VEGFR2-PI3K-Akt and VEGFR2-ERK1/2 signaling pathways [5].

PAAD, like other pancreatic cancers, sustains its growth and survival through three metabolic adaptations. These include reprogramming intracellular metabolism for glucose, amino acids, and lipids; intricate cross-talk with components of the tumor microenvironment; and enhanced nutrient acquisition through scavenging and recycling mechanisms [2].

The binding between Adropin and its putative receptor, GPR19, further highlights the complex role of this pathway in cancer biology. In mesenchymal-like breast cancer, for example, overexpression of GPR19 stimulates E-Cadherin expression and induces an epithelial-like phenotype via the MAPK/ERK1/2 pathway, thereby contributing to carcinogenesis and metastasis. Paradoxically, other studies have reported that high-level Adropin can induce apoptosis in an MCF-7 breast cancer cell line [6]. Similarly, in colorectal cancer, decreased Adropin expression has been linked to disease progression, with the carcinoma cell expression of Adropin inversely correlated with macrophage infiltration. Moreover, high concentrations of Adropin appear to promote pro-tumorigenic activities by inhibiting inflammasome activation and favoring the induction of M2 macrophages. Conversely, the upregulation of Adropin in tumor-associated macrophages correlates with increased metastasis and invasion. At the same time, transfection of the *ENHO* gene into MC38 colon cancer cells has shown inhibition of tumor growth in vivo. Moreover, low-dose Adropin treatment may enhance antitumor functions by stimulating inflammasome activity and promoting M1 macrophage induction [7].

In the context of pancreatic ductal adenocarcinoma (PDA), the treatment of xenografts with Adropin has been observed to promote cancer cells' proliferation and migration, concomitant with the upregulation of P-VEGFR2, Ki67, Cyclin D1, and Matrix Metalloprotein 2 expression. In contrast, the knockdown of Adropin yields opposite effects, effectively limiting PDA growth both in vitro and in vivo [8].

Given *ENHO*'s gene's central role in regulating energy homeostasis and, by extension, the metabolic adaptations critical for PAAD survival, there is compelling evidence for investigating its clinical implications. In light of the paradoxical effects observed for *ENHO* and its product Adropin across different cancer types, this study aimed to delineate the genetic and transcriptomic landscape of *ENHO* in PAAD patients, elucidating its prognostic significance and association with the tumor microenvironment.

2. Methods

2.1. Patient Population

The Cancer Genome Atlas (TCGA) PAAD project (https://portal.gdc.cancer.gov/projects/TCGA-PAAD, accessed on 28 April 2024) contains 187 sequenced pancreatic adenocarcinoma tumor samples at different stages of disease. This included 183 patients with *ENHO* expression counts. We retrieved the mRNA and miRNA raw count data for all patients. All subsequent analyses were performed either directly on this dataset or via online webtools that utilize the same patient cohort.

2.2. Differential Gene and miRNA Expression

First, we compared *ENHO* expression in normal pancreatic tissue with that in pancreatic cancer tissue using TNMnet (https://tnmplot.com/analysis/, accessed on 28 April 2024) [9]. Further differential gene expression analysis based on *ENHO* expression was carried out by labeling the top and bottom 25% of *ENHO* gene expressors in the TCGA PAAD cohort as "high" and "low" expressors, respectively. Differential expression analysis for both genes and miRNA between these groups was conducted using the "DeSeq2" package in R v4.3.2 [10]. For this analysis, we considered a Log2 fold change greater than 0.25 and an FDR-adjusted p-value below 0.05 as statistically significant. Lastly, the 25% cut-off was used to provide an adequate number of samples while maintaining enough variability in *ENHO* expression to represent biologically meaningful differences.

2.3. Survival Analysis

To evaluate the prognostic significance of *ENHO* in PAAD, survival analysis was conducted using different statistical models. A univariate Cox proportional hazards model was generated using the R packages "survival" [11] and "survminer" [12], with optimal cut-off points defined for *ENHO* expression. In addition, multivariate Cox regression analysis was conducted using TIMER2.0 (http://timer.cistrome.org, accessed on 28 April 2024) [13] for the same cohort. To further strengthen the prognostic significance of *ENHO* findings, Gene Set Variation Analysis (GSVA) based survival analysis using both upregulated and downregulated gene sets was retrieved from GSCAlite (https://guolab.wchscu.cn/GSCA/#/, accessed on 28 April 2024) [14].

2.4. Mutation Analysis

The mutational landscape of *ENHO* was characterized by gene gains, amplifications, shallow deletions, and deep deletions. We also explored the correlation between *ENHO* expression and tumor mutational burden and metaploidy. These analyses were performed using TCGEx [15] and cBioportal [16–18].

2.5. Drug Sensitivity

To assess how *ENHO* expression might influence drug response in PAAD, we conducted a drug sensitivity analysis using GSCAlite. This tool utilizes the Cancer Therapeutics Response Portal (CTRP) and the Genomics of Drug Sensitivity in Cancer (GDSC) datasets [14], both of which are large consortia of drug perturbation data in cancer cell lines. Correlation between gene expression and drug resistance was retrieved and represented via bubble plots. A positive correlation indicates that increased gene expression is related to drug resistance, while a negative correlation indicates drug sensitivity.

2.6. Immune Infiltration

The relationship between *ENHO* expression and different immune cells' infiltration in PAAD was examined through the immune infiltration analysis. Immune infiltration data were obtained from GSCAlite [14], which uses the "ImmuCellAI" algorithm [19] to quantify the expression of 24 distinct immune cell types. Furthermore, correlations between *ENHO* and other immune cell types were analyzed using the CIBERSORT ABS algorithm provided by TIMER2.0 [13]. Lastly, the prognostic impact of these immune cells was evaluated using data from TCGEx [15].

2.7. Protein–Protein Interactions and Co-Expressed Genes

A protein–protein interaction (PPI) network was generated using STRING (https://string-db.org/, accessed on 28 April 2024) [20] to identify proteins interacting with *ENHO*. Additionally, co-expressed genes were extracted using cBioPortal [16–18], with a focus on correlations between *ENHO* and key chemokines, human leukocyte antigens (HLAs), immune checkpoints, and immunostimulatory genes, and visualized. These genes were specifically chosen in order to show how *ENHO* correlates with the immune environment within a bulk RNA dataset.

2.8. Gene Set Enrichment Analysis and Transcription Factor Activity

Gene set enrichment analysis (GSEA) was conducted on both upregulated and downregulated genes using Enrichr [21–23] to identify biological pathways associated with *ENHO* expression in PAAD. The top 10 enriched terms from Gene Ontology (GO) (biological processes, molecular functions, and cellular components), Reactome, MsigDB, and KEGG were extracted and visualized using the ggplot2 package in R v4.3.2. Lastly, we analyzed transcription factor (TF) expression and activity using the NetAct R package. This analysis was based on the top and bottom 10% of *ENHO* expressors in the TCGA PAAD, with the NetAct package quantifying the TFs' expression, and subsequently using differentially expressed TF targets to quantify their activation [24]. The top and bottom 10% of *ENHO* expressors were chosen to provide a balance between the number of patients and meaningful results. Specifically, the NetAct package was made to compare differences between wet-lab experiments, which usually have a lower number of samples but higher biological variation. Using the top and bottom 10% of expressors was able to impose similar results.

2.9. mRNA-miRNA Interactions

Validated interactions between differentially expressed miRNA and downregulated mRNA were retrieved from mirTarBase and Targetscan using the "MultiMiR" package in R v4.3.2. A network was then generated using CytoScape along with its Cytohubba add-on to assess network metrics. Furthermore, the correlation between miRNA and mRNA expression was validated in the TCGA PAAD cohort using TCGEx and LinkedOmics [15,25].

3. Results

3.1. Comprehensive Analysis of ENHO Gene Alterations, Expression, and Clinical Correlations

The study population comprised a total of 183 pancreatic cancer patients with available *ENHO* expression data, stratified into groups based on median (Med) and quartile (Q1, Q3) cutoffs for STAR count expression levels. The mean age at index was 65.01 years (SD ± 11.16), with patients in the lower median group significantly older than those in the higher median group (66.45 vs. 62.85 years, $p = 0.0287$). Consistently, patients in the lower quartile (≤Q1) were older than those in the upper quartile (≥Q3) (66.00 vs. 61.56 years, $p = 0.0411$). The cohort included 82 females (44.8%) and 101 males (55.2%). Race distribution was predominantly White (n = 161, 88%), followed by Asian (n = 12, 6.6%) and Black or African American (n = 6, 3.3%). Prior malignancy was reported in 19 patients (10.4%), and 105 participants (57.4%) reported a history of alcohol use.

Disease types were mainly ductal and lobular adenocarcinomas (n = 145, 79.2%), with a smaller proportion of adenomas/adenocarcinomas (n = 32, 17.5%) that were not further classified into ductal adenocarcinomas or other subtypes. The primary diagnosis had a significant association with *ENHO* expression groups (≥Med or <Med) ($p = 0.012$). Most tumors originated in the head of the pancreas (n = 131, 71.6%), and most samples were from primary tumor sites (n = 178, 97.3%), in contrast with only one sample (0.50%), which was metastatic.

Pathologic staging showed a predominance of stage IIB (n = 122, 66.7%) and T3 tumors (n = 147, 80.3%). Node involvement (N1) was common (n = 123, 67.2%), while distant metastases (M1) were rare (n = 5, 2.7%) (Table S2).

Smoking history varied, with a mean of 1.43 cigarettes/day and 23.39 years smoked. The tumor dimensions and weight at sampling showed large variation. Markedly, overall survival time differed significantly between expression groups, favoring higher *ENHO* expression: patients in the ≥Med group had a longer mean overall survival (667.53 vs. 454.45 days, Wilcoxon $p = 0.0006$), as did those in the ≥Q3 group compared to ≤Q1 (785.73 vs. 472.94 days, Wilcoxon $p = 0.0011$) (Table S3).

The prevalence of *ENHO* alteration was examined across samples, showing a high frequency of mRNA expression and gene amplification, while only a few samples showed downregulation of *ENHO*, as shown in Figure 1a,b. Despite these variations, it was found that *ENHO* is consistently downregulated in PAAD relative to normal pancreatic tissue (Figure 1c). Furthermore, a negative correlation was observed between *ENHO* expression and both mutation count (rho = −0.17, $p = 0.0434$) and tumor ploidy (rho = −0.17, $p = 0.038$), whereas no significant correlation between *ENHO* expression and TMB (rho = 0.03, $p = 0.767$) was found (Figure 1d–f).

3.2. ENHO Expression in Different Survival Outcomes

In order to assess the clinical relevance of *ENHO* expression in PAAD patients, extensive survival analysis was performed across four survival metrics: overall survival (OS), progression-free survival (PFS), disease-free interval (DFI), and disease-specific survival (DSS). Higher *ENHO* expression was consistently associated with better patient outcomes (Figure 2a). Moreover, a multivariate Cox regression model incorporating *ENHO*, Gender, Stage, and Age demonstrated a significant protective effect for *ENHO* (HR = 0.597, 95% CI: 0.419–0.852, $p < 0.01$) (Figure S4). Lastly, the prognostic role of the top 100 downregulated and top 100 upregulated genes based on high and low expression of *ENHO* in the TCGA PAAD cohort was explored. GSVA indicated that the top 100 downregulated genes were associated with poorer outcomes, whereas the upregulated genes exhibited a protective effect across all survival metrics, as illustrated by the bubble plot for OS, PFS, DSS, and DFI shown in Figure 2b,c.

3.3. ENHO Expression and Drug Sensitivity

ENHO's relationship to drug sensitivity was explored by utilizing two drug databases that provide information on the sensitivity of cancer cells to different drugs: the Genomics of Drug Sensitivity in Cancer (GDSC) database and Cancer Therapeutics Response Portal (CTRP) database. Figure 3 shows the correlation between *ENHO* expression and drug resistance to 5-Fluorouracil, Paclitaxel, and Gemcitabine, which are all drugs that are commonly used to treat pancreatic adenocarcinoma. The CTRP database showed that *ENHO* was not significantly associated with resistance to any of the three drugs. However, the GDSC database showed that ENHO was positively correlated with resistance to Paclitaxel (r = 0.17, $p = 0.03$) and Gemcitabine (r = 0.13, $p = 0.002$).

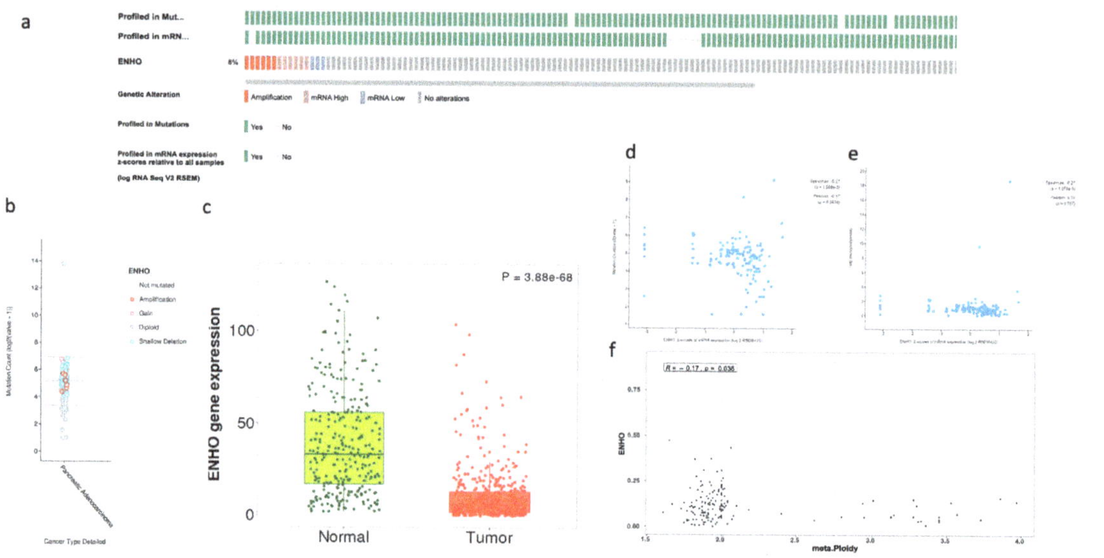

Figure 1. Complete mutational and expression landscape of *ENHO* in pancreatic adenocarcinoma. (**a**) shows onco-print showing the frequency of genetic alterations of *ENHO* in PAAD patients. (**b**) shows a further detailed box plot showing the types of mutations plotted against the mutation count. (**c**) shows the expression of *ENHO* in tumor vs. normal pancreatic tissue. (**d**) shows the correlation between *ENHO* mRNA expression and mutation count. (**e**) shows the correlation between *ENHO* mRNA expression and TMB. (**f**) shows the correlation between ENHO mRNA expression and aneuploidy of PAAD samples.

3.4. Immune Cell Infiltration

Given that PAAD is widely recognized as an immune desert, the role of *ENHO* in immune infiltration was examined. First, a correlation analysis was conducted between *ENHO* expression and the CIBERSORT absolute estimation of infiltration for nine different immune cell types. Increased *ENHO* expression was significantly correlated with higher infiltration of CD8+ T cells (rho = 0.345, $p < 0.001$), memory resting CD4+ T cells (rho = 0.377, $p < 0.001$), M2 macrophages (rho = 0.275, $p < 0.001$), and plasma B cells (rho = 0.23, $p = 0.0024$). Conversely, a significant negative correlation was observed between *ENHO* expression and the infiltration of M0 macrophages (rho = −0.283, $p < 0.001$) and resting NK cells (rho = −0.155, $p = 0.043$). Correlations with M1 macrophages, neutrophils, and activated CD4 memory cells did not reach statistical significance (Figure 4a).

To further strengthen our findings, an immune infiltration analysis was performed using the ImmuCellAI algorithm. The results were consistent with the previous findings, demonstrating positive correlations between *ENHO* expression and the infiltration of CD4+ T cells and CD8+ T cells, in addition to new associations with mucosal-associated invariant T cells (MAIT), NK cells, T follicular helper cells, and gamma delta T cells. Moreover, increased *ENHO* expression was associated with decreased infiltration of regulatory T cells (nTreg), monocytes, and dendritic cells (Figure 4b). The prognostic impact of each immune cell type in PAAD was also evaluated; however, none of the immune cell populations associated with *ENHO* expression had any significant prognostic effect (Figure 4c).

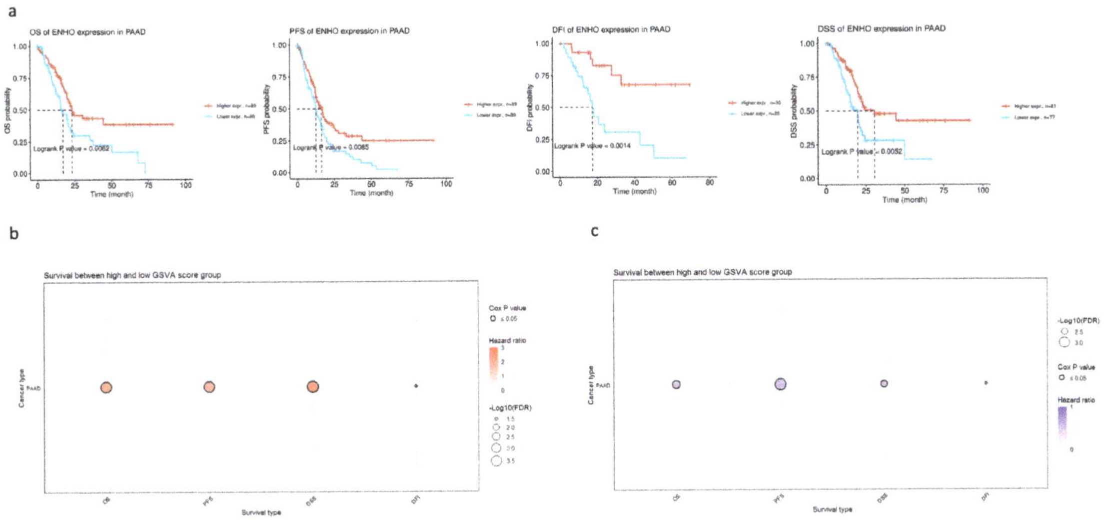

Figure 2. Prognostic role of *ENHO* in PAAD. (**a**) shows Kaplan–Meier plots splitting PAAD patients by their median *ENHO* expression into high and low groups for OS, PFS, DFI, and DSS. (**b**) shows the univariate cox-regression of the top 100 downregulated genes between high and low *ENHO* expressors. (**c**) shows the univariate Cox-regression of the top 100 upregulated genes between high and low *ENHO* expressors.

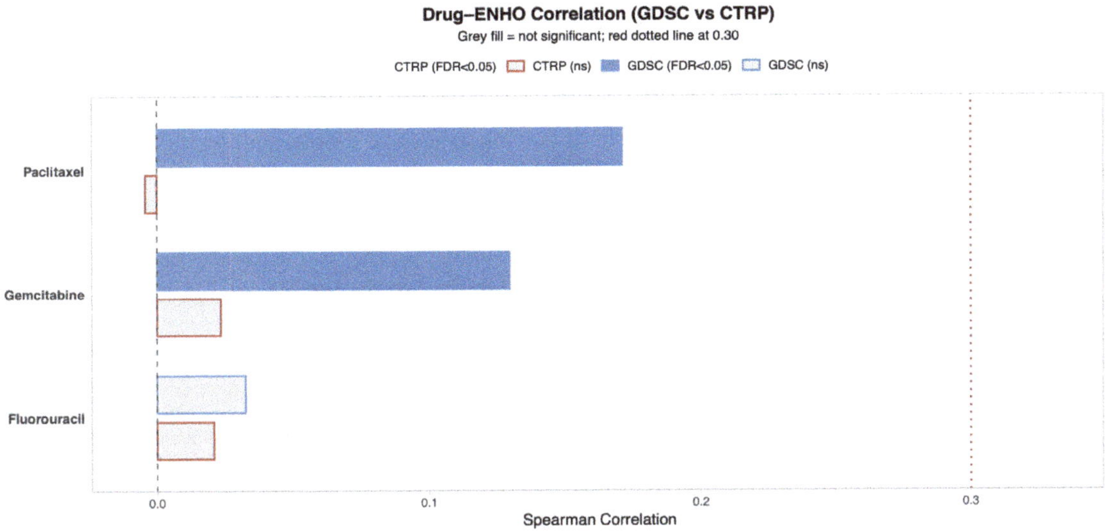

Figure 3. A comprehensive overview of the correlation between *ENHO* expression and drug sensitivity using both the GDSC and CTRP databases. Only drugs relevant to PAAD were included.

Finally, a correlation analysis was conducted to assess the association between *ENHO* expression and key immunological molecules, including chemokines, human leukocyte antigen (HLA), immune checkpoint inhibitors, and immunostimulatory genes. *ENHO* expression was positively co-expressed with chemokines such as CCL2, CCL4, CCL5, CCL14, CCL16, CCL19, CCL21, XCL2, and CXCL12 while being negative co-expression was noted with CCL20 and CXCL5. With regard to immunostimulatory molecules, positive co-expression was observed with CD27, CD40LG, IL6R, KLRG1, TNFRSF17, and CD48, whereas negative co-expression was detected with CD276 (B7-H3) and CD70, MICB and NT5E. In terms of antigen presentation, ENHO was positively co-expressed with HLA-DMA, HLA-DOA, HLA-DPA1, HLA-DPB1, and HLA-DRB1, which are integral to MHC class II-mediated antigen presentation and T cell activation, while negative co-expression with TAP1, TAP2, and TAPBP, which are genes involved in MHC class 1 antigen presentation. Lastly, ENHO was positively co-expressed with the immune checkpoint molecules PD-1 and LAG3 (Figure 5a).

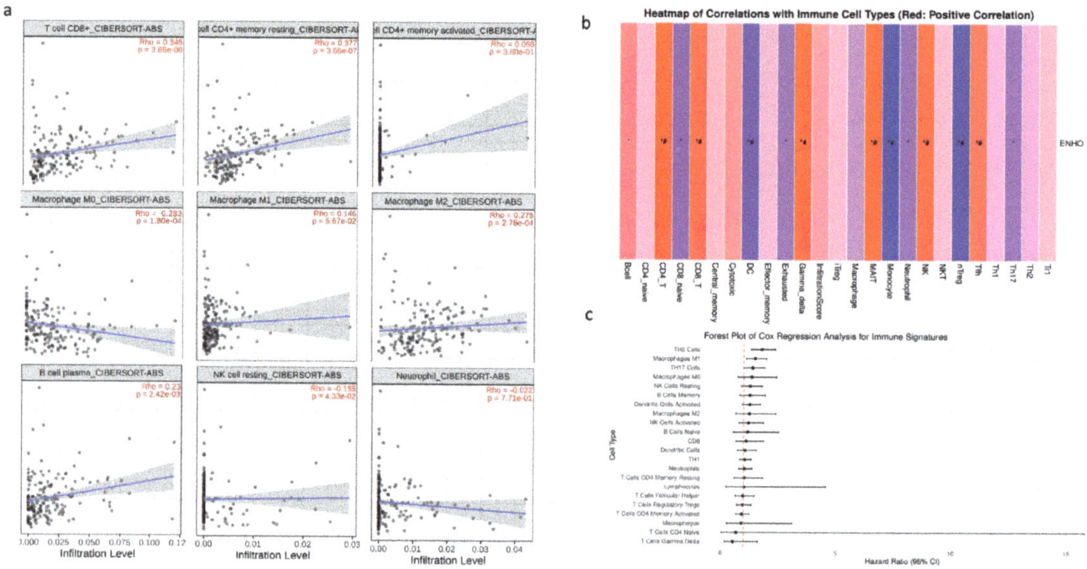

Figure 4. *ENHO* mRNA expression and immune cell infiltration analysis. (**a**) shows the infiltration of CD8+, resting CD4+, activated CD4+ T cells, M0, M1, and M2 macrophages, plasma B cells, resting NK cells, and neutrophils via the CIBERSORT ABS algorithm. (**b**) shows the infiltration of 24 different immune cell types by the ImmuCellAI algorithm. (**c**) shows a forest plot showing a multivariate Cox regression of all the immune cell types in pancreatic adenocarcinoma. * = $p < 0.05$, # = FDR < 0.05.

3.5. Gene Set Enrichment and Variation Analysis

GSE was performed on both upregulated and downregulated genes to elucidate the biological processes underlying *ENHO* expression patterns. The upregulated genes mainly showed enrichment in pathways associated with cellular homeostasis and neuronal regulation. Terms such as "Neuronal system", "Neuron projection", and "Ionotropic glutamate receptor complex" were enriched. In addition, pathways related to potassium and calcium channel activities, as well as those involved in the regulation of insulin and pancreatic secretion, were concomitantly enriched (Figure 5b). We also noted the upregulation of terms related to insulin secretion and pancreatic beta cell function. In contrast, the downregulated gene set was primarily enriched for terms related to extracellular matrix function and regulation. Enriched terms included "collagen formation", "extracellular structure organization", "external encapsulating structure organization", "extracellular matrix organization", and "collagen biosynthesis and modifying enzymes". Moreover, processes such as epithelial to mesenchymal transition (EMT), platelet-derived growth factor, hypoxia, and insulin-like growth factor 2 mRNA binding proteins were also enriched (Figure 5c).

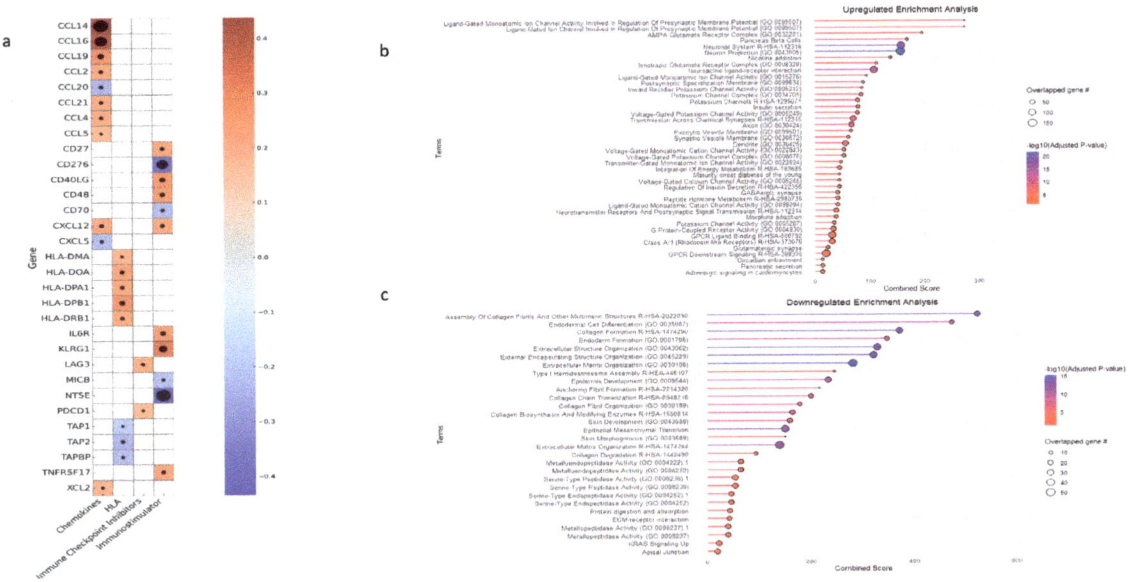

Figure 5. An elucidation of *ENHO*'s immune role, alongside a gene set enrichment analysis for the differentially expressed upregulated and downregulated genes. (**a**) shows a heatmap of the correlations between *ENHO* expression and different chemokines, human leukocyte antigens (HLAs), immune checkpoint inhibitors, and immunostimulators. (**b**) GSEA of differentially expressed upregulated genes. (**c**) GSEA of differentially expressed downregulated genes. The black circles in (**a**) correlate with -log10(FDR), all FDR's are < 0.05.

Looking at the differentially expressed genes, we saw that genes related to proper phasic insulin secretion were upregulated in patients with higher *ENHO* expression. In particular, there was an upregulation of genes that are crucial to the normal functioning of insulin secretion and sensitivity in the body. These were *GLUT2* (*SLC2A2*), *GLUT4* (*SLC2A4*), and key beta cell ion channels such as *KCNJ11* and *CACNA1D*. Furthermore, we also saw the upregulation of key IGF buffers, such as *IGFBPL1*, *IGF2-AS*, and *IGFALS*.

On the other hand, genes related to the Warburg effect, such as *GLUT1* (*SLC2A1*) and *HK2*, were downregulated. This was accompanied by the downregulation of downstream targets of *HIF-1a*, a key transcription factor up-regulated in the Warburg effect, such as *ANGPTL4*. We also saw the decreased expression of *IGF2BP1*, *2*, *3*, and multiple members of the IGFL family of peptides, all of which act to increase the stability of IGF or mimic its function (Table S1).

Further investigation into the transcriptional landscape of high *ENHO* expressors was carried out using GSVA. A set of ten well-established cancer pathways was used as a benchmark for this evaluation and assessed the activity of these pathways in three groups of genes: upregulated, downregulated, and co-expressed genes. The analysis revealed that the upregulated genes showed a significant correlation with *TSC/mTOR* activation. In contrast, the downregulated genes were significantly correlated with both *PI3K/AKT* and *TSC/mTOR* pathways. Lastly, co-expressed genes showed a positive correlation with the *TSC/mTOR* and *PI3K/AKT* pathways, while showing a negative correlation with apoptosis (Figure 6b–d).

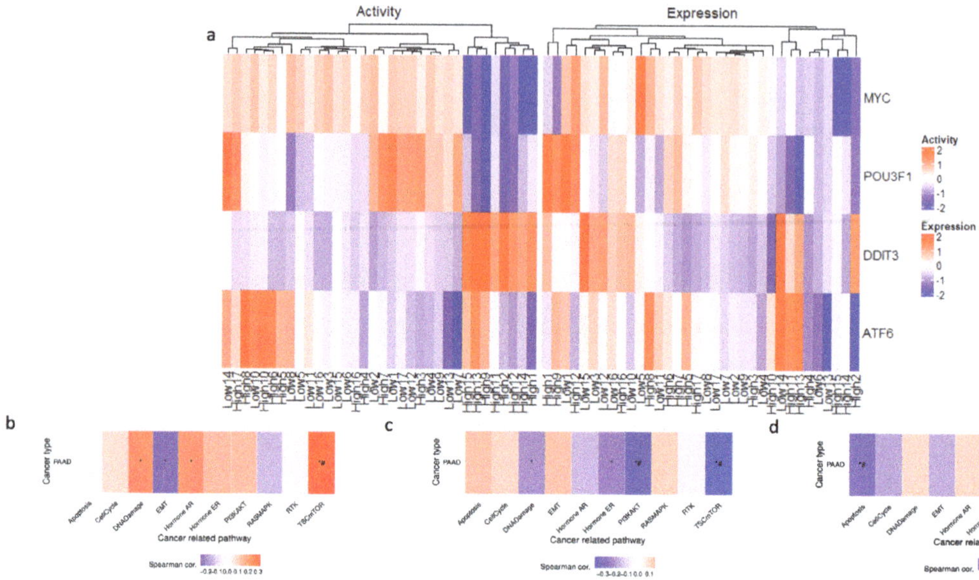

Figure 6. Exploring *ENHO*'s transcriptional landscape through transcription factor activity alongside Gene Set Variation Analysis of upregulated, downregulated, and co-expressed genes. (**a**) shows a heatmap that elucidates differential transcription factor expression and activity between the top and bottom 10% of *ENHO* expressors. (**b–d**) show the GSVA in 10 cancer-related pathways for differentially expressed (**b**) upregulated genes, (**c**) downregulated genes, and (**d**) co-expressed genes. * = $p < 0.05$, # = FDR < 0.05.

3.6. Transcription Factor Activity

Transcription factor activity analysis was performed in an attempt to uncover the underlying transcriptional network associated with high ENHO expressors. A heatmap (Figure 6a) was generated to display the differential activation of four activated transcription factors between high and low *ENHO* expressor groups. In particular, a cluster of high *ENHO* expressors was characterized by decreased activity of MYC and POU3F1, coupled with increased activity of DDIT3. Lastly, a small subset of five high expressors and two low expressors demonstrated increased activity of ATF6 (Figure 6a).

3.7. miRNA Differential Expression and miRNA-mRNA Interaction Networks

To further characterize the transcriptomic landscape of *ENHO* expressors, miRNA differential expression analysis was performed between high and low *ENHO* expressors. A total of 145 miRNAs were identified as significantly differentially expressed (FDR-adjusted p-value < 0.05). Subsequently, miRNA-mRNA interactions between differentially expressed miRNAs and genes were identified. In order to better understand miRNA function in the context of *ENHO*, we linked important enriched terms such as KRAS signaling, epithelial to mesenchymal transition, MET promotes cell motility, signaling by MET, and PI3K/AKT signaling pathway and their differentially expressed genes were integrated with the miRNA profiles, resulting in the miRNA-mRNA-function network illustrated in Figure 7.

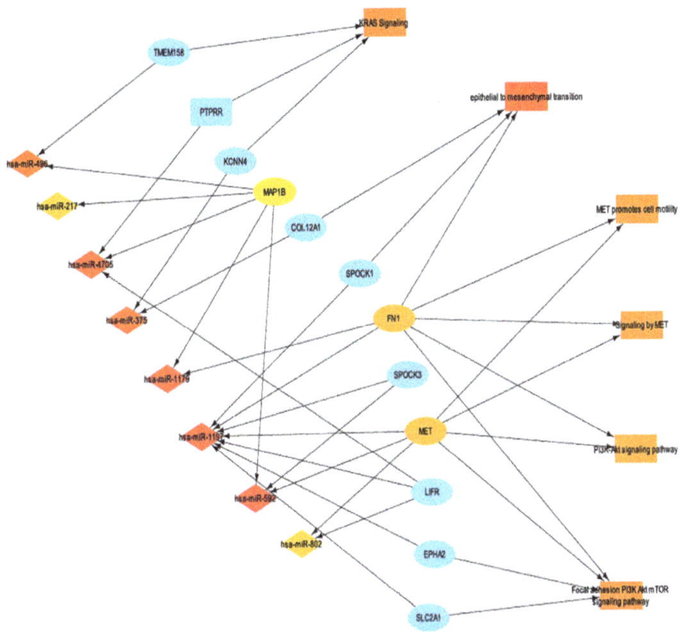

Figure 7. mRNA-mRNA interaction network with functionally enriched terms. It shows a subset of the network that contains the top 30 most connected nodes via maximum clique centrality (MCC).

Notably, two miRNAs stood out as particularly significant: hsa-miR-1179 (log2FC = 3.784, FDR p value < 0.001) and hsa-miR-375 (log2FC = 2.905, FDR p value < 0.001). Hsa-miR-1179 had validated interactions with *FN1*, a gene involved in EMT and MET signaling. Furthermore, hsa-miR-1179 had a positive correlation with *ENHO* expression (R = 0.57, $p < 0.0001$), while negative correlations were noted with both *FN1* (R = −0.35, $p < 0.0001$) and MET (R = −0.58, $p < 0.0001$) expression (Figure 8d–f). Hsa-miR-1179 also demonstrated a significant favorable prognostic effect ($p = 0.0035$) as shown by Figure 8h. Similarly, hsa-miR-375 was also associated with a favorable prognostic effect ($p = 0.033$) and primarily interacted with two genes: *KCCN4* and *COL12A1*, which are implicated in KRAS signaling and EMT, respectively (Figure 8g). Hsa-miR-375 was also positively correlated with *ENHO* (R = 0.42, $p < 0.0001$), and negatively correlated with *KCCN4* (R = −0.46, $p < 0.0001$) and *COL12A1* (R = −0.48, $p < 0.0001$) (Figure 8a–c).

In addition, hsa-miR-1197 and hsa-miR-592 were found to be positively co-expressed with *ENHO*, and negatively co-expressed with MET and *FN1*, albeit with associations that were less robust compared with the aforementioned miRNAs (Figures S1 and S2). A comprehensive list of differentially expressed miRNA and their respective fold change is provided in Table S4 Lastly, protein-protein interaction networks and their overall effect and tie in with ENHO are found in Figure S3.

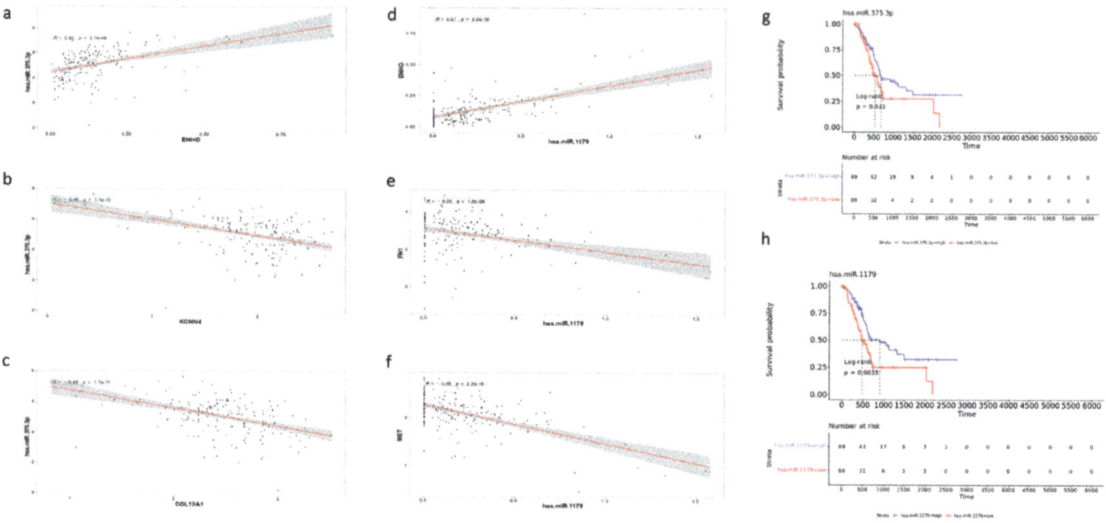

Figure 8. Validation of the role of different miRNAs in PAAD. The figure shows the correlation of MiR-375.3p with (**a**) *ENHO*, (**b**) *KCNN4*, and (**c**) *COL12A1*. Furthermore, the figure shows the correlation between MiR-1179 and (**d**) *ENHO*, (**e**) *FN1*, and (**f**) *MET*. (**g**) Kaplan–Meier of OS for MiR-375.3.p. (**h**) Kaplan–Meier of OS for MiR-1179.

4. Discussion

4.1. ENHO Dysregulation in Pancreatic Cancer

PAAD is an aggressive cancer associated with a 5-year survival rate of only around 13%, primarily due to its late-stage detection, a strong metastatic potential, and limited response to standard treatments [26]. Addressing this clinical challenge requires identifying novel biomarkers to enhance prognostication and guide therapeutic strategies. In the present study, we observed that *ENHO* expression was significantly lower in tumor tissues compared with normal pancreatic tissues ($p = 3.88 \times 10^{-68}$). This marked reduction suggests that *ENHO* dysregulation is a likely contributor to the development and progression of pancreatic cancer.

Further analysis revealed that *ENHO*'s upregulation in advanced stages of PAAD correlates with better overall survival (HR: 0.597, 95% CI: 0.419–0.852, $p < 0.01$), as well as improved PFS, DFI, and DSS. These findings highlight the clinical relevance of *ENHO* as a potential prognostic biomarker that could allow clinicians to stratify PAAD patients based on their survival risk, and is consistent with our previously reported results [27]. Specifically, patients with lower *ENHO* levels might be identified as higher-risk and could benefit from more intensive monitoring and treatment strategies. Conversely, higher *ENHO* levels could indicate a less aggressive disease course, thus aiding clinicians in treatment planning and patient counseling.

Pathway enrichment analysis further supported *ENHO*'s potential tumor-suppressive role in PAAD. High *ENHO* expression was negatively correlated with pro-oncogenic pathways such as PI3K/AKT, suggesting that *ENHO* may hinder tumor growth by suppressing these pathways. Conversely, low *ENHO* expression was associated with the activation of pathways related to epithelial-mesenchymal transition (EMT), extracellular matrix organization, and cancer metastasis. These findings shed light on *ENHO*'s potential as a protective factor in PAAD by potentially reducing invasiveness and metastatic potential.

Additionally, high *ENHO* expression is associated with a unique transcriptional landscape, characterized by the increased activity of *DDIT3*, a gene involved in integrated stress response pathways that code for pro-apoptotic transcription factors [28]. Concurrently, the transcription factors MYC and POU3F1, both known for driving cell proliferation and oncogenic signaling, were downregulated. Additionally, miRNA analysis revealed that hsa-miR-592 positively correlated with *ENHO* expression and was linked with the downregulation of oncogenes such as *MET* (a receptor tyrosine kinase that promotes cell growth and metastasis) and *HMGA2* (a transcriptional regulator involved in tumor progression and EMT). This negative correlation further highlights its potential tumor-suppressive function.

Similarly, the analysis also identified hsa-miR-1179 and hsa-miR-1197 as miRNAs that are positively associated with *ENHO* expression. These miRNAs also exhibited tumor-suppressive roles by negatively correlating with key oncogenes such as *FN1* and *MET*. Notably, both hsa-miR-592 and hsa-miR-1179 were significantly upregulated in high *ENHO* expressors, showing positive fold changes compared to low *ENHO* expressors. Moreover, hsa-miR-375 was also upregulated in high *ENHO* expressors and negatively correlated with *KCCN4* and *COL12A1*, genes linked to KRAS signaling and EMT, respectively. Together, these findings support the notion that *ENHO* expression has a protective role, potentially contributing to a less invasive and metastatic tumor PAAD phenotype. Furthermore, survival analysis revealed that high expression of hsa-miR-1179 (log-rank $p = 0.0035$) and hsa-miR-375 (log-rank $p = 0.033$) was associated with improved overall survival, further underscoring their role in tumor progression. These data collectively suggest that *ENHO*'s regulation of miRNAs might contribute to its potential as a biomarker and a key player in suppressing aggressive tumor behavior in PAAD.

4.2. *ENHO and Tumor Microenvironment (TME)*

The immunomodulatory role of *ENHO* in the PAAD tumor microenvironment was examined. High *ENHO* expression was observed to be positively correlated with immune infiltration, notably with increased levels of CD8+ T cells, CD4+ T cells, plasma B cells, and M2 macrophages. A positive co-expression of *ENHO* with *TNFRSF17*, a B-cell maturation factor, suggests that *ENHO* may facilitate the recruitment of more mature B cells into the tumor microenvironment, thereby contributing to anti-tumor effects. Additionally, *ENHO* was positively co-expressed with MHC class II presentation genes (including *HLA-DMA*, *HLA-DOA*, *HLA-DPA1*, *HLA-DPB1*, and *HLA-DRB1*), supporting its role in promoting anti-tumor immunity. In contrast, *ENHO* exhibited negative co-expression with MHC class I-related genes (*TAP1*, *TAP2*, and *TAPBP*), which may reflect a tumor-driven mechanism aimed at evading cytotoxic T cell-mediated immune surveillance. Moreover, a positive association between *ENHO* expression and chemokines such as *CCL14* and *CCL16* further indicates that ENHO may be associated with immune cell recruitment within PAAD's microenvironment.

ENHO also demonstrated negative correlations with immune checkpoint molecules *CD276* (B7-H3) and *CD70*, both of which are associated with immune suppression and adverse outcomes in cancer [29,30]. The observed downregulation of B7-H3 in conjunction with high *ENHO* levels suggests a diminished capacity for immune evasion, particularly given *B7-H3*'s known role in promoting tumor progression in pancreatic cancer.

Preclinical studies have further underscored the therapeutic significance of these findings, showing enhanced CAR-T efficacy when targeting CD276 and CD70 simultaneously [31]. Additionally, a modest positive co-expression between *ENHO* and *PDCD1* (PD-1) as well as *LAG3* indicates the potential for effective immunotherapy through immune checkpoint inhibition in patients with high *ENHO* expression.

The data also implies that *ENHO* is involved in a dual state of immunomodulation, where immune activation is promoted yet counteracted by tumor escape mechanisms. For instance, the positive correlation between *ENHO* and *CD27*, along with the negative correlation with its ligand *CD70*, suggests a protective immune response driven by *ENHO*, even as tumor strategies, such as upregulating immune checkpoints like PD-1 and *LAG3* or suppression of MHC-I antigen presentation via the downregulation of *TAP1*, *TAP2*, and *TAPBP*, counterbalance this effect. Moreover, *ENHO*'s negative correlations with other immune checkpoint molecules, such as *CD276* (B7-H3) and *NT5E* (CD73), which are implicated in immune escape by suppressing T-cell activity and promoting regulatory T-cell (Treg) responses [29,32], further reinforce its potential anti-tumor role. These observations are consistent with the findings of Li et al. [33], which highlight the contribution of such immune checkpoints to the progression of PAAD.

Although Xiao et al. reported that *TAP1* and *TAP2* are consistently upregulated in interferon-gamma-dominant PAAD subtypes, underscoring their role in MHC-1 antigen loading and presentation to cytotoxic T-cells [34], the analysis emphasized the downregulation of *TAP1* and *TAP2* as a tumor-mediated strategy for immune evasion. Overall, a more proficient adaptive immune response was observed in association with high *ENHO* expression, which appears to coexist with a tumor-driven attenuation of cytotoxic T cell responses due to the dysregulation of MHC-I and immune checkpoint molecules. These findings suggest that ENHO levels may serve as an indicator of patient response to immune checkpoint blockade in PAAD, although further clinical research is warranted to substantiate this potential.

4.3. Drug Sensitivity and Clinical Implications

The analysis of drug sensitivity, using data from the GDSC and CTRP databases, revealed an intriguing and somewhat paradoxical relationship between *ENHO* expression and the efficacy of multiple chemotherapeutic agents. It was observed that higher *ENHO* expression was linked to increased resistance to Paclitaxel and Gemcitabine, which together make up the drug regimen GemTaxol. GemTaxol is used in patients with pancreatic adenocarcinoma and is better tolerated than its more aggressive counterpart, the FOLFIRINOX regimen, which is usually reserved for younger, more fit patients. Despite this, several studies have noted that both regimens offer no difference in overall survival benefit [35].

ENHO's association with increased resistance toward both drugs used in GemTaxol could indicate clinical utility as a resistance biomarker; however, more robust biomarker validation studies are needed to confirm this observation.

4.4. Consistencies and Discrepancies with Prior Research

A review of the literature on *ENHO* and its genetic product, Adropin, in the context of PAAD reveals that the analysis may both contextualize and extend the findings of earlier studies. Although research in this area remains limited, the study by Hu et al. represents the only prior investigation of *ENHO*'s role in PAAD. Their in vitro experiments demonstrated that elevated Adropin levels in PANC-1 and CFPAC-1 cell lines enhanced proliferation, migration, and the expression of *p-VEGFR2*, *Ki67*, *cyclin D1*, and *MMP2*. Cells were treated with 50 nM recombinant Adropin (amino acids 34–76), a concentration selected based on preliminary dose-response testing, and assessed 96 h post-lentiviral infection. Mechanistically, Adropin's pro-tumorigenic effects were mediated via sustained activation of the *VEGFR2* signaling pathway, as shown by the reversal of these effects upon treatment with 16 μM Apatinib, a *VEGFR2* inhibitor. In vivo, Hu et al. established cell-derived xenografts (CDX) in nude mice injected subcutaneously with 1×10^6 PANC-1 cells. Daily intraperitoneal administration of 450 nmol/kg recombinant Adropin resulted in significantly accelerated tumor growth, increased microvessel density (CD31+), and elevated *VEGFR2* pathway activation. Conversely, tumors derived from Adropin-knockdown cells showed reduced growth and angiogenesis [8]. In contrast, the present study found that enhanced *ENHO* expression correlated with improved survival outcomes across multiple metrics, suggesting a potentially protective role. This apparent discrepancy highlights the need for further investigation to clarify the context-specific functions of *ENHO* and Adropin in PAAD.

This divergence from the findings of Hu et al. potentially arises from a combination of contributing factors. PANC-1, CFPAC-1 cell lines, and BALB/c nude mouse xenografts lack a functionally mature immune system and may not accurately emulate the complexity of the human tumor microenvironment [36]. This implication limits the applicability of their findings to human immunity, especially considering that *ENHO*'s antitumor effects appear to be mediated by immunomodulation within the tumor microenvironment. In contrast, our analysis captures the natural course of *ENHO* expression in patient tumors, within an intact immunometabolic setting, and examines how endogenous levels correlate with clinical outcomes, rather than testing the effects of recombinant Adropin administration. Furthermore, Hu et al. used supraphysiologic doses of recombinant Adropin (450 nmol/kg), which exceed physiologic serum concentrations (0.222–2.222 nmol/kg) [37]. Adropin's effects on the immune system are possibly dose dependent, as shown by Jia et al., high doses may promote tumor progression while small doses (<100 ng/mL) amplify antitumor functions [7].

In addition, the literature on *ENHO*'s role in other cancers has produced conflicting findings that appear to be context dependent, varying by cancer type and Adropin dosage. For example, the work of Jia et al. indicated that the overall effect of Adropin effect in MC38 colorectal cancer depends on the administered dose: high doses were shown to promote pro-tumor activities by inhibiting inflammasome activation and inducing M2 macrophages, whereas low doses (<100 ng/mL) enhance antitumor macrophage functions via the stimulation of the inflammasome and induction of M1 macrophage. Furthermore, the upregulation of Adropin in carcinoma cells was negatively associated with macrophage infiltration and positively associated with metastasis and invasion in tumor-associated macrophages. Moreover, the Adropin overexpressing MC38 cells also exhibited increased CD8+ T cell infiltration [7]. These findings are in line with our immune infiltration analysis, where we demonstrated that although *ENHO* expression was associated with increased M2 macrophages, it also correlated with an elevated infiltration of CD8+ T cells, CD4+ T cells, and plasma B cells, thereby indicating a more hostile microenvironment in PAAD patients.

Stelcer et al. reported that exposure to Adropin in HAC15 adrenal carcinoma cell lines stimulates long-lasting proliferation through AKT-mediated pathways, with the proliferative effect being completely abolished by PI3K/AKT inhibitors [38]. In contrast, the pathway analysis presented herein suggested that the gene expression patterns associated with high *ENHO* expression in PAAD were linked to the suppression of PI3K/AKT signaling. Although direct co-expression analysis indicated a positive correlation between *ENHO* and genes involved in PI3K/AKT signaling, the overall data support the notion that while exogenous Adropin may exert pro-tumorigenic effects, endogenous *ENHO* expression plays a more nuanced role in determining patient outcomes.

The study by Tuna et al. found that increased serum Adropin concentrations, induced by chronic or intermittent caloric restriction in an MMTV-TGFa breast cancer mouse model, were associated with a lower incidence of mammary tumors compared to mice with lower serum Adropin levels. Moreover, treatment of MCF-7 and MDA-MB231 breast cancer cells with Adropin significantly reduces cellular proliferation [39]. These findings are consistent with the present study, which found that increased *ENHO* expression was indicative of a less aggressive disease course and improved survival outcomes.

Rao et al. showed that Adropin binding to GPR19 upregulated E-cadherin via the ERK pathway, a process critical for EMT in MCF-7 and MDA-MB-231 breast cancer cells. This mechanism was posited to promote metastasis while also facilitating mesenchymal-epithelial transition, thereby contributing to the homing of primary tumor cells to secondary sites [40]. In this current analysis, upregulation of genes such as *CAV3*, *CAVIN2*, *SGCZ*, *DAG1*, *SNTG1*, and *SNTG2* in high *ENHO* expressors suggested an involvement in maintaining an epithelial phenotype. Yet, contrary to what was presented by Rao et al., it appears that this epithelial phenotype might be protective in PAAD patients, a finding further supported by the downregulation of *OVOL1*, a transcription factor known to drive EMT [41]. These results suggest a pleiotropic relationship between *ENHO* and cancer aggressiveness.

The findings of Nergiz et al., which reported reduced circulating Adropin levels in patients with endometrial cancer, closely parallel the present observation of downregulated *ENHO* expression in PAAD [42]. Both studies underscore the potential diagnostic utility of *ENHO* and Adropin in distinguishing cancer patients from healthy individuals, with the high sensitivity and specificity of Adropin in endometrial cancer reinforcing its role as a clinically relevant biomarker.

The study by Lin et al. demonstrated that the downregulation of miR-1179 in pancreatic cancer promotes cell proliferation through the silencing of E2F transcription factor 5 and that ectopic expression of miR-1179 suppresses migration, invasion, and proliferation by inducing G_0/G_1 cell cycle arrest [43]. These findings are consistent with the present, which showed the upregulation of miR-1179 in patients with high ENHO expression. With respect to hsa-miR-592 and has-miR-375-3p, the literature is sparse regarding their role in PAAD; however, the current findings suggest that these miRNAs may exhibit protective effects by targeting genes involved in *MET* signaling and EMT.

Lastly, we hypothesize that *ENHO*'s reflection of an overall favorable tumor microenvironment might come from its direct effect of regulating glucose metabolism and promoting the utilization of glucose in oxidative phosphorylation rather than aerobic glycolysis. The Warburg effect is a phenomenon that occurs when cancer cells shuttle glucose from oxidative phosphorylation to aerobic glycolysis to generate more cellular building blocks integral to their rapid proliferation [44]. Previous literature has shown that Adropin is a known regulator of insulin sensitivity and glucose utilization, where multiple pre-clinical studies have shown increased insulin sensitivity, decreased hepatic gluconeogenesis, and more efficient oxidative phosphorylation when treating multiple diseases such as coronary atherosclerosis and diabetes in mouse models [4]. A similar trend of insulin sensitivity and more physiological control of insulin was apparent in our study. Several upregulated genes, such as *GLUT4*, *GLUT2*, *KCNJ11*, and *CACNA1D*, indicate preserved insulin sensitivity and a more likely phasic secretion of insulin, indicating better insulin regulation. Furthermore, several genes integral to the Warburg effect were downregulated. This included *GLUT1* and *HK2*, which have been previously shown to significantly increase aerobic glycolysis in pancreatic cancer and are induced by *KRAS* and *STAT3*, respectively [45,46]. This, alongside the previous discussion about *ENHO*'s immunomodulatory role, is a plausible explanation for why increased *ENHO* expression is associated with better overall survival in pancreatic adenocarcinoma patients.

4.5. Limitations

While this study provides valuable insights into the potential role of *ENHO* as a prognostic biomarker in pancreatic adenocarcinoma (PAAD), several limitations should be noted. First, this bioinformatics-based analysis relied entirely on publicly available datasets, which—despite their comprehensiveness—may not fully capture the heterogeneity of real-world patient populations. Potential biases in sample selection, cohort composition, and data preprocessing could limit the generalizability of the findings.

Second, the study lacks experimental validation of key computational predictions. In particular, the inferred miRNA-mRNA interactions involving *ENHO*, the observed associations with immune infiltration, and its links to oncogenic signaling pathways require confirmation through in vitro and in vivo studies. Such validation is essential for establishing causality, determining *ENHO*'s role in PAAD progression and exploring its therapeutic potential at the transcriptomic and genomic levels.

Third, the use of bulk-RNA sequencing data does not allow for assessment of *ENHO* in specific cell types within the tumor microenvironment, potentially leading to incomplete conclusions. Fourth, no stratified analyses were conducted based on demographic or clinical factors such as age, sex, tumor stage, or comorbidities. These variables could influence *ENHO* expression and function, and should be examined in future research to better assess its utility across diverse patient subgroups.

Fourth, certain hypotheses generated in this study require more substantial evidence. For example, the hypotheses regarding ENHO's net protective effect against the Warburg effect need to be tested in pre-clinical models. Furthermore, insulin levels and pancreatic function in relation to ENHO need to be tested in vivo and possibly in pancreatic adenocarcinoma patients.

Finally, while comparisons with other cancers provide useful context, discrepancies in the literature highlight the need for further research to clarify *ENHO*'s role across different malignancies. Despite these limitations, the results highlight the translational potential of *ENHO* as a biomarker for patient stratification or therapeutic response prediction in PAAD. Advancing toward clinical application will require rigorous experimental validation and prospective studies to confirm its diagnostic, prognostic, and predictive value.

5. Conclusions

The discrepancies between the literature and the present analysis indicated that exogenous Adropin and endogenous *ENHO* expression may not overlap functionally in PAAD. Although Adropin, as the genetic product of the *ENHO* gene, appears to have an overall pro-tumorigenic effect when administered exogenously, by activating VEGFR2 and PI3K/AKT signaling pathways, the upregulation of ENHO in situ appears to confer a net protective effect in pancreatic adenocarcinoma. This protective effect is likely due to *ENHO*'s role in immune modulation, wherein it promotes immune infiltration and fosters a tumor microenvironment that is hostile to tumor growth. Furthermore, the metabolic reprogramming that *ENHO* is known for might play a role in modulating the metabolic utility of glucose in the context of cancer, favoring oxidative phosphorylation over aerobic glycolysis. It is further hypothesized that the protective network associated with *ENHO* upregulation, as evidenced by favorable immune signatures and miRNA interactions, cannot be fully recapitulated by exogenous Adropin treatment.

In summary, it is speculated that serum Adropin levels, which reflect *ENHO* expression within the tumor microenvironment, may more accurately represent the true role of *ENHO* in cancer, particularly in PAAD patients. Further research, through preclinical studies utilizing cancer models that better represent the tumor microenvironment and clinical studies assessing the levels of serum Adropin in pancreatic cancer patients, is warranted to confirm these findings and explore the relationship between serum Adropin levels, tissue *ENHO* expression, and patient outcomes.

Supplementary Materials: The following supporting information can be downloaded at https://www.mdpi.com/article/10.3390/cancers17132139/s1, Figure S1 shows the correlation of mir-1197 with its network interaction in Figure 7. (a) Shows the correlation between mir-1197 and ENHO. (b) Shows the correlation between mir-1197 and SLC2A1. (c) Shows the correlation between mir-1197 and EPHA2. (d) Shows the correlation between mir-1197 and MET. (e) Shows the correlation between mir-1197 and SPOCK1. (f) Shows the correlation between mir-1197 and FN1; Figure S2 validates the association between ENHO and MiR-592. (a) Shows the correlation between ENHO and MiR-592. (b) Shows the correlation between HMGA2 and MiR-592. (c) Shows the correlation between MET and MiR-592. (d) Kaplan Meier plot of OS for MiR-592; Figure S3 shows the Protein-to-protein interaction network for ENHO. (a) Shows the PPI network extracted from STRING. (b) Represents the GSVA pathway enrichment of the 13 differentially expressed genes. (c) Shows a dotplot of the prognostic outcomes of each of the 13 differentially expressed genes linked to ENHO; Figure S4 shows the multivariate forest plot for ENHO expression while accounting for Stage, Age, and Gender; Table S1 shows the Log Fold Change of multiple genes that were differentially expressed between high and low ENHO expressors; Table S2. *Distribution of clinical and pathological variables by expression quartiles and median groups, with Monte Carlo-derived p-values.* * *$p < 0.05$; NR: Not Reported. Expression metric: STAR Count.* Note: Frequencies and column-wise percentages are shown for each category under <Med vs. ≥Med and ≤Q1 vs. ≥Q3 *Adropin* expression groups. *p*-values were calculated using Monte Carlo permutation tests with 1000 simulations per variable. *p*-values are omitted (N/A) where statistical testing was not applicable due to insufficient data or zero counts; Table S3. *Comparison of Continuous Variables Across Median and Quartile Groups Using Wilcoxon Rank-Sum Test. Expression metric: STAR Count.* This table presents the comparison of continuous clinical and sample-related variables stratified by the median (Med) and quartiles (Q1 and Q3). Mean ± standard deviation (SD) values are shown for each group. *p*-values are derived from the Wilcoxon rank-sum test, assessing differences between high vs. low median groups and between upper (≥Q3) and lower (≤Q1) quartile Adropin expression groups. Asterisks (*) indicate statistically significant differences ($p < 0.05$). Variation in sample sizes ("n") across comparisons reflects missing values ("NA") excluded from analyses. Quantile cutoffs were based on all samples with reported expression data (n = 183); Table S4 Shows differentially expressed miRNA between high and low ENHO expressors.

Author Contributions: O.M.Y. conceived and designed the study. O.M.Y., F.B.Q., J.A.Y. and A.E.S. acquired and analyzed the data. O.M.Y., Z.K.A.-S., A.E.S. and T.N. interpreted the results. All authors drafted the manuscript. A.S. and Y.A.I. substantively revised the manuscript. All authors have read and agreed to the published version of the manuscript.

Funding: This research received no external funding.

Institutional Review Board Statement: All human data used in this project were from previously published data, where ethics approval and consent were published with the accompanied manuscript.

Informed Consent Statement: All data used are public access and can be used for research purposes.

Data Availability Statement: All the data used in this paper can be accessed publicly via the TCGA at the genomic data commons (https://portal.gdc.cancer.gov/, accessed on 28 April 2024) or through the online analysis webtools mentioned within the methods section of this article.

Conflicts of Interest: Anwaar Saeed reports advisory board role with AstraZeneca, Bristol-Myers Squibb, Merck, Exelixis, Pfizer, Xilio therapeutics, Taiho, Amgen, Autem therapeutics, KAHR medical, and Daiichi Sankyo; institutional research funding from AstraZeneca, Bristol-Myers Squibb, Merck, Clovis, Exelixis, Actuate therapeutics, Incyte Corporation, Daiichi Sankyo, Five prime therapeutics, Amgen, Innovent biologics, Dragonfly therapeutics, Oxford Biotherapeutics, Arcus therapeutics, and KAHR medical; and participation as a data safety monitoring board chair for Arcus therapeutics. The remaining authors have no relevant financial interests to disclose.

References

1. Siegel, R.L.; Giaquinto, A.N.; Jemal, A. Cancer statistics, 2024. *CA Cancer J. Clin.* **2024**, *74*, 12–49. [CrossRef] [PubMed]
2. Qin, C.; Yang, G.; Yang, J.; Ren, B.; Wang, H.; Chen, G.; Zhao, F.; You, L.; Wang, W.; Zhao, Y. Metabolism of pancreatic cancer: Paving the way to better anticancer strategies. *Mol. Cancer* **2020**, *19*, 50. [CrossRef]
3. Siegel, R.L.; Kratzer, T.B.; Giaquinto, A.N.; Sung, H.; Jemal, A. Cancer statistics, 2025. *CA A Cancer J. Clin.* **2025**, *75*, 10–45. [CrossRef]
4. Ali, I.I.; D'Souza, C.; Singh, J.; Adeghate, E. Adropin's Role in Energy Homeostasis and Metabolic Disorders. *Int. J. Mol. Sci.* **2022**, *23*, 8318. [CrossRef]
5. Lovren, F.; Pan, Y.; Quan, A.; Singh, K.K.; Shukla, P.C.; Gupta, M.; Al-Omran, M.; Teoh, H.; Verma, S. Adropin is a novel regulator of endothelial function. *Circulation* **2010**, *122*, S185–S192. [CrossRef]
6. Jasaszwili, M.; Billert, M.; Strowski, M.Z.; Nowak, K.W.; Skrzypski, M. Adropin as A Fat-Burning Hormone with Multiple Functions-Review of a Decade of Research. *Molecules* **2020**, *25*, 549. [CrossRef]
7. Jia, L.; Liao, L.; Jiang, Y.; Hu, X.; Lu, G.; Xiao, W.; Gong, W.; Jia, X.; Xiaoqin, J. Low-dose adropin stimulates inflammasome activation of macrophage via mitochondrial ROS involved in colorectal cancer progression. *BMC Cancer* **2023**, *23*, 1042. [CrossRef]
8. Hu, J.; Wu, Q.; Ding, Q.; Wu, W.; Li, Q.; Zheng, Z. High Level of Adropin Promotes the Progression of Pancreatic Ductal Adenocarcinoma. *Curr. Cancer Drug Targets* **2024**, *24*, 629–641. [CrossRef]
9. Bartha, Á.; Győrffy, B. TNMplot.com: A Web Tool for the Comparison of Gene Expression in Normal, Tumor and Metastatic Tissues. *Int. J. Mol. Sci.* **2021**, *22*, 2622. [CrossRef]
10. Love, M.I.; Huber, W.; Anders, S. Moderated estimation of fold change and dispersion for RNA-seq data with DESeq2. *Genome Biol.* **2014**, *15*, 550. Available online: https://pubmed.ncbi.nlm.nih.gov/25516281/ (accessed on 17 September 2024). [CrossRef]
11. Therneau, T.M.; Grambsch, P.M. *Modeling Survival Data: Extending the Cox Model*; Springer: New York, NY, USA, 2000.
12. Kassambara, A.; Kosinski, M.; Biecek, P. Survminer: Drawing Survival Curves Using "ggplot2" [Internet]. 2021. Available online: https://github.com/kassambara/survminer (accessed on 30 April 2024).
13. Li, T.; Fu, J.; Zeng, Z.; Cohen, D.; Li, J.; Chen, Q.; Li, B.; Liu, X.S. TIMER2.0 for analysis of tumor-infiltrating immune cells. *Nucleic Acids Res.* **2020**, *48*, W509–14. [CrossRef] [PubMed]
14. GSCA: Gene Set Cancer Analysis [Internet]. Available online: https://guolab.wchscu.cn/GSCA/#/ (accessed on 14 December 2024).
15. TCGExplorer [Internet]. Available online: https://tcgex.iyte.edu.tr/ (accessed on 14 December 2024).
16. Gao, J.; Aksoy, B.A.; Dogrusoz, U.; Dresdner, G.; Gross, B.E.; Sumer, S.O.; Sun, Y.; Jacobsen, A.; Sinha, R.; Larsson, E.; et al. Integrative Analysis of Complex Cancer Genomics and Clinical Profiles Using the cBioPortal. *Sci. Signal* **2013**, *6*, pl1. Available online: https://pubmed.ncbi.nlm.nih.gov/23550210/ (accessed on 23 August 2024). [CrossRef] [PubMed]
17. de Bruijn, I.; Kundra, R.; Mastrogiacomo, B.; Tran, T.N.; Sikina, L.; Mazor, T.; Li, X.; Ochoa, A.; Zhao, G.; Lai, B.; et al. Analysis and Visualization of Longitudinal Genomic and Clinical Data from the AACR Project GENIE Biopharma Collaborative in cBioPortal. *Cancer Res.* **2023**, *83*, 3861–3867. [CrossRef] [PubMed]
18. Cerami, E.; Gao, J.; Dogrusoz, U.; Gross, B.E.; Sumer, S.O.; Aksoy, B.A.; Jacobsen, A.; Byrne, C.J.; Heuer, M.L.; Larsson, E.; et al. The cBio Cancer Genomics Portal: An Open Platform for Exploring Multidimensional Cancer Genomics Data. *Cancer Discov.* **2012**, *2*, 401–404. Available online: https://pubmed.ncbi.nlm.nih.gov/22588877/ (accessed on 23 August 2024). [CrossRef]
19. Miao, Y.R.; Zhang, Q.; Lei, Q.; Luo, M.; Xie, G.Y.; Wang, H.; Guo, A.Y. ImmuCellAI: A Unique Method for Comprehensive T-Cell Subsets Abundance Prediction and its Application in Cancer Immunotherapy. *Adv. Sci.* **2020**, *7*, 1902880. [CrossRef]
20. Szklarczyk, D.; Franceschini, A.; Wyder, S.; Forslund, K.; Heller, D.; Huerta-Cepas, J.; Simonovic, M.; Roth, A.; Santos, A.; Tsafou, K.P.; et al. STRING v10: Protein-Protein Interaction Networks, Integrated Over the Tree of Life. *Nucleic Acids Res.* **2015**, *43*, D447–D452. Available online: https://pubmed.ncbi.nlm.nih.gov/25352553/ (accessed on 23 August 2024). [CrossRef]
21. Xie, Z.; Bailey, A.; Kuleshov, M.V.; Clarke, D.J.B.; Evangelista, J.E.; Jenkins, S.L.; Lachmann, A.; Wojciechowicz, M.L.; Kropiwnicki, E.; Jagodnik, K.M.; et al. Gene Set Knowledge Discovery with Enrichr. *Curr. Protoc.* **2021**, *1*, e90. Available online: https://pubmed.ncbi.nlm.nih.gov/33780170/ (accessed on 23 August 2024). [CrossRef]
22. Kuleshov, M.V.; Jones, M.R.; Rouillard, A.D.; Fernandez, N.F.; Duan, Q.; Wang, Z.; Koplev, S.; Jenkins, S.L.; Jagodnik, K.M.; Lachmann, A.; et al. Enrichr: A Comprehensive Gene Set Enrichment Analysis Web Server 2016 Update. *Nucleic Acids Res.* **2016**, *44*, W90–W97. Available online: https://pubmed.ncbi.nlm.nih.gov/27141961/ (accessed on 23 August 2024). [CrossRef]
23. Chen, E.Y.; Tan, C.M.; Kou, Y.; Duan, Q.; Wang, Z.; Meirelles, G.V.; Clark, N.R.; Ma'Ayan, A. Enrichr: Interactive and Collaborative HTML5 Gene List Enrichment Analysis Tool. *BMC Bioinform.* **2013**, *14*, 128. Available online: https://bmcbioinformatics.biomedcentral.com/articles/10.1186/1471-2105-14-128 (accessed on 23 August 2024). [CrossRef]
24. Su, K.; Katebi, A.; Kohar, V.; Clauss, B.; Gordin, D.; Qin, Z.S.; Karuturi, R.K.M.; Li, S.; Lu, M. NetAct: A Computational Platform to Construct Core Transcription Factor Regulatory Networks Using Gene Activity. *Genome Biol.* **2022**, *23*, 270. Available online: https://genomebiology.biomedcentral.com/articles/10.1186/s13059-022-02835-3 (accessed on 14 December 2024). [CrossRef]
25. LinkedOmics Suite [Internet]. Available online: https://www.linkedomics.org/#/ (accessed on 14 December 2024).

26. Manojlovic, N.; Savic, G.; Manojlovic, S. Neoadjuvant treatment of pancreatic ductal adenocarcinoma: Whom, when and how *World J. Gastrointest. Surg.* **2024**, *16*, 1223–1230. [CrossRef] [PubMed]
27. Younis, O.M.; Yasin, J.A.; Saeed, A.; Qubbaj, F.B.; Al-Sharif, Z.K.; Saeed, A. ENHO's Protective Role in Pancreatic Adenocarcinoma In Proceedings of the ESMO Gastrointestinal Cancers Congress 2024, Munich, Germany, 26–29 June 2024. [CrossRef]
28. Labbé, K.; LeBon, L.; King, B.; Vu, N.; Stoops, E.H.; Ly, N.; Lefebvre, A.E.Y.T.; Seitzer, P.; Krishnan, S.; Heo, J.-M.; et al. Specific activation of the integrated stress response uncovers regulation of central carbon metabolism and lipid droplet biogenesis *Nat. Commun.* **2024**, *15*, 8301. [CrossRef] [PubMed]
29. Flieswasser, T.; Eynde, A.V.D.; Van Audenaerde, J.; De Waele, J.; Lardon, F.; Riether, C.; de Haard, H.; Smits, E.; Pauwels, P Jacobs, J. The CD70-CD27 axis in oncology: The new kids on the block. *J. Exp. Clin. Cancer Res.* **2022**, *41*, 12. [CrossRef]
30. Getu, A.A.; Tigabu, A.; Zhou, M.; Lu, J.; Fodstad, Ø.; Tan, M. New frontiers in immune checkpoint B7-H3 (CD276) research and drug development. *Mol. Cancer* **2023**, *22*, 43. [CrossRef]
31. Yang, M.; Tang, X.; Zhang, Z.; Gu, L.; Wei, H.; Zhao, S.; Zhong, K.; Mu, M.; Huang, C.; Jiang, C.; et al. Tandem CAR-T cells targeting CD70 and B7-H3 exhibit potent preclinical activity against multiple solid tumors. *Theranostics* **2020**, *10*, 7622–7634 [CrossRef]
32. Kordaß, T.; Osen, W.; Eichmüller, S.B. Controlling the immune suppressor: Transcription factors and microRNAs regulating CD73/NT5E. *Front. Immunol.* **2018**, *9*, 813. [CrossRef]
33. Li, Y.; Su, Z.; Wei, B.; Qin, M.; Liang, Z. Bioinformatics analysis identified MMP14 and COL12A1 as immune-related biomarkers associated with pancreatic adenocarcinoma prognosis. *Math. Biosci. Eng. MBE* **2021**, *18*, 5921–5942. [CrossRef]
34. Xiao, H.N.; Zhao, Z.Y.; Li, J.P.; Li, A.Y. Comprehensive pan-cancer analysis: Essential role of ABCB family genes in cancer *Transl. Cancer Res.* **2024**, *13*, 1642–1664. [CrossRef]
35. Riedl, J.M.; Posch, F.; Horvath, L.; Gantschnigg, A.; Renneberg, F.; Schwarzenbacher, E.; Moik, F.; Barth, D.A.; Rossmann, C.H. Stotz, M.; et al. Gemcitabine/nab-Paclitaxel versus FOLFIRINOX for palliative first-line treatment of advanced pancreatic cancer A propensity score analysis. *Eur. J. Cancer* **2021**, *151*, 3–13. [CrossRef]
36. Chen, J.; Liao, S.; Xiao, Z.; Pan, Q.; Wang, X.; Shen, K.; Wang, S.; Yang, L.; Guo, F.; Liu, H.-F.; et al. The development and improvement of immunodeficient mice and humanized immune system mouse models. *Front. Immunol.* **2022**, *13*, 1007579 [CrossRef]
37. Zhang, S.; Chen, Q.; Lin, X.; Chen, M.; Liu, Q. A review of Adropin as the medium of dialogue between energy regulation and immune regulation. *Oxid. Med. Cell. Longev.* **2020**, *2020*, 3947806. [CrossRef] [PubMed]
38. Stelcer, E.; Milecka, P.; Komarowska, H.; Jopek, K.; Tyczewska, M.; Szyszka, M.; Lesniczak, M.; Suchorska, W.; Bekova, K. Szczepaniak, B.; et al. Adropin Stimulates Proliferation and Inhibits Adrenocortical Steroidogenesis in the Human Adrenal Carcinoma (HAC15) Cell Line. *Front. Endocrinol.* **2020**, *11*, 561370. [CrossRef] [PubMed]
39. Tuna, B.G.; Atalay, P.B.; Altunbek, M.; Kalkan, B.M.; Dogan, S. Effects of Chronic and Intermittent Calorie Restriction on Adropin Levels in Breast Cancer. *Nutr. Cancer* **2017**, *69*, 1003–1010. [CrossRef]
40. Rao, A.; Herr, D.R. G protein-coupled receptor GPR19 regulates E-cadherin expression and invasion of breast cancer cells *Biochim. Biophys. acta. Mol. Cell Res.* **2017**, *1864*, 1318–1327. [CrossRef]
41. Roca, H.; Hernandez, J.; Weidner, S.; McEachin, R.C.; Fuller, D.; Sud, S.; Schumann, T.; Wilkinson, J.E.; Zaslavsky, A.; Li, H.; et al Transcription factors OVOL1 and OVOL2 induce the mesenchymal to epithelial transition in human cancer. *PLoS ONE* **2013** *8*, e76773. [CrossRef]
42. Nergiz, S.; Altinkaya, S.O.; Kurt Ömürlü, İ.; Yuksel, H.; Küçük, M.; Demircan Sezer, S. Circulating adropin levels in patients with endometrium cancer. *Gynecol. Endocrinol. Off. J. Int. Soc. Gynecol. Endocrinol.* **2015**, *31*, 730–735. [CrossRef]
43. Lin, C.; Hu, Z.; Yuan, G.; Su, H.; Zeng, Y.; Guo, Z.; Zhong, F.; Jiang, K.; He, S. MicroRNA-1179 inhibits the proliferation, migration and invasion of human pancreatic cancer cells by targeting E2F5. *Chem.-Biol. Interact.* **2018**, *291*, 65–71. [CrossRef]
44. Liberti, M.V.; Locasale, J.W. The Warburg Effect: How Does it Benefit Cancer Cells? *Trends Biochem. Sci.* **2016**, *41*, 211–218 [CrossRef]
45. Chang, X.; Liu, X.; Wang, H.; Yang, X.; Gu, Y. Glycolysis in the progression of pancreatic cancer. *Am. J. Cancer Res.* **2022**, *12* 861–872.
46. Zheng, D.; Deng, Y.; Deng, L.; He, Z.; Sun, X.; Gong, Y.; Shi, B.; Lu, D.; Yu, C. CDCA7 enhances STAT3 transcriptional activity to regulate aerobic glycolysis and promote pancreatic cancer progression and gemcitabine resistance. *Cell Death Dis.* **2025**, *16*, 68 [CrossRef]

cancers

Article

Ultrasound as a New Method for the Release and Identification of Novel microRNAs and Proteins as Candidate Biomarkers in Pancreatic Cancer

Veronica Zelli [1], Alessandra Corrente [1], Chiara Compagnoni [1,*], Francesco Colaianni [1], Martina Sara Miscione [1], Monica Di Padova [1], Daria Capece [1], Gaetano Barbato [2,3], Edoardo Alesse [1], Francesca Zazzeroni [1] and Alessandra Tessitore [1,*]

[1] Department of Biotechnological and Applied Clinical Sciences, University of L'Aquila, 67100 L'Aquila, Italy; veronica.zelli@univaq.it (V.Z.); alessandra.corrente@graduate.univaq.it (A.C.); francesco.colaianni1@graduate.univaq.it (F.C.); martinasara.miscione@graduate.univaq.it (M.S.M.); monica.dipadova@univaq.it (M.D.P.); daria.capece@univaq.it (D.C.); edoardo.alesse@univaq.it (E.A.); francesca.zazzeroni@univaq.it (F.Z.)

[2] Inno-Sol srl, 00165 Rome, Italy; gaetano.barbato@inno-sol.it

[3] Department of Biology, School of Pharmacy, University of Rome Tor Vergata, 00133 Rome, Italy

* Correspondence: chiara.compagnoni@univaq.it (C.C.); alessandra.tessitore@univaq.it (A.T.); Tel.: +39-0862433518 (A.T.); Fax: +39-0862433131 (A.T.)

Simple Summary: The identification of highly sensitive and specific biomarkers for the early diagnosis of pancreatic cancer (PC) is a fundamental goal to improve the outcome and treatment options for PC patients. In this context, microRNAs and proteins released from the tumor microenvironment into body fluids represent promising non-invasive candidates for early cancer detection. Here, we employed an innovative ultrasound (US)-based instrument to promote and amplify the release of molecules from PC cell lines in order to identify novel putative diagnostic PC biomarkers. A preliminary validation of these findings using publicly available datasets of PC patients was also performed. Overall, the results of this study highlight the suitability and utility of US-based methodologies for the identification of novel molecules to be considered as candidate non-invasive biomarkers in PC.

Abstract: Background/Objectives: Pancreatic cancer (PC) is among the most aggressive malignancies, often diagnosed at late stages. MicroRNAs (miRNAs) and proteins released from the tumor microenvironment into body fluids represent promising non-invasive biomarkers for early cancer detection. In this study, we took advantage of an innovative ultrasound (US)-based instrument (SonoWell®, Inno-Sol srl, Rome, Italy) to treat PC cells in order to promote and amplify the release of molecules, with the aim of identifying novel putative diagnostic PC biomarkers. **Methods:** Three human pancreatic adenocarcinoma cell lines (T3M-4, Panc02.03, and PaCa-44) and a non-cancerous pancreatic epithelial line (HPanEPic) were subjected to US using the SonoWell instrument. MiRNAs released in the supernatants were profiled by TaqMan-based qRT-PCR microfluidic cards, while proteins were analyzed by antibody arrays. Publicly available datasets of circulating miRNAs in PC patients were also reviewed. **Results:** Expression levels of 22 miRNAs in T3M-4 cells, 11 in Panc02.03, and 22 in PaCa-44, none of which were identified in the non-cancerous cell line profiling, were increased in the supernatant of US-treated as opposed to control cells. Among the statistically significant miRNAs or miRNAs common to at least two tumor cell lines, the expression levels of miR-155-5p, miR-320a, miR-32-5p, and miR-93-5p were also found to be significantly upregulated in sera from PC patients compared to the results for healthy controls. With regard to proteins released after sonication, several molecules

 https://doi.org/10.3390/cancers17121979

were identified as candidate biomarkers in cancer US supernatants (Beta-2 microglobulin, CA125, CA19-9, CEA, CRP, Galectin-3, TIMP-1, uPA, and VEGF-A). **Conclusions:** We demonstrated that US-mediated sonoporation can promote and amplify the release of small molecules, miRNAs, and proteins into cell culture supernatants for consideration as putative biomarkers, thus encouraging further studies aimed at directly validating their expression levels in sera/plasma from PC patients and at deepening their role in the treatment of PC.

Keywords: pancreatic cancer; biomarkers; microRNA; early diagnosis; ultrasounds

1. Introduction

Pancreatic cancer (PC) is one the most fatal malignancies, being diagnosed at the unresectable or metastatic stage in approximately 80% of patients [1]. The detection delay is attributable to the absence of specific clinical symptoms in the early stages, thus contributing to very poor 5-year and overall survival rates (5–15% and 6%, respectively in the United States). More than 90% of PCs are exocrine adenocarcinomas arising from pancreatic ductal cells, and several risk factors (e.g., smoking, alcohol consumption, diabetes, obesity, chronic pancreatitis, family history) have been described [2]. Multidetector computed tomography (MDCT), abdominal magnetic resonance imaging (MRI)/magnetic resonance cholangiopancreatography (MRCP), and to a lesser extent, ultrasonography, are used to ascertain the presence of a suspected adenocarcinoma [3]. Several minimally invasive blood tests, such as liver function tests, especially in presence of jaundice, or tumor marker levels (CA19-9, CEA), can be used to aid pancreatic cancer diagnosis, but unfortunately, these lack the necessary diagnostic specificity, sensitivity, and accuracy [4]. Overall, invasive procedures (percutaneous or endoscopic biopsy, surgery with subsequent histological analysis) remain the definitive methods to confirm diagnosis [5]. In this context, the identification of new non-invasive biomarkers to support PC diagnosis at an earlier stage could revolutionize patients' clinical prognosis and treatment.

Therefore, the most important challenge to date is identifying novel molecules for early PC detection that can be distinguished from the physiological noise, with high specificity and sensitivity [6].

Small molecules physiologically released from the tumor microenvironment through biological membranes, such as nucleic acids (cfDNA, ctDNA, microRNA) or peptides/small proteins, are considered promising liquid biopsy-based biomarkers [6].

MicroRNAs (miRNAs) are short, non-coding RNAs able to specifically regulate the expression of target genes at the post-transcriptional level. They act by fine-tuning key physiological processes (e.g., cell proliferation, apoptosis, inflammation, metastasis), and miRNA expression dysregulation has been extensively described in several high-impact diseases (e.g., cardiovascular and neurodegenerative diseases, diabetes, cancer) [7–9]. MiRNAs can also be released by active or passive mechanisms from diseased tissues into the bloodstream, where they are stable and resistant to endogenous RNase [10–12], offering a potential source of non-invasive diagnostic, prognostic, and predictive biomarkers. Moreover, circulating miRNAs can be detected at very low concentrations in serum/plasma, thanks to the sensitive methods (e.g., quantitative PCR) available.

Ultrasound (US) and focused ultrasound (FUS) at low/moderate energy levels have been applied for diagnostic purposes due to their ability to overcome biological barriers and favor the release of small molecules, with negligible cell death, in in vitro and in vivo preclinical models [13–16]. This is attributable to the phenomenon of acoustic cavitation, generating cavities within biological membranes [17]. US waves are characterized by frequency and pressure amplitude, the latter with positive or negative values causing tissue compression or expansion, respectively. Negative pressure applied to a fluid induces cavitation bubbles (few μm in diameter) arising from gas dissolved within the medium, which can expand and shrink in size and then collapse, producing consequent mechanical stress and heating [18]. The cavitation responses associated with the rupture of biologic barriers can include five phases, with reversible or even irreversible effects in terms of cell viability, including membrane retraction, sonoporation, endo/exocytosis, membrane blebbing, and apoptosis, depending on the acoustic parameters. Membrane retraction seems to contribute to drug delivery and biomarker release due to the enlargement of cell–cell junctions [19]; sonoporation can induce the formation of pores within the lipid bilayer, mediating a bi-directional transport and leading to resealing; endocytosis and exocytosis can show protective effects against mechanical tension [20].

US-based technology has proven to be a useful tool to identify miRNAs of potential clinical utility by increasing a bidirectional flux that facilitates the release of low-molecular-weight molecules to be considered as potential biomarkers [16,21]. In this work, we used an ultrasound-based instrument for cellular research to promote and amplify the physiological process of small molecule release from PC human cell lines, thus increasing their concentration in culture supernatants and allowing for the identification of novel putative biomarkers, which were further validated on publicly available human datasets.

2. Materials and Methods

2.1. Cell Lines

Three pancreatic adenocarcinoma cell lines (T3M-4, Panc02.03, and PaCa-44) were purchased from ATCC (Manassas, VA, USA). Specifically, the T3M-4 metastatic (lymph node-derived) cells, isolated from a 64-year-old Asian male, were characterized by an epithelial-like morphology and the ability to produce the tumor marker CEA. At the molecular level, this cell line harbors the KRAS p.Gln61His and the TP53 p.Tyr220Cys oncogenic alterations. Panc02.03 and PaCa-44 are primary tumor-derived cell lines, obtained from a 70-year-old Caucasian female and a male of unspecified age, respectively. Regarding their main oncogenic alterations, Panc02.03 cells carry the KRAS p.Gly12Asp, TP53 p.Arg248Gln, CDKN2A p.Tyr44fs*1, and SMAD4 p.Arg135* variants, while the PaCa-44 cells exhibit the KRAS p.Gly12Val and TP53 p.Cys176Ser variants (https://www.cellosaurus.org/index.html and related databases, accessed on 3 June 2025).

The cells were cultured in RPMI-1640 (EuroClone, Milan, Italy) supplemented with exosome-free FBS (10%), L-glutamine (2 μm), and penicillin-streptomycin (0.05 U/mL) and were maintained at 37 °C with 5% CO_2. As a control, a normal pancreatic epithelial cell line (HPanEpic, P10475, Innoprot, Derio, Spain) was cultured under the same conditions by using the specific EpiCM medium (Innoprot), supplemented with exosome-free FBS (2%), epithelial growth supplements (1%, Innoprot), and penicillin-streptomycin (1%, Innoprot). At 80% confluency, the cells were treated with trypsin, counted with an automatic cell counter (Cyto Smart, Corning Life Sciences, Durham, NC, USA), transferred in a Falcon 24-well plate (cod 353047, Corning Incorporated, Corning, NY, USA) (per well: 80,000 T3M-4 cells, 150,000 Panc02.03, PaCa-44, and HPanEpic cells, in 500 μL of medium) and cultured at 37 °C with 5% CO_2 for 24 h.

2.2. US Treatment

After 24 h, the medium was removed, the cells were washed three times with PBS, and 300 μL of fresh serum-free medium was added to each well. Plate-wells, maintained at 37 °C, were subjected to US treatment (one single well at a time) using the SonoWell®

instrument (Inno-Sol srl, Rome, Italy) at 1 MHz frequency and a 460 kPa acoustic pressure (AP) negative peak. Total burst duration (TBD), duty cycle (DC), total sonication duration (SD), and thus, the corresponding acoustic energy intensity deposited (I_{sppa} and I_{spta}) were adapted to each cell line: T3M-4 (TBD 6 ms, 30% DC, SD 30 min, I_{sppa} 6.995 W/cm^2, I_{spta} 2.099 W/cm^2); Panc02.03 and HPanEpic (TBD 2 ms, 10% DC, SD 1 h, I_{sppa} 6.995 W/cm^2, I_{spta} 0.699 W/cm^2); PaCa-44 (TBD 2 ms, 10% DC, SD 40 + 40 min interspersed with 10 min pause without US, I_{sppa} 6.995 W/cm^2, I_{spta} 0.699 W/cm^2).

Measurements of the AP were performed following suggestions of the ITRUSST consensus, where applicable, to the in-vitro measurements [22], and we also adopt their suggested nomenclature for the acoustic parameters. A manufacturer-calibrated hydrophone (Precision Acoustic, Dorchester, UK), equipped with a 0.2 mm diameter needle-type tip, detected the acoustic pressure in the far field, positioning the fully submerged well-plate on top of the 1 MHz flat transducer (12 mm diameter) at the distance of the near/far field plane, 1 mm from the well bottom. The same z-coordinate was used during subsequent experiments. The measurements determined the maximum peak of intensity by scanning the x–y plane with the hydrophone at 12 fixed z-coordinates, exploring the volume within the well. Signal detection was obtained using a Picoscope 3204A (Pico Technology, St. Neots, UK).

All sonication parameters were set up to prevent any alteration in cell morphology and to maintain over 85% cell viability. Following US treatment, cells were incubated at 37 °C and 5% CO_2 for 10 min. Morphological alterations were evaluated by optical microscopy analysis. Cell viability was then assessed using an automatic cell counter (Cyto Smart, Corning Life Sciences) and Trypan Blue staining. The same washing, temperature, and timing conditions were applied to the untreated control samples, cultured in parallel within an incubator. Each supernatant was collected and centrifuged for 20 min at 4 °C and 1500× *g* to remove cellular debris. Samples were stored at −80 °C and used for downstream applications, as described below.

Further information on the SonoWell instrument and experimental reproducibility is available in the Supplementary Materials.

2.3. RNA Extraction and miRNA Expression Analysis

Total RNA, including fractions less than 200 nucleotides in length, was extracted from the US and control supernatants (300 µL) using the Plasma/Serum RNA Purification Mini kit (Norgen Biotek, Thorold, ON, Canada), following the manufacturer's instructions. Before extraction, cel-miR-39-3p was added as exogenous control at a 5 fmol/mL final concentration. RNA quantity and quality were measured using NanoDrop 2000 spectrophotometry (Thermo Fisher, San Diego, CA, USA).

To assess the release of molecules, as a priority, we considered the expression levels of miR-23b-3p and miR-7 in the US and control supernatants from adenocarcinoma and HPanEpic cells, respectively. For this purpose, we used Thermo Fisher TaqMan small RNA assays (#245306 and #005723, respectively). RNAs were briefly retrotranscribed (TaqMan MicroRNA Reverse Transcription Kit, Applied Biosystems, Foster City, CA, USA) and analyzed (7500 Fast Real Time PCR System, Applied Biosystems) using the $2^{-\Delta\Delta Ct}$ method by considering the spiked-in cel-miR-39-3p as an exogenous control and comparing US vs. untreated control samples. Each experiment was repeated at least three times. Once the miRNAs' release after sonication was ascertained, the RNAs were retrotranscribed again (TaqMan advanced miRNA cDNA synthesis kit, Applied Biosystems) and analyzed with TaqMan Advanced miRNA Human/Serum Plasma cards (Applied Biosystems) using a ViiA7 instrument (Applied Biosystems). The experiments were repeated at least three times. MiRNA expression levels were assessed using a comparative assay ($2^{-\Delta\Delta Ct}$), and the data were normalized using the global normalization method. RT-qPCR data were analyzed by Quant Studio and Expression Suite v1.3 software (Thermo Fisher). A manual check focused on PCR amplification plot profiles was also performed, and only miRNAs with good amplification curves were retained. Differentially expressed miRNAs, showing relative quantification (RQ) ≥ 2 in the sonicated compared to the control samples, were considered for further analyses. *p*-values were calculated using the Expression Suite software using a Student's *t*-test, and a *p*-value < 0.05 was considered statistically significant.

2.4. Protein Extraction and Analysis

Proteins from the US and control supernatants, obtained from single wells as previously described, were extracted using phosphatase inhibitor (0.1 mM PMSF, 1 μg/mL aprotinin, 10 mM NaF, 0.1 M Na3VO4) and a Complete-Mini protease inhibitor cocktail tablet (Roche Molecular Biochemicals, Basel, Switzerland) and centrifuged at 1500× *g* for 20 min at 4 °C. The protein concentration was quantified using the Pierce BCA protein assay kit (Thermo Fisher) at 562 nm, according to the manufacturer's instructions. Protein expression levels were analyzed using the Human Cancer Discovery Array C3 (RayBiotech, Peachtree Corners, GA, USA), based on the manufacturer's instructions, allowing us to evaluate the expression profile of 30 proteins involved in cancer biology. Chemiluminescent signals were collected using ImageQuant LAS 4000 (GE Healthcare, Tokyo, Japan), and densitometric analysis was performed using ImageJ software v 1.53e, based on the RayBiotech algorithm.

Proteins with a fold increase ≥ 1.3 (signal increase $\geq 30\%$) in US-treated tumor cells compared to that of the controls were considered upregulated. The analyses were performed in duplicate, and only results confirmed in both experiments were considered.

2.5. Publicly Available Datasets for Results Validation

Four publicly available datasets, EXP00529 (GSE106817) [23], EXP00620 (GSE112264) [24], EXP00609 (GSE113740) [25], and EXP00538 (GSE113486) [26], from the Database of Differentially Expressed miRNAs in Human Cancers (dbDEMC, https://www.biosino.org/dbDEMC/index, accessed on 20 January 2025), were used to validate the expression levels of miRNAs released in the US supernatants in the PC patients and healthy controls (Supplementary Table S1).

Notably, in these studies, miRNA profiling was performed on serum samples from cancer patients and healthy controls. Data were filtered based on a log2 fold change (FC) ≥ 0.58 and an adjusted *p*-value (padj) ≤ 0.05.

GSE106817 and GSE112264 datasets were also used to perform receiver operating characteristic (ROC) curve analysis in order to estimate the miRNAs' diagnostic value (individually or in combination) in discriminating PC cases from non-cancer samples, as well as from other cancer types, using the CombiROC R package [27]. The analysis was performed using R software v 4.3.1 (www.r-project.org).

2.6. Network and Pathway-Based Analysis

The multiple query module of the miRNet 2.0 tool (https://www.mirnet.ca/, accessed on 3 June 2025), which allows for the loading different input types (in this case, miRNAs and proteins), was used to identify the most relevant connections among the biomarkers emerging in this study. The STRING v10 protein–protein interaction (PPI) database was also considered to obtain a more comprehensive overview of the biological context of the identified miRNAs and proteins. Starting from the first-order network, a minimal subnetwork that maximally connects the seed nodes was extracted, thereby simplifying and focusing the network analysis. MiRNA enrichment analysis was performed using the explorer function of the miRNet tool, while the pathway analysis of all proteins in the network was conducted using the Database for Annotation, Visualization, and Integrated Discovery (DAVID) (https://davidbioinformatics.nih.gov/; accessed on 3 June 2025), based on the Kyoto Encyclopedia of Genes and Genomes (KEGG) and Reactome Pathway databases. An adjusted p-value ≤ 0.05 was applied to filter statistically significant terms.

3. Results

3.1. Assessment of Effective Molecule Release After US Treatment

Due to both the biological and technical variability in the cell response to US treatment, related to factors such as cell type, cell cycle phase, ultrasound parameters, and environmental culture conditions [16,28], the efficacy of US treatment was verified by evaluating the expression levels of miR-23b-3p and miR-7, which are known to be expressed in both PC and normal pancreatic cells, respectively [29–31]. The expression levels of these two miRNAs were evaluated in the US-treated and control supernatants from adenocarcinoma and HPanEpic cells, respectively, and only samples in which US-mediated release was confirmed (RQ $\geq$ 2) were considered for miRNA/protein profiling analysis (Figure 1A).

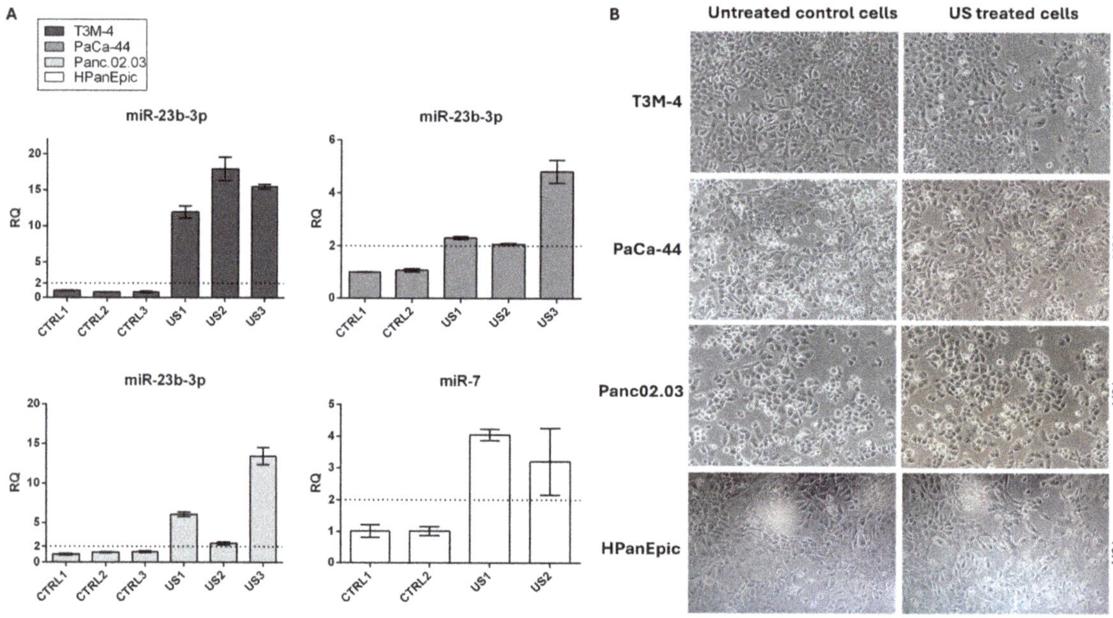

Figure 1. US parameter settings and validation. (**A**) miR-23b-3p and miR-7 expression levels in US-treated (US) compared to control (CTRL) supernatants from adenocarcinoma (T3M-4, PaCa-44, and Panc02.03) and HPanEpic cells, respectively, confirming US-mediated miRNA release (RQ $\geq$ 2, $p < 0.05$); each experiment was performed in triplicate under the same conditions. (**B**) US treatment parameters were set up to produce no morphological changes and more than 85% viable cells. Abbreviations: relative quantification (RQ).

Optical microscopy showed that the US parameters employed did not induce any significative alterations in cell morphology or adhesion properties (Figure 1B). Moreover, automatic cell count and Trypan Blue staining revealed more than 85% viable cells, demonstrating that US promoted miRNA release, without significant changes in cell morphology or viability, thus confirming the suitability of the experimental conditions.

3.2. MiRNA Profiling in US Supernatants

In the US supernatants of T3M-4 and PaCa-44 cells, eight (miR-19a-3p, -151a-3p, -382-5p, -93-3p, -93-5p, -652-3p, -155-5p, -425-5p) and one (miR-99b-5p) significantly differentially expressed miRNAs were identified, respectively. None of these miRNAs were detected in supernatants from normal HPanEpic cells. In addition, we extended the analysis to the released non-significant miRNAs: in this case, 22 miRNAs in T3M-4 cells, 11 miRNAs in Panc02.03, and 22 miRNAs in PaCa-44, none of which were identified in supernatants from the non-cancerous cell line, were found to be overexpressed after US (Figure 2A–C, Supplementary Table S2). Among them, we further focused on the analyses of 15 miRNAs that were statistically significant (miR-19a-3p, -151a-3p, -382-5p, -93-3p, -93-5p, -652-3p, -155-5p, -425-5p and -99b-5p) or non-significant, but common to at least two tumor cell lines (miR-32-3p, -486-5p, -339-3p, -320a, -18a-3p, and -502-3p) (Figure 2D).

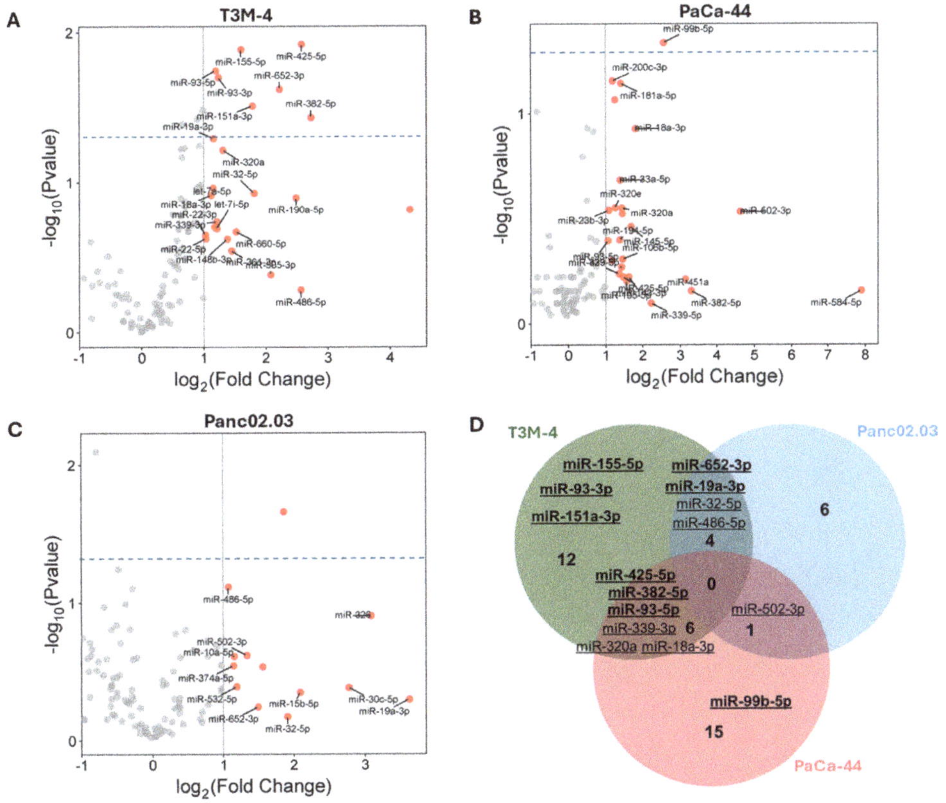

Figure 2. Profiling of PC US-released miRNAs. Volcano plots of miRNAs released from T3M-4 (**A**), PaCa-44 (**B**) and Panc02.03 (**C**) cells after sonication; only miRNAs identified in cancer cell lines but not in non-cancerous HPanEpic cells are labeled. (**D**) Venn diagram showing the eight and one statistically significant miRNAs in T3M-4 and PaCa-44 cells, respectively (highlighted in bold), as well as non-significant upregulated miRNAs (RQ $\geq$ 2) common to at least two tumor cell lines (n = 6), for a total of 15 miRNAs considered for further analysis.

3.3. In Silico Validation of Differentially Expressed miRNAs

In order to preliminarily validate miRNAs as putative PC biomarkers, an in silico analysis of publicly available datasets obtained from the Database of Differentially Expressed miRNAs in Human Cancers (dbDEMC) was performed (Table 1). According to our results, significant upregulation of miR-151a-3p, -155-5p, -320a, -32-5p, -339-3p, -652-3p, -93-3p, -93-5p, and -502-3p was observed in sera from PC patients. In particular, miR-155-5p, miR-320a, miR-32-5p, and miR-93-5p emerged as the most interesting, being differentially expressed in at least two out of four datasets investigated (Table 1).

Table 1. Studies from dbDEMC (https://www.biosino.org/dbDEMC/index, (accessed on 20 January 2025)) reporting statistically significant differences (log2FC $\geq$ 0.58; adj *p*-value < 0.05) in serum of PC samples compared to normal samples for the 15 selected miRNAs; among them, miR-155-5p, miR-320a, miR-32-5p, and miR-93-5p emerged as the most interesting, as they were found to be deregulated in more than one dataset.

				EXP00529 (GSE106817)		**EXP00620 (GSE112264)**		**EXP00609 (GSE113740)**		**EXP00538 (GSE113486)**	
miRNA	**T3M-4**	**Pnc02.03**	**PaCa-44**	**log2FC**	**adj *p*-Value**	**log2FC**	**adj *p*-Value**	**log2FC**	**adj *p*-Value**	**log2FC**	**adj *p*-Value**
hsa-miR-151a-3p	0.031					1.466	0.005				
hsa-miR-155-5p	0.013			1.502	1.15×10^{-13}	1.337	0.0006				
hsa-miR-18a-3p											
hsa-miR-19a-3p	0.050										
hsa-miR-320a				1.907	5.62×10^{-129}	1.795	5.808×10^{-23}	1.572	2.93×10^{-15}	1.643	4.848×10^{-21}
hsa-miR-32-5p				1.719	2.932×10^{-14}	2.420	9.082×10^{-7}			1.358	0.003
hsa-miR-339-3p				1.014	6.419×10^{-8}						
hsa-miR-382-5p	0.037										
hsa-miR-425-5p	0.012										
hsa-miR-486-5p											
hsa-miR-652-3p	0.024			0.959	1.773×10^{-7}						
hsa-miR-93-3p	0.020			0.977	1.12×10^{-5}						
hsa-miR-93-5p	0.018			0.721	0.003	1.527	0.001				
hsa-miR-502-3p				0.583	0.002						
hsa-miR-99b-5p			0.046								

The CombiROC R package was used to estimate the diagnostic value of miR-155-5p, miR-320a, miR-32-5p, and miR-93-5p in discriminating PC from non-cancer samples, as well as from other cancer types, using the two publicly available datasets GSE106817 and GSE112264 (Figure 3A). Notably, the two datasets include different samples (female and male patients, respectively) from the same study series, analyzed using the same method [23,24]. Therefore, by using the CombiROC package separately with each dataset or with the merged dataset, we obtained similar results.

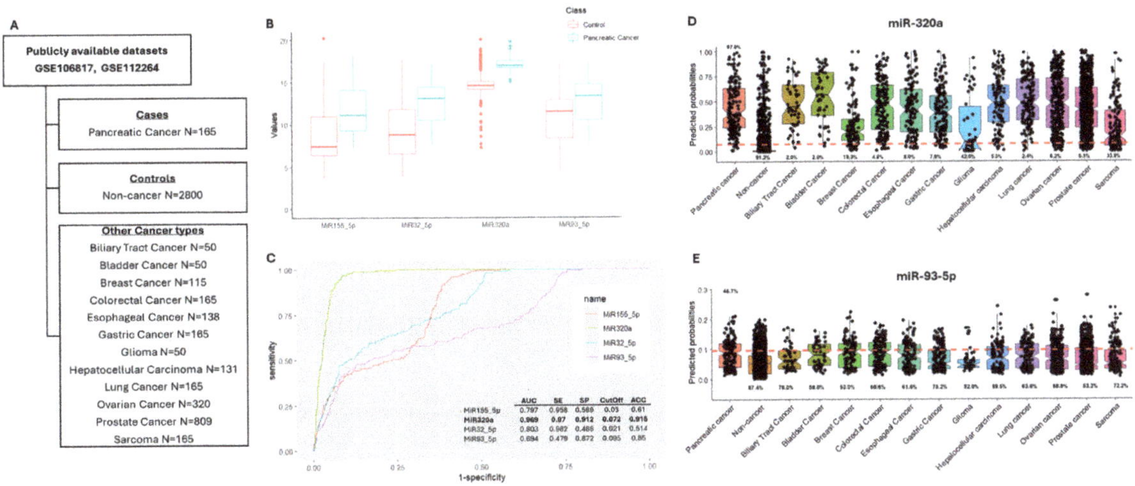

Figure 3. Evaluation of diagnostic potential of miR-155-5p, miR-320a, miR-32-5p, and miR-93-5p. (**A**) Study series analyzed. (**B**) Boxplots of the distribution of each miRNA in pancreatic cancer and non-cancer controls; the corresponding ROC curves and performance parameters are reported in (**C**). The ability of miR-320a (**D**) and miR-93-5p (**E**) to correctly distinguish PC patients, not only from non-cancer controls but also from the other cancer types, is displayed. The red dotted line indicates the optimal cutoff based on ROC curve analysis for PC cases and non-cancer controls. Abbreviations: area under the curve (AUC); sensitivity (SE); specificity (SP); accuracy (ACC); receiver operating characteristic (ROC).

Based on ROC curve analysis, miR-320a showed the highest diagnostic potential, with an AUC value of 0.969, a sensitivity of 0.97, a specificity of 0.912, and accuracy of 0.915, highlighting the ability of this miRNA to distinguish PC cases from healthy controls, with good efficiency (Figure 3B,C).

However, using the predicted probability function to classify the other cancer types according to the optimal cutoff obtained from the previously described ROC curves (PC cases vs. healthy controls), the results revealed the low specificity of the model in discriminating PC cases from other cancers (Figure 3D).

Similar results were observed using different miRNA combinations (Supplementary Table S3, Supplementary Figure S1)

On the other hand, although miR-93-5p showed moderate diagnostic potential in discriminating PC cases from non-cancer controls (AUC 0.694, sensitivity 0.479, specificity 0.872, and accuracy 0.85), mainly due to low sensitivity (Figure 3C), this miRNA performed better than miR-320a in terms of specificity when other tumor types were considered (Figure 3E).

3.4. US Protein Secretome Analysis

To evaluate protein factors to be considered as putative PC biomarkers, the release of which was promoted and amplified by US, proteins were also extracted from supernatants and analyzed by antibody arrays. A total of nine factors were found to be more highly expressed in US-treated compared to non-treated cell supernatants, none of which were observed in non-cancerous cell line profiling. These include well-known tumor markers (e.g., CA19-9, CEA, and CA125), as well as proteins more recently described as potential novel biomarkers for the detection of PC (e.g., Beta-2 microglobulin (B2M), TIMP-1, CRP, Galectin-3, uPA, and VEGF-A) (Figure 4).

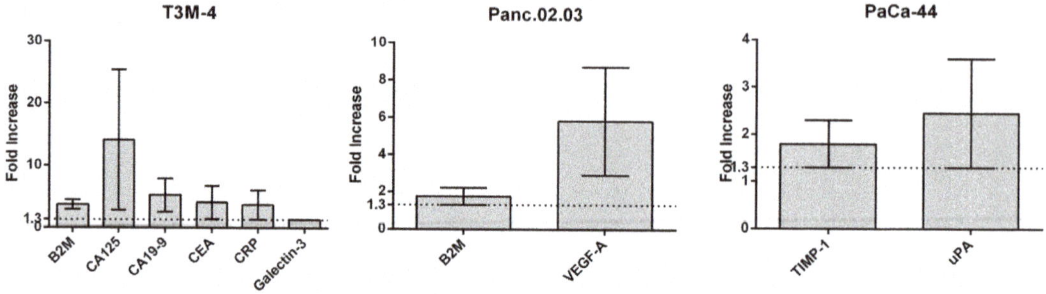

Figure 4. Profiling of PC US-released proteins. Bar plots showing proteins released from the three tumor cell lines after sonication compared to the results for the control cells.

3.5. Analysis of the Biological Role and Molecular Interactions of the Identified Biomarkers

To determine the potential molecular interactions and biological relevance of the identified miRNAs and proteins, a network was created and pathway-based analysis was performed, as described in the methods section.

Overall, a network comprising a total of 122 nodes (miRNAs/proteins) was obtained (Figure 5A). Pathway analysis revealed overlapping biological processes involving both miRNAs and proteins, including immune regulation and angiogenesis. Protein enrichment analysis also highlighted pathways of interest known to be involved in PC development and progression, such as the Ras signaling pathway and the RAF/MAP kinase cascade, the p53 signaling pathway, and signaling by TGFB family members (Figure 5B).

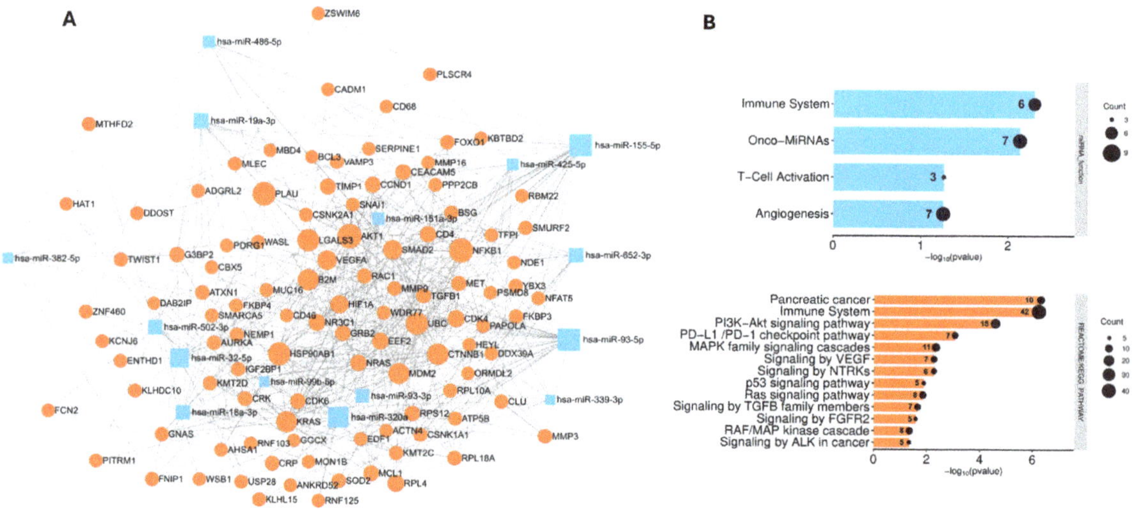

Figure 5. Network and pathway-based analysis of miRNAs (n = 15) and proteins (n = 9) identified in the present study, further enriched using a STRING v10 protein–protein interaction (PPI) database. MiRNA–protein and protein–protein interactions were derived from a minimal sub-network that maximally connects the different seed nodes (**A**), and related enrichment analysis was performed separately for miRNAs (n = 15) and all proteins (n = 107). Only the terms considered as the most representative and interesting among the significant expressions are reported. The miRNA and protein counts for each pathway are shown within the bars (**B**).

4. Discussion

PC is one of the most aggressive type of tumors, typically characterized by late-stage diagnosis and poor prognosis due in part to the lack of early symptoms and the absence of routine screening programs [1]. This highlights the urgent need to identify new biomarkers, characterized by high sensitivity and specificity, to improve the outcome and clinical management of PC patients. In this study, using SonoWell®, an innovative US-based instrument designed for cellular studies on well-plates to promote and amplify the release of small molecules in PC cell lines, we identified novel putative miRNAs/proteins as non-invasive biomarkers for the early detection of PC.

The different cellular effects triggered by US, ranging from sonoporation/endo-exocytosis to apoptosis/necrosis, are highly dependent on the physical and biophysical parameters of the US applied [32]. Exploiting US waves to transiently permeabilize cell membranes can facilitate the uptake of molecules while maintaining cell viability, and the use of US as a new therapeutic tool in cancer has garnered great attention in recent years due to its potential to improve drug delivery [32]. Sonication can also be effective in amplifying the release of small intracellular molecules in body fluids, suggesting that this technique could be considered useful for earlier detection of cancer lesions, for example, in the presence of precancerous lesions or for the identification of prognostic biomarkers [14,33]. In this scenario, the on-site application of US waves in cancer patients, with the following quantification of released biomarkers, could represent an additional tool for a more precise diagnosis/prognosis, for which additional specific preclinical and clinical studies are required. However, it is important to emphasize that using an US-based approach in this context would require the application of FUS with low power, without any ablation, to a precise target area of the body characterized by a known lesion and only to superficial organs accessible to FUS; these are just some of the current limitations to its use in a clinical setting. In this study, we proposed the use of US as a research method to guide the identification of potential biomarkers suitable for supporting PC diagnosis. Therefore, the translational applicability is mainly related to the analysis of such molecules, identified in the in vitro models, in serum/plasma from cancer patients in order to confirm their expression level modulation and diagnostic potential.

Among the miRNAs identified here and validated in external publicly available datasets, miR-155-5p, -320a, -32-5p, and 93-5p emerged as the most interesting putative biomarkers for PC diagnosis.

MiR-155, in both its -5p and -3p forms, is considered an oncogenic miRNA widely studied for its role in promoting cell survival, proliferation, migration, and invasiveness [34,35]. A recent meta-analysis showed that tissue miR-155 is a valuable diagnostic and prognostic biomarker in most solid tumors, including PC [36]. Moreover, several studies observed the upregulation of miR-155-5p in the plasma/serum of PC patients compared to levels in healthy controls, also highlighting the possible assessment of this miRNA, alone or in combination with other miRNAs/proteins, as a biomarker for early PC diagnosis [37–40].

In contrast, miR-32-5p was predominantly described as a tumor suppressor in different cancer types [41–43], and few data are currently available regarding its expression levels and putative role as a circulating biomarker in cancer.

MiRNA-93-5p is involved in gemcitabine resistance in PC through targeting the PTEN-mediated PI3K/Akt signaling pathway [44]. Circulating levels of miR-93-5p emerged as relevant indicators in various cancer types, particularly PC and colorectal cancers, where high miR-93-5p expression has been correlated with disease and progression, suggesting its possible consideration as a diagnostic and prognostic biomarker [45,46]. However, the diagnostic value of miR-93-5p was found to be quite moderate, being able to discriminate PC patients from healthy controls with a sensitivity and specificity of 60% and 77%, respectively [45].

Conflicting data are available regarding the role of miR-320a in human cancers, suggesting that the oncogenic or suppressive function of this miRNA is context-dependent [47]. MiR-320a was mainly downregulated and described as a tumor suppressor in cancers such as colorectal, breast, lung, and gastric cancer [48–53]. However, in malignant pleural mesothelioma, Costa et al. reported that the upregulation of miR-320a in cell lines promotes cell proliferation, viability, and migration, whereas its stable silencing resulted in contradictory effects [47]. Similarly, Yao et al. found that miR-320a/c/d ectopic expression increased the migration and invasion of hepatocarcinoma cells [54]. Wang et al. showed that the upregulation of miR-320a promotes the proliferation, migration, and invasion of PC cells, thereby reducing 5-FU sensitivity [55].

Interestingly, in analyzing the expression levels of a panel of 17 circulating miRNAs, miR-320a and miR-93-5p emerged among the miRNAs with the highest ability to discriminate PC patients and individuals with preneoplastic lesions from healthy controls, with AUC results of 0.85 and 0.80, respectively. Furthermore, using the combination of miR-33a-3p+miR-320a+CA19.9, an AUC value of 0.95, a sensitivity of 93%, and a specificity of 85% were achieved, suggesting that this combination could represent a significant biomarker signature for the non-invasive early diagnosis of PC [56].

MiR-320a and miR-93-5p are the two miRNAs that emerged as the most promising in our study: miR-320a showed high diagnostic potential to discriminate PC cases from healthy controls (AUC of 0.969, sensitivity of 0.97, specificity of 0.912, and accuracy of 0.915), but low specificity for PC compared to other tumor cases. On the other hand, miR-93-5p showed worse performance parameters, in particular, lower sensitivity, in distinguishing PC cases from non-cancerous controls (AUC of 0.694, sensitivity of 0.479, specificity of 0.872, and accuracy of 0.85), but higher specificity for a subset of PC (~47%) compared to other cancer types.

The differences in circulating biomarkers based on molecular cancer subtypes are significant, particularly in breast cancer, where distinct profiles can inform about diagnosis, prognosis, and treatment strategies. Studies indicate that circulating biomarkers, including proteins, metabolites, and microRNAs, can vary across molecular subtypes, reflecting the underlying biological heterogeneity of cancers [57,58]. Although PC subtypes do not currently guide the clinical management of patients, increasing evidence based on omics analysis is currently defining PC subgroups with distinct biology and potential subtype-specific therapeutic vulnerabilities, offering the opportunity to define new possible clinically applicable molecular classification [59]. Therefore, it can be hypothesized that the complexity of cancer biology, including that of PC, underscores the need for further investigation into the implications and utility of circulating biomarkers, considering factors such as molecular subtypes. Notably, to date, no data is available regarding specific biomarkers associated with PC molecular subtypes. However, considering the only partially overlapping (common) miRNAs identified across the three cell lines, we can hypothesize that differences observed may be in part explained by the distinct molecular characteristics of each cell line.

We also analyzed protein factors released in the supernatants of US-treated cancer cells, detecting well-known tumor markers (e.g., CA19-9, CEA, and CA125) [4], as well as proteins as candidate novel biomarkers for the detection of PC, particularly B2M, CRP, TIMP1, and Galectin-3 [60].

CA19-9 is currently the most widely used non-invasive biomarker for PC diagnosis, and although several studies have recommended the combination of CA19-9, CA-125, and

CEA as a routine screening method for PC detection, these factors are ineffective as early markers due to their low specificity [60].

Among the novel suggested protein biomarkers, B2M (in this study, common to two PC cell lines) and CRP were recently included in a PC diagnostic panel comprising 11 candidate factors which demonstrated significant performance in terms of specificity and sensitivity in discriminating PC from control samples [61]; CRP has also been suggested as a PC prognostic factor in combination with CA19-9 [62].

Similarly, TIMP-1 has been reported as a potential biomarker for the early detection of PC [60], particularly in familial PC in association with LCN2 [63], while Galectin-3 was described as a putative biomarker for screening and diagnosis, as well as an independent prognostic indicator in PC [64].

In the supernatants of US-treated cancer cells, we also detected upregulated levels of uPA and VEGF-A, the first of which has been reported to be positively associated with increased PC severity and poor clinical outcome [65], while the latter is generally found to be significantly elevated in cancer patients, including those with PC, compared to the results for healthy individuals [66].

Interestingly, the network and pathway analysis of identified miRNAs and proteins highlighted their involvement in key biological processes related to PC development and progression, which are closely associated with oncogenic driver alterations that mainly affect the *KRAS*, *TP53*, *CDKN2A*, and *SMAD4* genes [67]. Indeed, among the most representative and relevant pathways, the Ras signaling pathway and the RAF/MAP kinase cascade, the p53 signaling pathway, and signaling by TGFB family members emerged, in addition to the modulation of VEGF signaling/angiogenesis and the modulation of the immune system. These findings suggest that molecules identified in this study may function not only as diagnostic biomarkers, but also as active contributors to PC tumorigenesis. However, further investigations are required to elucidate their role in PC pathogenesis.

Overall, due to the complexity of tumor biology and the heterogeneity of cancers, our results, in agreement with data reported in the literature, show that the most successful strategy for the identification of biomarkers of clinical utility could be a combination of factors (e.g., miRNA/proteins), also taking into account the possible pathological and/or molecular features of tumors.

Studies have shown that biomarker panels outperform single biomarkers [68,69], suggesting that the factors identified here could be part of such effective combinations.

This leads to the main limitations of the present study, which, in addition to the imbalance in the number of cases and controls in the publicly available datasets queried, relate to the inability to directly analyze our own PC study series to test the diagnostic potential of the different combinations of miRNA/protein described.

5. Conclusions

In conclusion, we demonstrated the suitability of US-mediated sonoporation to promote and amplify the release of miRNAs and proteins in PC cell lines, highlighting the use of this method to identify candidate circulating biomarkers. This study introduces novel molecules to be considered as non-invasive biomarkers in PC (e.g., miR-320a, miR-93-5p, B2M, CRP, and TIMP-1), encouraging further studies, including those of a prospective nature, aimed at deepening the understanding of their role in PC and to support the validation of different miRNA/protein combinations directly in the sera/plasma of PC patients for early diagnostic and prognostic purposes. Advances in high-throughput sequencing, the development of standardized protocols, and analysis of large well-characterized series are essential to improve the identification of non-invasive molecular biomarkers of clinical relevance.

Supplementary Materials: The following supporting information can be downloaded at: https://www.mdpi.com/article/10.3390/cancers17121979/s1, Table S1: Publicly available datasets; Table S2: List of released miRNAs identified in PC cell line; Table S3: Evaluation of the diagnostic potential of the most interesting emerging miRNAs; Figure S1: Overview of the diagnostic potential of the best performing miRNA combinations, along with additional information on SonoWell instrument specifications and experimental reproducibility.

Author Contributions: Conceptualization, V.Z., C.C., G.B., and A.T.; methodology, validation and formal analysis, A.C., F.C., and M.S.M.; investigation, V.Z. and C.C.; resources and data curation, V.Z., C.C., M.D.P., D.C., E.A., F.Z., and A.T.; writing—original draft preparation, V.Z., C.C., and A.T.; writing—review and editing, G.B., M.D.P., D.C., E.A., and F.Z.; supervision, project administration and funding acquisition, A.T. All authors have read and agreed to the published version of the manuscript.

Funding: This research was funded by the DISCAB GRANT 2024 (07_DG_2024_22) awarded to A.T. by the Department of Biotechnological and Applied Clinical Sciences, University of L'Aquila. This work was supported by the European Union—NextGenerationEU under the Italian Ministry of University and Research (MUR) National Innovation Ecosystem [ECS00000041—VITALITY]. V.Z. is supported by MIUR funding (DM 737/2021, code DM 737.PNRR_DISCAB). A.C. and M.S.M. are supported by the PON 2014–2020 Research and Innovation PhD program. F.C. is supported by the PNRR PhD program.

Institutional Review Board Statement: Not applicable.

Informed Consent Statement: Not applicable.

Data Availability Statement: The original contributions presented in the study are included in the article. Further inquiries can be directed to the corresponding author. Publicly available datasets analyzed in this study are available in the dbDEMC database (https://www.biosino.org/dbDEMC/index (accessed on 20 January 2025)) and GEO repository (https://www.ncbi.nlm.nih.gov/geo/query/acc.cgi?acc=GSE106817, (accessed on 20 January 2025), https://www.ncbi.nlm.nih.gov/geo/query/acc.cgi?acc=GSE112264 (accessed on 20 January 2025)).

Acknowledgments: The authors wish to thank Saloni Mudholkar for her contribution in critically reading the manuscript and providing English language editing.

Conflicts of Interest: G.B. is the Scientific Director and CEO of Inno-Sol srl and declares no conflict of interest. All other authors declare no conflicts of interest.

Abbreviations

The following abbreviations are used in this manuscript:

ACC	Accuracy
AP	Acoustic Pressure (negative peak)
AUC	Area Under the Curve
B2M	Beta-2 microglobulin
dbDEMC	Database of Differentially Expressed miRNAs in Human Cancers
DC	Duty Cycle
FC	Fold Change
FUS	Focused Ultrasound
I_{sppa}	Intensity of Spatial Peak Pressure Average
I_{spta}	Intensity of Spatial Peak Time Average
miRNA	microRNA
PC	Pancreatic Cancer
ROC	Receiver Operating Characteristic
RQ	Relative Quantification
SE	Sensitivity
SP	Specificity
TBD	Tone Burst Duration
US	Ultrasound

References

1. Mizrahi, J.D.; Surana, R.; Valle, J.W.; Shroff, R.T. Pancreatic Cancer. *Lancet* **2020**, *395*, 2008–2020. [CrossRef]
2. Puckett, Y.; Garfield, K. Pancreatic Cancer. In *StatPearls*; StatPearls Publishing: Treasure Island, FL, USA, 2025.
3. Scialpi, M.; Reginelli, A.; D'Andrea, A.; Gravante, S.; Falcone, G.; Baccari, P.; Manganaro, L.; Palumbo, B.; Cappabianca, S. Pancreatic Tumors Imaging: An Update. *Int. J. Surg.* **2016**, *28* (Suppl. 1), S142–S155. [CrossRef]
4. Poruk, K.E.; Gay, D.Z.; Brown, K.; Mulvihill, J.D.; Boucher, K.M.; Scaife, C.L.; Firpo, M.A.; Mulvihill, S.J. The Clinical Utility of CA 19-9 in Pancreatic Adenocarcinoma: Diagnostic and Prognostic Updates. *Curr. Mol. Med.* **2013**, *13*, 340–351. [CrossRef]
5. Zofia Rogowska, A. Ultrasound-Guided Percutaneous Core-Needle Biopsy of Focal Pancreatic Lesions—Practical Aspectss. *J. Ultrason.* **2022**, *22*, 117–120. [CrossRef]
6. Ignatiadis, M.; Sledge, G.W.; Jeffrey, S.S. Liquid Biopsy Enters the Clinic—Implementation Issues and Future Challenges. *Nat. Rev. Clin. Oncol.* **2021**, *18*, 297–312. [CrossRef] [PubMed]
7. Juźwik, C.A.; Drake, S.S.; Zhang, Y.; Paradis-Isler, N.; Sylvester, A.; Amar-Zifkin, A.; Douglas, C.; Morquette, B.; Moore, C.S.; Fournier, A.E. microRNA Dysregulation in Neurodegenerative Diseases: A Systematic Review. *Prog. Neurobiol.* **2019**, *182*, 101664. [CrossRef]
8. Zhou, S.-S.; Jin, J.-P.; Wang, J.-Q.; Zhang, Z.-G.; Freedman, J.H.; Zheng, Y.; Cai, L. miRNAS in Cardiovascular Diseases: Potential Biomarkers, Therapeutic Targets and Challenges. *Acta Pharmacol. Sin.* **2018**, *39*, 1073–1084. [CrossRef]
9. Peng, Y.; Croce, C.M. The Role of MicroRNAs in Human Cancer. *Signal Transduct. Target. Ther.* **2016**, *1*, 15004. [CrossRef]
10. Arroyo, J.D.; Chevillet, J.R.; Kroh, E.M.; Ruf, I.K.; Pritchard, C.C.; Gibson, D.F.; Mitchell, P.S.; Bennett, C.F.; Pogosova-Agadjanyan, E.L.; Stirewalt, D.L.; et al. Argonaute2 Complexes Carry a Population of Circulating microRNAs Independent of Vesicles in Human Plasma. *Proc. Natl. Acad. Sci. USA* **2011**, *108*, 5003–5008. [CrossRef]
11. Vickers, K.C.; Palmisano, B.T.; Shoucri, B.M.; Shamburek, R.D.; Remaley, A.T. MicroRNAs Are Transported in Plasma and Delivered to Recipient Cells by High-Density Lipoproteins. *Nat. Cell Biol.* **2011**, *13*, 423–433. [CrossRef]
12. Sun, Z.; Shi, K.; Yang, S.; Liu, J.; Zhou, Q.; Wang, G.; Song, J.; Li, Z.; Zhang, Z.; Yuan, W. Effect of Exosomal miRNA on Cancer Biology and Clinical Applications. *Mol. Cancer* **2018**, *17*, 147. [CrossRef] [PubMed]
13. D'Souza, A.L.; Tseng, J.R.; Pauly, K.B.; Guccione, S.; Rosenberg, J.; Gambhir, S.S.; Glazer, G.M. A Strategy for Blood Biomarker Amplification and Localization Using Ultrasound. *Proc. Natl. Acad. Sci. USA* **2009**, *106*, 17152–17157. [CrossRef]
14. D'Souza, A.L.; Chevillet, J.R.; Ghanouni, P.; Yan, X.; Tewari, M.; Gambhir, S.S. Tumor Characterization by Ultrasound-Release of Multiple Protein and microRNA Biomarkers, Preclinical and Clinical Evidence. *PLoS ONE* **2018**, *13*, e0194268. [CrossRef]
15. Zhu, L.; Nazeri, A.; Pacia, C.P.; Yue, Y.; Chen, H. Focused Ultrasound for Safe and Effective Release of Brain Tumor Biomarkers into the Peripheral Circulation. *PLoS ONE* **2020**, *15*, e0234182. [CrossRef] [PubMed]
16. Cornice, J.; Capece, D.; Di Vito Nolfi, M.; Di Padova, M.; Compagnoni, C.; Verzella, D.; Di Francesco, B.; Vecchiotti, D.; Flati, I.; Tessitore, A.; et al. Ultrasound-Based Method for the Identification of Novel MicroRNA Biomarkers in Prostate Cancer. *Genes* **2021**, *12*, 1726. [CrossRef]
17. Krasovitski, B.; Frenkel, V.; Shoham, S.; Kimmel, E. Intramembrane Cavitation as a Unifying Mechanism for Ultrasound-Induced Bioeffects. *Proc. Natl. Acad. Sci. USA* **2011**, *108*, 3258–3263. [CrossRef] [PubMed]
18. Azhari, H. *Basics of Biomedical Ultrasound for Engineers*; John Wiley & Sons: Hoboken, NJ, USA, 2010; pp. 313–314. [CrossRef]
19. Beekers, I.; Vegter, M.; Lattwein, K.R.; Mastik, F.; Beurskens, R.; van der Steen, A.F.W.; de Jong, N.; Verweij, M.D.; Kooiman, K. Opening of Endothelial Cell-Cell Contacts Due to Sonoporation. *J. Control Release* **2020**, *322*, 426–438. [CrossRef]
20. Hu, Y.; Wei, J.; Shen, Y.; Chen, S.; Chen, X. Barrier-Breaking Effects of Ultrasonic Cavitation for Drug Delivery and Biomarker Release. *Ultrason. Sonochem.* **2023**, *94*, 106346. [CrossRef]
21. Forbrich, A.; Paproski, R.; Hitt, M.; Zemp, R. Comparing Efficiency of Micro-RNA and mRNA Biomarker Liberation with Microbubble-Enhanced Ultrasound Exposure. *Ultrasound. Med. Biol.* **2014**, *40*, 2207–2216. [CrossRef]
22. Martin, E.; Aubry, J.-F.; Schafer, M.; Verhagen, L.; Treeby, B.; Pauly, K.B. ITRUSST Consensus on Standardised Reporting for Transcranial Ultrasound Stimulation. *Brain Stimul.* **2024**, *17*, 607–615. [CrossRef]
23. Yokoi, A.; Matsuzaki, J.; Yamamoto, Y.; Yoneoka, Y.; Takahashi, K.; Shimizu, H.; Uehara, T.; Ishikawa, M.; Ikeda, S.-I.; Sonoda, T.; et al. Integrated Extracellular microRNA Profiling for Ovarian Cancer Screening. *Nat. Commun.* **2018**, *9*, 4319. [CrossRef] [PubMed]
24. Urabe, F.; Matsuzaki, J.; Yamamoto, Y.; Kimura, T.; Hara, T.; Ichikawa, M.; Takizawa, S.; Aoki, Y.; Niida, S.; Sakamoto, H.; et al. Large-Scale Circulating microRNA Profiling for the Liquid Biopsy of Prostate Cancer. *Clin. Cancer Res.* **2019**, *25*, 3016–3025. [CrossRef] [PubMed]
25. Yamamoto, Y.; Kondo, S.; Matsuzaki, J.; Esaki, M.; Okusaka, T.; Shimada, K.; Murakami, Y.; Enomoto, M.; Tamori, A.; Kato, K.; et al. Highly Sensitive Circulating MicroRNA Panel for Accurate Detection of Hepatocellular Carcinoma in Patients with Liver Disease. *Hepatol. Commun.* **2019**, *4*, 284–297. [CrossRef] [PubMed]
26. Usuba, W.; Urabe, F.; Yamamoto, Y.; Matsuzaki, J.; Sasaki, H.; Ichikawa, M.; Takizawa, S.; Aoki, Y.; Niida, S.; Kato, K.; et al. Circulating miRNA panels for specific and early detection in bladder cancer. *Cancer Sci.* **2019**, *110*, 408–419. [CrossRef]

27. Mazzara, S.; Rossi, R.L.; Grifantini, R.; Donizetti, S.; Abrignani, S.; Bombaci, M. CombiROC: An Interactive Web Tool for Selecting Accurate Marker Combinations of Omics Data. *Sci. Rep.* **2017**, *7*, 45477. [CrossRef]
28. Tu, J.; Yu, A.C.H. Ultrasound-Mediated Drug Delivery: Sonoporation Mechanisms, Biophysics, and Critical Factors. *BME Front.* **2022**, *2022*, 9807347. [CrossRef]
29. Chen, D.; Wu, X.; Xia, M.; Wu, F.; Ding, J.; Jiao, Y.; Zhan, Q.; An, F. Upregulated Exosomic miR-23b-3p Plays Regulatory Roles in the Progression of Pancreatic Cancer. *Oncol. Rep.* **2017**, *38*, 2182–2188. [CrossRef]
30. Zhang, Y.; Chen, D.; Zhang, G.; Wu, X.; Zhou, L.; Lin, Y.; Ding, J.; An, F.; Zhan, Q. MicroRNA-23b-3p Promotes Pancreatic Cancer Cell Tumorigenesis and Metastasis via the JAK/PI3K and Akt/NF-κB Signaling Pathways. *Oncol. Lett.* **2020**, *20*, 160. [CrossRef]
31. López-Beas, J.; Capilla-González, V.; Aguilera, Y.; Mellado, N.; Lachaud, C.C.; Martín, F.; Smani, T.; Soria, B.; Hmadcha, A. miR-7 Modulates hESC Differentiation into Insulin-Producing Beta-like Cells and Contributes to Cell Maturation. *Mol. Ther. Nucleic Acids* **2018**, *12*, 463–477. [CrossRef]
32. Przystupski, D.; Ussowicz, M. Landscape of Cellular Bioeffects Triggered by Ultrasound-Induced Sonoporation. *Int. J. Mol. Sci.* **2022**, *23*, 11222. [CrossRef]
33. Chevillet, J.R.; Khokhlova, T.D.; Giraldez, M.D.; Schade, G.R.; Starr, F.; Wang, Y.-N.; Gallichotte, E.N.; Wang, K.; Hwang, J.H.; Tewari, M. Release of Cell-Free MicroRNA Tumor Biomarkers into the Blood Circulation with Pulsed Focused Ultrasound: A Noninvasive, Anatomically Localized, Molecular Liquid Biopsy. *Radiology* **2017**, *283*, 158–167. [CrossRef] [PubMed]
34. Madadjim, R.; An, T.; Cui, J. MicroRNAs in Pancreatic Cancer: Advances in Biomarker Discovery and Therapeutic Implications. *Int. J. Mol. Sci.* **2024**, *25*, 3914. [CrossRef] [PubMed]
35. Calatayud, D.; Dehlendorff, C.; Boisen, M.K.; Hasselby, J.P.; Schultz, N.A.; Werner, J.; Immervoll, H.; Molven, A.; Hansen, C.P.; Johansen, J.S. Tissue MicroRNA Profiles as Diagnostic and Prognostic Biomarkers in Patients with Resectable Pancreatic Ductal Adenocarcinoma and Periampullary Cancers. *Biomark. Res.* **2017**, *5*, 8. [CrossRef]
36. Wu, Y.; Hong, Q.; Lu, F.; Zhang, Z.; Li, J.; Nie, Z.; He, B. The Diagnostic and Prognostic Value of miR-155 in Cancers: An Updated Meta-Analysis. *Mol. Diagn. Ther.* **2023**, *27*, 283–301. [CrossRef]
37. Nakamura, S.; Sadakari, Y.; Ohtsuka, T.; Okayama, T.; Nakashima, Y.; Gotoh, Y.; Saeki, K.; Mori, Y.; Nakata, K.; Miyasaka, Y.; et al. Pancreatic Juice Exosomal MicroRNAs as Biomarkers for Detection of Pancreatic Ductal Adenocarcinoma. *Ann. Surg. Oncol.* **2019**, *26*, 2104–2111. [CrossRef]
38. Wnuk, J.; Strzelczyk, J.K.; Gisterek, I. Clinical Value of Circulating miRNA in Diagnosis, Prognosis, Screening and Monitoring Therapy of Pancreatic Ductal Adenocarcinoma-A Review of the Literature. *Int. J. Mol. Sci.* **2023**, *24*, 5113. [CrossRef]
39. Lee, J.; Lee, H.S.; Park, S.B.; Kim, C.; Kim, K.; Jung, D.E.; Song, S.Y. Identification of Circulating Serum miRNAs as Novel Biomarkers in Pancreatic Cancer Using a Penalized Algorithm. *Int. J. Mol. Sci.* **2021**, *22*, 1007. [CrossRef]
40. Xue, J.; Jia, E.; Ren, N.; Lindsay, A.; Yu, H. Circulating microRNAs as Promising Diagnostic Biomarkers for Pancreatic Cancer: A Systematic Review. *Onco Targets Ther.* **2019**, *12*, 6665–6684. [CrossRef] [PubMed]
41. Zhang, J.-X.; Yang, W.; Wu, J.-Z.; Zhou, C.; Liu, S.; Shi, H.-B.; Zhou, W.-Z. MicroRNA-32-5p Inhibits Epithelial-Mesenchymal Transition and Metastasis in Lung Adenocarcinoma by Targeting SMAD Family 3. *J. Cancer* **2021**, *12*, 2258–2267. [CrossRef]
42. Liu, Y.-J.; Zhou, H.-G.; Chen, L.-H.; Qu, D.-C.; Wang, C.-J.; Xia, Z.-Y.; Zheng, J.-H. MiR-32-5p Regulates the Proliferation and Metastasis of Cervical Cancer Cells by Targeting HOXB8. *Eur. Rev. Med. Pharmacol. Sci.* **2019**, *23*, 87–95. [CrossRef]
43. Yuan, P.; Tang, C.; Chen, B.; Lei, P.; Song, J.; Xin, G.; Wang, Z.; Hui, Y.; Yao, W.; Wang, G.; et al. miR-32-5p Suppresses the Proliferation and Migration of Pancreatic Adenocarcinoma Cells by Targeting TLDC1. *Mol. Med. Rep.* **2021**, *24*, 752. [CrossRef] [PubMed]
44. Wu, Y.; Xu, W.; Yang, Y.; Zhang, Z. miRNA-93-5p Promotes Gemcitabine Resistance in Pancreatic Cancer Cells by Targeting the PTEN-Mediated PI3K/Akt Signaling Pathway. *Ann. Clin. Lab. Sci.* **2021**, *51*, 310–320. [PubMed]
45. Mądro, A.; Kazimierak, W.; Grenda, A.; Krawczyk, P. Circulating microRNAs as a Potential Diagnostic Marker in Chronic Pancreatitis, Pancreatic Cancer and Colorectal Cancer. *Oncol. Clin. Pract.* **2023**, *19*, 34–42. [CrossRef]
46. Despotović, J.; Bogdanović, A.; Dragičević, S.; Galun, D.; Krivokapić, Z.; Nikolić, A. Prognostic Potential of Circulating miR-93-5p in Patients with Colorectal Cancer Liver Metastases. *Neoplasma* **2022**, *69*, 430–442. [CrossRef]
47. Costa, C.; Indovina, P.; Mattioli, E.; Forte, I.M.; Iannuzzi, C.A.; Luzzi, L.; Bellan, C.; De Summa, S.; Bucci, E.; Di Marzo, D.; et al. Correction: P53-Regulated miR-320a Targets PDL1 and Is Downregulated in Malignant Mesothelioma. *Cell Death Dis.* **2020**, *11*, 867. [CrossRef] [PubMed]
48. Sun, J.-Y.; Huang, Y.; Li, J.-P.; Zhang, X.; Wang, L.; Meng, Y.-L.; Yan, B.; Bian, Y.-Q.; Zhao, J.; Wang, W.-Z.; et al. MicroRNA-320a Suppresses Human Colon Cancer Cell Proliferation by Directly Targeting β-Catenin. *Biochem. Biophys. Res. Commun.* **2012**, *420*, 787–792. [CrossRef]
49. Wang, B.; Yang, Z.; Wang, H.; Cao, Z.; Zhao, Y.; Gong, C.; Ma, L.; Wang, X.; Hu, X.; Chen, S. MicroRNA-320a Inhibits Proliferation and Invasion of Breast Cancer Cells by Targeting RAB11A. *Am. J. Cancer Res.* **2015**, *5*, 2719–2729. [CrossRef]
50. Yang, H.; Yu, J.; Wang, L.; Ding, D.I.; Zhang, L.; Chu, C.; Chen, Q.; Xu, Z.; Zou, Q.; Liu, X. miR-320a Is an Independent Prognostic Biomarker for Invasive Breast Cancer. *Oncol. Lett.* **2014**, *8*, 1043–1050. [CrossRef]

51. Wang, J.; Shi, C.; Wang, J.; Cao, L.; Zhong, L.; Wang, D. MicroRNA-320a Is Downregulated in Non-Small Cell Lung Cancer and Suppresses Tumor Cell Growth and Invasion by Directly Targeting Insulin-like Growth Factor 1 Receptor. *Oncol. Lett.* **2017**, *13*, 3247–3252. [CrossRef]
52. Zhao, W.; Sun, Q.; Yu, Z.; Mao, S.; Jin, Y.; Li, J.; Jiang, Z.; Zhang, Y.; Chen, M.; Chen, P.; et al. MiR-320a-3p/ELF3 Axis Regulates Cell Metastasis and Invasion in Non-Small Cell Lung Cancer via PI3K/Akt Pathway. *Gene* **2018**, *670*, 31–37. [CrossRef]
53. Ge, X.; Cui, H.; Zhou, Y.; Yin, D.; Feng, Y.; Xin, Q.; Xu, X.; Liu, W.; Liu, S.; Zhang, Q. miR-320a Modulates Cell Growth and Chemosensitivity via Regulating ADAM10 in Gastric Cancer. *Mol. Med. Rep.* **2017**, *16*, 9664–9670. [CrossRef] [PubMed]
54. Yao, J.; Liang, L.-H.; Zhang, Y.; Ding, J.; Tian, Q.; Li, J.-J.; He, X.-H. GNAI1 Suppresses Tumor Cell Migration and Invasion and Is Post-Transcriptionally Regulated by Mir-320a/c/d in Hepatocellular Carcinoma. *Cancer Biol. Med.* **2012**, *9*, 234–241. [CrossRef] [PubMed]
55. Wang, W.; Zhao, L.; Wei, X.; Wang, L.; Liu, S.; Yang, Y.; Wang, F.; Sun, G.; Zhang, J.; Ma, Y.; et al. MicroRNA-320a Promotes 5-FU Resistance in Human Pancreatic Cancer Cells. *Sci. Rep.* **2016**, *6*, 27641. [CrossRef]
56. Vila-Navarro, E.; Duran-Sanchon, S.; Vila-Casadesús, M.; Moreira, L.; Ginès, À.; Cuatrecasas, M.; Lozano, J.J.; Bujanda, L.; Castells, A.; Gironella, M. Novel Circulating miRNA Signatures for Early Detection of Pancreatic Neoplasia. *Clin. Transl. Gastroenterol.* **2019**, *10*, e00029. [CrossRef]
57. Zelli, V.; Compagnoni, C.; Capelli, R.; Cannita, K.; Sidoni, T.; Ficorella, C.; Capalbo, C.; Zazzeroni, F.; Tessitore, A.; Alesse, E. Circulating MicroRNAs as Prognostic and Therapeutic Biomarkers in Breast Cancer Molecular Subtypes. *J. Pers. Med.* **2020**, *10*, 98. [CrossRef]
58. Martini, R.; Amankwah, M.; Sahler, J.; Stonaker, B.; Sadullozoda, M.; Radzio, P.; August, A.; Newman, L.; Davis, M. Abstract C009: Race- and TNBC-Specific Circulating Biomarker Profiles among Breast Cancer Patients. *Cancer Epidemiol. Biomark. Prev.* **2023**, *32*, C009. [CrossRef]
59. Collisson, E.A.; Bailey, P.; Chang, D.K.; Biankin, A.V. Molecular Subtypes of Pancreatic Cancer. *Nat. Rev. Gastroenterol. Hepatol.* **2019**, *16*, 207–220. [CrossRef] [PubMed]
60. Liou, G.-Y.; Byrd, C.J. Diagnostic Bioliquid Markers for Pancreatic Cancer: What We Have vs. What We Need. *Cancers* **2023**, *15*, 2446. [CrossRef] [PubMed]
61. Kim, H.; Kang, K.N.; Shin, Y.S.; Byun, Y.; Han, Y.; Kwon, W.; Kim, C.W.; Jang, J.-Y. Biomarker Panel for the Diagnosis of Pancreatic Ductal Adenocarcinoma. *Cancers* **2020**, *12*, 1443. [CrossRef]
62. Nurmi, A.M.; Mustonen, H.K.; Stenman, U.-H.; Seppänen, H.E.; Haglund, C.H. Combining CRP and CA19-9 in a Novel Prognostic Score in Pancreatic Ductal Adenocarcinoma. *Sci. Rep.* **2021**, *11*, 781. [CrossRef]
63. Slater, E.P.; Fendrich, V.; Strauch, K.; Rospleszcz, S.; Ramaswamy, A.; Mätthai, E.; Chaloupka, B.; Gress, T.M.; Langer, P.; Bartsch, D.K. LCN2 and TIMP1 as Potential Serum Markers for the Early Detection of Familial Pancreatic Cancer. *Transl. Oncol.* **2013**, *6*, 99–103. [CrossRef] [PubMed]
64. Yi, N.; Zhao, X.; Ji, J.; Xu, M.; Jiao, Y.; Qian, T.; Zhu, S.; Jiang, F.; Chen, J.; Xiao, M. Serum Galectin-3 as a Biomarker for Screening, Early Diagnosis, Prognosis and Therapeutic Effect Evaluation of Pancreatic Cancer. *J. Cell. Mol. Med.* **2020**, *24*, 11583–11591. [CrossRef] [PubMed]
65. Kumar, A.A.; Buckley, B.J.; Ranson, M. The Urokinase Plasminogen Activation System in Pancreatic Cancer: Prospective Diagnostic and Therapeutic Targets. *Biomolecules* **2022**, *12*, 152. [CrossRef]
66. Pistol-Tanase, C.; Raducan, E.; Dima, S.O.; Albulescu, L.; Alina, I.; Marius, P.; Cruceru, L.M.; Codorean, E.; Neagu, T.M.; Popescu, I. Assessment of Soluble Angiogenic Markers in Pancreatic Cancer. *Biomark. Med.* **2008**, *2*, 447–455. [CrossRef] [PubMed]
67. Kamisawa, T.; Wood, L.D.; Itoi, T.; Takaori, K. Pancreatic Cancer. *Lancet* **2016**, *388*, 73–85. [CrossRef]
68. Zhou, Y.; Tao, L.; Qiu, J.; Xu, J.; Yang, X.; Zhang, Y.; Tian, X.; Guan, X.; Cen, X.; Zhao, Y. Tumor Biomarkers for Diagnosis, Prognosis and Targeted Therapy. *Signal Transduct. Target. Ther.* **2024**, *9*, 132. [CrossRef]
69. Felekkis, K.; Papaneophytou, C. The Circulating Biomarkers League: Combining miRNAs with Cell-Free DNAs and Proteins. *Int. J. Mol. Sci.* **2024**, *25*, 3403. [CrossRef]

cancers

MDPI

Article

Impact of Long-Term Chemotherapy on Outcomes in Pancreatic Ductal Adenocarcinoma: A Real-World UK Multi-Centre Study

Umair Mahmood [1,2], Joanna Lynch [3], Simran Kaur Sandhu [3], Zahir Amin [4], John Bridgewater [1,5], Daniel Hochhauser [1,5], Kai-Keen Shiu [1,5], Paul Miller [2], Elizabeth C. Smyth [2] and Khurum Khan [1,5,*]

1 Department of Gastrointestinal Oncology, University College London Hospitals NHS Foundation Trust, London NW1 2BU, UK; umair.mahmood1@nhs.net (U.M.); john.bridgewater@nhs.net (J.B.); daniel.hochhauser@nhs.net (D.H.); kaikeen.shiu@nhs.net (K.-K.S.)
2 Department of Oncology, Oxford University Hospitals NHS Foundation Trust, Oxford OX3 7LE, UK; paul.miller@ouh.nhs.uk (P.M.); elizabeth.smyth@ouh.nhs.uk (E.C.S.)
3 HCA Healthcare UK, London W1G 6AF, UK; joanna.lynch@hcahealthcare.co.uk (J.L.); simran.kaursandhu@hcahealthcare.co.uk (S.K.S.)
4 Department of Radiology, University College Hospital NHS Foundation Trust (UCLH), London NW1 2BU, UK; zahir.amin@nhs.net
5 University College London Cancer Institute, London WC1E 6DD, UK
* Correspondence: khurum.khan1@nhs.net

Simple Summary: Traditional chemotherapy for pancreatic ductal adenocarcinoma has limited effectiveness and high toxicity, with poor survival outcomes after diagnosis. While best supportive care is often used after initial treatment failure, younger, healthier patients may benefit from extended chemotherapy using alternative regimens. This multi-centre retrospective study examined long-term chemotherapy use in pancreatic ductal adenocarcinoma, finding that patients receiving more treatment lines and longer therapy—potentially due to better tolerance in younger patients—had improved survival. Localised treatment in select patients also contributed to improved survival. Notably, the duration of first-line chemotherapy interruptions, rather than their frequency, was associated with better outcomes in localised cases. Although toxicity remains a concern, managing treatment delays carefully may allow more patients to benefit from extended chemotherapy. Following validation of our results in future studies, our findings may help guide clinicians in selecting patients for long-term treatment and adapting chemotherapy plans to improve survival in this challenging clinical population.

Abstract: Background: We reviewed outcomes of short and long-term chemotherapy with or without breaks in pancreatic ductal adenocarcinoma (PDAC) patients. **Methods:** PDAC patients receiving $\geq$3 chemotherapy cycles between 2019 and 2024 at three institutions were included. Progression-free survival after first-line chemotherapy (PFS1), overall survival (OS) and best overall response (BOR) to chemotherapy were assessed using the Wilcoxon test, Kaplan–Meier test, and univariate and multivariate Cox regression models. **Results:** We screened 237 patients, and 135 patients met the study criteria. Among these patients, 25 had resectable disease, and 110 had unresectable/metastatic disease (13% borderline resectable (BRPC), 20% locally advanced (LAPC), 10% localised developing metastases, 57% de novo metastatic). Ten patients (7%) underwent genetic profiling; *KRAS* aberrations (N = 4), actionable *PLAB2/BRCA2/FGFR2* mutations (N = 3), *ATM/BRIP1* alteration (N = 1). Two patients were managed with PARP inhibitors after receiving multiple lines of chemotherapy. Median PFS1 and OS were concordant with the published literature, but select patient groups achieved prolonged survival outcomes. Among the 36 BRPC/LAPC patients, we observed >1-year PFS1 in 9 (25%) patients and >2-year OS in 3 (8%) patients. Among the 63 de novo metastatic patients, we observed >1-year PFS1 and

>2-year OS in 6 (10%) patients. Among patients with localised disease, smoking history was a poor prognostic factor with respect to OS ($p = 0.03$). Improved PFS1 and OS was associated with ≥6 cycles of first-line chemotherapy, its duration of ≥3.66 months, and local treatment after first chemotherapy ($p < 0.05$ for all). Stereotactic body radiotherapy following first-line chemotherapy was delivered in N = 6 (27%) and N = 1 (7%) of patients with LAPC and BRPC, respectively. Chemotherapy interruption duration, but not number, was associated with PFS1 and OS only in the localised cohort ($p < 0.05$). In patients with de novo metastatic disease, prevalence of type 2 diabetes was adversely associated with OS ($p = 0.03$). Improved PFS and OS was associated with ≥6 cycles of first-line chemotherapy, its duration of ≥4.37 months, and BOR to it (only in this cohort) ($p < 0.05$ for all). A favourable OS was associated with >1 line of chemotherapy ($p = 0.003$). **Conclusion:** Despite challenges, extended chemotherapy and multiple treatment lines may improve survival, with localised treatments benefiting select patients.

Keywords: pancreatic ductal adenocarcinoma; long-term chemotherapy; prolonged survival

1. Introduction

Conventional chemotherapy for pancreatic ductal adenocarcinoma (PDAC) has limited efficacy, significant toxicity, and drug resistance, highlighting the need for new treatment approaches to meet this major unmet clinical need [1–3]. PDAC is the third leading cause of cancer death [4], with median overall survival (OS) ranging from 8.5 months with nab-paclitaxel/gemcitabine [5] to 11.1 months with FOLFIRINOX [6]. NICE guidelines recommend first-line FOLFIRINOX for locally advanced or metastatic PDAC with an Eastern Cooperative Oncology Group (ECOG) performance status of 0–1 [7], typically for 12 cycles over 6 months. However, many patients can only tolerate first-line therapy and die within 6–10 months of their diagnosis. Best supportive care is typically considered to maintain quality of life following disease progression after 6 months of chemotherapy. In younger patients with a good performance status, physicians may continue treatment beyond progression by switching to alternative chemotherapeutic regimens to prolong survival. However, there is a paucity of data on outcomes in patients treated with long-term chemotherapy.

We conducted a multi-institutional review of PDAC patients treated with chemotherapy to determine if long-term chemotherapy improves outcomes compared to shorter courses with or without treatment breaks. The study assessed treatment response, progression-free survival (PFS), and OS and sought to identify clinicopathological factors associated with PFS and OS to refine patient selection for chemotherapy. We aimed to identify patients who would benefit most from extended chemotherapy, given the potential for long-term survival benefit in this challenging population.

2. Material and Methods

2.1. Patient Selection

We screened adult individuals diagnosed with PDAC to identify eligible subjects treated with any type of chemotherapy between 1 January 2019 and 30 June 2024 across three UK healthcare institutions. Patients must have received at least 3 cycles of first-line chemotherapy as standard of care treatment exclusive of participation in an interventional chemotherapy-related clinical trial. We abstracted data from patient medical records including clinician's notes, radiology, radiation oncology, and operative and pathology reports, as well as clinical reports regarding next-generation sequencing.

2.2. Statistical Considerations

Primary outcome measures included progression-free survival following first-line systemic chemotherapy treatment (PFS1) due to the availability of an adequate sample size. PFS1 was defined as the time between the first dose of chemotherapy until radiological/clinical evidence of disease progression, date of last follow-up, or death. We also evaluated OS in our complete cohort. Best overall response (BOR) was evaluated based on the individual physician assessment of chemotherapy response.

Median and interquartile range were used to summarise continuous variables of age, number of cycles, and duration of treatment with chemotherapy, as well as number and duration of chemotherapy interruptions. Frequency tables summarised categorical variables including gender, smoking status, ECOG performance status, stage at initial diagnosis, anatomic site of metastasis, pre-existing co-morbidities, prior surgical treatment, type of chemotherapies received by patients, BOR to each chemotherapy, nature of chemotherapy continuity, common reasons for chemotherapy treatment interruptions, and patterns of systemic treatment change. Outcomes were analysed using Kaplan–Meier actuarial survival methods and Cox proportional-hazards models. Analysis was also performed using univariate and multivariate methods. The Wilcoxon test was used to compare treatment subgroups. Statistical significance was defined as $p < 0.05$ using log-rank tests to identify associations between patient and treatment variables with PFS1 and OS. Patients with missing data were excluded from analysis. All data analysis was performed using R (version 4.2.3) in RStudio (version 2022.12.0.353) and Microsoft Excel (version 16.75) software.

3. Results

3.1. Clinical and Molecular Profile of PDAC Patient Population

We screened 237 patients and identified 135 (57%) eligible subjects who received chemotherapy for pancreatic ductal adenocarcinoma. The median age at PDAC diagnosis was 65 years, and most patients were female (n = 72, 53%) and were non-smokers (n = 73, 54%) (Table 1). We note a relative higher incidence of patients with an ECOG performance status 0–1 prior to commencing first-line chemotherapy (n = 83, 61%) (Table 1). Most patients presented with de novo metastatic disease at initial diagnosis (n = 63, 47%), primarily in the liver (n = 44, 70%) (Table 1). A limited number of subjects in our cohort were previously managed surgically, mainly individuals presenting with resectable disease (n = 14, 10%) (Table 1). In terms of pre-existing co-morbidities prior to PDAC diagnosis, approximately half the cohort was composed of patients with an abnormal body weight (n = 64, 48%) (Table 1).

Table 1. Baseline characteristics of the complete cohort (N = 135).

	Total Number of Subjects	
	N	%
Age at commencing first-line chemotherapy following PDAC diagnosis (years)		
Median	65	
Range	33–85	
Interquartile range	60–73	
Gender		
Male	63	47
Female	72	53

Table 1. *Cont.*

	Total Number of Subjects	
	N	%
Smoking status		
Non-smoker	73	54
Current smoker	13	10
Former smoker	38	28
Unknown	11	8
ECOG performance status		
ECOG 0	39	29
ECOG 0–1	2	1
ECOG 1	42	31
ECOG 1–2	6	4
ECOG 2	7	5
Unknown	39	29
Stage at initial diagnosis		
Resectable PDAC	14	10
Borderline resectable PDAC	14	10
Locally advanced PDAC	22	16
Localised disease followed by distant metastases *	22	16
De novo metastatic disease	63	47
Anatomic site of disease for de novo metastatic patients		
Lung	18	29
Liver	44	70
Brain	1	2
Bone	3	5
Lymph node	12	19
Peritoneum	6	10
Other **	14	22
Prior surgical treatment ***		
Resectable PDAC	14	10
Borderline resectable PDAC	2	1
Locally advanced PDAC	1	1
Localised disease followed by distant metastases	11	8
De novo metastatic disease	2	1
Pre-existing co-morbidities prior to PDAC diagnosis		
Type 2 diabetes mellitus	23	17
Chronic pancreatitis	3	2
Abnormal body weight		
Overweight	32	24
Obese	32	24
None	47	35
Unknown	24	18

Abbreviations: ECOG, Eastern Cooperative Oncology Group; PDAC, pancreatic ductal adenocarcinoma. * Refers to patients receiving chemotherapy both at the time of initial localised disease and subsequently after metastatic progression. ** Omental metastasis (N = 3), adrenal gland (N = 2), spleen (N = 2), mesentery of the small bowel and omentum (N = 1), appendical mass (N = 1), gallbladder (N = 1), ovary (N = 1), lesion located inferior to the third part of the duodenum (N = 1), stomach (N = 1), colon (N = 1). *** None of the evaluated patients received radiotherapy prior to commencing first-line chemotherapy.

There were 10 patients (7%) who underwent genetic profiling on patient request or previous clinical trial screening for exploratory analysis; *KRAS* aberrations (N = 4), actionable *PLAB2/BRCA2/FGFR2* mutations (N = 3), *ATM/BRIP1* alteration (N = 1). Tumour mutational burden was available for a total of six patients; zero mutations per megabase in two patients, three mutations per megabase in one patient, and four mutations per megabase for the remaining three subjects.

We evaluated our patients up to three lines of chemotherapy. First-, second-, and third-line chemotherapy were received by 135, 44, and 9 patients, respectively. The vast majority of our patients received FOLFIRINOX (n = 85, 63%) as their first line of systemic treatment, followed by gemcitabine and nab-paclitaxel in the second-line setting (n = 18, 41%) and fluorouracil and liposomal irinotecan (n = 5, 56%) as the third-line treatment (Supplementary Table S1).

A variable pattern of chemotherapy reception and treatment interruptions was noted across the three systemic treatment lines (Supplementary Table S2A–C). Accumulation of chemotoxicities was the major cause of treatment interruptions in the first (n = 69, 51%) and second treatment line settings (n = 11, 26%) (Supplementary Table S2A,B). Acquiring a COVID-19 infection served as the main cause of third-line chemotherapy interruption (n = 2, 67%) (Supplementary Table S2C). Patterns of chemotherapy change were influenced by the development of progressive disease in our cohort, resulting in a treatment switch to another chemotherapy regimen in the first- (n = 46, 34%) and third-line settings (n = 4, 44%) or systemic treatment discontinuation in the second-line chemotherapy setting (n = 11, 25%) (Supplementary Table S2A–C).

3.2. *Survival Outcomes of Patients with Unresectable or Metastatic Disease*

Our cohort included 25 patients with resectable disease who were excluded from analysis. Among these patients, 10 remained relapse-free after adjuvant chemotherapy, and 9 were alive at 2 years follow-up surveillance. The final analysis included 110 patients with unresectable or metastatic disease (13% borderline resectable, 20% locally advanced, 10% localised disease that developed metastases, and 57% de novo metastatic). As expected, de novo metastatic patients had lower median PFS1 and OS compared to those with localised disease (Table 2).

Table 2. Survival outcomes in major diagnostically staged unresectable cohorts (N = 110).

	Median PFS1 *months* **(95% CI)**	**Median OS** *months* **(95% CI)**
Localised disease * (N = 36)	8.28 (5.98–19.02)	15.15 (11.20–NR)
Localised disease followed by distant metastases (N = 11)	8.15 (2.56–NR)	18.27 (17.38–NR)
De novo metastatic disease (N = 63)	6.41 (5.98–8.18)	9.30 (8.05–12.81)

Abbreviations: CI, confidence interval; NR, not reached; OS, overall survival; PFS1, progression-free survival while on first-line chemotherapy. * Refers to patients diagnosed with borderline resectable and locally advanced pancreatic ductal adenocarcinoma.

3.3. *Treatment Response and Survival Outcomes in the Localised Disease Cohort*

Our localised disease cohort included patients with borderline resectable or locally advanced PDAC receiving chemotherapy. A trend towards treatment response or disease stabilisation was noted primarily in the first-line setting (Supplementary Table S3A), with reduced clinical benefit in subsequent lines due to limited patient numbers in these advanced treatment cohorts (Supplementary Table S3B,C).

Multivariate analysis did not demonstrate any association between PFS1 and age ($p = 0.83$), gender ($p = 0.46$), smoking history ($p = 0.72$), ECOG performance status ($p = 1.00$), history of type 2 diabetes ($p = 0.68$), overweight ($p = 0.37$), and obesity ($p = 0.12$) (Table 3). All these patient-specific factors were not associated with OS, with the exception of smoking history ($p = 0.03$) (Table 3).

Table 3. Associations with PFS1 and OS for patients with localised disease (i.e., borderline resectable and locally advanced disease settings).

	PFS1				OS			
	Univariate HR (95% CI)	***p*-Value**	**Multivariate HR (95% CI) ***	***p*-Value**	**Univariate HR (95% CI)**	***p*-Value**	**Multivariate HR (95% CI) ***	***p*-Value**
Age at commencing first chemotherapy (<75 years vs. ≥75 years)	0.65 (0.21–1.97)	0.45	0.88 (0.28–2.79)	0.83	0.39 (0.14–1.09)	0.07	0.49 (0.16–1.45)	0.20
Gender (male vs. Female)	0.69 (0.26–1.82)	0.46	0.68 (0.25–1.88)	0.46	0.96 (0.38–2.41)	0.93	0.94 (0.35–2.53)	0.90
Smoking status (current or former smoker vs. never smoker)	1.30 (0.56–3.00)	0.54	1.19 (0.46–3.07)	0.72	2.52 (1.00–6.34)	0.05	3.46 (1.10–10.86)	0.03
ECOG performance status at commencing first chemotherapy (ECOG 0 vs. ECOG 1 or higher)	0.00 (0.00–Inf)	1.00	0.00 (0.00–Inf)	1.00	0.00 (0.00–Inf)	1.00	0.00 (0.00–Inf)	1.00
History of type 2 diabetes (prevalent vs. non-prevalent)	0.84 (0.28–2.50)	0.76	1.28 (0.39–4.17)	0.68	1.02 (0.30–3.50)	0.97	1.81 (0.47–6.98)	0.39
History of abnormal body weight								
None	-	-	-	-	-	-	-	-
Overweight	1.34 (0.42–4.25)	0.62	1.89 (0.47–7.62)	0.37	1.53 (0.48–4.86)	0.47	1.72 (0.52–5.65)	0.37
Obese	2.06 (0.65–6.49)	0.22	2.98 (0.75–11.84)	0.12	2.36 (0.74–7.51)	0.15	2.52 (0.75–8.44)	0.14
Number of chemotherapy lines (>1 vs. 1)	N/A	N/A	N/A	N/A	0.87 (0.29–2.59)	0.80	0.63 (0.19–2.04)	0.44
Number of first-line chemotherapy cycles (≥6 vs. <6 cycles)	0.32 (0.14–0.72)	0.006	0.23 (0.09–0.63)	0.004	0.34 (0.14–0.83)	0.02	0.22 (0.06–0.77)	0.02
Duration of first-line chemotherapy (≥3.66 months vs. <3.66 months) **	0.37 (0.15–0.88)	0.02	0.21 (0.08–0.57)	0.002	0.30 (0.12–0.75)	0.01	0.30 (0.11–0.78)	0.01
Number of first-line chemotherapy interruptions (≤2 vs. >2 treatment interruptions)	1.00 (0.41–2.42)	0.99	1.72 (0.58–5.16)	0.33	1.55 (0.56–4.28	0.39	1.67 (0.54–5.11)	0.37
Duration of first-line chemotherapy interruptions (≤28 vs. >28 interrupted days)	2.22 (0.90–5.47)	0.08	3.48 (1.20–10.09)	0.02	3.93 (1.26–12.27)	0.02	13.48 (2.90–62.60)	<0.001
Best overall response on first-line chemotherapy (responders vs. non-responders)	0.36 (0.14–0.90)	0.03	0.39 (0.15–1.02)	0.05	0.30 (0.11–0.84)	0.02	0.41 (0.14–1.19)	0.10
Local treatment after commencing first-line chemotherapy (recipients vs. non-recipients)	0.10 (0.03–0.34)	<0.001	0.09 (0.03–0.32)	<0.001	0.19 (0.07–0.51)	<0.001	0.19 (0.07–0.50)	<0.001

* Adjusted analysis by age at commencing first chemotherapy, gender, local stage at diagnosis, and radiotherapy and/or surgical treatment after commencing first-line chemotherapy. ** Refers to chemotherapy duration while excluding total treatment interruptions. Abbreviations: CI, confidence interval; ECOG, Eastern Cooperative Oncology Group; HR, hazard ratio; N/A, not applicable; OS, overall survival; PFS1, progression-free survival while on first-line chemotherapy.

Patients receiving a greater number of chemotherapy treatment lines were not associated with OS in the localised disease cohort ($p = 0.44$) (Table 3). However, in the first-line setting, a multivariate assessment of treatment-specific factors revealed that an improved PFS1 was associated with ≥6 cycles of first-line chemotherapy ($p = 0.004$), as well as OS

($p = 0.02$) (Figure 1A,B, Table 3). We also observed an association between the median duration of first-line chemotherapy exceeding 3.66 months and PFS1 ($p = 0.002$) as well as OS ($p = 0.01$) (Figure 1C,D, Table 3). During first-line treatment, the median number of chemotherapy interruptions was not associated with PFS1 ($p = 0.33$) or OS ($p = 0.37$) (Table 3). However, we note that patients with a shorter duration of chemotherapy interruption (≤ 28 days) were associated with poor PFS1 ($p = 0.02$) and OS outcomes in the adjusted models ($p < 0.001$) (Table 3). There was no association between BOR on first-line chemotherapy and PFS1 ($p = 0.05$) or OS ($p = 0.10$) in the adjusted analysis (Table 3). Lastly, we observed an association between local treatment after commencing first-line chemotherapy and PFS1 ($p < 0.001$) as well as OS ($p < 0.001$) (Supplementary Figure S1A,B, Table 3). Given the limited number of patients receiving variable types of localised therapies, caution is warranted while interpreting this hypothesis-generating finding.

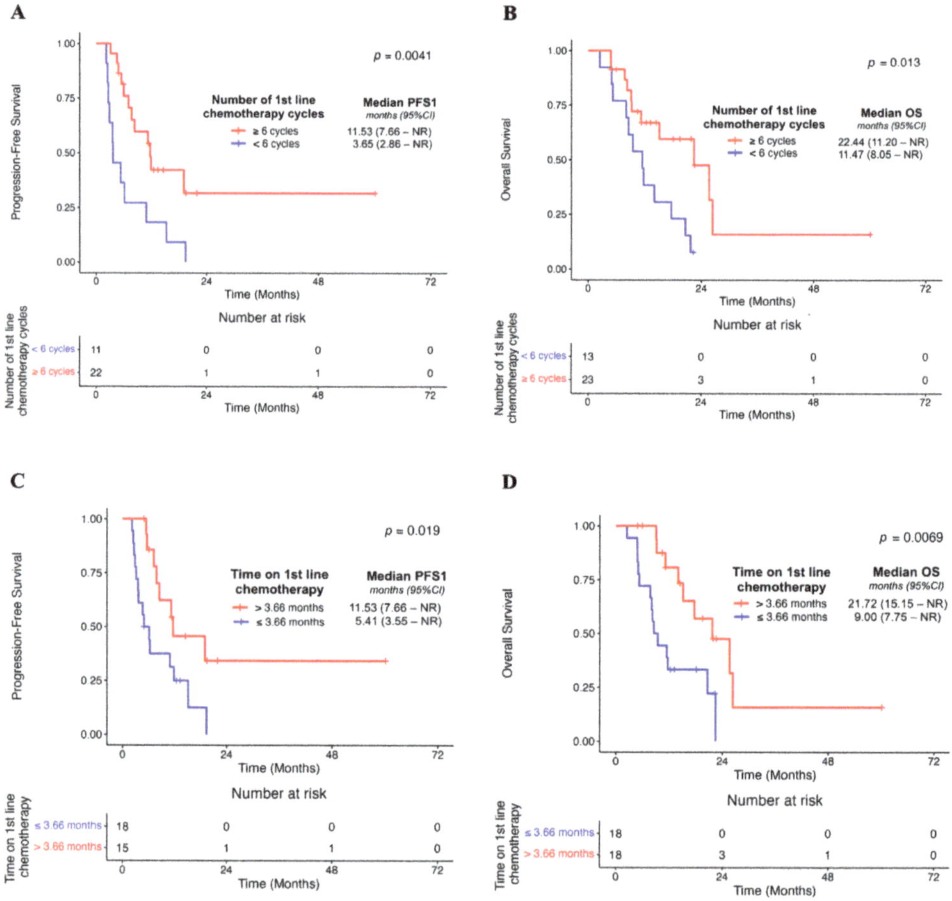

Figure 1. Associations between the number of first-line chemotherapy cycles in the localised disease cohort and PFS1 (**A**) and OS (**B**), respectively. The median value of 6 cycles was used to divide subjects in this disease setting. Associations were also evaluated between the time of first-line chemotherapy in the localised disease cohort and PFS1 (**C**) and OS (**D**), respectively. The median value of 3.66 months was used to divide subjects in this instance.

3.4. Treatment Response and Survival Outcomes in the De Novo Metastatic Disease Cohort

In the de novo metastatic disease cohort, a trend towards decreasing treatment response and disease stabilisation rate was noted while transitioning towards subsequent systemic chemotherapy lines (Supplementary Table S3A–C).

Additionally, our multivariate analysis of patient-specific characteristics revealed no associations between PFS1 and age ($p = 0.09$), gender ($p = 0.78$), smoking history ($p = 0.72$), ECOG performance status ($p = 0.31$), history of type 2 diabetes ($p = 0.37$), overweight ($p = 0.33$), and obesity ($p = 0.69$) (Table 4). Likewise, these factors also did not demonstrate an association with OS, except for a history of type 2 diabetes ($p = 0.03$) (Table 4).

Table 4. Associations with PFS1 and OS in the de novo metastatic disease cohort.

	PFS1				OS			
	Univariate HR (95% CI)	p-Value	Multivariate HR (95% CI) *	p-Value	Univariate HR (95% CI)	p-Value	Multivariate HR (95% CI) *	p-Value
Age at commencing first chemotherapy (<75 years vs. ≥75 years)	0.64 (0.33–1.23)	0.18	0.54 (0.26–1.11)	0.09	0.52 (0.27–0.99)	0.05	0.55 (0.27–1.15)	0.11
Gender (male vs. female)	1.24 (0.71–2.16)	0.44	0.91 (0.48–1.74)	0.78	1.22 (0.68–2.21)	0.50	1.02 (0.51–2.02)	0.96
Smoking status (current or former smoker vs. never smoker)	1.51 (0.79–2.89)	0.21	1.14 (0.56–2.32)	0.72	1.74 (0.89–3.41)	0.10	1.14 (0.56–2.36)	0.71
ECOG performance status at commencing first chemotherapy (ECOG 0 vs. ECOG 1 or higher)	1.00 (0.51–1.96)	1.00	1.46 (0.71–3.02)	0.31	0.87 (0.44–1.74)	0.70	0.88 (0.41–1.87)	0.74
History of type 2 diabetes (prevalent vs. non-prevalent)	0.84 (0.37–1.90)	0.67	1.54 (0.60–3.95)	0.37	1.34 (0.59–3.03)	0.49	2.94 (1.13–7.63)	0.03
History of abnormal body weight								
None	-	-	-	-	-	-	-	-
Overweight	0.65 (0.28–1.51)	0.31	0.63 (0.25–1.60)	0.33	0.78 (0.34–1.81)	0.56	0.56 (0.23–1.36)	0.20
Obese	0.95 (0.48–1.87)	0.88	0.85 (0.39–1.86)	0.69	1.05 (0.52–2.13)	0.90	0.74 (0.34–1.61)	0.45
Number of chemotherapy lines (>1 vs. 1)	N/A	N/A	N/A	N/A	0.37 (0.18–0.73)	0.004	0.31 (0.14–0.67)	0.003
Number of first-line chemotherapy cycles (≥6 vs. <6 cycles)	0.24 (0.13–0.45)	<0.001	0.26 (0.12–0.56)	<0.001	0.28 (0.15–0.51)	<0.001	0.40 (0.20–0.80)	0.01
Duration of first-line chemotherapy (≥4.37 months vs. <4.37 months) **	0.25 (0.14–0.45)	<0.001	0.11 (0.05–0.26)	<0.001	0.28 (0.15–0.52)	<0.001	0.23 (0.12–0.45)	<0.001
Number of first-line chemotherapy interruptions (≤2 vs. >2 treatment interruptions)	1.30 (0.69–2.44)	0.42	1.38 (0.70–2.74)	0.35	1.39 (0.72–2.69)	0.32	1.30 (0.65–2.58)	0.46
Duration of first-line chemotherapy interruptions (≤34 vs. >34 interrupted days)	0.99 (0.52–1.86)	0.96	0.99 (0.51–1.93)	0.97	1.14 (0.59–2.21)	0.69	1.39 (0.70–2.75)	0.35
Best overall response on first-line chemotherapy (responders vs. non-responders)	0.32 (0.17–0.59)	<0.001	0.40 (0.21–0.79)	0.008	0.27 (0.14–0.52)	<0.001	0.35 (0.17–0.71)	0.004

*Adjusted analysis by age at commencing first chemotherapy, gender, and local treatment after commencing first-line chemotherapy. ** Refers to chemotherapy duration while excluding total treatment interruptions. Abbreviations: CI, confidence interval; ECOG, Eastern Cooperative Oncology Group; HR, hazard ratio; N/A, not applicable; OS, overall survival; PFS1, progression-free survival while on first-line chemotherapy.

However, patients receiving more than a single line of chemotherapy were associated with improved OS outcomes (p = 0.003) (Figure 2 and Table 4). Patients receiving a median number of ≥6 cycles of first-line chemotherapy achieved improved PFS1 (p < 0.001) and OS (p = 0.01) (Supplementary Figure S2A,B and Table 4). Subjects receiving ≥6 cycles of first chemotherapy were younger than patients tolerating fewer cycles (median age 59.84 vs. 72.25 years) (p < 0.001) (Supplementary Figure S2C). We also noted that subjects receiving first-line chemotherapy for a period greater than the median duration of 4.37 months experienced prolongation of their PFS1 (p < 0.001) and OS (p < 0.001) as compared to individuals receiving chemotherapy for ≤4.37 months (Supplementary Figure S3A,B and Table 4). Conversely, PFS1 was not associated with the median number of chemotherapy interruptions (p = 0.35) or the duration of such interruptions (p = 0.97) in a first-line setting (Table 4). These two factors were also not associated with OS; p = 0.46 and p = 0.35, respectively (Table 4). Finally, we observed an association between PFS1 and BOR on first-line chemotherapy (p = 0.008), as well as OS (p = 0.004) (Supplementary Figure S4A,B and Table 4).

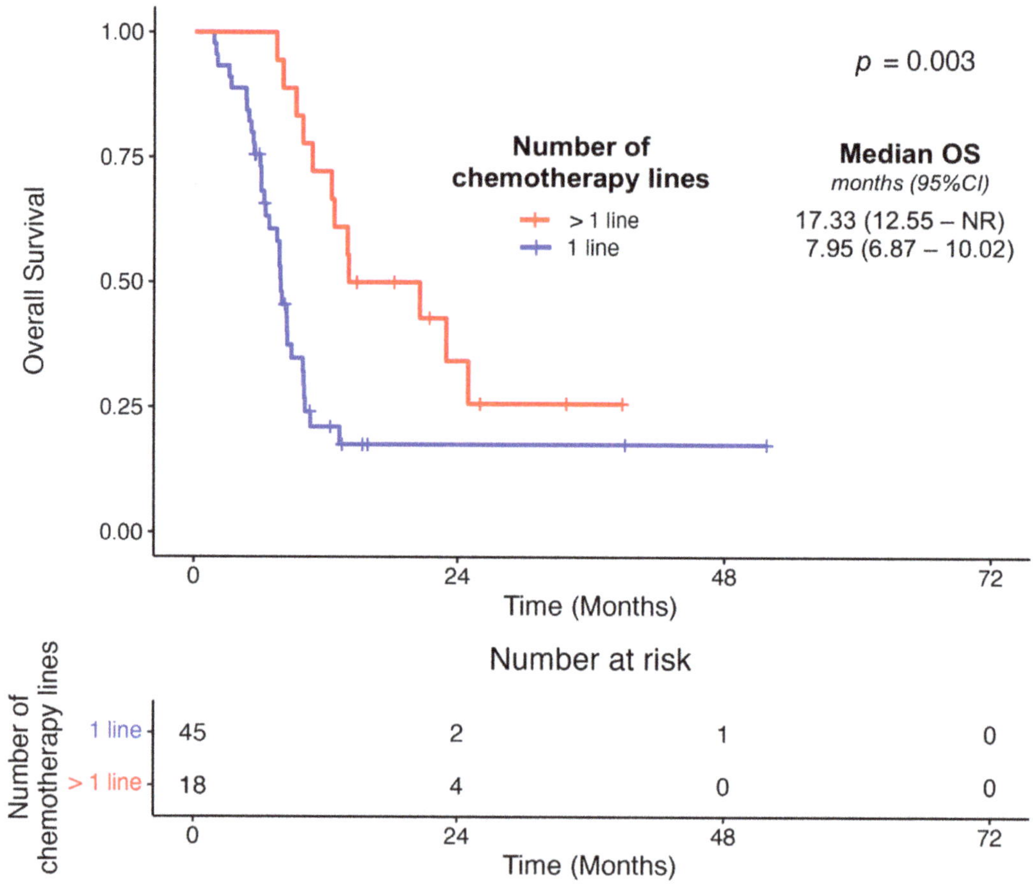

Figure 2. Association between the number of sequential systemic lines of chemotherapy in the de novo metastatic cohort and OS.

3.5. Long-Term Chemotherapy Promotes Instances of Exceptional Responses and Prolongation of OS

We observed three subjects who attained an exceptional treatment response and survival outcomes following clinical management of their underlying PDAC with long-term chemotherapeutic regimens.

Patient #135 is a 73-year-old male who completed 6 months of capecitabine and gemcitabine treatment following R1 resection of his pancreatic primary in July 2022. He then completed 12 cycles of FOLFIRINOX for his local disease recurrence in July 2023. This remained stable until January 2024 where the patient was then treated with radiotherapy for his second local recurrence. The subject experienced peritoneal relapse in June 2024 for which the patient received a PARP inhibitor owing to *ATM S28822** and *BRIP1 W448** mutations, with continued disease stabilisation as of February 2025. Therefore, clinical management using a combination of localised treatment options and multiple lines of systemic therapies (predominantly chemotherapy) resulted in an OS of over 39 months in this patient.

Subject #68 is a 59-year-old male initially diagnosed with localised PDAC who received surgical resection of the primary tumour following completion of 12 cycles of first-line FOLFIRINOX and achieved complete radiographic response (Supplementary Figure S5A,B). The patient subsequently developed disease progression in the liver and was managed with radiotherapy and multiple lines of chemotherapy, resulting in long-term survival exceeding 31 months.

Patient #113 is a 33-year-old female with metastatic liver lesions who achieved a significant treatment response following completion of 13 cycles of modified FOLFIRINOX as first-line chemotherapy (Supplementary Figure S6A,B). She then developed disease progression in a single liver lesion which was managed with radiofrequency ablation and further lines of chemotherapy, resulting in an OS of over 21 months.

In the localised disease cohort, we observed 17 patients whose OS exceeded 12 months, 3 of whom had an OS beyond 24 months. In addition to management with local radiotherapy and surgery after commencing first-line chemotherapy, this improvement in 1-year OS outcomes could have been promoted by the prescription of long-term chemotherapy in a first-line setting composed of a median number of seven cycles and a treatment duration of 5.06 months. Similarly, in the de novo metastatic disease group, 20 subjects had an OS surpassing 12 months, including 6 patients who lived for more than 24 months. This improvement in 1-year OS outcomes can be partially explained by the use of extended first-line chemotherapy, with a median of 12 cycles and a chemotherapy duration of 5.19 months.

4. Discussion

Locally advanced or metastatic PDAC represents an important avenue of ongoing clinical investigations to bridge a major unmet clinical need via establishment of treatment standards ensuring optimum survival outcomes. Long-term chemotherapy can improve symptom management, quality of life, disease control, overall survival, and future clinical trial opportunities. We endeavoured to evaluate clinical outcomes of extended chemotherapy in PDAC patients, as data on this population is limited.

Most of our cohort had an ECOG performance status ≤ 1 and received first-line FOLFIRINOX. The PRODIGE-4 trial demonstrated that FOLFIRINOX outperforms gemcitabine in metastatic PDAC, with a median OS increase of 4.3 months (11.1 vs. 6.8 months) [6]. This is partly due FOLFIRINOX patients tolerating more chemotherapy cycles (median 10 vs. 6, $p < 0.001$), but they also experienced more grade 3/4 neutropenia, febrile neutropenia, thrombocytopenia, diarrhoea, and sensory neuropathy. Chemotherapy interruptions did not correspond with survival in our de novo metastatic cohort, suggesting that maintenance chemotherapy, rather than dose density, might be more important and influences survival outcomes. This signifies the importance of active dose interruptions and timely reductions to ensure durable efficacy of extended chemotherapy. Together with PRODIGE-4, our data supports prolonged chemotherapy, with judicious consideration of chemotoxicities, as a prudent first-line approach in metastatic PDAC, preferably in younger patients with ECOG performance status 0–1 as per ESMO guidelines [8].

Neoadjuvant chemotherapy for locally advanced PDAC (LAPC) has gained momentum in recent years [9,10]. Previous real-world evidence demonstrates that most patients with LAPC completing 6 months of neoadjuvant chemotherapy had a median OS not reached in resectable cases and 15.4 months in unresectable cases [11]. Further studies utilising total neo-adjuvant therapy for borderline resectable or locally advanced PDAC have demonstrated that treatment with ≥6 cycles of chemotherapy is an independently associated factor with survival [12]. Given the increasing interest in neoadjuvant treatments, it would be important to further explore the utility of extended chemotherapy within this disease setting using prospectively designed studies.

The low incidence of actionable genetic alterations in PDAC (0.5–7%) [13] often obviates the need for comprehensive genomic profiling in standard clinical practice. Limited profiling in our cohort was driven by patient request or previous clinical trial screening. However, KRAS alterations are noted in 80–93% of PDAC cases in previous studies [14,15], prompting exploration of RAS inhibitors in ongoing clinical trials. Successful developments originating from these initiatives would confer a paradigm shift in management of PDAC patients owing to a synergistic effect by combining extended chemotherapy treatment plans with targeted agents to improve patient outcomes.

Our study is limited by heterogeneity in metastatic anatomic sites and variability in treatment types, doses, and schedules. Subgroup sample sizes were limited precluding further stratification in our analysis accounting for additional variables, and multiple testing adjustments were not performed. Genomic profiling was performed on a limited number of samples, and the results were exploratory in nature. We intended to limit selection of patients receiving ≥3 cycles of first-line chemotherapy to allow for adequate follow-up time to perform PFS analysis and treatment response assessment. However, this patient selection strategy might have also influenced our results by overestimating our survival outcomes. We observed a relatively lower median age of patients who commenced first-line FOLFIRINOX/modified FOLFIRINOX (N = 79) vs. other chemotherapy regimens (N = 31) (64 years vs. 75 years). Hence, selection of younger patients who were able to better tolerate FOLFIRINOX/modified FOLFIRINOX could have impacted our study findings. It was also challenging to account for chemotherapy dose adjustments as well as reductions between full-dose and milder regimens as these can tend to vary between institutions. Most patients received the outdated FOLFIRINOX regimen, associated with greater side effects, poor compliance, and higher treatment discontinuation, leading to suboptimal outcomes [16–18]. With the recent shift towards modified FOLFIRINOX, we would anticipate better survival outcomes than observed in our study due to improved chemotolerance, a hypothesis that warrants further investigation in future studies. Our study did not include detailed characterisation of patients receiving localised therapies. Such characterisation and further evaluation of localised therapies impacting outcomes in the context of PDAC management is an important concept which should be explored in future studies specifically designed for this purpose.

5. Conclusions

Our data supports consideration of extended chemotherapy for both localised and de novo metastatic PDAC patients. Promising outcomes were seen in patients receiving more chemotherapy lines and longer treatment, potentially due to better tolerance in younger patients. Achieving systemic response contributes to favourable PFS and OS outcomes. While limited genomic profiling was performed, localised treatments in carefully selected patients may improve survival. Chemotherapy-related toxicity is a concern, but careful treatment delays may allow PDAC patients to remain on treatment and derive the clinical benefits associated with long-term chemotherapy. Despite limitations of a retrospective analysis, our findings could help guide clinicians to aid patient selection for long-term chemotherapy or encourage modification of chemotherapy plans to optimise clinical outcomes in this challenging patient population. Future investigations could further explore our findings in larger prospectively designed clinical trials to further validate our results.

Supplementary Materials: The following supporting information can be downloaded at: https://www.mdpi.com/article/10.3390/cancers17111896/s1, Supplementary Figure S1: Associations between local treatment after commencing 1st line chemotherapy in the localised disease cohort and PFS1 (A) and OS (B), respectively. Supplementary Figure S2: Associations between the number of 1st line chemotherapy cycles in the de novo metastatic cohort and PFS1 (A) and OS (B), respectively. The median value of 6 cycles was used to divide subjects in this disease setting. A boxplot of patient's age at the time of initiating 1st line chemotherapy in the de novo metastatic cohort with respect to the number of 1st line chemotherapy treatment cycles (C). Supplementary Figure S3: Associations between time on 1st line chemotherapy among de novo metastatic patients and PFS1 (C) and OS (D), respectively. The median value of 4.37 months was used to divide subjects in this instance. Supplementary Figure S4: Associations between best overall response (BOR) on 1st line chemotherapy in the de novo metastatic cohort and PFS1 (A) and OS (B), respectively. Responders achieved partial or complete response as their BOR, while non-responders had stable or progressive disease as their BOR on 1st line chemotherapy. Supplementary Figure S5: Pre-treatment baseline scan for subject # 68 from February 2022 demonstrated a pancreatic primary with largest axial measurement of 25.1 mm (A). Patient achieved complete radiographic response in December 2022 after completing 12 cycles of FOLFIRINOX (B). Supplementary Figure S6: Pre-treatment baseline scan of Subject # 113 from December 2022 demonstrates liver metastases with largest axial measurement of 15.36 mm (A). Patient achieved partial radiographic response in March 2023 while on 1st line modified FOLFIRINOX, which demonstrated the greatest regression in liver tumour volume in July 2023 limited to 2.94 mm (B). Supplementary Table S1: Systemic treatment types stratified by treatment lines among evaluated patients (N = 135). Supplementary Table S2: (A) Systemic treatment details for patients on 1st line chemotherapy (N = 135). (B) Systemic treatment details for patients on 2nd line chemotherapy (N = 44). (C) Systemic treatment details for patient on 3rd line chemotherapy (N = 9). Supplementary Table S3: (A) Best overall response amongst unresectable patients following 1st line treatment with chemotherapy stratified by stage at initial diagnosis (N = 110). (B) Best overall response amongst unresectable patients following 2nd line treatment with chemotherapy stratified by stage at initial diagnosis (N = 33). (C) Best overall response amongst unresectable patient following 3rd line treatment with chemotherapy stratified by stage at initial diagnosis (N = 7).

Author Contributions: Conceptualization, U.M., E.C.S. and K.K.; Methodology, U.M. and K.K.; Formal analysis, U.M.; Investigation, U.M.; Resources, E.C.S. and K.K.; Data curation, U.M., J.L., S.K.S. and Z.A.; Writing—original draft, U.M., J.L., S.K.S., Z.A., J.B., D.H., K.-K.S., P.M., E.C.S. and K.K. All authors have read and agreed to the published version of the manuscript.

Funding: This work was supported by the University College London Hospital Cancer Fund.

Institutional Review Board Statement: The study was conducted in accordance with the Declaration of Helsinki and approved by the Ethics Committee of Oxford University Hospitals, HCA Healthcare UK, and the University College London Hospital (protocol code 281124 and 25 June 2024).

Informed Consent Statement: Patient consent was waived due to the retrospective nature of this study.

Data Availability Statement: The original contributions presented in this study are included in the article/Supplementary Materials; further inquiries can be directed to the corresponding author.

Conflicts of Interest: J.B. Consulting or Advisory Role—AstraZeneca; Basilea; Bayer; Bristol-Myers Squibb; Incyte; Roche; Taiho Oncology. Speakers' Bureau—Incyte; SERVIER. Research Funding—Incyte (Inst) Travel, Accommodations, Expenses—SERVIER. D.H. Stock and Other Ownership Interests—Moderna Therapeutics; Novartis; Roche. K.-K.S. Honoraria—Bayer; Bristol-Myers Squibb; Merck Serono; MSD Oncology; SERVIER. Consulting or Advisory Role—Bristol-Myers Squibb; GlaxoSmithKline; Mirati Therapeutics; MSD Oncology; Nouscom; Roche; Seagen; Takeda Research Funding—AstraZeneca (Inst); BioNTech SE (Inst); MSD Oncology (Inst); Nouscom (Inst); Roche (Inst). E.C.S. Employment—HCA International (I) Honoraria—Bristol-Meyer Squibb; Novartis; Pfizer; SERVIER Consulting or Advisory Role—Amal Therapeutics; Amgen; AstraZeneca; BeiGene; Bristol-Myers Squibb; Merck Serono; Novartis; Roche; SERVIER; Turning Point Therapeutics; Viracta Therapeutics; Zymeworks Research Funding—Bristol-Meyers Squibb (Inst) Travel, Accommodations, Expenses—Amgen. K.K. Honoraria—Bayer; Bristol Myers Squibb Foundation; Nouscom; SERVIER; Takeda Consulting or Advisory Role—Bayer Health Research Funding—Nouscom. All remaining authors declare no conflict of interest.

References

1. Amrutkar, M.; Gladhaug, I.P. Pancreatic Cancer Chemoresistance to Gemcitabine. *Cancers* **2017**, *9*, 157. [CrossRef] [PubMed]
2. Kang, M.-J.; Li, H.-X.; Gan, Y.; Fang, C.; Yang, X.-L.; Li, B.; Su, S. Efficacy and safety of first-line chemotherapies for patients with advanced pancreatic ductal adenocarcinoma: A systematic review and network meta-analysis. *Heliyon* **2024**, *10*, e27679. [CrossRef] [PubMed]
3. Carvalho, T.M.A.; Di Molfetta, D.; Greco, M.R.; Koltai, T.; Alfarouk, K.O.; Reshkin, S.J.; Cardone, R.A. Tumor Microenvironment Features and Chemoresistance in Pancreatic Ductal Adenocarcinoma: Insights into Targeting Physicochemical Barriers and Metabolism as Therapeutic Approaches. *Cancers* **2021**, *13*, 6135. [CrossRef] [PubMed]
4. Siegel, R.L.; Miller, K.D.; Wagle, N.S.; Jemal, A. Cancer statistics, 2023. *CA Cancer J. Clin.* **2023**, *73*, 17–48. [CrossRef] [PubMed]
5. Von Hoff, D.D.; Ervin, T.; Arena, F.P.; Chiorean, E.G.; Infante, J.; Moore, M.; Seay, T.; Tjulandin, S.A.; Ma, W.W.; Saleh, M.N.; et al. Increased survival in pancreatic cancer with nab-paclitaxel plus gemcitabine. *N. Engl. J. Med.* **2013**, *369*, 1691–1703. [CrossRef] [PubMed]
6. Conroy, T.; Desseigne, F.; Ychou, M.; Bouché, O.; Guimbaud, R.; Bécouarn, Y.; Adenis, A.; Raoul, J.-L.; Gourgou-Bourgade, S.; de la Fouchardière, C.; et al. FOLFIRINOX versus gemcitabine for metastatic pancreatic cancer. *N. Engl. J. Med.* **2011**, *364*, 1817–1825. [CrossRef] [PubMed]
7. Recommendations | Pancreatic Cancer in Adults: Diagnosis and Management | Guidance | NICE. Available online: https://www.nice.org.uk/guidance/ng85/chapter/Recommendations#managing-unresectable-pancreatic-cancer (accessed on 15 February 2025).
8. Conroy, T.; Pfeiffer, P.; Vilgrain, V.; Lamarca, A.; Seufferlein, T.; O'Reilly, E.M.; Hackert, T.; Golan, T.; Prager, G.; Haustermans, K.; et al. Pancreatic cancer: ESMO Clinical Practice Guideline for diagnosis, treatment and follow-up☆. *Ann. Oncol.* **2023**, *34*, 987–1002. [CrossRef] [PubMed]
9. Mahmood, U.; Carrier, E.; Khan, K. Neoadjuvant management of locally advanced pancreatic ductal adenocarcinoma—Heading towards a promising change in treatment paradigm. *Cancer Treat. Rev.* **2024**, *127*, 102750. [CrossRef] [PubMed]
10. Davis, C.H.; Beane, J.D.; Gazivoda, V.P.; Grandhi, M.S.; Greenbaum, A.A.; Kennedy, T.J.; Langan, R.C.; August, D.A.; Alexander, H.R.; Pitt, H.A. Neoadjuvant Therapy for Pancreatic Cancer: Increased Use and Improved Optimal Outcomes. *J. Am. Coll. Surg.* **2022**, *234*, 436. [CrossRef] [PubMed]
11. Rose, J.B.; Rocha, F.G.; Alseidi, A.; Biehl, T.; Moonka, R.; Ryan, J.A.; Lin, B.; Picozzi, V.; Helton, S. Extended Neoadjuvant Chemotherapy for Borderline Resectable Pancreatic Cancer Demonstrates Promising Postoperative Outcomes and Survival. *Ann. Surg. Oncol.* **2014**, *21*, 1530–1537. [CrossRef] [PubMed]

2. Truty, M.J.; Kendrick, M.L.; Nagorney, D.M.; Smoot, R.L.; Cleary, S.P.; Graham, R.P.; Goenka, A.H.; Hallemeier, C.L.; Haddock, M.G.; Harmsen, W.S.; et al. Factors Predicting Response, Perioperative Outcomes, and Survival Following Total Neoadjuvant Therapy for Borderline/Locally Advanced Pancreatic Cancer. *Ann. Surg.* **2021**, *273*, 341. [CrossRef]
3. Targeted Therapy for Pancreatic Cancer. Pancreat Cancer Action Netw n.d. Available online: https://pancan.org/facing-pancreatic-cancer/treatment/treatment-types/targeted-therapy/ (accessed on 15 February 2025).
4. Cowzer, D.; Zameer, M.; Conroy, M.; Kolch, W.; Duffy, A.G. Targeting KRAS in Pancreatic Cancer. *J. Pers. Med.* **2022**, *12*, 1870. [CrossRef] [PubMed]
5. Biankin, A.V.; Waddell, N.; Kassahn, K.S.; Gingras, M.-C.; Muthuswamy, L.B.; Johns, A.L.; Miller, D.K.; Wilson, P.J.; Patch, A.-M.; Wu, J.; et al. Pancreatic cancer genomes reveal aberrations in axon guidance pathway genes. *Nature* **2012**, *491*, 399–405. [CrossRef] [PubMed]
6. Trieu, V.N.; Qazi, S.; Fein, S.H.; Maida, A.E.; Joh, T. Meta-analysis comparing the incidence of serious adverse events, overall survival, and progression-free survival in patients with pancreatic adenocarcinoma harboring unresectable tumors treated with modified FOLFIRINOX or FOLFIRINOX regimen. *J. Clin. Oncol.* **2024**, *42*, e16318. [CrossRef]
7. Yoshida, K.; Iwashita, T.; Uemura, S.; Maruta, A.; Okuno, M.; Ando, N.; Iwata, K.; Kawaguchi, J.; Mukai, T.; Shimizu, M. A multicenter prospective phase II study of first-line modified FOLFIRINOX for unresectable advanced pancreatic cancer. *Oncotarget* **2017**, *8*, 111346–111355. [CrossRef] [PubMed]
8. Gotfrit, J.; Marginean, H.; Ko, Y.-J.; Ghafoor, A.; Kavan, P.; Chalchal, H.; Ahmed, S.; Mulder, K.; Tang, P.; Goodwin, R. Administration of FOLFIRINOX for Advanced Pancreatic Cancer: Physician Practice Patterns During Early Use. *Curr. Oncol.* **2025**, *32*, 128. [CrossRef] [PubMed]

cancers

MDPI

Article

The RAGE Inhibitor TTP488 (Azeliragon) Demonstrates Anti-Tumor Activity and Enhances the Efficacy of Radiation Therapy in Pancreatic Cancer Cell Lines

Kumari Alka [1], Jacob F. Oyeniyi [1], Ghulam Mohammad [1], Yi Zhao [1], Stephen Marcus [2] and Prakash Chinnaiyan [1,3,*]

1 Department of Radiation Oncology, Corewell Health William Beaumont University Hospital, Royal Oak, MI 48076, USA; kumari.alka@corewellhealth.org (K.A.); jacob.oyeniyi@corewellhealth.org (J.F.O.); ghulam.mohammad@corewellhealth.org (G.M.); yi.zhao@corewellhealth.org (Y.Z.)
2 Cantex Pharmaceuticals, Weston, FL 33326, USA
3 Radiation Oncology, Oakland University William Beaumont School of Medicine, Rochester, MI 48309, USA
* Correspondence: prakash.chinnaiyan@corewellhealth.org

Simple Summary: Pancreatic cancer is a leading cause of cancer-related deaths in the U.S. The receptor for advanced glycation end products (RAGE) plays a key role in this disease by promoting tumor growth, treatment resistance, and suppressing immune response. This study investigated TTP488 (Azeliragon), a RAGE inhibitor, both alone and combined with radiation therapy (RT) in models of pancreatic cancer. In laboratory and animal tests, Azeliragon blocked RAGE-related pathways, reduced tumor growth, enhanced RT response, and modulated the immune-suppressive tumor microenvironment in pancreatic cancer. These findings suggest that Azeliragon, used alone or in combination with RT, could be a valuable treatment approach for pancreatic cancer and warrants further investigation.

Abstract: Pancreatic cancer is the third leading cause of cancer-related mortality in the United States, with rising incidence and mortality. The receptor for advanced glycation end products (RAGE) and its ligands significantly contribute to pancreatic cancer progression by enhancing cell proliferation, fostering treatment resistance, and promoting a pro-tumor microenvironment via activation of the nuclear factor-kappa B (NF-κB) signaling pathways. This study validated pathway activation in human pancreatic cancer and evaluated the therapeutic efficacy of TTP488 (Azeliragon), a small-molecule RAGE inhibitor, alone and in combination with radiation therapy (RT) in preclinical models of pancreatic cancer. Human (Panc1) and murine (Pan02) pancreatic cancer cell lines exhibited elevated levels of RAGE and its ligands compared to normal pancreatic tissue. In vitro, Azeliragon inhibited RAGE-mediated NF-κB activation and ligand-mediated cell proliferation in pancreatic cancer cell lines. Target engagement of Azeliragon was confirmed in vivo, as determined by decreased NF-κB activation. Azeliragon demonstrated significant growth delay in mouse models of pancreatic cancer and additive effects when combined with RT. Additionally, Azeliragon modulated the immune suppressive tumor microenvironment in pancreatic cancer by reducing immunosuppressive cells, including M2 macrophages, regulatory T cells, and myeloid-derived suppressor cells, while enhancing CD8+ T cell infiltration. These findings suggest that Azeliragon, by inhibiting RAGE-mediated signaling and modulating immune response, may serve as an effective anti-cancer agent in pancreatic cancer.

Keywords: pancreatic cancer; RAGE; Azeliragon; NF-κB; immunosuppressive microenvironment; radiation therapy

1. Introduction

Pancreatic cancer is the third leading cause of cancer deaths in the United States, contributing to 3% of cancer incidence and 8% of cancer mortality, with an expected increase in incidence and mortality over the next decade. It is projected to become the second leading cause of cancer-related death by 2030 [1,2]. The five-year survival rate for patients with pancreatic cancer has improved marginally over the past two decades and is currently estimated to be 10%, 3%, 15%, and 36% for all stages, metastatic, regional, and localized disease, respectively [1]. The tumor microenvironment has been attributed to the observed therapeutic resistance in this malignancy, wherein hypoxia, immunosuppression, and the accumulation of anti-apoptotic proteins are predominant features [3–5]. Novel treatment strategies, including those aimed at modulating the tumor microenvironment, hold promise for achieving clinical gains in this aggressive malignancy.

The receptor for advanced glycation end products (RAGE) is a transmembrane receptor belonging to the immunoglobulin superfamily that has been implicated in various pathological processes, including cancer, diabetes, and neurodegenerative conditions such as Alzheimer's disease [6–9]. It binds to a diverse array of ligands, such as advanced glycation end products (AGE), Mac-1, S100 proteins, HMGB1, glycosaminoglycans, and amyloid-β-proteins. The activation of RAGE by these ligands triggers diverse signaling pathways, which vary based on factors including the ligand type, concentration, and cellular context [6,7]. This versatility in ligand recognition has led to RAGE being classified as a pattern recognition receptor. Additionally, because many RAGE ligands are linked to tissue damage and stress, RAGE is also described as a receptor for damage-associated molecular patterns (DAMPs), and upregulated RAGE protein in human tumors portends a higher histological grade and poorer clinical outcomes in multiple cancers [10–15].

RAGE has been implicated in the development, advancement, and treatment resistance of pancreatic cancer. DiNorcia et al. demonstrated that deletion of the RAGE gene inhibits pancreatic tumor development and significantly prolongs survival in a mouse model [16]. RAGE has been shown to promote growth and survival in pancreatic cancer cells via multiple mechanisms, including sustaining autophagy, limiting apoptosis, and providing protection against oxidative stress, both in vivo and in vitro. Additionally, RAGE enhances tumor cell ATP production, proliferation, and migration [17–19]. Similarly, up-regulation of RAGE in pancreatic cancer cells has been shown to differentially promote cell proliferation and migration [20].

In addition to the receptor itself, RAGE ligands such as S100P and high mobility group box 1 (HMGB1) have been widely investigated for their roles in pancreatic cancer [21–23]. S100P has been shown to enhance cell proliferation and migration in pancreatic cancer Panc-1 cells through a RAGE-dependent mechanism. Elevated levels of S100P correlate with increased proliferation, survival, migration, and invasion in both in vitro and in vivo models, and these effects were inhibited by a RAGE antagonist peptide [21]. Interactions between RAGE and its ligands activate multiple signaling pathways, including MAP kinase and p38 mitogen-activated protein kinase, Ras kinase, Cdc42/Rac, and stress-activated protein kinase, ultimately inducing a sustained NF-κB response [24–27]. NF-κB is a transcription factor that upregulates anti-apoptotic genes such as A1, A20, XIAP, Bcl-2, and Bcl-XL, leading to the overexpression of anti-apoptotic proteins and the activation of the cellular antioxidant defense system [28–30]. This NF-κB-mediated mechanism is particularly relevant in response to ionizing radiation, as it reduces cell death and contributes to radiation resistance. Furthermore, the constitutive activation of NF-κB genes in malignant cells has been linked to increased resistance to radiation therapy [31].

RAGE inhibitors, primarily through direct inhibition of the RAGE ligand S100P, have shown antitumor activity in preclinical models of pancreatic cancer [32,33]. TTP488 (Azeliragon; Figure 1), an orally bioavailable small-molecule RAGE inhibitor that binds directly to RAGE and blocks its interaction with all ligands, has been thoroughly investigated in human clinical trials and demonstrated excellent safety in patients with Alzheimer's disease [34,35]. In preclinical animal models of breast cancer, Azeliragon demonstrated efficacy via RAGE inhibition [36]. This compound is currently undergoing phase I/II clinical studies in patients with metastatic pancreatic cancer refractory to prior treatments, as well as phase Ib/II studies in combination with standard chemoradiation in patients with newly diagnosed glioblastoma [37,38]. Based on the multiple ways the RAGE pathway has been implicated in the progression of pancreatic cancer and its capacity to modulate radiation response, we evaluated both the anti-tumor activity of the RAGE inhibitor Azeliragon and its potential to enhance radiation response in pancreatic cancer preclinical models.

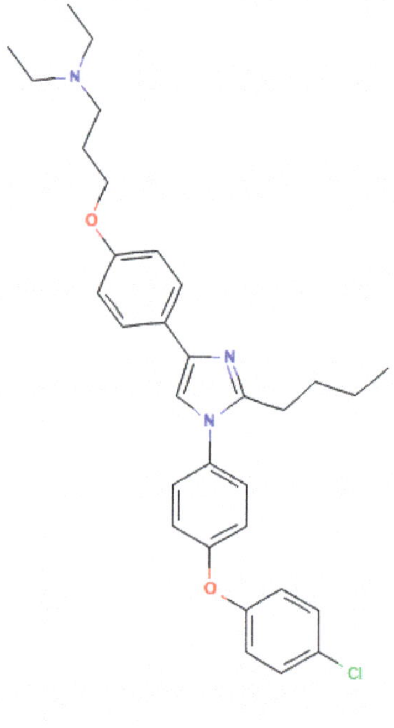

Figure 1. Chemical Structure of Azeliragon (retrieved from PubChem) [34].

2. Materials and Methods

2.1. Cell Lines

The murine pancreatic adenocarcinoma cell line Panc02 was obtained from the National Cancer Institute (NIH, MD, USA) and was cultured in RPMI-1640 medium supplemented with 10% FBS, 100 units/mL penicillin, and 100 µg/mL streptomycin. (Gibco-Thermofisher, Grand Island, NY, USA). The human Panc1 adenocarcinoma cell line was obtained from the American Type Culture Collection (ATCC, Manassas, VA, USA) and was cultured in DMEM medium supplemented with 10% FBS, 100 units/mL penicillin, and 100 µg/mL streptomycin (Gibco, Thermo Fisher Scientific, Inc., Waltham, MA, USA). Both cell lines were cultured and maintained in a humidified atmosphere containing 5% CO_2/95% air at 37 °C. Human pancreas extract (Santa Cruz Biotechnology, TX, USA) and murine pancreas lysate (collected from the pancreas of female C57BL/6NJ mouse) were used as normal pancreas samples.

2.2. Cell Proliferation

Cells (10^5) were plated for 24 h before Azeliragon was added in serial dilution (0.05–3 μM) to the culture medium. Viable cells were counted at the indicated timepoint using trypan blue (Corning/VWR, Chicago, IL, USA). Azeliragon (Cantex Pharmaceuticals, FL, USA) was dissolved in cell culture-grade dimethyl sulfoxide (DMSO, Sigma-Aldrich, St. Louis, MO, USA) and diluted with PBS for in vitro/in vivo studies.

2.3. Tumor Model

Female C57BL/6NJ and NU/J mice (5-week-old) were purchased from The Jackson Laboratory (ME, USA). A total of 2×10^6 Pan02 or Panc1 cells suspended in PBS were subcutaneously injected into the left flank of each mouse. Animals were monitored daily, and tumors were measured with a caliper twice a week. Mice were randomized to four groups (n = 5 per group): (1) control; (2) radiation alone; (3) Azeliragon alone; (4) and radiation + Azeliragon. On day 14 post-tumor implantation, the mice were treated with AZ (1 mg/kg) intraperitoneally or vehicular control, and one day later, RT treatment was initiated. AZ treatment continued daily till the mice survived. Before radiation treatment, each mouse was anesthetized and shielded using a lead box to ensure that only the flank was irradiated. Faxitron model CP160 (Faxitron XRay Corp., Wheeling, IL, USA) was used to irradiate mice at a dose of 2 Gy daily for 5 days. Mice were euthanized upon reaching endpoint criteria (1000 mm^3 for C57BL/6NJ mice and 1500 mm^3 for NU/J mice). For correlative studies, flank tumors (2×10^6 Pan02 or Panc1 cells) were implanted in different sets of mice (Female C57BL/6NJ and NU/J mice), which were randomly selected when the tumor volume reached approximately 150 mm^3 and divided into the indicated groups. Azeliragon (1 mg/kg, i.p.) or vehicle control was started on day 14 post-tumor implantation. Mice were euthanized at day 24 post-tumor implantation, and tumors were harvested for further studies. All in vivo experiments were performed according to institutional guidelines and approved by the Institutional Animal Care and Use Committee of Corewell Health.

2.4. Clonogenic Assay

Cells (10^5) were seeded into six-well tissue culture plates. After 24 h, cells were treated with Azeliragon (1μM) for 24 h and exposed to radiation at various doses (2Gy, 4Gy, 6Gy) using the CIX2, XSTRAHL Cabinet Irradiator (Camberley, UK). Plates were incubated for 10 to 14 days for colony formation, and the medium was left unchanged during the duration of the experiment. Colonies were stained with crystal violet, and the number of colonies was calculated.

2.5. Western Blot

Western blot was performed using established methods. Briefly, proteins in the whole-cell lysate were resolved on 4–12% Criterion XT Bis-Tris gels (Bio-Rad, CA, USA) and transferred to a nitrocellulose membrane. After blocking, the membrane was incubated overnight at 4 °C with various primary antibodies. This was followed by incubation with a secondary antibody (goat anti-rabbit or goat anti-mouse antibody, Cell Signaling Technology, Beverly, MA, USA). The blot was visualized with a chemiluminescence substrate (Thermo Scientific, Massachusetts, NY, USA), and images were captured using an Odyssey infrared imaging system by Li-Cor (Lincoln, NE, USA) and analyzed with ImageJ software. Antibodies against RAGE (216329), HMGB1 (79823), S100P (133554), S100A2 (109494), pNF-kB (76302), and NF-kB (16502) were purchased from Abcam (Cambridge, MA, USA). Antibodies against vinculin were purchased from Cell Signaling Technology (Danvers, MA, USA). For Western blot, the primary antibodies were used at a dilution of 1:1000.

Western blot bands were quantified using densitometric analysis with ImageJ software. Data were normalized to the loading control (vinculin) and presented as mean ± SD from three independent experiments.

2.6. Flow Cytometric Analysis

Tumors harvested from mice were dissociated into single-cell suspensions using a combination of DNase I and Collagenase IV (Sigma Aldrich, St Louis, MO, USA). The resulting cell suspensions were washed in FACS buffer, which consisted of PBS supplemented with 0.2% BSA and 0.01% NaN3. Fluorochrome-conjugated monoclonal antibodies were used for staining, along with a mouse Fc receptor blocking agent (clone: 93). Fixation and permeabilization were performed using an eBioscience/Thermo Fisher kit. Flow cytometric analysis was conducted to identify specific cell populations, including M2 macrophages (CD45+CD11b+F4/80+CD206+), myeloid-derived suppressor cells (MDSCs, CD45+CD11b+Gr1+), regulatory T cells (Tregs, CD45+CD4+FoxP3+CD25+), and CD8+ T cells (CD45+CD11b−CD8+). A BD FACS Canto II flow cytometer (Becton Dickinson, Mountain View, CA, USA) was utilized for this analysis, and data were processed using FlowJo V.10 software (FlowJo, LLC, Ashland, OR, USA). Antibodies used in the experiments included CD45 (clone 30-F11; 1:400 dilution), CD4 (clone GK1.5; 1:300 dilution), CD8a (clone 53-6.7; 1:400 dilution), CD25 (clone PC61; 1:300 dilution), CD11b (clone M1/70; 1:500 dilution), Gr1 (clone RB6-8C5; 1:400 dilution), CD69 (clone H1.2F3; 1:400 dilution), F4/80 (clone BM8; 1:500 dilution), and CD68 (clone FA-11; 1:400 dilution), all obtained from Biolegend (San Diego, CA, USA). For FoxP3 staining, a Foxp3 staining buffer set and FoxP3 antibody (clone 150D/E4) from eBioscience/Thermo Fisher (Grand Island, NY, USA) were used.

2.7. Statistical Analysis

All quantitative data were presented as mean ± SD and statistical significance (p) was calculated by a two-tailed Student's t-test. For comparisons involving more than one group, a one-way ANOVA was performed, followed by Tukey's multiple comparisons test.

3. Results

3.1. RAGE Pathway Activation in Pancreatic Cancer

As an initial investigation, we sought to determine the relative expression of RAGE and its associated ligands in pancreatic cancer. Using data from pancreatic cancer patient samples from The Cancer Genome Atlas (TCGA), we demonstrated that although there was no change in the expression of RAGE, the RAGE ligands, S100P and S100A2, were significantly increased in pancreatic tumors when compared to normal pancreatic tissue (Figure 2A). We next determined if the RAGE pathway was implicated in a specific subtype of pancreatic cancer. An integrated genomic analysis of 456 pancreatic ductal adenocarcinomas identified four subtypes, with the squamous and pancreatic progenitor subtypes representing subtypes with the highest incidence and worst prognosis. These subtypes correlated with distinct histopathological characteristics and differential survival [39]. The squamous subtype was linked to squamous and adenosquamous histology, while the pancreatic progenitor subtype was associated with mucinous non-cystic adenocarcinomas and carcinomas arising from intraductal papillary mucinous neoplasms (IPMN). Notably, the squamous subtype was an independent poor prognostic factor [39]. Interestingly, using this database to evaluate the relative expression of RAGE-related proteins, clear clustering was observed, suggesting these two subtypes used distinct mechanisms for activating the RAGE pathway (Figure 2B). Variable importance plot (VIP) analysis identified S100A2, HMGA2, S100A9, and S100A8 as the primary ligands utilized by the pancreatic progenitor subtype, while S100P and S100A1 were the top ligands overexpressed in the squamous subtype (Figure 2C).

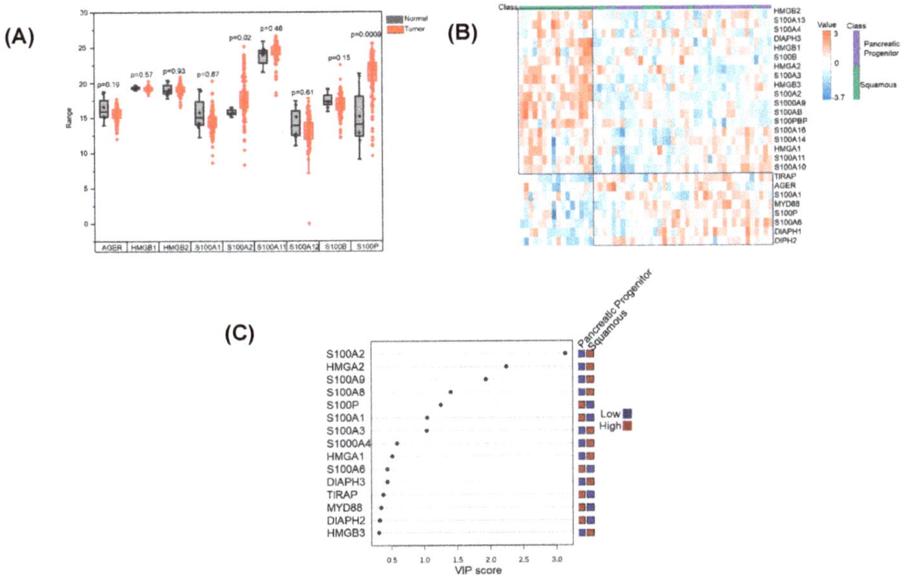

Figure 2. Expression and clustering of RAGE (AGER) and its ligands in pancreatic cancer: (**A**) Expression levels of RAGE (Receptor for Advanced Glycation End Products (encoded by the AGER gene)) and its ligands in pancreatic cancer patient samples obtained from The Cancer Genome Atlas (TCGA) database; (**B**) Clustering of RAGE ligands and activators within distinct pancreatic cancer subtypes (progenitor and squamous subtypes) as described by Bailey et al. [35]; (**C**) Variable Importance Plot (VIP) analysis highlights key ligands (e.g., S100A2, HMGA2) that differentiate the pancreatic progenitor and squamous subtypes. Red indicates upregulated genes, while blue indicates downregulated genes, underscoring subtype-specific mechanisms of RAGE pathway activation.

3.2. Azeliragon Inhibits RAGE Pathway Activation in Pancreatic Cancer Cell Lines

We next sought to determine if preclinical models of pancreatic cancer recapitulated the aberrant expression of RAGE pathway mediators observed in human tumors. Western blot analysis was done to evaluate the expression of RAGE and its associated ligands in both human (Panc1) and murine (Pan02) pancreatic cancer cell lines compared to normal pancreas. As shown in Figure 3A, in addition to RAGE expression, the expression of the RAGE ligands HMGB1, S100A2, and S100P was significantly upregulated in both human and murine pancreatic cancer cell lines when compared to normal pancreas. As we established the RAGE pathway is active in pancreatic cell lines grown in vitro, we next evaluated the potential for the RAGE inhibitor Azeliragon to modulate this pathway. Azeliragon demonstrated a dose-dependent inhibition of NF-κB phosphorylation, which represents a downstream mediator for RAGE pathway activation, with significant inhibition being observed at a drug concentration of 1 μM after 3 h in both Panc1 (Figure 3B) and Pan02 (Figure 3C) cell lines. We next performed a time course study in Panc1 cells, demonstrating pathway inhibition of Azeliragon (1 μM) as early as 3 h and was sustained for 24 h (Figure 3D). Pathway inhibition was also sustained for 24 h in the Pan02 line (Figure 3E), confirming the ability of Azeliragon to disrupt RAGE-mediated NF-κB activation in pancreatic cancer cell lines.

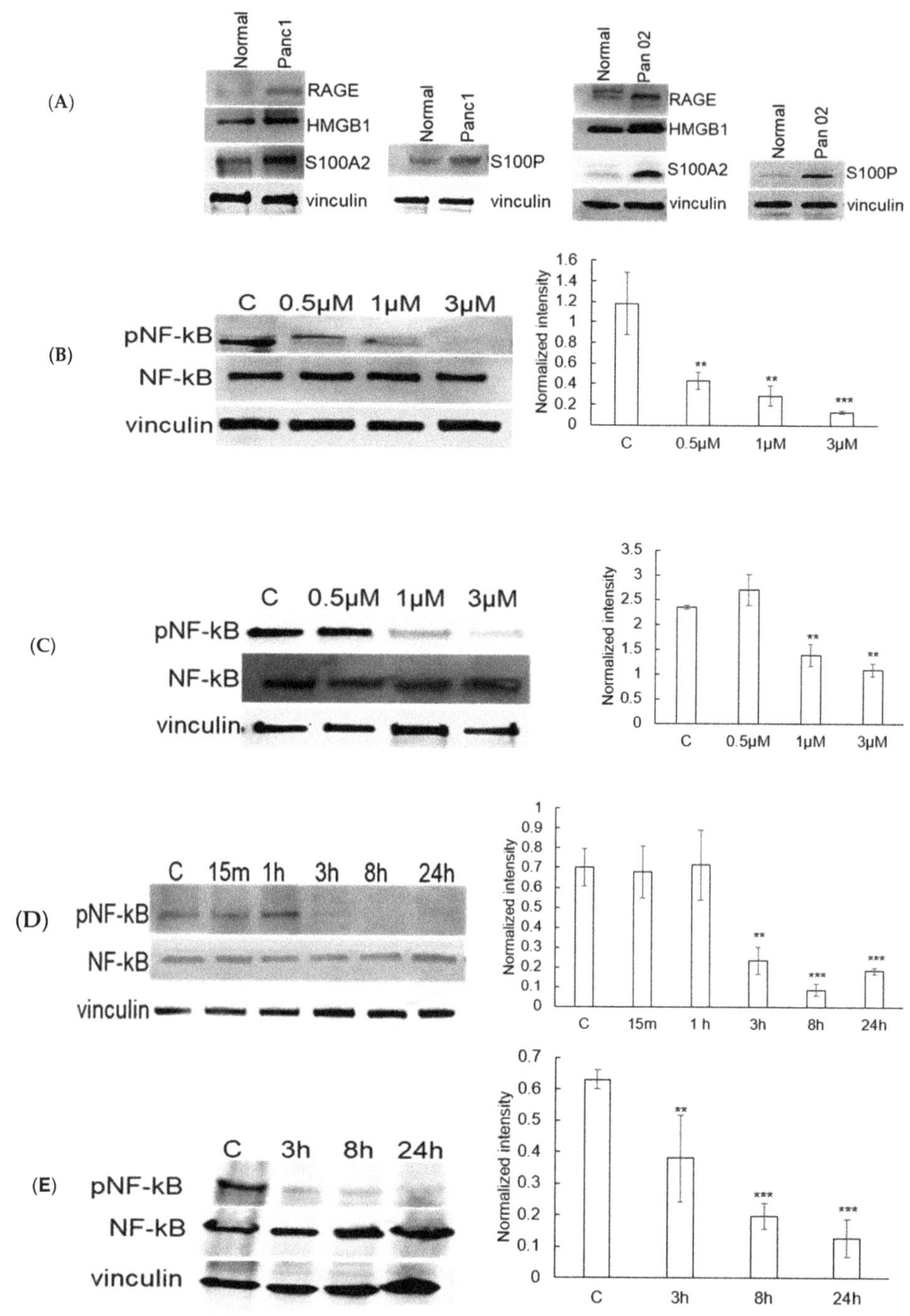

Figure 3. Expression of RAGE and its ligands in pancreatic cancer cell lines and the inhibitory effect of Azeliragon on RAGE signaling: (**A**) Expression levels of RAGE (Receptor for Advanced Glycation End Products) and its ligands—S100P, S100A2, and HMGB1—in human (Panc1) and murine (Pan02) pancreatic cancer cell lines; (**B–E**) Azeliragon (AZ), a RAGE inhibitor, inhibits the downstream signaling pathway of RAGE in pancreatic cancer cell lines: (**B**,**C**) Expression levels of

phosphorylated NF-κB (pNF-κB) in Panc1 (**B**) and Pan02 (**C**) cells treated with indicated concentrations of AZ for 3 h; (**D**,**E**) Expression levels of pNF-κB in Panc1 (**D**) and Pan02 (**E**) cells treated with 1 μM AZ at indicated time points. Statistical significance: ** $p < 0.01$, *** $p < 0.001$ compared to the control group. The corresponding uncropped blots are provided in Supplementary Figures S2 and S3.

Next, we evaluated if Azeliragon-mediated inhibition of RAGE demonstrated anti-tumor activity in pancreatic cell lines in vitro. Despite potent inhibition of RAGE-mediated NF-κB activation, Azeliragon (1–3 μM) only led to modest inhibition of cell proliferation in both pancreatic cell lines tested (Figure 4A). In addition, no sensitization of radiation response was observed in these culture conditions (Figure 4B). We hypothesized that typical culture conditions when growing these cancer cell lines in vitro may not recapitulate the observed RAGE pathway activation in vivo. Specifically, RAGE ligands and their associated pathway activation may not be as pronounced when these lines are grown in standard culture conditions [40]. To test this, we stimulated cells with RAGE ligands observed to be upregulated in human pancreatic cancer, including S100P, S100A2, and HMGB1. Ligand stimulation led to potent NF-κB phosphorylation in Panc1 cells, which was completely attenuated when treated with Azeliragon (Figure 4C). When evaluating for proliferation, ligand stimulation led to an increase in proliferation, which, similar to western blot, was attenuated by Azeliragon (Figure 4D). Similar results were observed in the Pan02 line (Figure 4E). Collectively, we demonstrate the capacity of Azeliragon to inhibit the RAGE pathway in pancreatic cancer cell lines. However, determining the biological consequence of this pathway in vitro may be limited, which is likely attributed to the important role the tumor microenvironment plays in activating this pathway in vivo.

(**A**)

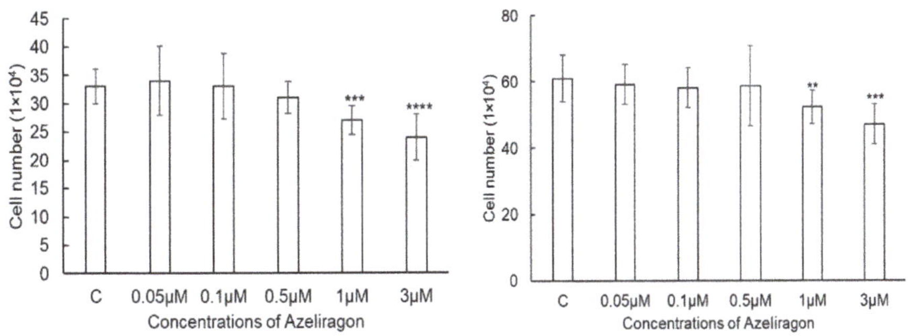

(**B**)

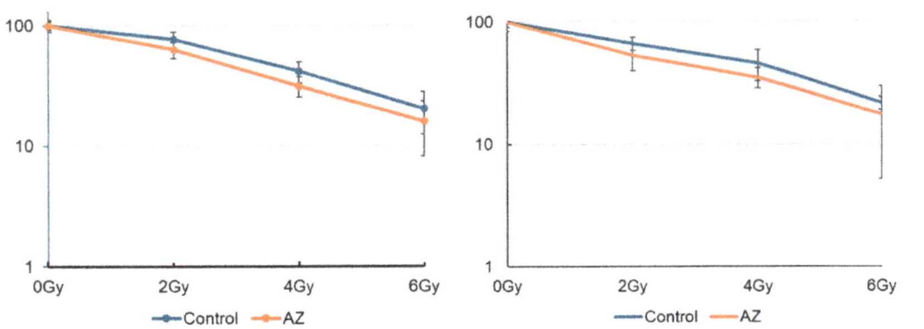

Figure 4. *Cont.*

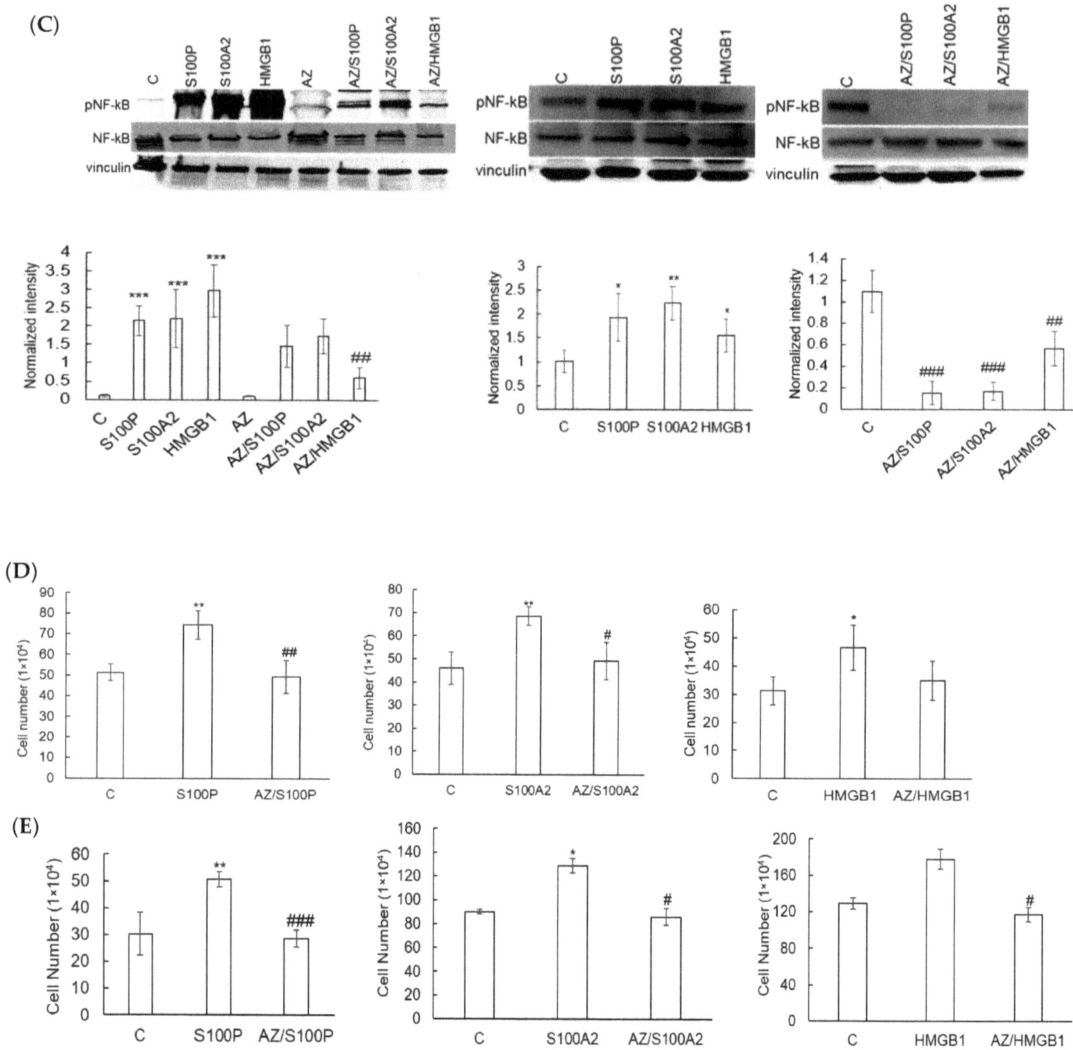

Figure 4. Azeliragon inhibits proliferation and NF-κB activation in pancreatic cancer cell lines: (**A**,**B**) Azeliragon (AZ) suppresses proliferation in pancreatic cancer cell lines: (**A**) Proliferation was determined by treating human Panc1 (left) and murine Pan02 (right) cells with indicated concentrations of AZ for 24 h. Live cells were counted using the trypan blue exclusion; (**B**) Clonogenic assay of Panc1 (left) and Pan02 (right) cells treated with 1 μM AZ for 24 h, followed by exposure to radiation doses of 2 Gy, 4 Gy, and 6 Gy. Results are representative of at least three independent experiments. Data represent mean ± standard deviation (SD). Significant results are indicated as: ** $p = 0.01$; *** $p = 0.001$; **** $p < 0.001$; (**C**) Azeliragon inhibits RAGE ligand-induced expression of phosphorylated NF-κB (pNF-κB). Expression level of pNF-κB in Panc1 (left) and Pan02 (right) cells stimulated with RAGE ligands (S100P, S100A2, HMGB1; 0.1 μM) for 24 h then treated with Azeliragon (1 μM AZ for 24 h). (**D**,**E**) Azeliragon inhibits RAGE ligand-induced cell proliferation. Effect of RAGE ligand stimulation (0.1 μM ligands for 24 h) on the proliferation of Panc1 (**D**) and Pan02 (**E**) cells with and without Azeliragon treatment (1 μM AZ for 24 h). Data represent mean ± SD of three or more independent experiments. Statistical significance: * $p < 0.05$, ** $p < 0.01$, *** $p < 0.001$ for ligands compared to the control group; # $p = 0.05$, ## $p < 0.01$, ### $p = 0.001$ for AZ-treated groups compared to their respective ligand-treated groups. The corresponding uncropped blots are provided in Supplementary Figure S4.

3.3. *Azeliragon Demonstrates Anti-Tumor Activity and Modulates the Immune Microenvironment in Pancreatic Cancer Cell Lines In Vivo*

In vivo studies were conducted to assess the anti-tumor activity of Azeliragon, both alone and in combination with radiation therapy (RT), in pancreatic cancer mouse models. Panc1 cells were injected into the flank of NU/NU mice, and treatment with Azeliragon (1 mg/kg, i.p.) was initiated 14 days post-tumor implantation. Daily RT (2 Gy × 5 days) began one day after Azeliragon treatment. Azeliragon was well tolerated in mice and did not result in significant weight loss (Supplementary Figure S1). Mice treated with Azeliragon alone ($p < 0.05$) or RT alone ($p < 0.01$) exhibited tumor growth delay compared to controls (Figure 5A). The combination of Azeliragon and RT led to an additive tumor growth delay when compared to control or either treatment alone ($p < 0.001$ for RT+AZ vs. control, $p < 0.01$ for RT + AZ vs. AZ alone, $p < 0.01$ for RT + AZ vs. RT alone). Mice treated with Azeliragon and RT survived beyond day 50, while all control mice reached endpoint criteria by day 35. Correlative studies demonstrated target inhibition of Azeliragon in vivo, determined by decreased NF-κB phosphorylation (Figure 5B). Similar findings were observed when we extended these studies to the murine pancreatic cancer cell line Pan02 (Figure 5C,D). Using this model, we went on to determine the immune consequences of Azeliragon. Interestingly, Azeliragon-mediated RAGE inhibition modulated several tumor-supportive, immune-suppressive cells within the pancreatic cancer microenvironment (Figure 5E). This included a reduction in M2 macrophages and Tregs, which were further diminished when combined with RT. The combination of Azeliragon and RT led to a decrease in MDSCs. This reduction in immune suppression was coupled with an increase in immune activation in Azeliragon-treated mice, which was determined by an increase in CD8+ T cells. Collectively, these findings support the role Azeliragon plays in targeting both pancreatic cancer cells and this tumor's immune suppressive microenvironment.

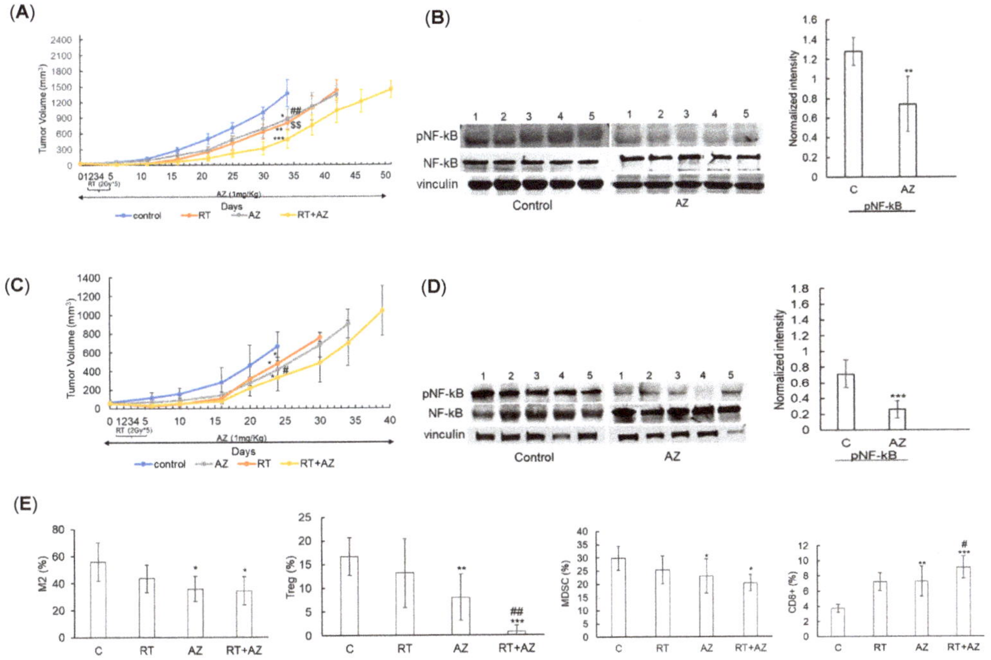

Figure 5. The in vivo antitumor activity of Azeliragon in pancreatic cancer mouse models: (**A**,**B**) Panc1 cells were injected into the flank of NU/NU mice. On day 14 post-tumor implantation, AZ treatment (1 mg/kg, i.p.) was initiated, and one day later, RT treatment (2 Gy X 5 days) was initiated. AZ treatment

continued daily: (**A**) Tumor growth curves of mice. Data represent mean ± SD. Statistical significance calculated on day 34: * $p < 0.05$, ** $p < 0.01$, *** $p < 0.001$ compared to the control group; ## $p < 0.01$ RT + AZ significantly different from the AZ group; $$ $p < 0.01$ RT + AZ significantly different from the RT group. For correlative studies, mice were euthanized 10 days after the first day of treatment, and tumors were harvested for further analysis; (**B**) Expression levels of phosphorylated NF-κB (pNF-κB) in tumors in indicated treatment groups; (**C–E**): Pan02 cells were injected subcutaneously into the flank of C57BL/6 mice. On day 14 post-tumor implantation, AZ treatment (1 mg/kg) was initiated, and one day later, RT treatment (2 Gy X 5 days) was initiated. AZ treatment continued daily until the mice met the criteria requiring euthanization; (**C**) Tumor growth of C57BL/6 mice. Data represents mean ± SD. Statistical significance as calculated on day 24: * $p < 0.01$ significantly different from the control group. # $p < 0.05$ RT + AZ significantly different from RT group. For correlative studies, tumors were harvested 24 days post-tumor implantation; (**D**) Expression of pNF-kB in tumors in indicated treatment groups; (**E**) Immune profiling of tumors was performed using flow cytometry. Data represents mean ± SD. * $p < 0.05$, ** $p < 0.01$, *** $p < 0.001$ significantly different from control group. # $p < 0.05$, ## $p < 0.01$ significantly different from RT group. The corresponding uncropped blots are provided in Supplementary Figure S4.

4. Discussion

Our study demonstrates that RAGE inhibition using Azeliragon leads to anti-tumor and immunomodulatory effects in preclinical models of pancreatic cancer, with an additive growth delay observed when combined with radiation therapy. Pancreatic cancer is highly resistant to standard therapies, largely due to overexpression of anti-apoptotic proteins and an immunosuppressive microenvironment, mechanisms that promote cancer cell survival and spread [3–5]. These characteristics are closely associated with NF-κB activation, a downstream target of RAGE signaling. In our study, Azeliragon effectively inhibited RAGE-mediated NF-κB activation, thus impacting key pathways associated with tumor progression and therapeutic resistance.

Consistent with prior literature, we observed significantly elevated levels of RAGE ligands—HMGB1, S100A2, and S100P—in both human and murine pancreatic cancer cell lines relative to normal pancreatic tissue [21]. Azeliragon effectively suppressed RAGE-mediated NF-κB activation in both in vitro and in vivo settings. Although the drug exhibited only a modest impact on cell proliferation and radiosensitivity in standard in vitro culture, stimulation with RAGE ligands under in vitro conditions led to increased proliferation, which was completely inhibited by Azeliragon. This suggests that the modest impact observed in traditional culture conditions may stem from the lack of a complex microenvironment typically present in vivo. Our in vivo studies underscored Azeliragon's anti-tumor efficacy, both as monotherapy and in combination with RT. Mice treated with both Azeliragon and RT demonstrated delayed tumor growth and an extended survival beyond 50 days, compared to control mice, which succumbed by day 35. While other RAGE inhibitors, such as cromolyn and a S100P-derived inhibitor, have shown anti-tumor effects in pancreatic cancer models, their mechanisms are often limited to binding specifically to S100P, which restricts their utility against other RAGE ligands involved in pancreatic cancer progression [15,32,33]. In contrast, Azeliragon's ability to bind directly to RAGE and inhibit multiple ligands of RAGE offers a broader inhibition of the RAGE pathway, which is advantageous given that multiple ligands are implicated in promoting tumor growth, migration, and resistance to therapy via the RAGE pathway [7,18,21,34].

A notable aspect of Azeliragon's mechanism is its immune-modulatory capacity. Pancreatic cancer is characterized by a highly immunosuppressive environment, populated by Tregs, MDSCs, and M2 macrophages that support tumor growth and hinder immune-mediated tumor destruction [5]. In our study, Azeliragon treatment notably reduced these suppressive cell populations while increasing cytotoxic CD8+ T cell infiltration, thereby reshaping the immune environment towards a pro-inflammatory, anti-tumor state. Although our study did not directly explore the mechanism by which Azeliragon modulates the tumor immune microenvironment, this effect is likely mediated through the inhibition of RAGE-driven NF-κB signaling. NF-κB has been shown to influence the recruitment and differentiation of immune cells, including driving the polarization of macrophages toward the M2 phenotype [41–44]. Additionally, RT promotes immunogenic cell death and increases CD8+ T cell infiltration, and thus, the combined use of Azeliragon and RT synergistically creates a tumor microenvironment potentially more amenable to immune-mediated eradication [36,45,46].

The clinical implications of these findings suggest that Azeliragon, through its dual targeting of the RAGE pathway and immune-suppressive microenvironment, could be a promising candidate in the treatment of pancreatic cancer. Given that Azeliragon has shown safety in human trials for Alzheimer's disease, its repurposing for pancreatic cancer could expedite clinical translation. Our findings support further clinical studies to confirm Azeliragon's efficacy as a monotherapy and in combination with RT in patients with pancreatic cancer. Additionally, given the immunomodulatory effects observed, it may be valuable to explore Azeliragon in combination with immune checkpoint inhibitors to further enhance T cell-mediated anti-tumor activity.

While the current study focuses on the role of Azeliragon in pancreatic cancer, the involvement of RAGE in other cancers, such as colorectal and lung cancer, suggests that Azeliragon could have broader therapeutic applications [14,47]. Future studies should explore its effectiveness in these cancers to determine its potential clinical utility across malignancies and evaluate whether cross-cancer side effects might arise. Such investigations could further inform the safety profile and optimize the use of Azeliragon in oncology. Additionally, as the only RAGE inhibitor currently cleared for human use, Azeliragon presents a unique opportunity to benchmark its therapeutic advantages against other agents targeting RAGE, both in preclinical and clinical settings. Such comparisons would not only elucidate its distinctive benefits but also contribute to optimizing treatment regimens for pancreatic cancer.

Although the findings of this study provide evidence of Azeliragon's therapeutic potential in pancreatic cancer, some limitations are acknowledged. First, while the use of murine models allows for the controlled study of Azeliragon's effects on tumor growth and the tumor microenvironment, the generalizability of these results to human patients requires further validation in clinical settings. The complexities of human pancreatic cancer, including genetic heterogeneity and patient-specific tumor microenvironment dynamics, may influence treatment efficacy. Second, long-term studies are needed to evaluate its sustained efficacy and potential toxicity, including possible off-target effects and side effects that may arise with chronic use. While Azeliragon has demonstrated a favorable safety profile in clinical trials for Alzheimer's disease, with patients receiving the drug for up to 18 months, its safety in the context of cancer therapy, particularly when combined with radiation or other treatments, warrants further investigation [48].

5. Conclusions

Our study demonstrates the therapeutic potential of Azeliragon, a RAGE inhibitor, as an adjunctive treatment in pancreatic cancer. Azeliragon effectively inhibited NF-κB signaling, a pathway critical to RAGE-mediated tumor progression and therapeutic resistance, resulting in significant tumor growth delay alone and when combined with radiation therapy in preclinical models. Additionally, Azeliragon displayed immunomodulatory effects within the tumor microenvironment, reducing immune-suppressive cells while enhancing CD8+ T cell infiltration. This dual action of direct tumor inhibition and immune modulation suggests that Azeliragon holds promise for improving pancreatic cancer outcomes. Clinical studies are warranted to validate these findings and explore Azeliragon's integration into treatment regimens to improve pancreatic cancer outcomes.

Supplementary Materials: The following supporting information can be downloaded at: https://www.mdpi.com/article/10.3390/cancers17010017/s1, Figure S1: Body weight monitoring of mice during study. Figure S2: Uncropped western blots showing expression of RAGE and its ligands in pancreatic cancer cell (Figure 3A in manuscript). Figure S3: Uncropped western blots showing the inhibitory effect of Azeliragon on RAGE signaling (Figure 3B-E in manuscript). Figure S4: Uncropped western blots showing antitumor activity of Azeliragon in vitro and in vivo (Figures 4C and 5B&D in manuscript).

Author Contributions: Conceptualization, P.C and K.A.; methodology, P.C., K.A., G.M. and Y.Z.; data acquisition, K.A., G.M. and Y.Z.; formal analysis, K.A.; resources, P.C. and S.M.; writing—original draft preparation, P.C., K.A. and J.F.O.; writing—review and editing, K.A., J.F.O., G.M. and Y.Z., S.M. and P.C.; supervision, P.C.; funding acquisition, P.C. All authors have read and agreed to the published version of the manuscript.

Funding: This research was funded, in part, by a Research Grant provided by Cantex Pharmaceuticals, grant 3000671. P.C. is funded by the National Institute of Health (NIH)/National Institute of Neurological Disorders and Stroke (NINDS) grants R01NS110838 and R01NS129744.

Institutional Review Board Statement: This study does not contain any studies involving human participants. All animal studies were performed in an AAALAC-accredited facility located at Beaumont Research Institute, Royal Oak, MI. All animal experiments were approved by the IACUC at Beaumont Research Institute and performed in accordance with animal protocols: AL-23-01 (date of approval–10 April 2023).

Informed Consent Statement: Not applicable.

Data Availability Statement: Data are available on request from the corresponding author.

Conflicts of Interest: S.M. serves as CEO of Cantex Pharmaceuticals, whose Research Grant helped fund this study. The funders had no role in the design of the study; in the collection, analyses, or interpretation of data; in the writing of the manuscript; or in the decision to publish the results. The remainder of the authors declare no conflicts of interest.

References

1. Siegel, R.L.; Miller, K.D.; Fuchs, H.E.; Jemal, A. Cancer Statistics, 2021. *CA Cancer J. Clin.* **2021**, *71*, 7–33. [CrossRef] [PubMed]
2. Rahib, L.; Smith, B.D.; Aizenberg, R.; Rosenzweig, A.B.; Fleshman, J.M.; Matrisian, L.M. Projecting Cancer Incidence and Deaths to 2030: The Unexpected Burden of Thyroid, Liver, and Pancreas Cancers in the United States. *Cancer Res.* **2014**, *74*, 2913–2921. [CrossRef] [PubMed]
3. Quiñonero, F.; Mesas, C.; Doello, K.; Cabeza, L.; Perazzoli, G.; Jimenez-Luna, C.; Rama, A.R.; Melguizo, C.; Prados, J. The Challenge of Drug Resistance in Pancreatic Ductal Adenocarcinoma: A Current Overview. *Cancer Biol. Med.* **2019**, *16*, 688–699. [CrossRef] [PubMed]
4. Espona-Fiedler, M.; Patthey, C.; Lindblad, S.; Sarró, I.; Öhlund, D. Overcoming Therapy Resistance in Pancreatic Cancer: New Insights and Future Directions. *Biochem. Pharmacol.* **2024**, *229*, 116492. [CrossRef]
5. Li, Y.; Xiang, S.; Pan, W.; Wang, J.; Zhan, H.; Liu, S. Targeting Tumor Immunosuppressive Microenvironment for Pancreatic Cancer Immunotherapy: Current Research and Future Perspective. *Front. Oncol.* **2023**, *13*, 1166860. [CrossRef] [PubMed]
6. Schmidt, A.M.; Hofmann, M.; Taguchi, A.; Yan, S.D.; Stern, D.M. RAGE: A Multiligand Receptor Contributing to the Cellular Response in Diabetic Vasculopathy and Inflammation. *Semin. Thromb. Hemost.* **2000**, *26*, 485–493. [CrossRef] [PubMed]
7. Logsdon, C.D.; Fuentes, M.K.; Huang, E.H.; Arumugam, T. RAGE and RAGE Ligands in Cancer. *Curr. Mol. Med.* **2007**, *7*, 777–789. [CrossRef]
8. Bierhaus, A.; Humpert, P.M.; Morcos, M.; Wendt, T.; Chavakis, T.; Arnold, B.; Stern, D.M.; Nawroth, P.P. Understanding RAGE, the Receptor for Advanced Glycation End Products. *J. Mol. Med.* **2005**, *83*, 876–886. [CrossRef] [PubMed]

9. Sparvero, L.J.; Asafu-Adjei, D.; Kang, R.; Tang, D.; Amin, N.; Im, J.; Rutledge, R.; Lin, B.; Amoscato, A.A.; Zeh, H.J.; et al. RAGE (Receptor for Advanced Glycation Endproducts), RAGE Ligands, and Their Role in Cancer and Inflammation. *J. Transl. Med.* **2009**, *7*, 17. [CrossRef] [PubMed]
10. Chavakis, T.; Bierhaus, A.; Al-Fakhri, N.; Schneider, D.; Witte, S.; Linn, T.; Nagashima, M.; Morser, J.; Arnold, B.; Preissner, K.T.; et al. The Pattern Recognition Receptor (RAGE) Is a Counterreceptor for Leukocyte Integrins: A Novel Pathway for Inflammatory Cell Recruitment. *J. Exp. Med.* **2003**, *198*, 1507–1515. [CrossRef]
11. Foell, D.; Wittkowski, H.; Vogl, T.; Roth, J. S100 Proteins Expressed in Phagocytes: A Novel Group of Damage-Associated Molecular Pattern Molecules. *J. Leukoc. Biol.* **2007**, *81*, 28–37. [CrossRef]
12. Hsieh, H.-L.; Schäfer, B.W.; Sasaki, N.; Heizmann, C.W. Expression Analysis of S100 Proteins and RAGE in Human Tumors Using Tissue Microarrays. *Biochem. Biophys. Res. Commun.* **2003**, *307*, 375–381. [CrossRef] [PubMed]
13. Ishiguro, H.; Nakaigawa, N.; Miyoshi, Y.; Fujinami, K.; Kubota, Y.; Uemura, H. Receptor for Advanced Glycation End Products (RAGE) and Its Ligand, Amphoterin Are Overexpressed and Associated with Prostate Cancer Development. *Prostate* **2005**, *64*, 92–100. [CrossRef] [PubMed]
14. Kuniyasu, H.; Chihara, Y.; Takahashi, T. Co-Expression of Receptor for Advanced Glycation End Products and the Ligand Amphoterin Associates Closely with Metastasis of Colorectal Cancer. *Oncol. Rep.* **2003**, *10*, 445–448. [CrossRef] [PubMed]
15. Faruqui, T.; Khan, M.S.; Akhter, Y.; Khan, S.; Rafi, Z.; Saeed, M.; Han, I.; Choi, E.-H.; Yadav, D.K. RAGE Inhibitors for Targeted Therapy of Cancer: A Comprehensive Review. *Int. J. Mol. Sci.* **2022**, *24*, 266. [CrossRef] [PubMed]
16. DiNorcia, J.; Lee, M.K.; Moroziewicz, D.N.; Winner, M.; Suman, P.; Bao, F.; Remotti, H.E.; Zou, Y.S.; Yan, S.F.; Qiu, W.; et al. RAGE Gene Deletion Inhibits the Development and Progression of Ductal Neoplasia and Prolongs Survival in a Murine Model of Pancreatic Cancer. *J. Gastrointest. Surg.* **2012**, *16*, 104–112; discussion 112. [CrossRef]
17. Kang, R.; Loux, T.; Tang, D.; Schapiro, N.E.; Vernon, P.; Livesey, K.M.; Krasinskas, A.; Lotze, M.T.; Zeh, H.J. The Expression of the Receptor for Advanced Glycation Endproducts (RAGE) Is Permissive for Early Pancreatic Neoplasia. *Proc. Natl. Acad. Sci. USA* **2012**, *109*, 7031–7036. [CrossRef] [PubMed]
18. Kang, R.; Tang, D.; Schapiro, N.E.; Loux, T.; Livesey, K.M.; Billiar, T.R.; Wang, H.; Van Houten, B.; Lotze, M.T.; Zeh, H.J. The HMGB1/RAGE Inflammatory Pathway Promotes Pancreatic Tumor Growth by Regulating Mitochondrial Bioenergetics. *Oncogene* **2014**, *33*, 567–577. [CrossRef] [PubMed]
19. Kang, R.; Tang, D.; Livesey, K.M.; Schapiro, N.E.; Lotze, M.T.; Zeh, H.J. The Receptor for Advanced Glycation End-Products (RAGE) Protects Pancreatic Tumor Cells against Oxidative Injury. *Antioxid. Redox Signal.* **2011**, *15*, 2175–2184. [CrossRef] [PubMed]
20. Swami, P.; Thiyagarajan, S.; Vidger, A.; Indurthi, V.S.K.; Vetter, S.W.; Leclerc, E. RAGE Up-Regulation Differently Affects Cell Proliferation and Migration in Pancreatic Cancer Cells. *Int. J. Mol. Sci.* **2020**, *21*, 7723. [CrossRef]
21. Arumugam, T.; Simeone, D.M.; Van Golen, K.; Logsdon, C.D. S100P Promotes Pancreatic Cancer Growth, Survival, and Invasion. *Clin. Cancer Res.* **2005**, *11*, 5356–5364. [CrossRef]
22. Arumugam, T.; Ramachandran, V.; Gomez, S.B.; Schmidt, A.M.; Logsdon, C.D. S100P-Derived RAGE Antagonistic Peptide Reduces Tumor Growth and Metastasis. *Clin. Cancer Res.* **2012**, *18*, 4356–4364. [CrossRef] [PubMed]
23. Swami, P.; O'Connell, K.A.; Thiyagarajan, S.; Crawford, A.; Patil, P.; Radhakrishnan, P.; Shin, S.; Caffrey, T.C.; Grunkemeyer, J.; Neville, T.; et al. Inhibition of the Receptor for Advanced Glycation End Products Enhances the Cytotoxic Effect of Gemcitabine in Murine Pancreatic Tumors. *Biomolecules* **2021**, *11*, 526. [CrossRef] [PubMed]
24. Lander, H.M.; Tauras, J.M.; Ogiste, J.S.; Hori, O.; Moss, R.A.; Schmidt, A.M. Activation of the Receptor for Advanced Glycation End Products Triggers a P21(Ras)-Dependent Mitogen-Activated Protein Kinase Pathway Regulated by Oxidant Stress. *J. Biol. Chem.* **1997**, *272*, 17810–17814. [CrossRef] [PubMed]
25. Huttunen, H.J.; Fages, C.; Kuja-Panula, J.; Ridley, A.J.; Rauvala, H. Receptor for Advanced Glycation End Products-Binding COOH-Terminal Motif of Amphoterin Inhibits Invasive Migration and Metastasis. *Cancer Res.* **2002**, *62*, 4805–4811. [PubMed]
26. Kang, R.; Tang, D.; Schapiro, N.E.; Livesey, K.M.; Farkas, A.; Loughran, P.; Bierhaus, A.; Lotze, M.T.; Zeh, H.J. The Receptor for Advanced Glycation End Products (RAGE) Sustains Autophagy and Limits Apoptosis, Promoting Pancreatic Tumor Cell Survival. *Cell Death Differ.* **2010**, *17*, 666–676. [CrossRef] [PubMed]
27. Taguchi, A.; Blood, D.C.; del Toro, G.; Canet, A.; Lee, D.C.; Qu, W.; Tanji, N.; Lu, Y.; Lalla, E.; Fu, C.; et al. Blockade of RAGE-Amphoterin Signalling Suppresses Tumour Growth and Metastases. *Nature* **2000**, *405*, 354–360. [CrossRef] [PubMed]
28. Bierhaus, A.; Schiekofer, S.; Schwaninger, M.; Andrassy, M.; Humpert, P.M.; Chen, J.; Hong, M.; Luther, T.; Henle, T.; Klöting, I.; et al. Diabetes-Associated Sustained Activation of the Transcription Factor Nuclear Factor-KappaB. *Diabetes* **2001**, *50*, 2792–2808. [CrossRef]
29. Huttunen, H.J.; Fages, C.; Rauvala, H. Receptor for Advanced Glycation End Products (RAGE)-Mediated Neurite Outgrowth and Activation of NF-KappaB Require the Cytoplasmic Domain of the Receptor but Different Downstream Signaling Pathways. *J. Biol. Chem.* **1999**, *274*, 19919–19924. [CrossRef] [PubMed]

30. Wang, W.; Abbruzzese, J.L.; Evans, D.B.; Larry, L.; Cleary, K.R.; Chiao, P.J. The Nuclear Factor-Kappa B RelA Transcription Factor Is Constitutively Activated in Human Pancreatic Adenocarcinoma Cells. *Clin. Cancer Res.* **1999**, *5*, 119–127. [PubMed]
31. Singh, V.; Gupta, D.; Arora, R. NF-KB as a Key Player in Regulation of Cellular Radiation Responses and Identification of Radiation Countermeasures. *Discoveries* **2015**, *3*, e35. [CrossRef] [PubMed]
32. Camara, R.; Ogbeni, D.; Gerstmann, L.; Ostovar, M.; Hurer, E.; Scott, M.; Mahmoud, N.G.; Radon, T.; Crnogorac-Jurcevic, T.; Patel P.; et al. Discovery of Novel Small Molecule Inhibitors of S100P with In Vitro Anti-Metastatic Effects on Pancreatic Cancer Cells *Eur. J. Med. Chem.* **2020**, *203*, 112621. [CrossRef]
33. Arumugam, T.; Ramachandran, V.; Logsdon, C.D. Effect of Cromolyn on S100P Interactions with RAGE and Pancreatic Cancer Growth and Invasion in Mouse Models. *J. Natl. Cancer Inst.* **2006**, *98*, 1806–1818. [CrossRef]
34. National Center for Biotechnology PubChem Compound Summary for CID 11180124, Azeliragon. Available online: https //pubchem.ncbi.nlm.nih.gov/compound/Azeliragon (accessed on 19 December 2024).
35. Burstein, A.H.; Sabbagh, M.; Andrews, R.; Valcarce, C.; Dunn, I.; Altstiel, L. Development of Azeliragon, an Oral Small Molecule Antagonist of the Receptor for Advanced Glycation Endproducts, for the Potential Slowing of Loss of Cognition in Mild Alzheimer's Disease. *J. Prev. Alzheimers Dis.* **2018**, *5*, 149–154. [CrossRef]
36. Magna, M.; Hwang, G.H.; McIntosh, A.; Drews-Elger, K.; Takabatake, M.; Ikeda, A.; Mera, B.J.; Kwak, T.; Miller, P.; Lippman, M.E.; et al. RAGE Inhibitor TTP488 (Azeliragon) Suppresses Metastasis in Triple-Negative Breast Cancer. *NPJ Breast Cancer* **2023**, *9*, 59. [CrossRef] [PubMed]
37. ClinicalTrials.gov. Azeliragon and Chemoradiotherapy in Newly Diagnosed Glioblastoma. Available online: https://clinicaltrials gov/study/NCT05635734?intr=azeliragon&rank=3 (accessed on 19 December 2024).
38. ClinicalTrials.gov. Study of Effect of Azeliragon in Patients Refractory to First-Line Metastatic Pancreatic Cancer. Available online: https://clinicaltrials.gov/study/NCT05766748?intr=azeliragon&rank=2 (accessed on 19 December 2024).
39. Bailey, P.; Chang, D.K.; Nones, K.; Johns, A.L.; Patch, A.-M.; Gingras, M.-C.; Miller, D.K.; Christ, A.N.; Bruxner, T.J.C.; Quinn, M.C.; et al. Genomic Analyses Identify Molecular Subtypes of Pancreatic Cancer. *Nature* **2016**, *531*, 47–52. [CrossRef] [PubMed]
40. Gu, A.; Li, J.; Qiu, S.; Hao, S.; Yue, Z.-Y.; Zhai, S.; Li, M.-Y.; Liu, Y. Pancreatic Cancer Environment: From Patient-Derived Models to Single-Cell Omics. *Mol. Omics* **2024**, *20*, 220–233. [CrossRef] [PubMed]
41. Gebhardt, C.; Riehl, A.; Durchdewald, M.; Németh, J.; Fürstenberger, G.; Müller-Decker, K.; Enk, A.; Arnold, B.; Bierhaus, A.; Nawroth, P.P.; et al. RAGE Signaling Sustains Inflammation and Promotes Tumor Development. *J. Exp. Med.* **2008**, *205*, 275–285 [CrossRef]
42. Lawrence, T. The Nuclear Factor NF-KappaB Pathway in Inflammation. *Cold Spring Harb. Perspect. Biol.* **2009**, *1*, a001651 [CrossRef] [PubMed]
43. Mancino, A.; Lawrence, T. Nuclear Factor-KappaB and Tumor-Associated Macrophages. *Clin. Cancer Res.* **2010**, *16*, 784–789 [CrossRef] [PubMed]
44. Liu, T.; Zhang, L.; Joo, D.; Sun, S.-C. NF-KB Signaling in Inflammation. *Signal Transduct. Target. Ther.* **2017**, *2*, 17023. [CrossRef] [PubMed]
45. Fujiwara, K.; Saung, M.T.; Jing, H.; Herbst, B.; Zarecki, M.; Muth, S.; Wu, A.; Bigelow, E.; Chen, L.; Li, K.; et al. Interrogating the Immune-Modulating Roles of Radiation Therapy for a Rational Combination with Immune-Checkpoint Inhibitors in Treating Pancreatic Cancer. *J. Immunother. Cancer* **2020**, *8*, e000351. [CrossRef]
46. Demaria, S.; Bhardwaj, N.; McBride, W.H.; Formenti, S.C. Combining Radiotherapy and Immunotherapy: A Revived Partnership. *Int. J. Radiat. Oncol. Biol. Phys.* **2005**, *63*, 655–666. [CrossRef] [PubMed]
47. Chen, M.-C.; Chen, K.-C.; Chang, G.-C.; Lin, H.; Wu, C.-C.; Kao, W.-H.; Teng, C.-L.J.; Hsu, S.-L.; Yang, T.-Y. RAGE Acts as an Oncogenic Role and Promotes the Metastasis of Human Lung Cancer. *Cell Death Dis.* **2020**, *11*, 265. [CrossRef] [PubMed]
48. Galasko, D.; Bell, J.; Mancuso, J.Y.; Kupiec, J.W.; Sabbagh, M.N.; van Dyck, C.; Thomas, R.G.; Aisen, P.S. Alzheimer's Disease Cooperative Study Clinical Trial of an Inhibitor of RAGE-Aβ Interactions in Alzheimer Disease. *Neurology* **2014**, *82*, 1536–1542. [CrossRef] [PubMed]

cancers MDPI

Article

Obesity Is Associated with Distal Migration of Pancreatic Adenocarcinoma to Body and Tail: A Multi-Center Study

Wisam Sbeit [1,2], Gil Gershovitz [1,2], Amir Shahin [1,2], Shhady Shhadeh [1,2], Mahmoud Salman [3], Maamoun Basheer [1,2] and Tawfik Khoury [1,2,*]

1 Gastroenterology Department, Galilee Medical Center, Nahariya 22100, Israel; wisams@gmc.gov.il (W.S.); gil.ggarshowitz@live.biu.ac.il (G.G.); amir.schahin@gmail.com (A.S.); sh7ady.it91@gmail.com (S.S.); maamon.basheer@mail.huji.ac.il (M.B.)

2 Azrieli Faculty of Medicine, Bar-Ilan University, Safed 1311502, Israel

3 Department of Surgery, Shaare Zedek Medical Center, Jerusalem 91120, Israel; dr.mahmoud88@hotmail.com

* Correspondence: tawfikkhoury1@hotmail.com; Tel.: +972-50-987-0611

Simple Summary: Pancreatic adenocarcinoma (PAC) is one of the most lethal types of cancer. Most cases of PAC occur in the head of the pancreas. This study aimed to identify predictors of non-head PAC. We showed that obesity represents a significant clinical predictor of distal PAC. To the best of our knowledge, this association has not been previously described in the English literature. We found a relatively high occurrence of distal PAC in our cohort, with a potential role of obesity in the development of distal PAC. We suggest proper intervention to possibly minimize the risk of the disease. Awareness of patients' complaints regarding unexplained abdominal pain is crucial to avoid misdiagnosis of distal PAC, which tends to present at later clinical stages and may aid in improving outcomes.

Abstract: (1) Background: Pancreatic adenocarcinoma (PAC) is one of the most lethal types of cancer. Most cases of PAC occur in the head of the pancreas. Given the proximity of the pancreatic head to the bile duct, most patients present clinically during early stages of the disease, while distally located PAC could have delayed clinical presentation. (2) Aims: To assess predictors of non-head PAC. (3) Methods: A retrospective multicenter study was conducted, including all patients who had endoscopic ultrasound (EUS) for pancreatic masses and who had histologic confirmation of PAC. (4) Results: Of the 151 patients included, 92 (60.9%) had pancreatic head cancer, and 59 (39.1%) had distal pancreatic cancer. PAC at body was the most common location in the distal PAC group (31 patients (52.5%)). Logistic regression analysis demonstrated a significant association of obesity with distal migration of PAC (OR 4.44, 95% CI 1.15–17.19, $p = 0.03$), while none of the other assessed parameters showed a significant association. Notably, abdominal pain was more significantly associated with distal PAC vs. head location (OR 2.85, 95% CI 1.32–6.16, $p = 0.008$). (5) Conclusions: Obesity shows a significant association as a clinical predictor of distal PAC. Further studies are needed to better explore this association.

Keywords: pancreas; pancreatic adenocarcinoma; distal migration

1. Introduction

The global burden of pancreatic cancer has increased dramatically over the past few decades and is expected to continue to represent a leading cause of cancer-related mortality. The past two decades have seen a doubling in the global annual number of pancreatic cancers diagnosed. Pancreatic adenocarcinoma (PAC) is a lethal disease constituting the seventh highest cause of death from cancer in developed countries worldwide [1]. The incidence of PAC is continuously rising, as it is estimated to be the second leading cause of cancer-related mortality by the end of 2030 [2]. The etiopathogenesis of the disease is multifactorial and has an association with smoking [3] and family history [4]. In addition, the disease has been associated with physical inactivity, alcohol consumption and several medical conditions including chronic pancreatitis, diabetes mellitus and obesity [5]. Prognosis of PAC is extremely poor, with a typical 1-year survival rate of 24% and a 5-year survival rate of only 9% following disease diagnosis [6]. During the early stages of PAC, patients are usually asymptomatic [7], and the site of the malignancy is the leading factor determining clinical presentation with disease advancement [6]. About 85% of cases of PAC occur in the head of the pancreas, while 15% occur in the pancreatic body and tail [8]. Survival and prognoses differ between adenocarcinoma of the pancreatic head vs. adenocarcinoma of the body and tail due to later clinical presentation and, therefore, advanced stages of the disease in the body and tail vs. the head [9,10]. To date, there is controversy about whether the pancreatic cancer site affects patients' prognosis and survival, as the data in this field have yielded conflicting results. However, a recent systematic review and meta-analysis demonstrated that patients with pancreatic head vs. body and tail adenocarcinoma had a 5% reduced risk of mortality [11]. Assuming that one of the main factors affecting disease prognosis is the location of the lesion in the pancreas [9,12], the identification of predicting factors, both clinical and demographic, of distal PAC locations while still asymptomatic may contribute to earlier diagnosis of the disease. Therefore, the aim of our study was to identify variables that may predict distal migration (body and tail) of PAC.

2. Methods

We performed an analytical observational retrospective multi-center study that included all patients diagnosed with PAC at two medical centers in Israel (Galilee Medical Center and Shaare Zedek Medical Center) from 2015–2020. Inclusion criteria were patients aged 18 years and above who had undergone endoscopic ultrasound (EUS) and were diagnosed with PAC, with histologic confirmation that was obtained by endoscopic-ultrasound fine needle biopsy. Exclusion criteria were patients diagnosed with non-adenocarcinoma pancreatic neoplasms, such as neuroendocrine neoplasms and metastatic cancer to the pancreas, a family history of cancers, or patients with a hereditary/genetic predisposition for PAC. The variables that were assessed were demographic data for each patient including age, sex and ethnic background, clinical parameters including body mass index (BMI), background diseases and clinical presentations, and data regarding the location of the tumor and prognosis. These data were obtained from the medical centers' electronic medical records. The study protocol conformed to the ethical guidelines of the 1975 declaration of Helsinki and was approved by the human research committee (approval number NHR-21-0027). Written informed consent was waived by the ethics committees due to the retrospective non-interventional nature of the study.

Statistical Analysis

Continuous variables with normal distribution were represented with informative statistics as arhythmical averages and standard deviation (±SD) or with median and interquartile range for variables that are not normally distributed. Categorical variables were represented in incidence and percentage tables. Several indices were collected, including age, gender, weight, ethnicity, obesity smoking, metabolic syndrome, alcohol consumption, BMI, and background diseases. Following data collection, a logistic regression model was constructed to anticipate distal migration (migration yes/no) according to the indices described. A minimal statistical significance of 5% was set, along with a statistical power of 80%. Statistical analyses were completed using the Statistical Package for Social Science (SPSS version 24.0, IBM, Chicago, IL, USA).

3. Results

3.1. Demographics and Baseline Characteristics

Of the continuous variables, only BMI was normally distributed according to the Kolmogorov–Smirnov test and was reported by mean ± SD; the other continuous parameters were not normally distributed and were thus reported by median ± IQR. Overall, 151 patients were included in the study. Of these, 92 patients (60.9%) had pancreatic head cancer (group A), and 59 patients (39.1%) had distal pancreatic cancer (group B). The most common location in group B was the pancreatic body in 31 patients (52.5%), followed by the pancreatic tail in 17 patients (28.8%) and the pancreatic neck in 11 patients (18.7%) (Figure 1).

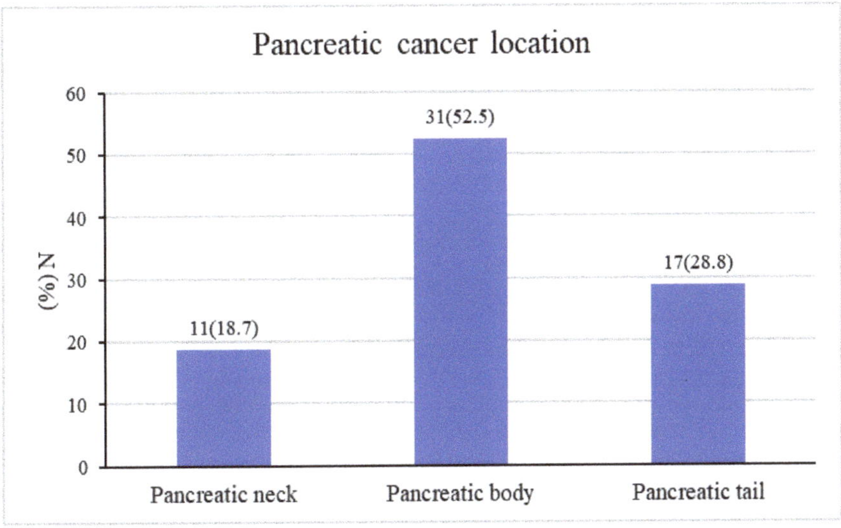

Figure 1. Distribution of non-head pancreatic cancer.

The median ± IQR for age was 72.5 ± 19 years in group A vs. 69 ± 18 years in group B. The male/female ratio was almost similar in the two groups. Similarly, the distribution of Arab and Jewish patients was similar. Of note, there was no difference in the rate of background diseases between the two groups. The rates of smoking, metabolic syndrome, active alcohol drinkers, diabetes mellitus and hypertension were 28.3%, 1.1%, 6.5%, 50% and 58.7% in group A vs. 16.9%, 0, 5.1%, 61% and 66.1% in group B, respectively. Table 1 shows the demographics and baseline characteristics.

Table 1. Demographics and baseline characteristics.

	Group A	Group B	p Value
Number	92	59	-
Age, median ± IQR (years)	72.5 ± 19	69 ± 18	0.29
Gender, N (%)			
• Male	52 (56.5)	31 (52.5)	0.63
• Female	40 (43.5)	28 (47.5)	
Ethnicity			
• Arab	30 (32.6)	19 (32.2)	0.95
• Jewish	62 (67.4)	40 (67.8)	

Table 1. *Cont.*

	Group A	Group B	*p* Value
Weight, median ± IQR (kg)	68 ± 15	67 ± 21	0.14
Body mass index, mean ± SD	25.03 ± 3	24.9 ± 4.2	0.42
Obesity, N (%)	4 (4.3)	8 (13.6)	0.04
Smoking, N (%)	26 (28.3)	10 (16.9)	0.11
Metabolic syndrome, N (%)	1 (1.1)	0	0.75
Alcohol, N (%)	6 (6.5)	3 (5.1)	0.72
Overweight, N (%)	39 (42.4)	21 (35.6)	0.4
Diabetes mellitus, N (%)	46 (50)	36 (61)	0.18
Ischemic heart disease, N (%)	15 (16.3)	8 (13.6)	0.65
Hypertension, N (%)	54 (58.7)	39 (66.1)	0.36
Obstructive lung disease, N (%)	9 (9.8)	3 (5.1)	0.3
Renal failure, N (%)	6 (6.5)	0	0.17
Congestive heart disease, N (%)	8 (8.7)	4 (6.8)	0.67
Hyperlipidemia, N (%)	44 (47.8)	33 (55.9)	0.33

3.2. Clinical Presentations among the Study Cohort

The most common clinical presentation for the entire cohort was abdominal pain followed by weight loss. Between the two groups, abdominal pain was more prevalent in group B (81.4%) than in group A (59.8%). On the other hand, jaundice and pruritus were more prevalent in group A (52.2% and 9.8%) as compared to group B (1.7% and 0), respectively, while weight loss did not differ between the two groups. Notably, distant metastasis was found at the time of diagnosis in 31.5% of patients in group A as compared to 45.7% of patients in group B. Figure 2 shows the clinical presentations.

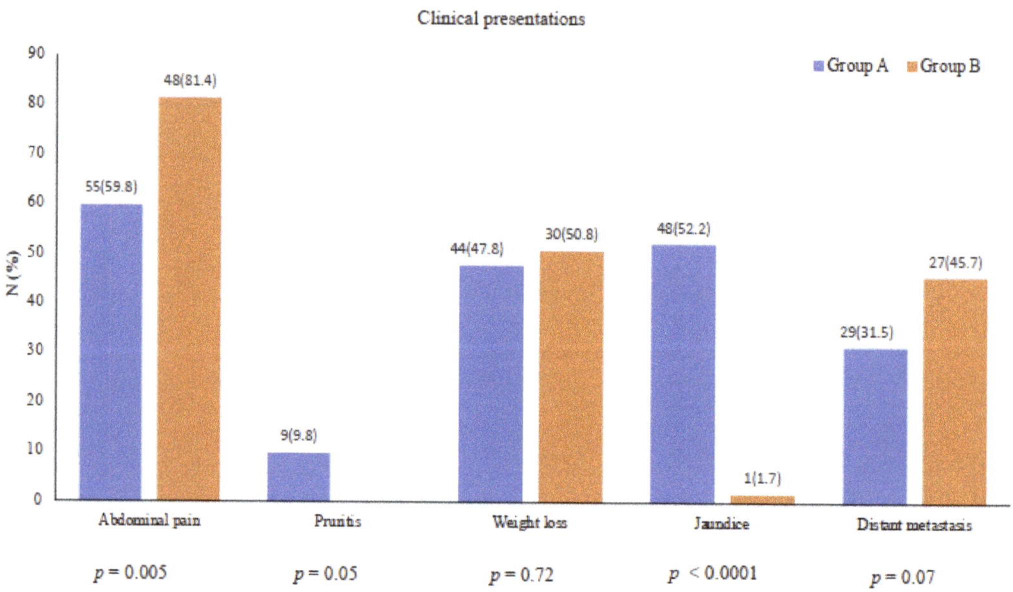

Figure 2. Clinical presentations of the study cohort.

3.3. Logistic Regression Analysis to Identify Parameters Associated with Distal Migration of Pancreatic Cancer

Performing univariate logistic regression analysis of demographics and baseline parameters to investigate the association with distal migration of PAC, we found that only obesity was significantly associated with distal migration of PAC (OR 4.44, 95% CI 1.15–17.19, $p = 0.03$). We could not identify any other clinical parameter associated with distal migration, including age (OR 0.99, 95% CI 0.97–1.02, $p = 0.58$), male gender (OR 0.85, 95% CI 0.44–1.64, $p = 0.63$), smoking (OR 0.55, 95% CI 0.24–1.26, $p = 0.16$) and diabetes mellitus (OR 1.55, 95% CI 0.80–3.01, $p = 0.19$). Table 2 shows the logistic regression analysis of the demographics and baseline characteristics. With regard to clinical presentation, abdominal pain was significantly associated with distal PAC location (OR 2.85, 95% CI 1.32–6.16, $p = 0.008$). As can be expected, jaundice showed a lower association with distal location (OR 0.02, 95% CI 0.004–0.13, $p < 0.0001$). Moreover, there was no difference in the rate of distant metastasis upon presentation (OR 1.79, 95% CI 0.91–3.52, $p = 0.09$) (Table 3).

Table 2. Univariate logistic regression analysis of baseline parameters associated with distal migration.

	OR	95% CI	*p* Value
Age	0.99	0.97–1.02	0.58
Male gender	0.85	0.44–1.64	0.63
Ethnicity	1.01	0.50–2.04	0.97
Smoking	0.55	0.24–1.26	0.16
Metabolic syndrome	0.49	0.005–48.20	0.76
Alcohol	0.82	0.20–3.38	0.79
Overweight	0.68	0.34–1.39	0.29
Diabetes mellitus	1.55	0.80–3.01	0.19
Ischemic heart disease	0.82	0.33–2.08	0.68
Hypertension	1.36	0.69–2.68	0.37
Obstructive lung disease	0.54	0.14–2.04	0.37
Renal failure	0.11	0.005–2.54	0.17
Congestive heart failure	0.81	0.23–2.78	0.73
Hyperlipidemia	1.38	0.71–2.66	0.34
Obesity	4.44	1.15–17.19	0.03

Table 3. Logistic regression analysis of clinical presentations associated with distal migration.

	OR	95% CI	*p* Value
Abdominal pain	2.85	1.32–6.16	0.008
Weight loss	1.13	0.59–2.17	0.72
Jaundice	0.02	0.004–0.13	<0.0001
Pruritus	0.07	0.004–1.51	0.09
Distant metastasis	1.79	0.91–3.52	0.09

4. Discussion

Pancreatic tumors remain a leading cause of death worldwide, with pancreatic adenocarcinoma contributing to most cases of pancreatic malignancies [13,14]. An overall increase in incidence and incidence-based mortality due to PAC has recently been demonstrated [15], and it is expected that PAC will become the second most common cause of death from cancer by the year 2040 [16]. Surgical resection is the only chance of a cure from the disease; however, given the late disease presentation, only 15–20% of patients have a resectable disease upon presentation [17].

Previous studies describing the distribution of tumors within the pancreas have shown that the most common site of PAC is in the head of the pancreas (ranging between 67% to 84% of cases), followed by the distal parts (neck, body, and tail) of the pancreas (ranging between 13% to 17% of cases) [18–20]. This distribution has a great consequential impact on the presentation, management, outcome, and prognosis of the disease. Given the high lethality rate of PAC, our study aimed to assess predictors of distal migration of PAC that are believed to be associated with late clinical presentation, advanced disease, poor prognosis, and survival.

Our work also found that the pancreatic head is the most common location of PAC, but with a relatively different ratio compared with distal parts of the pancreas. We found a higher proportion of distal PAC (39.1%) compared to studies prevailing in the literature (up to 17%) [18–20]. Our findings of an increase in the rate of distal (body, tail) PAC is in line with a previous study reporting the Surveillance, Epidemiology, and End Results Program (SEER) registry (including 85,715 cases from 1973–2014), which showed a steady decrease in the proportion of head PAC from 75.1 to 63.7% and a consistent gradual increase in the rate of distal body/tail PAC from 24.9 to 36.3% [21].

Several studies have suggested that the anatomic location of pancreatic tumors represents a potential determinant of survival [22,23]. A previous systematic review and meta-analysis of a total of 93 studies including 254,429 patients showed that the long-term prognosis of head cancers was better than that of body/tail cancers (HR = 0.96, 95% CI: 0.92–0.99; $p = 0.02$) and that pancreatic head adenocarcinoma was an independent prognostic factor for increased survival [11].

This led us to investigate potential predictors of distal migration of PAC to the pancreatic body and tail as well as the precipitants of such events. Our study found that obesity, defined as BMI > 30, is associated with a statistically significant association with distal migration of PAC. The association between obesity and the development of several comorbidities, including cancer, has been extensively studied and proven and has been specifically shown to be a risk factor for PAC [24,25]. Investigation of the underlying mechanisms of such a correlation has been carried out and has shown that fat deposition in the pancreas ("fatty pancreas") serves as a mediator between obesity and the development of pancreatic cancer, and several molecular pathways have been linked to the pathophysiology and carcinogenesis of this process [26–28]. The other mechanisms include: (1) insulin resistance and hyperinsulinemia, which is associated with amplified digestive enzyme protein translation, inducing local inflammation followed by recurrent and chronic pancreatitis, which is considered a major risk factor for pancreatic intra-epithelial neoplasia and PAC [29]; (2) gut microbiota. Recently, the complex effects of gut microbiota have been elucidated as being a major risk factor in the development and progression of PAC [30]. A previous prospective study revealed a decline in gut microbiome diversity and a specific microbial profile in Chinese patients with pancreatic cancer [31]. An imbalance in the distribution of gut microbiota, named intestinal dysbiosis, can lead to the initiation of chronic inflammation that is mediated by a bacterial translocation component, such as lipopolysaccharide, which activates Toll-like receptors, inducing innate immunity and enhancing cancer progression [32]. Additionally, lipopolysaccharide plays an important role in the initiation of a pro-inflammatory cascade by activating the nuclear factor-κappa B (NF-κB) pathway, leading to the production of pro-inflammatory cytokines [tumor necrosis factor alpha (TNF-α), interleukin (IL)-6, and IL-1] and leading to oxidative stress and an inflammatory state [33]; and (3) pancreatic microbiota, as a previous study demonstrated the presence of various bacterial taxa in the pancreatic tissue, and some of these bacteria were found to be inhabitants in the oral cavity [34]. Del Castillo et al. found a lower level of Lactobacillus bacteria and a relative abundance of oro-dental-related bacteria in patients with PAC as compared to non-cancer controls [34]. Moreover, Geller et al. found that pathogenic bacteria colonize the cancerous pancreatic tissue and are a component in the cancer microenvironment; they thus lead to a change in tumor course and might impact tumor sensitivity to chemotherapy [35].

To date, no one has attempted to elaborate on predictors for distal migration of PAC. Further studies are needed to exactly define the site of fatty infiltration within the pancreatic portions and to correlate it with the development of head or distal PAC.

The association between certain risk factors, such as smoking or diabetes mellitus, and the development of pancreatic cancer remains unclear. Several studies reported a link between smoking [3,36] and diabetes [37,38] and the development of PAC; however, these data are contradicted by other studies reporting no such link [39]. Our work revealed no significant association of smoking and diabetes with distal vs. head PAC.

To the best of our knowledge, no other published study in the English literature has focused specifically on the analysis of this association, and we believe that this association needs to be further explored, given the size of our study population, to determine if such a relation does in fact exist. Not surprisingly, clinical presentation of PAC may vary broadly depending on the location of the tumor. As expected, the results of our study showed that jaundice is more strongly associated with tumors in the pancreatic head. Previous studies have shown similar results, with pancreatic head cancer presenting at earlier clinical stages with clinical features of obstructive jaundice [18,40]. This can be explained by the mechanical obstruction of the common bile duct caused by the tumor, based on the size of the lesion and alteration of normal anatomy. Malignancies located more distally in the pancreas are less likely to inflict such anatomical consequences, and jaundice was therefore less common in these patients. However, in patients with distal PAC, abdominal pain was found to be more prominent in our study. This finding has been previously demonstrated, and the characterization of the pain has been described [10,41]. Therefore, our results may emphasize the importance of physicians' awareness of complaints exhibited by patients regarding unexplained abdominal pain, especially in obese patients. In these cases, we advocate that one proceed with a radiological investigation of the pancreas, to avoid the possibility of misdiagnosing distal PAC. The appropriate timing for making a diagnosis may enable us to offer the appropriate treatment, which has important prognostic value because late diagnosis may lead to locally advanced or metastatic disease [11]. Therefore, we highly urge caregivers to remain aware of pancreatic adenocarcinoma and proceed with appropriate investigations in obese patients with complaints of abdominal pain.

Notably, in our study we found that distant metastasis was more common in distally located pancreatic adenocarcinoma (45.7%) as compared to pancreatic head adenocarcinoma (31.5%), with no statistical significance ($p = 0.09$). Distal pancreatic adenocarcinomas usually do not cause jaundice by obstructing the common bile duct, thus reducing the opportunity for early diagnosis when compared to adenocarcinoma of the pancreatic head. This difference may explain the worse prognosis of body and tail adenocarcinoma compared to that in the head location [31]. A previous study showed that pancreatic head adenocarcinoma had a significantly lower risk of distant metastasis as compared to pancreatic body and tail adenocarcinoma [42]. The relatively small sample size in our study probably yielded a higher rate of distant metastasis, but without statistical significance. Therefore, a larger cohort study is warranted to precisely assess the effect of the PAC location on the distant metastasis rate.

Potential limitations of our study are the size of the research population and its retrospective design. We believe a larger study population may yield improved results and aid in determining more risk factors associated with distal migration of PAC. Additionally, characterizing the exact pancreatic portions of fatty infiltration will enable us to assess two points: first, whether obesity causes diffuse pancreatic fatty infiltration, and second, whether the association of obesity with distal PAC is related to the infiltration of fat within the distal part of the pancreas.

5. Conclusions

Obesity shows a significant association as a clinical predictor of distal PAC. We found a relatively high occurrence of distal PAC in our cohort, with a potential role for obesity in the development of distal PAC. We suggest proper intervention to possibly minimize the risk of the disease. Awareness of patients' complaints regarding unexplained abdominal pain is crucial to avoid misdiagnosis of distal PAC, which tends to present at later clinical stages, and this may aid in improving outcomes.

Author Contributions: W.S. and T.K. contributed to the conception and design; W.S. and T.K. contributed to the development of the methodology and acquisition of data; G.G., A.S., M.S. and S.S., contributed to data collection; All the authors contributed to analysis and interpretation of data; W.S., G.G. and T.K. contributed to manuscript writing; W.S., M.B. and T.K. contributed to reviewing or editing the manuscript; W.S. and T.K. contributed to administrative, technical, or material support; and W.S. and T.K. supervised the study. All authors have read and agreed to the published version of the manuscript.

Funding: This research received no external funding.

Institutional Review Board Statement: The study was approved on 18 May 2021 by the local ethics committee at Galilee medical center, Israel (approval number NHR-21-0027). The analysis of the data from our electronic medical record database was performed under the oversight of the ICH guidelines for good clinical practice.

Informed Consent Statement: Written informed consent was waived by the ethics committees due to the retrospective non-interventional nature of the study.

Data Availability Statement: Data are available from the authors upon reasonable request. The data are found at the Gastroenterology Department at Galilee Medical Center, Nahariya, Israel and will be available upon reasonable request.

Conflicts of Interest: The authors declare that they have no conflict of interest.

Abbreviations

PAC: Pancreatic adenocarcinoma; EUS: endoscopic ultrasound; BMI: body mass index.

References

1. Bray, F.; Ferlay, J.; Soerjomataram, I.; Siegel, R.L.; Torre, L.A.; Jemal, A. Global cancer statistics 2018: GLOBOCAN estimates of incidence and mortality worldwide for 36 cancers in 185 countries. *CA Cancer J. Clin.* **2018**, *68*, 394–424. [CrossRef] [PubMed]
2. Rahib, L.; Smith, B.D.; Aizenberg, R.; Rosenzweig, A.B.; Fleshman, J.M.; Matrisian, L.M. Projecting cancer incidence and deaths to 2030: The unexpected burden of thyroid, liver, and pancreas cancers in the United States. *Cancer Res.* **2014**, *74*, 2913–2921. [CrossRef] [PubMed]
3. Bosetti, C.; Lucenteforte, E.; Silverman, D.T.; Petersen, G.; Bracci, P.M.; Ji, B.T.; Negri, E.; Li, D.; Risch, H.A.; Olson, S.; et al. Cigarette smoking and pancreatic cancer: An analysis from the International Pancreatic Cancer Case-Control Consortium (Panc4). *Ann. Oncol.* **2012**, *23*, 1880–1888. [CrossRef] [PubMed]
4. Klein, A.P.; Brune, K.A.; Petersen, G.M.; Goggins, M.; Tersmette, A.C.; Offerhaus, G.J.; Griffin, C.; Cameron, J.; Yeo, C.; Kern, S.; et al. Prospective risk of pancreatic cancer in familial pancreatic cancer kindreds. *Cancer Res.* **2004**, *64*, 2634–2638. [CrossRef] [PubMed]
5. Simoes, P.K.; Olson, S.H.; Saldia, A.; Kurtz, R.C. Epidemiology of pancreatic adenocarcinoma. *Chin. Clin. Oncol.* **2017**, *6*, 24. [CrossRef] [PubMed]
6. Rawla, P.; Sunkara, T.; Gaduputi, V. Epidemiology of Pancreatic Cancer: Global Trends, Etiology and Risk Factors. *World J. Oncol.* **2019**, *10*, 10–27. [CrossRef] [PubMed]
7. De La Cruz, M.S.; Young, A.P.; Ruffin, M.T. Diagnosis and management of pancreatic cancer. *Am. Fam. Physician* **2014**, *89*, 626–632.
8. Greenlee, R.T.; Murray, T.; Bolden, S.; Wingo, P.A. Cancer statistics, 2000. *CA Cancer J. Clin.* **2000**, *50*, 7–33. [CrossRef]
9. Brennan, M.F.; Moccia, R.D.; Klimstra, D. Management of adenocarcinoma of the body and tail of the pancreas. *Ann. Surg.* **1996**, *223*, 506–551. [CrossRef]
10. Watanabe, I.; Sasaki, S.; Konishi, M.; Nakagohri, T.; Inoue, K.; Oda, T.; Kinoshita, T. Onset symptoms and tumor locations as prognostic factors of pancreatic cancer. *Pancreas* **2004**, *28*, 160–165. [CrossRef]

1. Tomasello, G.; Ghidini, M.; Costanzo, A.; Ghidini, A.; Russo, A.; Barni, S.; Petrelli, F. Outcome of head compared to body and tail pancreatic cancer: A systematic review and meta-analysis of 93 studies. *J. Gastrointest. Oncol.* **2019**, *10*, 259–269. [CrossRef] [PubMed]
2. Wade, T.P.; Virgo, K.S.; Johnson, F.E. Distal pancreatectomy for cancer: Results in U.S. Department of Veterans Affairs hospitals, 1987–1991. *Pancreas* **1995**, *11*, 341–344. [CrossRef] [PubMed]
3. Hidalgo, M.; Cascinu, S.; Kleeff, J.; Labianca, R.; Lohr, J.M.; Neoptolemos, J.; Real, F.X.; Laethem, J.; Heinemann, V. Addressing the challenges of pancreatic cancer: Future directions for improving outcomes. *Pancreatology* **2015**, *15*, 8–18. [CrossRef] [PubMed]
4. Collisson, E.A.; Bailey, P.; Chang, D.K.; Biankin, A.V. Molecular subtypes of pancreatic cancer. *Nat. Rev. Gastroenterol. Hepatol.* **2019**, *16*, 207–220. [CrossRef] [PubMed]
5. Saad, A.M.; Turk, T.; Al-Husseini, M.J.; Abdel-Rahman, O. Trends in pancreatic adenocarcinoma incidence and mortality in the United States in the last four decades; A SEER-based study. *BMC Cancer* **2018**, *18*, 688. [CrossRef] [PubMed]
6. Rahib, L.; Wehner, M.R.; Matrisian, L.M.; Nead, K.T. Estimated Projection of US Cancer Incidence and Death to 2040. *JAMA Netw. Open* **2021**, *4*, e214708. [CrossRef] [PubMed]
7. Allen, P.J.; Kuk, D.; Castillo, C.F.; Basturk, O.; Wolfgang, C.L.; Cameron, J.L.; Lilemoe, K.D.; Ferrone, C.; Morales, V.; He, J.; et al. Multi-institutional Validation Study of the American Joint Commission on Cancer (8th Edition) Changes for T and N Staging in Patients With Pancreatic Adenocarcinoma. *Ann. Surg.* **2017**, *265*, 185–191. [CrossRef]
8. Winer, L.K.; Dhar, V.K.; Wima, K.; Morris, M.C.; Lee, T.C.; Shah, S.A.; Syed, A.; Ahmad, A.; Patel, S.H. The Impact of Tumor Location on Resection and Survival for Pancreatic Ductal Adenocarcinoma. *J. Surg. Res.* **2019**, *239*, 60–66. [CrossRef]
9. Van Erning, F.N.; Mackay, T.M.; van der Geest, L.G.M.; Groot Koerkamp, B.; van Laarhoven, H.W.M.; Bonsing, B.A.; Wilmink, J.W.; Santvoort, H.C.; Geelen, J.; Eijck, C.; et al. Association of the location of pancreatic ductal adenocarcinoma (head, body, tail) with tumor stage, treatment, and survival: A population-based analysis. *Acta Oncol.* **2018**, *57*, 1655–1662. [CrossRef]
10. Birnbaum, D.J.; Bertucci, F.; Finetti, P.; Birnbaum, D.; Mamessier, E. Head and Body/Tail Pancreatic Carcinomas Are Not the Same Tumors. *Cancers* **2019**, *11*, 497. [CrossRef]
11. Luo, G.; Jin, K.; Cheng, H.; Guo, M.; Gong, Y.; Fan, Z.; Yang, C.; Huang, Q.; Ni, Q.; Liu, C.; et al. Prognosis of distal pancreatic cancers controlled by stage. *Exp. Ther. Med.* **2020**, *20*, 1091–1097. [CrossRef]
12. Lau, M.K.; Davila, J.A.; Shaib, Y.H. Incidence and survival of pancreatic head and body and tail cancers: A population-based study in the United States. *Pancreas* **2010**, *39*, 458–462. [CrossRef] [PubMed]
13. Artinyan, A.; Soriano, P.A.; Prendergast, C.; Low, T.; Ellenhorn, J.D.; Kim, J. The anatomic location of pancreatic cancer is a prognostic factor for survival. *HPB* **2008**, *10*, 371–376. [CrossRef] [PubMed]
14. Bao, B.; Wang, Z.; Li, Y.; Kong, D.; Ali, S.; Banerjee, S.; Ahmad, A.; Sarkar, F.H. The complexities of obesity and diabetes with the development and progression of pancreatic cancer. *Biochim. Biophys. Acta* **2011**, *1815*, 135–146. [CrossRef]
15. Berrington de Gonzalez, A.; Sweetland, S.; Spencer, E. A meta-analysis of obesity and the risk of pancreatic cancer. *Br. J. Cancer* **2003**, *89*, 519–523. [CrossRef] [PubMed]
16. Chang, M.L. Fatty Pancreas-Centered Metabolic Basis of Pancreatic Adenocarcinoma: From Obesity, Diabetes and Pancreatitis to Oncogenesis. *Biomedicines* **2022**, *10*, 692. [CrossRef]
17. Gumbs, A.A. Obesity, pancreatitis, and pancreatic cancer. *Obes. Surg.* **2008**, *18*, 1183–1187. [CrossRef]
18. Preziosi, G.; Oben, J.A.; Fusai, G. Obesity and pancreatic cancer. *Surg. Oncol.* **2014**, *23*, 61–71. [CrossRef]
19. Zhang, A.M.Y.; Xia, Y.H.; Lin, J.S.H.; Chu, K.H.; Wang, W.C.K.; Ruiter, T.J.J.; Yang, J.; Chen, N.; Chhuor, J.; Patil, S.; et al. Hyperinsulinemia acts via acinar insulin receptors to initiate pancreatic cancer by increasing digestive enzyme production and inflammation. *Cell. Metab.* **2023**, *35*, 2119.e5–2135.e5. [CrossRef]
20. Li, Q.; Jin, M.; Liu, Y.; Jin, L. Gut Microbiota: Its Potential Roles in Pancreatic Cancer. *Front. Cell. Infect. Microbiol.* **2020**, *10*, 572492. [CrossRef]
21. Ren, Z.; Jiang, J.; Xie, H.; Li, A.; Lu, H.; Xu, S.; Zhou, L.; Zhang, H.; Cui, G.; Chen, X.; et al. Gut microbial profile analysis by MiSeq sequencing of pancreatic carcinoma patients in China. *Oncotarget* **2017**, *8*, 95176–95191. [CrossRef] [PubMed]
22. Gualtieri, P.; Cianci, R.; Frank, G.; Pizzocaro, E.; De Santis, G.L.; Giannattasio, S.; Merra, G.; Butturini, G.; Lorenzo, A.; Renzo, L. Pancreatic Ductal Adenocarcinoma and Nutrition: Exploring the Role of Diet and Gut Health. *Nutrients* **2023**, *15*, 4465. [CrossRef]
23. Darnaud, M.; Faivre, J.; Moniaux, N. Targeting gut flora to prevent progression of hepatocellular carcinoma. *J. Hepatol.* **2013**, *58*, 385–387. [CrossRef] [PubMed]
24. Del Castillo, E.; Meier, R.; Chung, M.; Koestler, D.C.; Chen, T.; Paster, B.J.; Charpentier, K.; Kelsey, K.; Izard, J.; Michaud, D. The Microbiomes of Pancreatic and Duodenum Tissue Overlap and Are Highly Subject Specific but Differ between Pancreatic Cancer and Noncancer Subjects. *Cancer Epidemiol. Biomark. Prev.* **2019**, *28*, 370–383. [CrossRef] [PubMed]
25. Geller, L.T.; Barzily-Rokni, M.; Danino, T.; Jonas, O.H.; Shental, N.; Nejman, D.; Gavert, N.; Zwang, Y.; Cooper, Z.; Shee, K.; et al. Potential role of intratumor bacteria in mediating tumor resistance to the chemotherapeutic drug gemcitabine. *Science* **2017**, *357*, 1156–1160. [CrossRef]
26. Blackford, A.; Parmigiani, G.; Kensler, T.W.; Wolfgang, C.; Jones, S.; Zhang, X.; Parsons, D.W.; Lin, J.; Leary, R.; Goggins, M. Genetic mutations associated with cigarette smoking in pancreatic cancer. *Cancer Res.* **2009**, *69*, 3681–3688. [CrossRef]
27. Li, D. Diabetes and pancreatic cancer. *Mol. Carcinog.* **2012**, *51*, 64–74. [CrossRef]
28. Khadka, R.; Tian, W.; Hao, X.; Koirala, R. Risk factor, early diagnosis and overall survival on outcome of association between pancreatic cancer and diabetes mellitus: Changes and advances, a review. *Int. J. Surg.* **2018**, *52*, 342–346. [CrossRef]

39. Crous-Bou, M.; Porta, M.; Lopez, T.; Jariod, M.; Malats, N.; Alguacil, J.; Morales, E. Lifetime history of tobacco consumption and K-ras mutations in exocrine pancreatic cancer. *Pancreas* **2007**, *35*, 135–141. [CrossRef]
40. Zhang, Q.; Zeng, L.; Chen, Y.; Lian, G.; Qian, C.; Chen, S.; Li, J.; Huang, K. Pancreatic Cancer Epidemiology, Detection, and Management. *Gastroenterol. Res. Pract.* **2016**, *2016*, 8962321. [CrossRef]
41. Freelove, R.; Walling, A.D. Pancreatic cancer: Diagnosis and management. *Am. Fam. Physician* **2006**, *73*, 485–492. [PubMed]
42. Lou, X.; Li, J.; Wei, Y.Q.; Jiang, Z.J.; Chen, M.; Sun, J.J. Comparable prevalence of distant metastasis and survival of different primary site for LN^+ pancreatic tumor. *J. Transl. Med.* **2020**, *18*, 266. [CrossRef] [PubMed]

cancers

MDPI

Article

Neutralization of p40 Homodimer and p40 Monomer Leads to Tumor Regression in Patient-Derived Xenograft Mice with Pancreatic Cancer

Monica Sheinin [1], Susanta Mondal [1] and Kalipada Pahan [1,2,*]

[1] Department of Neurological Sciences, Rush University Medical Center, Chicago, IL 60612, USA; susanta_mondal@rush.edu (S.M.)

[2] Division of Research and Development, Jesse Brown Veterans Affairs Medical Center, Chicago, IL 60612, USA

* Correspondence: kalipada_pahan@rush.edu

Simple Summary: Pancreatic ductal adenocarcinoma (PDAC) is one of the deadliest cancers, and immunotherapy could be one of the safest options to control PDAC. Although the p40 family of cytokines has four members comprising IL-12, p40 homodimer ($p40_2$), p40 monomer (p40), and IL-23, we found an increase in $p40_2$ and p40 and a decrease in IL-12 and IL-23 in serum of pancreatic cancer patients as compared to healthy controls. Similarly, human pancreatic cancer cells also produced greater levels of $p40_2$ and p40 and lower levels of IL-12 and IL-23 than normal human pancreatic cells. Accordingly, neutralization of $p40_2$ by a3-1d monoclonal antibody (mAb) and p40 by a3-3a mAb separately led to apoptosis of pancreatic cancer cells and tumor shrinkage in a patient-derived xenograft (PDX) mouse model of pancreatic cancer, highlighting the possible therapeutic potential of mAbs against $p40_2$ and p40 in pancreatic cancer.

Abstract: Pancreatic cancer is a highly aggressive cancer with a high mortality rate and limited treatment options. It is the fourth leading cause of cancer in the US, and mortality is rising rapidly, with a 12% relative 5-year survival rate. Early diagnosis remains a challenge due to vague symptoms, lack of specific biomarkers, and rapid tumor progression. Interleukin-12 (IL-12) is a central cytokine that regulates innate (natural killer cells) and adaptive (cytokine T-lymphocytes) immunity in cancer. We demonstrated that serum levels of IL-12p40 homodimer ($p40_2$) and p40 monomer (p40) were elevated and that of IL-12 and IL-23 were lowered in pancreatic cancer patients compared to healthy controls. Comparably, human PDAC cells produced greater levels of $p40_2$ and p40 and lower levels of IL-12 and IL-23 compared to normal pancreatic cells. Notably, neutralization of $p40_2$ by mAb a3-1d and p40 by mAb a3-3a induced the death of human PDAC cells, but not normal human pancreatic cells. Furthermore, we demonstrated that treatment of PDX mice with $p40_2$ mAb and p40 mAb resulted in apoptosis and tumor shrinkage. This study illustrates a new role of $p40_2$ and p40 monomer in pancreatic cancer, highlighting possible approaches against this deadly form of cancer with $p40_2$ and p40 monomer immunotherapies.

Keywords: pancreatic cancer; pancreatic ductal adenocarcinoma; IL-12p40 monomer; IL-12p40 homodimer; patient-derived xenograft mouse model; immunotherapy; IL-23; IL-12; apoptosis; cell death

1. Introduction

Pancreatic cancer is a highly malignant cancer commonly detected at advanced stages. It accounts for about 3% of cancers in the US, with the lowest 5-year relative survival rate at 12% [1]. Pancreatic ductal adenocarcinoma (PDAC) is the predominant neoplasm responsible for the majority of pancreatic cancer cases, and many patients have unresectable, advanced, or metastatic manifestation at diagnosis [2]. Current treatments including surgery, radiation, targeted therapy, and chemotherapy have shown inadequate improvement in survival [3]. Recently, studies have shown that immunotherapy is a worthwhile approach, which can enhance the immune system's capacity to identify and kill cancer cells [4,5]. Some limitations of existing therapies include chemoresistance, a dense desmoplastic tumor microenvironment, genetic heterogeneity across patients, and a lack of specific biomarkers [6,7].

The p40 family of cytokines has four members, p40 homodimer ($p40_2$), p40 monomer (p40), IL-12 (p40:p35), and IL-23 (p40:p19) [8]. IL-12 plays a crucial role in the early inflammatory response by producing T helper type 1 (Th1) cells [9,10]. It is believed that most effects are mediated by IFN-γ secretion [11]. Until recently, $p40_2$ and p40 were considered inactive partners of the IL-12 family [12–14]. Since all four members of the p40 family contain p40 in distinctive forms, a specific monoclonal antibody (mAb) is necessary to characterize these molecules. Monoclonal antibodies (mAbs) are immunoglobulins produced to target specific proteins and found to improve long-term outcomes of patients [15]. Antibody-mediated immunotherapy targets tumors using mAbs to inhibit oncogenic signaling, immune suppression, or immune checkpoint blockade [16]. Therefore, we have produced neutralizing mAbs against p40 and $p40_2$ [17] and, by using such mAbs, we have delineated that the level of p40 is higher in the serum of prostate [18] and breast cancer [19] patients as compared to healthy controls, and selective neutralization of p40 by mAb leads to tumor regression in mice [18,19]. On the other hand, the level of $p40_2$ is reduced in the serum of prostate and breast cancer patients in comparison with healthy controls [18,19], indicating the specificity of our finding.

In contrast to prior results, we found an increase in both $p40_2$ and p40 in the serum of pancreatic cancer patients when matched to healthy controls and in various human pancreatic cancer cells in comparison to normal human pancreatic duct epithelial cells. Furthermore, we demonstrated that selective neutralization of $p40_2$ by $p40_2$ mAb a3-1d and p40 by p40 mAb a3-3a stimulated death in human pancreatic cancer cells in culture and in vivo in PDX tumor tissue. This study highlights the role of $p40_2$ and p40 in the survival of pancreatic cancer cells and tissues that could be of therapeutic benefit for patients with pancreatic cancer.

2. Materials and Methods

2.1. Cell Culture and Reagents

Human pancreatic cancer cell lines were purchased from ATCC (Manassas, VA, USA). PANC-1 (CRL-1469) were cultured with DMEM (10-017-CV). BxPC-3 (CRL-1687) were cultured with RPMI-1640 (11875-093) (ThermoFisher Scientific, Waltham, MA, USA). Both cell lines were supplemented with 10% FBS obtained from Atlas Biologicals (Fort Collins, CO, USA) and antibiotic–antimycotic from ThermoFisher Scientific, Waltham, MA, USA). Human pancreatic duct epithelial cells HPDE-H6c7 (ECA001-FP) purchased from Kerafast (Boston, MA, USA) were cultured with Keratinocyte SFM (Invitrogen, Waltham, MA, USA) supplemented with EGF and bovine pituitary extract as well as antibiotic–antimycotic. All cell lines were cultured at 37 °C and 5% CO_2 in complete medium. When cells grew to 80% confluency, they were passaged. Phosphate-buffered solution (PBS) was added to the flasks to wash cells, then they were treated with 0.25% trypsin from Corning. Culture medium neutralized the trypsin, cells were resuspended then seeded into T75 flasks, and the cells from the logarithmic phase were utilized for experiments. Additional cell line details are included below (see Table 1).

Table 1. Cell lines for this project.

Cell Line	Diagnosis	Mutation	Cell Type	Tissue	Age	Sex	Manufacturer
HPDE-H6c7	Normal	wt p53 wt KRAS	Epithelial	Pancreatic duct	63	F	Kerafast
PANC-1	Epithelioid Carcinoma	mut p53 mut KRAS	Epithelial	Pancreatic duct	56	M	ATCC
BxPC-3	Adenocarcinoma	mut p53 wt KRAS	Epithelial	Pancreas	61	F	ATCC

2.2. Serum Samples of Pancreatic Cancer Patients

The serum samples of pancreatic cancer patients before drug treatment and some age-matched healthy controls were purchased from Discovery Life Sciences, Los Osos, CA, USA. Serum samples of the rest of the age-coordinated healthy individuals were obtained from Rush University Medical Center. Controls are defined as healthy individuals without significant medical history. Details are included below (see Table 2).

Table 2. Serum Samples used in this study.

Patient ID	Diagnosis	Age	Sex	Ethnicity	Manufacturer
Healthy Controls					
HC-130	Normal	39	F	White	DLS
HC-798	Normal	57	F	White	DLS
HC-144	Normal	65	F	White	DLS
HC-792	Normal	51	F	White	DLS
HC-594	Normal	37	F	American Indian	DLS
HC-806	Normal	34	F	White	RUMC
HC-593	Normal	63	M	White	RUMC
HC-810	Normal	63	M	White	RUMC
HC-900	Normal	54	M	Asian	RUMC
HC-901	Normal	32	F	Asian	RUMC
Pancreatic Cancer					
PC-416	Pancreatic Cancer	65	F	Black	DLS
PC-316	Adenocarcinoma	58	F	White	DLS
PC-716	Adenocarcinoma	68	M	Black	DLS
PC-617	Adenocarcinoma	78	M	White	DLS
PC-717	Pancreatic Cancer	71	M	White	DLS
PC-2617	Adenocarcinoma	52	M	White	DLS
PC-217	Adenocarcinoma	58	M	White	DLS
PC-417	Adenocarcinoma	57	F	Black	DLS
PC-110	Adenocarcinoma	74	F	White	DLS
PC-418	Adenocarcinoma	70	M	Black	DLS

Serum samples were purchased mainly from Discovery Life Sciences (DLS). Some normal samples were obtained from Rush University Medical Center (RUMC). Each sample was analyzed for p40, p40$_2$, and IL-12 three times by ELISA.

2.3. Sandwich ELISA

Sandwich ELISA was performed to quantify $p40_2$ and p40 as described by our laboratory [17,18,20]. Please see dilutions for $p40_2$ mAb and p40 mAb capture and biotinylated detection antibodies [19]. Concentrations of IL-12 and IL-23 were measured in patient serum or tissue homogenates via ELISA (eBioscience/Thermo Fisher (San Diego, CA, USA)), according to the manufacturer's guidelines as described previously [18].

2.4. Assessment of Cell Viability: MTT and LDH Assays

Cell viability was calculated using the 3-(4,5-dimethylthiazol-2-yl)-2,5-diphenyl tetrazolium bromide (MTT) method (Sigma) as delineated in previous experiments [18,19]. Cells were seeded in 12-well plates with 500 µL of DMEM and RPMI-1640 medium for 24 h then treated in serum-free medium. After cells were treated for 24 h, 100 µL supernatant was separated to be used for the LDH assay followed by addition of MTT reagent. To measure mitochondrial activity, formazan crystals were dissolved by adding equivalent volume of solubilization solution. After treatment, 300 µL of culture medium was removed from each well and 10 µL of MTT solution (5 mg/mL) was added and incubated for 30 min. Supernatant was added to a 96-well plate, then absorbance was measured at 595 nm with the Thermo Fisher Multiskan MCC plate reader. Lactate dehydrogenase (LDH) activity was measured using an LDH assay kit (Sigma, St. Louis, MO, USA) as outlined before [18,19].

2.5. Fragment End Labeling DNA—TUNEL Assay

Fragmented DNA was detected in cells and tissues by the terminal deoxynucleotide transferase (TdT)-facilitated binding to 3′OH ends of DNA fragments broken due to apoptotic signals, using a kit (TdT FragEL DNA Detection Kit) from Millipore Sigma (Burlington, MA, USA) as described previously [18,19]. PANC-1, BxPc-3 and HPDE cells were cultured to 70–80% confluence, and plated on coverslips, then fixed with chilled methanol (Fisher Scientific, Waltham, MA, USA) for an hour, followed by rinses with sterile PBS. Cells and tissues were treated as described by us in previous studies [21]. Coverslips were mounted, and dried overnight. Then, slides were imaged under the Olympus BX41 with an attached Hamamatsu ORCA-03G camera.

2.6. Flow Cytometry

For FACS analysis, single cells were resuspended and isolated using a cell strainer from PANC-1, BxPC-3, and HPDE cells. They were stained using an apoptosis kit for flow cytometry (Thermo Fisher, Waltham, MA, USA) as described previously [22]. Briefly, single-cell suspensions of PANC-1 and BxPC-3 cells were stained with Zombie Aqua™ Fixable Viability Kit (Biolegend, San Diego, CA, USA). Cells were washed with FACS buffer (Thermo Fisher), stained with PE-anti-human IFNγ antibody (Biolegend), and identified by FACS Canto II Flow cytometer (BD Biosciences) and analyzed using FlowJo Software (v10). Controls were composed of Annexin V, PI, and unstained cells.

2.7. Immunostaining

Coverslips containing PANC-1, BxPc-3, and HPDE cells were cultured to 70–80% confluence. The cells were fixed with chilled methanol (Fisher Scientific, Waltham, MA, USA) for one hour, then washed with filtered PBS. For tissue samples, antigen retrieval in heated sodium citrate buffer pH 6.0 multiple times was necessary [23]. A detailed procedure for immunostaining was previously outlined by us [21]. The primary antibodies used included IFN-γ (1:100; Thermo Fisher, Waltham, MA, USA), cleaved caspase 3 (1:400; Cell Signaling, Danvers, MA, USA), CA19-9 (1:500; Thermo Fisher, Waltham, MA, USA); they were incubated for 2 h on a shaker at RT (see Table 3). Cells and tissues were rinsed multiple times in filtered PBS, then incubated with Cy5-labeled secondary antibody (1:200; Jackson ImmunoResearch, West Grove, PA, USA) for 1 h. After three washes in PBS, cells were incubated for 5 min in 4′, 6′- diamindino-2-phenylindole (DAPI, 1:10,000; Millipore

Sigma, Burlington, MA, USA) followed by mounting, drying overnight, and observing under the Olympus BX41 equipped with a Hamamatsu ORCA-03G camera.

Table 3. Antibodies used in this study.

Antibody	Manufacturer	Catalog	Host	Application	Dilution
Cleaved caspase 3	Cell Signaling	#9661	rabbit	IF	1:1000
IFN-γ	Invitrogen	MA5-44024	mouse	IF	1:200
CA19-9	Invitrogen	MA5-12421	mouse	IF	1:200
Phospho-BAD	Santa-Cruz	sc-166932	mouse	WB	1:200
Bcl-2	Santa-Cruz	sc-7382	mouse	WB	1:200

IF, Immunofluorescence; WB, Western blotting.

2.8. Real-Time PCR

Real-time PCR was performed as described [20,22] in the ABI-Prism 7700 sequence detection system (Applied Biosystems, Foster City, CA, USA) using PowerUp SYBR green master mix (Thermo Fisher, Waltham, MA, USA). The mRNA expression of the targeted gene was standardized to the level of GAPDH mRNA. The following primers were used for human IFN-γ and GAPDH.

IFN-γ:
Sense: CGGCACAGTCATTGAAAGCC
Antisense: TGCATCCTTTTTCGCCTTGC
GAPDH:
Sense: GCATCTTCTTGTGCAGTGCC
Antisense: TACGGCCAAATCCGTTCACA

Immunoblotting

Immunoblotting was conducted as described by us [20,22]. The tissues were lysed and protein extracted using a detailed method described by us previously [21]. Protein concentration was analyzed from the lysed tissue supernatant, using the Bradford method (Bio-Rad, Hercules, CA, USA). Additional immunoblotting procedure was outlined by us in previous studies [21]. The membrane was blocked for 1 h in intercept blocking buffer (Li-COR, Lincoln, NE). After, the membranes were incubated overnight at 4 °C on a shaker in primary antibodies diluted in blocking buffer at indicated dilutions (see Table 3). Actin was run as a loading control. The following day, membranes were washed in PBS containing 0.1% Tween 20 (PBS-T) for 30 min (3× for 10 min), and incubated with secondary antibodies (Li-COR, Lincoln, NE; Dilution: 1:10,000) for 1 h at room temperature. Then, the blot was washed in PBST for 30 min and imaged using the Odyssey Infrared Imaging System (Li-COR, Lincoln, NE, USA).

2.9. Experimental Animals

Female NOD scid gamma (NSG) mice engrafted with patient-derived pancreatic cancer were generated by The Jackson Laboratory (#TM01212) [16,24,25]. Mice were engrafted subcutaneously in the right flank. All NSG mice were housed under immunocompromised conditions with autoclaved cages, water, and irradiated feed. Mice were treated with either $p40_2$ mAb or p40 mAb twice a week (2 mg/kg) via intraperitoneal injection. Control mice received only sterile saline. Mice were weighed one time per week, and observations were noted. Tumor size was measured three times per week as soon as the xenograft was palpable using a digital caliper and recorded in a lab notebook for each animal. To calculate tumor volume, we used the following formula:

$$V = (\text{length} \times \text{width}^2)/2$$

Tumor volume was measured until experimental endpoints were reached, and once control tumors reached about 20 mm. National Institutes of Health guidelines were followed for animal experiments. All animal experiments were approved by the Institutional Animal Care and Use Committee (IACUC) of the Rush University Medical Center.

2.9.1. Histopathology

IACUC protocol was followed to euthanize mice by carbon dioxide fixation followed by cervical dislocation. Mouse blood samples were taken via cardiac puncture and tumor tissue was excised post-euthanasia. Tumor tissue sections were fixed in 4% paraformaldehyde for at least 24 h, embedded in paraffin, and mounted on slides in 5 μm sections. Slides were stained with hematoxylin and eosin for additional morphological studies. The tumor area was analyzed as described by us in previous studies [21].

2.9.2. Statistical Analysis

For tumor regression, a repeated measure ANOVA was conducted, and quantitative data were presented as the mean ± SEM. Statistical significance was assessed via one-way ANOVA with Tukey post hoc analysis. All further data were expressed as means ± SD of three independent experiments. A p value of less than 0.05 was considered statistically significant. Analyses were completed by GraphPad Prism 7.02 software.

3. Results

3.1. Levels of $p40_2$, p40 and IL-12, IL-23 in Serum of Pancreatic Cancer Patients

Earlier, it was not possible to examine the roles of $p40_2$ and p40 in the pathogenesis of diseases due to the lack of specific neutralizing mAbs; therefore, we generated neutralizing mAbs against $p40_2$ and p40 [17] and developed an ELISA to detect and quantify $p40_2$ and p40 independently [17–20]. In previous studies, we found that levels of p40 are much higher in the serum of prostate cancer patients [18] and breast cancer patients [19] compared to healthy controls. In order to understand whether this observation is specific to prostate or breast cancer, we measured levels of $p40_2$, p40, IL-12, and IL-23 in the serum of pancreatic cancer patients (n = 10) and healthy controls (n = 10). We used the serum of pre-treated pancreatic cancer patients, to eliminate any influence of different treatments on cytokine levels. Compared to our previous research in prostate or breast cancer cases, we observed that $p40_2$ levels were substantially elevated in the serum of pancreatic cancer patients compared to healthy controls (Figure 1A). Similar to the observations in prostate or breast cancer, the level of p40 was also significantly higher in pancreatic cancer patients than in healthy controls (Figure 1B). Likewise, when comparing them to prostate and breast cancer cases, levels of IL-12 (Figure 1C) and IL-23 (Figure 1D) were also significantly lower in pancreatic cancer as compared to healthy controls.

To further understand the significance of our finding, we detected the levels of the p40 family of cytokines in human pancreatic cancer cell lines. Pancreatic cancer cells such as PANC-1 and BxPC-3 as well as normal human pancreatic duct epithelial (HPDE) [26] cells were cultured under serum-free conditions for 24 h, followed by measurements of $p40_2$, p40, IL-12, and IL-23 by sandwich ELISA. Similarly to the serum of pancreatic cancer patients, levels of $p40_2$ and p40 levels were higher in both PANC-1 and BxPC-3 pancreatic cancer cells as compared to normal HPDE cells (Figure 1E,F). In contrast, levels of IL-12 and IL-23 were remarkably lower in PANC-1 and BxPC-3 cells in comparison to HPDE cells (Figure 1G,H).

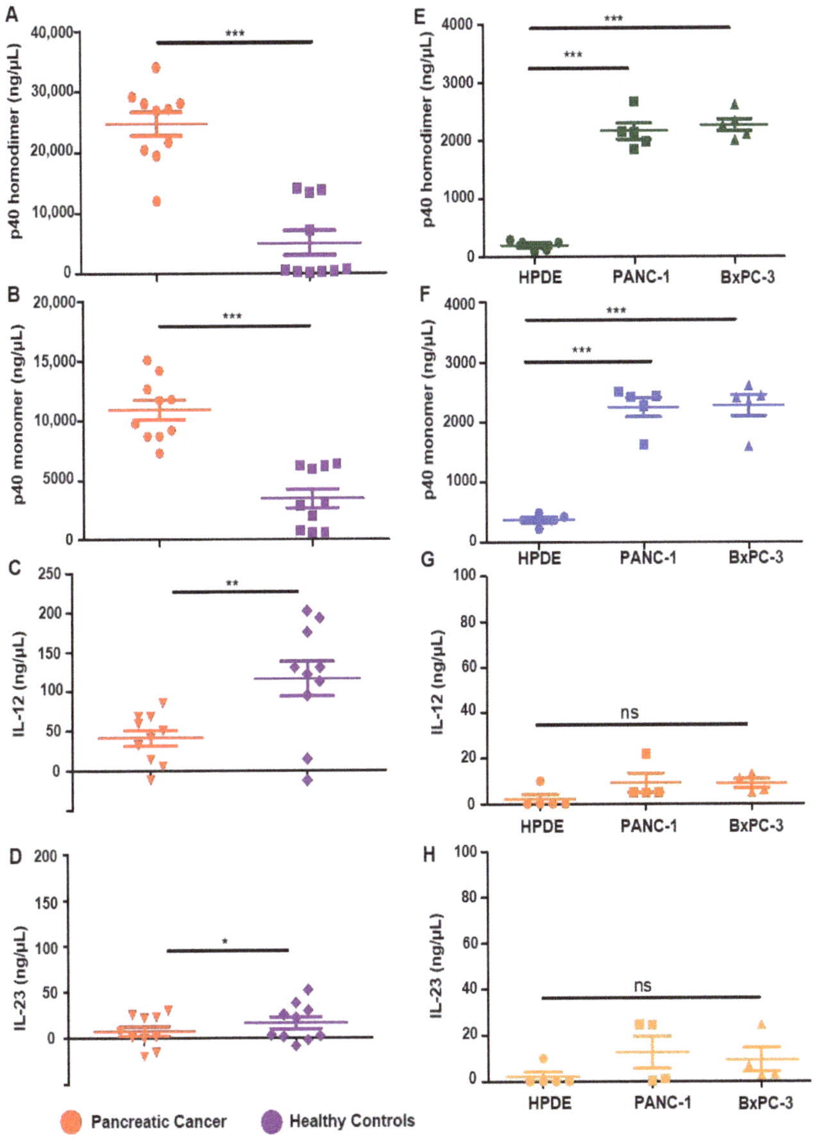

Figure 1. Levels of $p40_2$, p40, IL-12, and IL-23 in serum of pancreatic cancer patients and pancreatic cancer cells. We checked levels of the p40 (IL-12) family of cytokines in serum of pre-treated pancreatic cancer patients (n = 10) (red) and age-matched healthy controls (n = 10) (purple). The samples were purchased from Discovery Life Sciences (Los Osos, CA, USA) and were measured for $p40_2$ (**A**), p40 (**B**), IL-12 (**C**), and IL-23 (**D**) by sandwich ELISA. Supernatants of HPDE normal pancreatic cells compared to PANC-1 and BxPC-3 pancreatic cancer cells (**E**,**F**) were analyzed for levels of $p40_2$, and p40 by sandwich ELISA along with levels of IL-12 and IL-23 (**G**,**H**). Results are mean + SD of three different experiments. * $p < 0.05$; ** $p < 0.01$; *** $p < 0.001$.

3.2. Immunotherapies with mAbs against p40$_2$ and p40 Induces Death in Human Pancreatic Cancer Cells

Earlier in our studies, we examined the role of p40 in the survival of cancer cells, and found that in the p40 family of cytokines, only p40 monomer levels were observed to be higher than other subsets of this immune-modulating cytokine [18]. Contrary to prior observations, this study reveals the cytotoxic effects of p40$_2$ mAb in human PDAC cell lines. As seen in (Figure 2A,B), p40$_2$ mAb increased LDH [27] release in both PANC-1 and BxPC-3 cells, and a decrease in cell viability (Figure 2D,E), as shown by MTT metabolism, indicating the induction of cell death in PDAC cells by the neutralization of p40$_2$ by p40$_2$ mAb (a3-1d). This result is regarded as specific since control and hamster IgG had no effect on either LDH or MTT in human PDAC cells.

It is important to note that in HPDE cells (normal pancreatic cells), treatment with p40$_2$ mAb had no significant effects on either LDH (Figure 2C) or MTT (Figure 2F). To confirm our previous observation, we performed FACS double-labeling with AnnexinV and propidium iodide (PI) and found that p40$_2$ mAb treatment significantly increased apoptotic cells in both PANC-1 (Figure 2G) and BxPC-3 (Figure 2H) cells, followed by quantitative analyses (Figure 2J) and (Figure 2K). In comparison to the LDH and MTT results, treatment with p40$_2$ mAb in HPDE cells displayed no significant effects (Figure 2I) as demonstrated by quantitative analyses (Figure 2L). As indicated in other cancer cell types by previous studies [18,19], the p40 mAb (a3-3a) increased LDH release (Figure 3A,B) and decreased MTT (Figure 3D,E) in PDAC cells. Compared with the p40$_2$ mAb-treated cell results, p40 mAb also had no significant effects on normal pancreatic cells (Figure 3C,F).

Accordingly, FACS analysis with AnnexinV and PI in PANC-1 (Figure 3G) and BxPC-3 (Figure 3H) cells confirmed this observation and described that p40 mAb treatment also increased the level of apoptotic cells (Figure 3J,K) in PDAC cell lines. In line with previous results, treatment with p40 mAb in HPDE cells displayed no significant effects (Figure 3I,L). Moreover, TUNEL staining clearly showed that the population of TUNEL-positive cells in p40$_2$ mAb-treated PDAC cells (Figure 4A,B) was larger (Figure 4G–H) than in the control, IgG, or normal pancreatic cells (Figure 4C,I). In p40 mAb-treated PDAC cells (Figure 4D,E), our TUNEL results clearly indicated increased TUNEL bodies (Figure 4J,K) compared to the control, IgG, or normal pancreatic cells (Figure 4F), where no presence (Figure 4L) of TUNEL bodies was visualized. Overall, evidence illustrates that neutralization of p40$_2$ by p40$_2$ mAb and functional blocking of p40 by p40 mAb stimulates cell death in PDAC cell lines, not normal pancreatic cells.

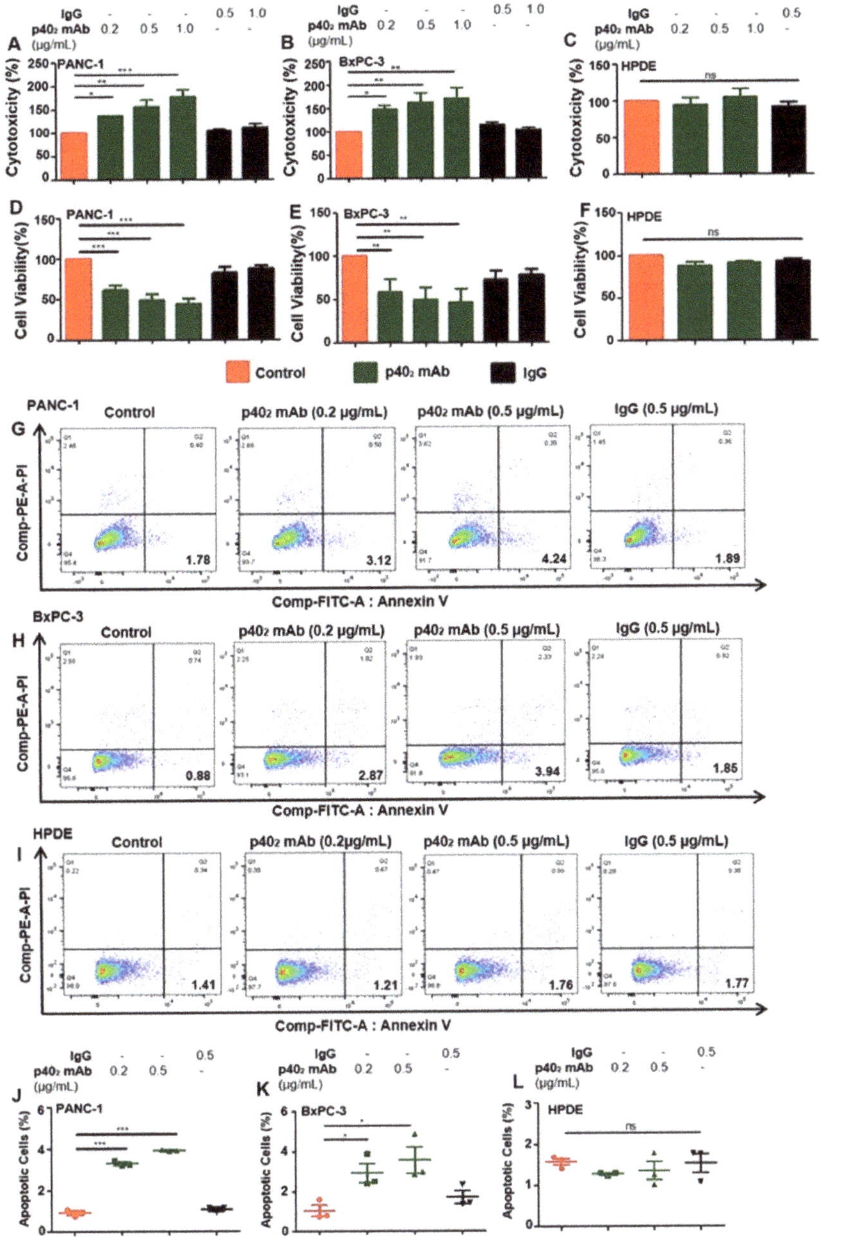

Figure 2. Monoclonal antibody-mediated neutralization of p40$_2$ by p40$_2$ mAb induces apoptosis in PANC-1 and BxPC-3 pancreatic cancer cells but not in normal pancreatic cells. Cells were treated for 24 h under serum-free condition followed by detecting LDH release (**A–C**) and MTT metabolism (**D–F**). Single-cell suspensions of pancreatic cancer cells and normal cells (**G–I**) were studied by dual FACS for Annexin V-FITC and propidium iodide (PI) using the FACS-Canto II system (BD Biosciences) followed by analysis using FlowJo Software (v10). Quantification of the percent of apoptotic cells (PI$^-$ Annexin V$^+$ early apoptotic) (**J–L**). Results are mean + SD of three different experiments. * $p < 0.05$; ** $p < 0.01$; *** $p < 0.001$.

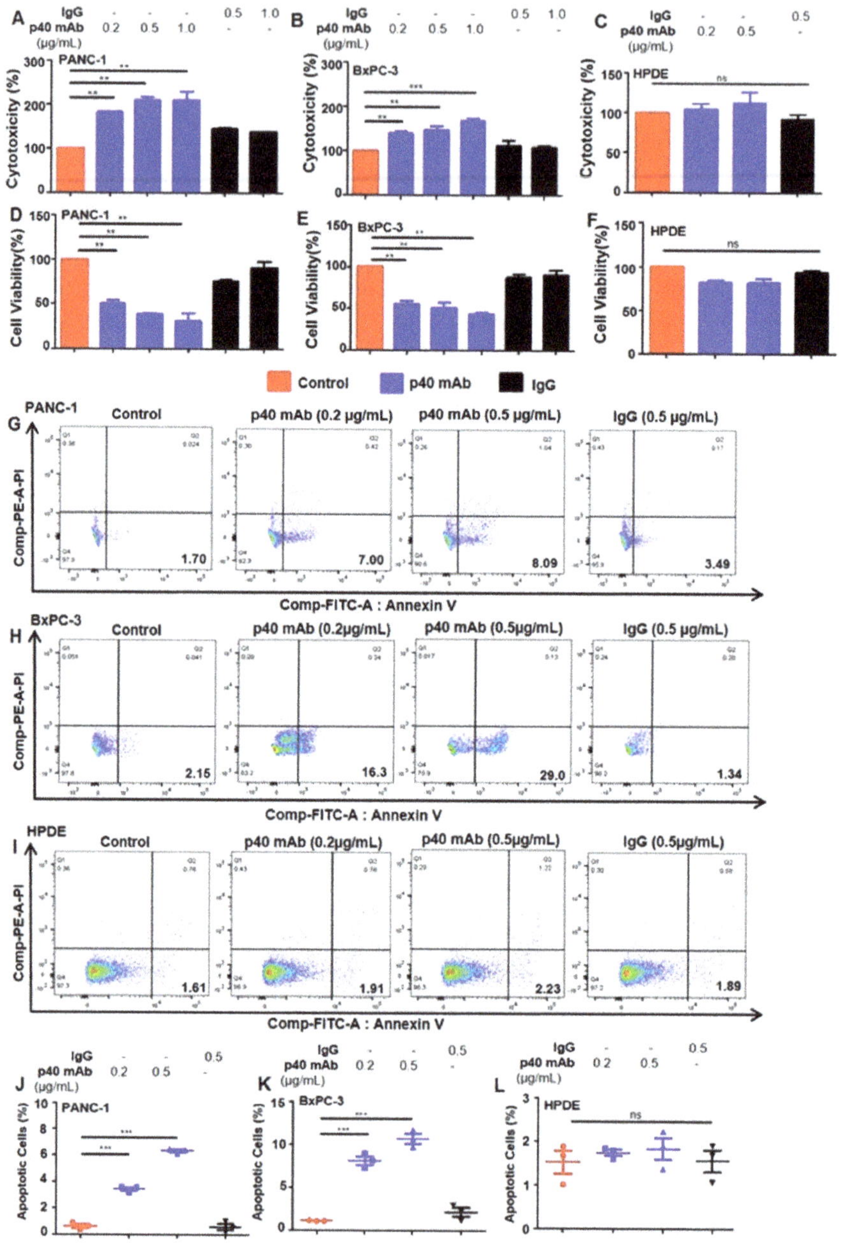

Figure 3. Monoclonal antibody-mediated neutralization of p40 by p40 mAb induces apoptosis in PANC-1 and BxPC-3 pancreatic cancer cells but not in normal pancreatic cells. Cells were treated for 24 h under serum-free condition followed by detecting LDH release (**A–C**) and MTT metabolism (**D–F**). Single-cell suspensions of pancreatic cancer cells and normal cells (**G–I**) were studied by dual FACS for Annexin V-FITC and propidium iodide (PI) using the FACS-Canto II system (BD Biosciences) followed by analysis using FlowJo Software (v10). Quantification of the percent of apoptotic cells (PI^- Annexin V^+ early apoptotic) (**J–L**). Results are mean + SD of three different experiments. ** $p < 0.01$; *** $p < 0.001$; ns, not significant.

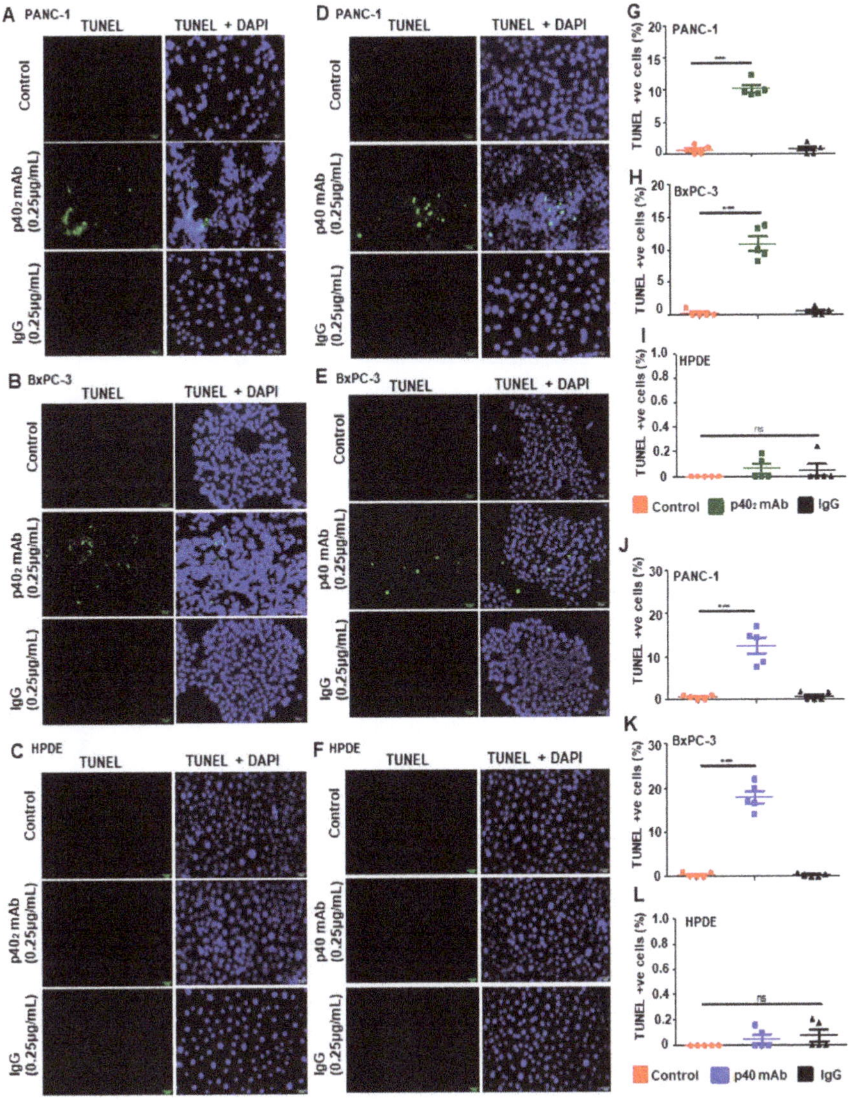

Figure 4. Increase in death response by p40 homodimer- and p40 monomer-treated pancreatic cancer cells but not in normal pancreatic cells. Cells were labeled for TUNEL in control cells and pancreatic cancer cells treated with IgG, p40 homodimer (**A**,**B**), and p40 monomer (**D**,**E**), and normal pancreatic cells (**C**,**F**). TUNEL-positive cells were counted and quantified in a 20× field in p40 homodimer-treated (**G**,**H**), in p40 monomer (**J**,**K**) -treated PDAC cells, and in normal pancreatic cells (**I**,**L**) as percent of control. TUNEL-positive cells were counted in 10 different images per group and plotted as a percentage of control. Results are mean + SD of three different experiments. *** $p < 0.001$; ns, not significant. Scale bar = 20 μm.

3.3. Upregulation of IFN-γ In Vitro in PDAC Cells after p40$_2$ mAb and p40 mAb Treatments

The IL-12 signaling pathway induces IFN-γ production in various cell types once activated [12,18,19]. We investigated the mechanisms by which p40$_2$ mAb and p40 mAb induced a death response in PDAC cancer cells. Earlier studies showed that higher expression of IFN-γ in p40 mAb-treated cancer cells was involved in cell death [28]. IFN-γ production is a confirmed therapeutic approach to stimulate cytotoxicity in cancer cells [29]. IFN-γ is a pleiotropic cytokine with antitumor and immunomodulatory functions; it plays a central role in orchestrating innate and adaptive immune responses [30]. IFN-γ production is controlled by IL-12-activated Th1 cells [31]. Although IFN-γ is a T-cell-derived cytokine, other cells such as epithelial cells [18] are capable of producing IFN-γ. Studies found that IFN-γ can induce apoptosis in tumor-specific T-cells, guiding antitumor immunity [32]. We examined if p40$_2$ mAb and p40 mAb treatment caused the upregulation of IFN-γ in PDAC cells. Immunostaining analysis clearly indicated that p40$_2$ mAb and p40 mAb treatments increased the level of IFN-γ in both PANC-1 (Figure 5A) and BxPC-3 (Figure 5B) cells, compared to either control cells or IgG-treated cells. Followed by counting of IFN-γ cells, quantitative analysis of both PANC-1 (Figure 5C) and BxPC-3 (Figure 5D) cells showed elevated levels of IFN-γ in p40$_2$ mAb- and p40 mAb-treated PDAC cells.

To further confirm, the mRNA expression of IFNγ was checked by real-time PCR. We found increased IFN-γ mRNA expression in PANC-1 (Figure 5E) and BxPC-3 (Figure 5F) cells that were treated with p40$_2$ mAb, but not control IgG. Likewise, p40 mAb, but not control IgG, upregulated IFN-γ mRNA expression in PANC-1 (Figure 5G) and BxPC-3 (Figure 5H) cells as compared to control untreated cells. To confirm it further, we performed dual FACS analysis with IFN-γ after live/dead cell exclusion and found that treatment with p40$_2$ mAb and p40 mAb markedly increased apoptotic cells in both PANC-1 (Figure 5I) and BxPC-3 (Figure 5J) cells. This was corroborated by quantitative analysis (PANC-1, Figure 5K; BxPC-3, Figure 5L). Collectively, these results suggest that neutralization of p40$_2$ by p40$_2$ mAb and p40 by p40 mAb is capable of inducing cell death in PDAC cells.

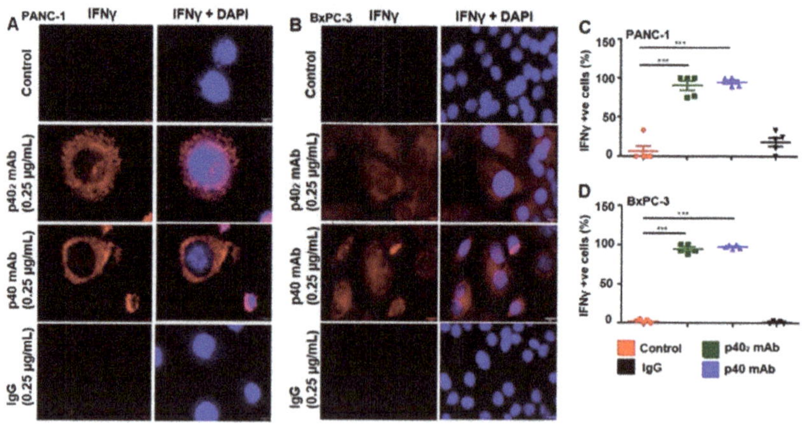

Figure 5. *Cont.*

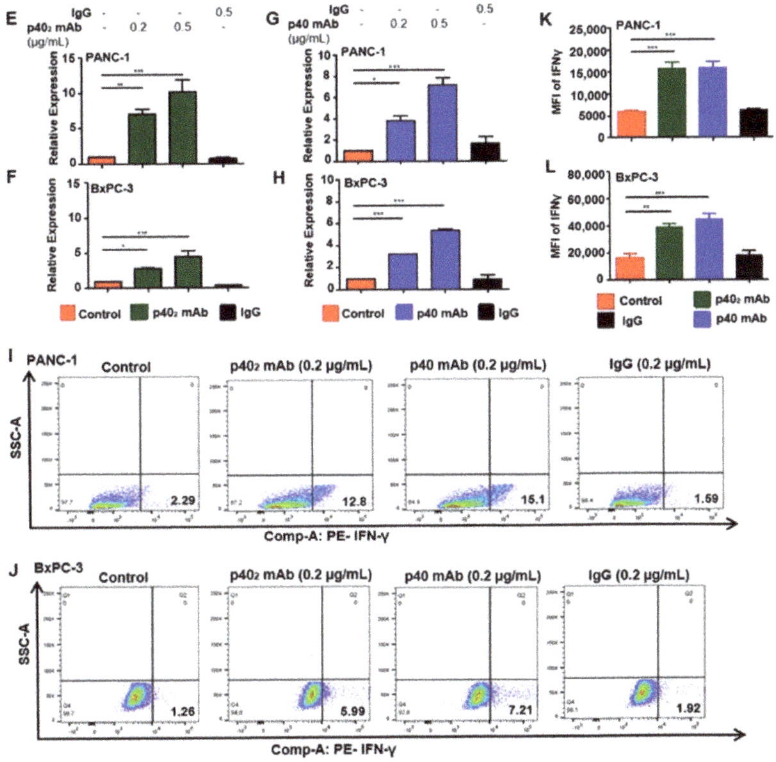

Figure 5. Neutralization of $p40_2$ and p40 increases levels of IFN-γ in pancreatic cancer cells. Immunohistochemical analysis at 60× magnification of PANC-1 (**A**) and BxPC-3 cells (**B**) treated with p40 homodimer or p40 monomer were labeled with IFN-γ (red). DAPI was used to stain the nuclei. Cells positive for IFN-γ were counted and quantified (5 images per slide) [33] (**C**,**D**). Real-time mRNA analysis of IFN-γ levels in pancreatic cancer cells treated with p40 homodimer (**E**,**F**) and p40 monomer (**G**,**H**). Single-cell suspensions isolated from PANC-1 (**I**) and BxPC-3 (**J**) cells were studied by dual FACS for IFN-γ and live/dead using the FACS Canto II system (BD Biosciences) followed by analysis using FlowJo Software (v10.8). PDAC cell quantification of early apoptotic cells (PI-Annexin V+) treated with $p40_2$ mAb and p40 mAb (**K**,**L**). Results are mean + SD of three different experiments. * $p < 0.05$; ** $p < 0.01$; *** $p < 0.001$. Scale bar = 10 μm.

3.4. Immunotherapies with $p40_2$ mAb and p40 mAb Lead to Tumor Regression in a Patient-Derived Xenograft (PDX) Mouse Model of Pancreatic Cancer

The PDX model, reliably developing tumors within a few weeks, recapitulates the spatial structure of cancer, the intratumoral heterogeneity of cancer, and the genomic features of cancer patients [34,35]. We used the PDX model (ID# TM01212; Jackson Lab) [36] for this study. In this particular model, cryopreserved tissue obtained from patients with pancreatic cancer was minced and implanted subcutaneously into the NOD scid gamma (NSG) mouse's fat pad. To examine the role of $p40_2$ and p40 in the progression of PDAC tumors, we investigated the effect of $p40_2$ mAb and p40 mAb on tumor size in PDX mice. Once palpable tumors were detected, they were measured three times weekly until experimental endpoints were reached.

Once tumors reached 0.5 cm^2 in area, mice were treated with $p40_2$ mAb (a3-1d) and p40 mAb (a3-3a) at a dose of 2 mg/kg body wt/week i.p. for 3.5 weeks (Figure 6A). When control or IgG tumors reached around 10% of mouse body weight, tumors were labeled with IR dye 800-conjugated 2-deoxyglucose via tail vein injection and imaged using a LI-

COR Odyssey infrared scanner (Figure 6B). This was corroborated by quantitative analysis (Figure 6C). Notably, we observed that treatment with p40$_2$ mAb and p40 mAb separately reduced tumor size as discerned from images of excised tumors (Figure 7A). Although we did not observe complete tumor regression of PDAC tumors with either p40$_2$ mAb or p40 mAb, our tumor measurements, seen in the tumor regression curve, clearly showed that the p40$_2$ mAb- and p40 mAb-treated mice had smaller tumors compared to either control or IgG-treated PDX mice (Figure 7B). H&E staining showed a substantial decrease in live cells and necrosis in both p40$_2$ mAb- and p40 mAb-treated mice compared to either untreated control or IgG-treated mice (Figure 7C). These results were corroborated by quantification of the tumor area (Figure 7D).

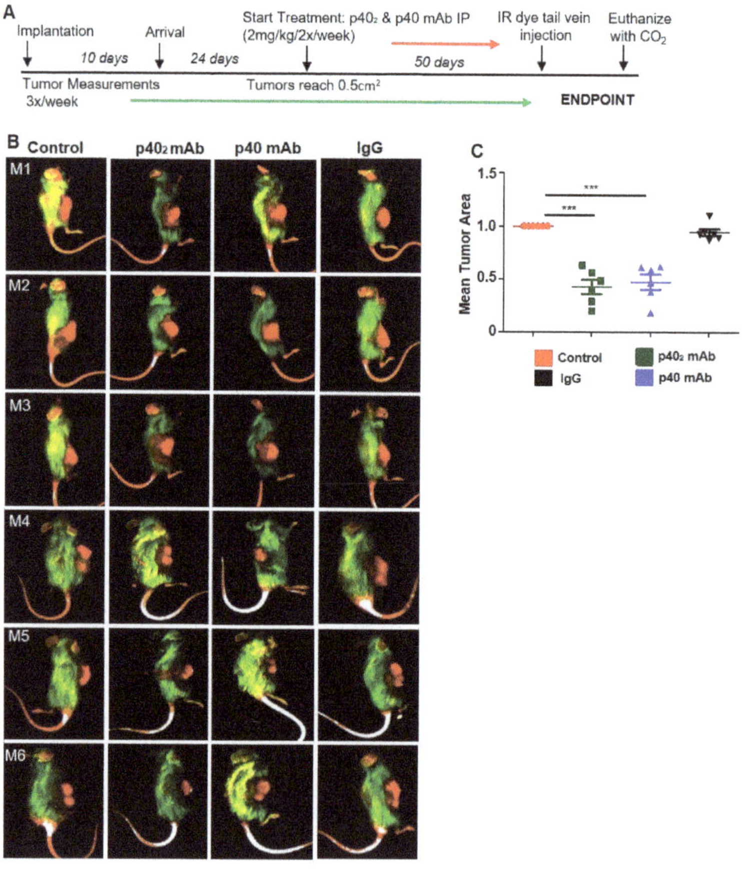

Figure 6. PDAC tumor regression in vivo in PDX mice treated with mAbs against p40 homodimer and p40 monomer. The experimental design is illustrated for PDAC PDX mice (**A**). Female 6–8-week-old NOD scid gamma (NSG) mice were engrafted with PDAC tumor fragments (TM01212) in the flank. When PDX mice (n = 6) tumors reached 0.5 cm^2, mice were treated with p40$_2$ and p40 mAbs and control hamster IgG at a dose of 2 mg/kg/body weight twice a week. After four weeks of treatment, tumors were labeled with Alexa800-2DG dye via tail vein injection and imaged using LICOR Odyssey infrared imaging system (**B**). This was corroborated by quantitative analysis (**C**). Six mice (n = 6) were included in each group. Results are mean + SD of three different experiments. *** $p < 0.001$.

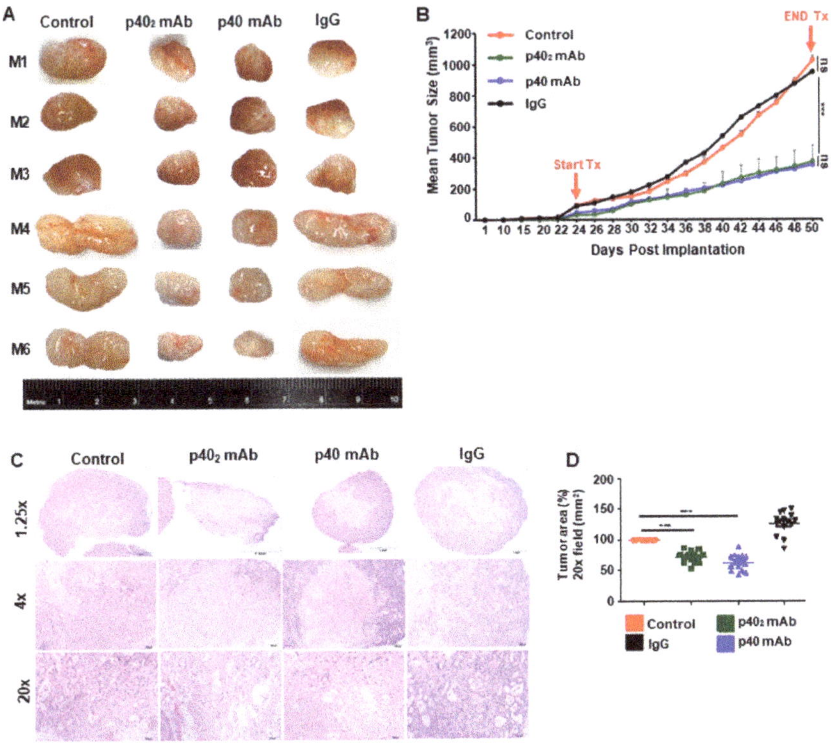

Figure 7. Results were compared with control and IgG groups. Tumors were surgically removed from the flanks of all mice. Six mice (n = 6) were included in each group (**A**). Tumor size was monitored every other day (**B**). Tumor sections were stained with H&E (**C**). The histological tumor area was quantified in a 20× field as percent of control (**D**). Results are mean + SD of three different experiments. *** $p < 0.001$; ns, not significant. Scale bar = 1 mm, 200 μm, and 50 μm.

3.5. Immunotherapies with p40$_2$ mAb and p40 mAb Induce a Death Response and Upregulation of IFN-γ in Tumor Tissues of PDX Mouse Model of Pancreatic Cancer

Cancer cells have a notorious property of evading cell death [37]. Accordingly, we monitored programmed cell death or apoptosis in tumor tissues by TUNEL assay. For better visualization of apoptosis, tumor sections were double-labeled for TUNEL and cleaved caspase 3, an apoptotic marker capable of propagating an apoptotic signal through enzymatic activity [38]. As expected, very few TUNEL-positive (Figure 8A,B) or cleaved caspase 3-positive (Figure 8A,C) cells were found in tumors of untreated PDX mice. However, we observed a significant increase in TUNEL-positive (Figure 8A,B) and cleaved caspase 3-positive (Figure 8A,C) cells in tumors of p40$_2$ mAb- and p40 mAb-treated PDX mice as compared to untreated PDX mice (Figure 8A). However, IgG treatment remained unable to stimulate either TUNEL-positive (Figure 8A,B) or cleaved caspase 3-positive (Figure 8A,C) cells in tumors of PDX mice (Figure 8A), indicating the specificity of treatment.

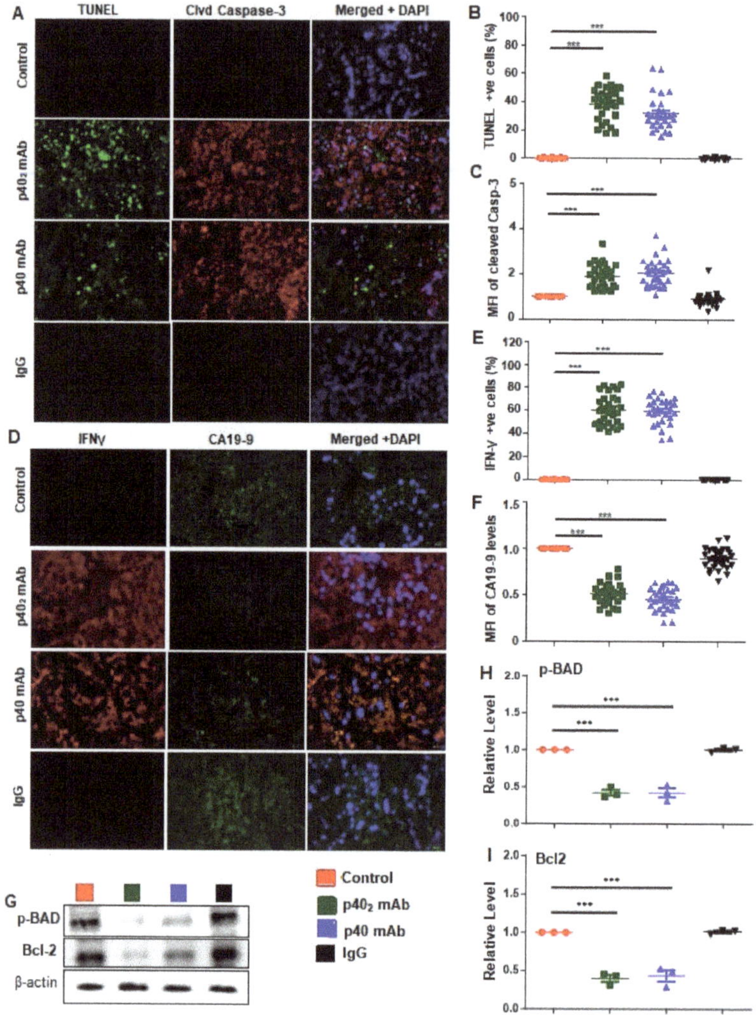

Figure 8. Stimulation of a death response and IFN-γ induction in PDAC tumors of PDX mice by $p40_2$ and p40 mAbs. After 4 weeks of treatment, tumor sections were double-labeled for TUNEL and cleaved caspase-3 (**A**) followed by counting TUNEL-positive cells in 5 sections of 6 mice per group (**B**), and mean fluorescent intensity (MFI) of cleaved caspase 3 (**C**) was quantified in a 40× field as percent of control. Tumor cross sections were double-immunolabeled for IFN-γ and CA19-9, a prognostic PDAC marker (**D**). Cells positive for IFN-γ (**E**) and with a MFI of CA19-9 (**F**) were quantified in a 60× field as percent of control was counted (5 images per mouse) of six different mice per group. DAPI was used to stain the nuclei. The stained tumor sections were quantified in a 40× field as percent of control. Tumor tissues were immunoblotted for survival proteins (phospho-BAD and Bcl-2) (**G**). Actin was run as a loading control. Results represent three independent experiments. Bands were scanned and values are presented as relative to control; the relative density of immunoblot analyses was normalized with β-actin (**H**,**I**). Results are mean + SD of three different experiments. *** $p < 0.001$. Scale bar = 40 μm.

Since upregulation of IFN-γ production is one of the key mechanisms in tumor regression, we monitored the levels of IFN-γ levels in PDAC tumors by double-labeling tumor tissues with IFNγ and CA19-9 (Figure 8D), a commonly used PDAC diagnostic marker used to detect pancreatic cancer treatment [39]. As expected, tumor tissues of untreated PDX mice expressed CA19-9 (Figure 8D,F), but not IFNγ (Figure 8D,E). On the other hand, treatment of PDX mice with both $p40_2$ mAb and p40 mAb led to a significant decrease in CA19-9 (Figure 8D,F) and a marked increase in IFNγ (Figure 8D,E) in tumor tissues, indicating an improvement in disease prognosis in comparison to either untreated control or IgG-treated PDX mice.

Several molecules such as Bcl-2 and a phosphorylated version of BAD are known to support cell survival and anti-apoptosis [40,41]. Therefore, to further confirm our findings on cell survival and death in tumor tissues of PDX mice, we performed immunoblot analyses of phospho-BAD and Bcl-2 (Figures 8G and S1) in tumors of in $p40_2$ mAb- and p40 mAb-treated PDX mice. For raw blots, please see . Consistent with the induction of apoptosis, we found a significant decrease in phospho-BAD (Figure 8G,H) and Bcl-2 (Figure 8G,I) in the tumor tissues of $p40_2$ mAb- and p40 mAb-treated PDX mice as compared to those of untreated PDX mice. Again, these results were specific, as IgG treatment remained unable to decrease the levels of phospho-BAD (Figure 8G,H) and Bcl-2 (Figure 8G,I) in the tumor tissues of PDX mice. Overall, these results suggest that, similarly to the observations in PDAC cells, $p40_2$ mAb and p40 mAb treatments are capable of inducing apoptosis in vivo in PDAC tumors in PDX mice.

4. Discussion

PDAC is the most common pancreatic neoplasm, accounting for more than 90% of all pancreatic cancers. The overall survival rate is 12%, and it remains the third leading cause of cancer deaths [42]. Treatment is largely determined by the stage of disease, and unfortunately, most cases present with locally advanced or non-resectable stages and metastases [43]. The current standard of care is surgical resection followed by adjuvant chemotherapy and/or radiation [1,3]. Monoclonal antibodies (mAbs) have proven effective at targeting solid tumors for decades [44]. Accordingly, although multiple immunotherapies such as anti-CTLA-4, or anti-PD-1 [45] are being used for PDAC treatment, there is an urgent need for the development of effective therapeutic strategies for PDAC.

The p40 family of cytokines, representing the first line of the immune response, plays a key role in coordinating the activities of innate and adaptive immune systems [8,18,20,22]. Recently, we have described an increase in p40 and decreases in $p40_2$, IL-12, and IL-23 in the serum of patients with prostate and breast cancers [18,19]. Accordingly, the selective neutralization of p40 by p40 mAb leads to the regression of prostate cancer and triple-negative breast cancer in mouse models [18,19]. Similarly to prostate and breast cancer cases, the present study highlights the upregulation of $p40_2$ in the serum of pancreatic cancer patients as compared to healthy controls and in supernatants of human PDAC cells in comparison to normal human HPDE pancreatic cells. This is the first demonstration of $p40_2$ upregulation in any cancer. In addition to $p40_2$ and similarly to prostate and breast cancer, we have also seen an increase in p40 in the serum of pancreatic cancer patients and human PDAC cells as compared to their respective controls, indicating the possible involvement of $p40_2$ and p40 in the pathogenesis of pancreatic cancer. *First*, the levels of $p40_2$ and p40 were significantly higher in human PDAC cells compared with IL-12, IL-23, and notably, normal pancreatic cells. *Second*, the neutralization of $p40_2$ and p40 induced cell death in PDAC cells, but more importantly, it did not in normal pancreatic cells. *Third*, our Annexin-V staining experiments demonstrated higher levels of death in PDAC cells compared to normal pancreatic cells. *Fourth*, our TUNEL staining also indicated the same findings. *Lastly*, intraperitoneal injection of $p40_2$ mAb and p40 mAb, but not IgG, significantly reduced the sizes of tumors grown in PDAC PDX mice. Overall, our study delineates an important role of $p40_2$ and p40 in the progression/regression of pancreatic cancer.

For accomplishing tumor regression, it is obligatory to stimulate apoptosis in tumor tissues. We demonstrated, from multiple approaches, the substantial death response in PDAC tumors after treatment with p40$_2$ mAb and p40 mAb. Our conclusions are based on the following observations: Initially, tumor growth in mice was measured, and visualized using IR dye. Then, H&E staining showed decreased tumor size, and a hollow core in p40$_2$ mAb- and p40 mAb-treated mice compared to untreated or control IgG-treated PDX mice. Next, the number of TUNEL-positive cells was much higher in tumors treated with p40$_2$ mAb and p40 mAb compared to either untreated control or IgG-treated PDX mice. Finally, in p40$_2$ mAb- and p40 mAb-treated tumors, we observed a decrease in anti-apoptotic markers, phospho-BAD, and Bcl-2, a common survival protein. Therefore, both p40$_2$ mAb and p40 mAb may be a considerable therapy for stimulating a cell death response in PDAC tumors.

While investigating mechanisms responsible for p40$_2$- and p40-mediated tumor cell death, we examined upregulation of IFN-γ, an important cytotoxic cytokine [46], when treated with p40$_2$ mAb. IFN-γ production is commonly motivated by IL-12, and elevated levels are indicative of tumor regression [12,47,48]. As observed in prostate [18] and breast cancer cells [12] with the p40 mAb, IFN-γ production was elevated when PDAC cells were treated with both p40$_2$ mAb and p40 mAb. It is likely that p40$_2$ mAb and p40 mAb mediated death in PDAC cells, and tumor tissue was stimulated by the cytotoxic quality of IFN-γ. The suppressed tumor growth in vivo validated that p40$_2$ mAb and p40 mAb induce PDAC cell death via IFN-γ. To monitor the effectiveness of p40$_2$ mAb and p40 mAb from another perspective, we observed the levels of carbohydrate antigen (CA19-9), a commonly used tumor marker for PDAC. This glycoprotein complex, produced by ductal cells in the pancreas, is expressed in both benign and malignant disorders [49]. It is currently used to monitor treatment response for resectability and prognosis [50]. We observed exceedingly decreased levels of CA19-9 in p40$_2$ mAb and p40 mAb tumor sections. Consistent with the cytotoxic nature of IFN-γ, our results further demonstrate that treatment with p40$_2$ mAb and p40 mAb induces cell death and apoptosis in PDAC.

5. Limitations

This therapeutic approach involves mAb treatment, and the efficacy may vary from patient to patient depending on the level of p40$_2$ and/or p40. At present, we do not know whether the neutralization of p40$_2$ and p40 will cause immune suppression or not. Like any other medications, there could be side effects, which are not known at present. Therefore, further studies are necessary to ascertain the safety profile over time. Moreover, there is a possibility that this therapy may interact with other medications. In that case, further data are necessary to determine additional contraindications.

6. Conclusions

To summarize, our studies demonstrated higher levels of p40$_2$ and p40 in the serum of pancreatic cancer patients and supernatants of human PDAC cells in comparison to their respective controls. Accordingly, functional blocking of p40$_2$ and p40 by p40$_2$ mAb and p40 mAb, respectively, caused apoptosis and cell death in human PDAC cells, but not in healthy pancreatic cells. In the PDX mouse model of pancreatic cancer, treatments with p40$_2$ mAb and p40 mAb, separately, also resulted in apoptosis and tumor regression. Although the PDX mouse model of pancreatic cancer may not perfectly reproduce the in vivo condition of a pancreatic adenocarcinoma tumor in human pancreatic cancer patients, our results suggest that the p40$_2$ mAb and p40 mAb may provide new immunotherapeutic options against pancreatic cancer.

Supplementary Materials: The following supporting information can be downloaded at: https://www.mdpi.com/article/10.3390/cancers15245796/s1, Figure S1: Raw Western Blots for Figure 8G.

Author Contributions: Conceptualization, K.P.; formal analysis, M.S.; investigation, M.S. and S.M.; resources, K.P.; writing—original draft preparation, M.S.; writing—review and editing, K.P.; supervision, K.P.; project administration, K.P.; funding acquisition, K.P. All authors have read and agreed to the published version of the manuscript.

Funding: This study was supported by the Pahan Family Foundation. Moreover, the Pahan Lab is funded by NIH grants (AT10980 and AG069229), and Dr. Pahan is also the recipient of a Research Career Scientist Award (1IK6 BX004982) from the Department of Veterans Affairs. However, the views expressed in this article are those of the authors and do not necessarily reflect the position or policy of the Department of Veterans Affairs or the United States government.

Institutional Review Board Statement: Animal protocol (22-007) was approved by the Rush University Medical Center Institutional Animal Care and Use Committee.

Informed Consent Statement: Not applicable.

Data Availability Statement: All data are present in this manuscript.

Conflicts of Interest: The authors declare no conflict of interest.

References

1. Siegel, R.L.; Miller, K.D.; Wagle, N.S.; Jemal, A. Cancer statistics, 2023. *CA Cancer J. Clin.* **2023**, *73*, 17–48. [CrossRef] [PubMed]
2. Sarantis, P.; Koustas, E.; Papadimitropoulou, A.; Papavassiliou, A.G.; Karamouzis, M.V. Pancreatic ductal adenocarcinoma: Treatment hurdles, tumor microenvironment and immunotherapy. *World J. Gastrointest. Oncol.* **2020**, *12*, 173–181. [CrossRef] [PubMed]
3. Werner, J.; Combs, S.E.; Springfeld, C.; Hartwig, W.; Hackert, T.; Buchler, M.W. Advanced-stage pancreatic cancer: Therapy options. *Nat. Rev. Clin. Oncol.* **2013**, *10*, 323–333. [CrossRef] [PubMed]
4. Lasek, W.; Zagozdzon, R.; Jakobisiak, M. Interleukin 12: Still a promising candidate for tumor immunotherapy? *Cancer Immunol. Immunother.* **2014**, *63*, 419–435. [CrossRef] [PubMed]
5. Morrison, A.H.; Byrne, K.T.; Vonderheide, R.H. Immunotherapy and Prevention of Pancreatic Cancer. *Trends Cancer* **2018**, *4*, 418–428. [CrossRef] [PubMed]
6. Bear, A.S.; Vonderheide, R.H.; O'Hara, M.H. Challenges and Opportunities for Pancreatic Cancer Immunotherapy. *Cancer Cell* **2020**, *38*, 788–802. [CrossRef] [PubMed]
7. Wang, P.; Li, X.; Wang, J.; Gao, D.; Li, Y.; Li, H.; Chu, Y.; Zhang, Z.; Liu, H.; Jiang, G.; et al. Re-designing Interleukin-12 to enhance its safety and potential as an anti-tumor immunotherapeutic agent. *Nat. Commun.* **2017**, *8*, 1395. [CrossRef]
8. Brahmachari, S.; Pahan, K. Role of cytokine p40 family in multiple sclerosis. *Minerva Med.* **2008**, *99*, 105–118.
9. Heinzel, F.P.; Hujer, A.M.; Ahmed, F.N.; Rerko, R.M. In vivo production and function of IL-12 p40 homodimers. *J. Immunol.* **1997**, *158*, 4381–4388. [CrossRef]
10. Hsieh, C.S.; Macatonia, S.E.; Tripp, C.S.; Wolf, S.F.; O'Garra, A.; Murphy, K.M. Development of TH1 CD4+ T cells through IL-12 produced by Listeria-induced macrophages. *Science* **1993**, *260*, 547–549. [CrossRef]
11. Tugues, S.; Burkhard, S.H.; Ohs, I.; Vrohlings, M.; Nussbaum, K.; Vom Berg, J.; Kulig, P.; Becher, B. New insights into IL-12-mediated tumor suppression. *Cell Death Differ.* **2015**, *22*, 237–246. [CrossRef] [PubMed]
12. Gately, M.K.; Renzetti, L.M.; Magram, J.; Stern, A.S.; Adorini, L.; Gubler, U.; Presky, D.H. The interleukin-12/interleukin-12-receptor system: Role in normal and pathologic immune responses. *Annu. Rev. Immunol.* **1998**, *16*, 495–521. [CrossRef] [PubMed]
13. Oppmann, B.; Lesley, R.; Blom, B.; Timans, J.C.; Xu, Y.; Hunte, B.; Vega, F.; Yu, N.; Wang, J.; Singh, K.; et al. Novel p19 protein engages IL-12p40 to form a cytokine, IL-23, with biological activities similar as well as distinct from IL-12. *Immunity* **2000**, *13*, 715–725. [CrossRef] [PubMed]
14. Vignali, D.A.; Kuchroo, V.K. IL-12 family cytokines: Immunological playmakers. *Nat. Immunol.* **2012**, *13*, 722–728. [CrossRef]
15. Fan, J.Q.; Wang, M.F.; Chen, H.L.; Shang, D.; Das, J.K.; Song, J. Current advances and outlooks in immunotherapy for pancreatic ductal adenocarcinoma. *Mol. Cancer* **2020**, *19*, 32. [CrossRef] [PubMed]
16. Banerjee, K.; Kumar, S.; Ross, K.A.; Gautam, S.; Poelaert, B.; Nasser, M.W.; Aithal, A.; Bhatia, R.; Wannemuehler, M.J.; Narasimhan, B.; et al. Emerging trends in the immunotherapy of pancreatic cancer. *Cancer Lett.* **2018**, *417*, 35–46. [CrossRef]
17. Dasgupta, S.; Bandopadhyay, M.; Pahan, K. Generation of functional blocking monoclonal antibodies against mouse interleukin-12 p40 homodimer and monomer. *Hybridoma* **2008**, *27*, 141–151. [CrossRef]
18. Kundu, M.; Roy, A.; Pahan, K. Selective neutralization of IL-12 p40 monomer induces death in prostate cancer cells via IL-12-IFN-gamma. *Proc. Natl. Acad. Sci. USA* **2017**, *114*, 11482–11487. [CrossRef]

19. Kundu, M.; Raha, S.; Roy, A.; Pahan, K. Regression of Triple-Negative Breast Cancer in a Patient-Derived Xenograft Mouse Mode by Monoclonal Antibodies against IL-12 p40 Monomer. *Cells* **2022**, *11*, 259. [CrossRef]
20. Mondal, S.; Kundu, M.; Jana, M.; Roy, A.; Rangasamy, S.B.; Modi, K.K.; Wallace, J.; Albalawi, Y.A.; Balabanov, R.; Pahan, K. IL-1 p40 monomer is different from other IL-12 family members to selectively inhibit IL-12Rβ1 internalization and suppress EAE. *Pro Natl. Acad. Sci. USA* **2020**, *117*, 21557–21567. [CrossRef]
21. Sheinin, M.; Jeong, B.; Paidi, R.K.; Pahan, K. Regression of Lung Cancer in Mice by Intranasal Administration of SARS-CoV- Spike S1. *Cancers* **2022**, *14*, 5648. [CrossRef] [PubMed]
22. Sheinin, M.; Mondal, S.; Roy, A.; Gorai, S.; Rangasamy, S.B.; Poddar, J.; Pahan, K. Suppression of Experimental Autoimmun Encephalomyelitis in Mice by beta-Hydroxy beta-Methylbutyrate, a Body-Building Supplement in Humans. *J. Immunol.* **202** *211*, 187–198. [CrossRef] [PubMed]
23. Kim, S.W.; Roh, J.; Park, C.S. Immunohistochemistry for Pathologists: Protocols, Pitfalls, and Tips. *J. Pathol. Transl. Med.* **2016**, *5* 411–418. [CrossRef]
24. Boyer, S.; Lee, H.J.; Steele, N.; Zhang, L.; Sajjakulnukit, P.; Andren, A.; Ward, M.H.; Singh, R.; Basrur, V.; Zhang, Y.; et al. Multiomi characterization of pancreatic cancer-associated macrophage polarization reveals deregulated metabolic programs driven by th GM-CSF-PI3K pathway. *eLife* **2022**, *11*, e73796. [CrossRef] [PubMed]
25. Vaziri-Gohar, A.; Cassel, J.; Mohammed, F.S.; Zarei, M.; Hue, J.J.; Hajihassani, O.; Graor, H.J.; Srikanth, Y.V.V.; Karim, S.A Abbas, A.; et al. Limited nutrient availability in the tumor microenvironment renders pancreatic tumors sensitive to allosteri IDH1 inhibitors. *Nat. Cancer* **2022**, *3*, 852–865. [CrossRef]
26. Ouyang, H.; Mou, L.; Luk, C.; Liu, N.; Karaskova, J.; Squire, J.; Tsao, M.S. Immortal human pancreatic duct epithelial cell line with near normal genotype and phenotype. *Am. J. Pathol.* **2000**, *157*, 1623–1631. [CrossRef]
27. Peacock, T.P.; Goldhill, D.H.; Zhou, J.; Baillon, L.; Frise, R.; Swann, O.C.; Kugathasan, R.; Penn, R.; Brown, J.C.; Sanchez David, R.Y.; et al. The furin cleavage site of SARS-CoV-2 spike protein is a key determinant for transmission due to enhance replication in airway cells. *BioRxiv.* **2020**. [CrossRef]
28. Gollob, J.A.; Murphy, E.A.; Mahajan, S.; Schnipper, C.P.; Ritz, J.; Frank, D.A. Altered interleukin-12 responsiveness in Th1 an Th2 cells is associated with the differential activation of STAT5 and STAT1. *Blood* **1998**, *91*, 1341–1354. [CrossRef]
29. Schroder, K.; Hertzog, P.J.; Ravasi, T.; Hume, D.A. Interferon-gamma: An overview of signals, mechanisms and function *J. Leukoc. Biol.* **2004**, *75*, 163–189. [CrossRef]
30. Mendoza, J.L.; Escalante, N.K.; Jude, K.M.; Sotolongo Bellon, J.; Su, L.; Horton, T.M.; Tsutsumi, N.; Berardinelli, S.J.; Haltiwange R.S.; Piehler, J.; et al. Structure of the IFNgamma receptor complex guides design of biased agonists. *Nature* **2019**, *567*, 56–6 [CrossRef]
31. Hu, X.; Ivashkiv, L.B. Cross-regulation of signaling pathways by interferon-gamma: Implications for immune responses an autoimmune diseases. *Immunity* **2009**, *31*, 539–550. [CrossRef] [PubMed]
32. Jorgovanovic, D.; Song, M.; Wang, L.; Zhang, Y. Roles of IFN-gamma in tumor progression and regression: A review. *Biomark Res.* **2020**, *8*, 49. [CrossRef]
33. Bertolotto, C.; Lesueur, F.; Giuliano, S.; Strub, T.; de Lichy, M.; Bille, K.; Dessen, P.; d'Hayer, B.; Mohamdi, H.; Remenieras, A.; et a Corrigendum: A SUMOylation-defective MITF germline mutation predisposes to melanoma and renal carcinoma. *Nature* **2016** *531*, 126. [CrossRef]
34. Nastala, C.L.; Edington, H.D.; McKinney, T.G.; Tahara, H.; Nalesnik, M.A.; Brunda, M.J.; Gately, M.K.; Wolf, S.F.; Schreiber, R.D. Storkus, W.J.; et al. Recombinant IL-12 administration induces tumor regression in association with IFN-gamma production *J. Immunol.* **1994**, *153*, 1697–1706. [CrossRef]
35. Abdolahi, S.; Ghazvinian, Z.; Muhammadnejad, S.; Saleh, M.; Asadzadeh Aghdaei, H.; Baghaei, K. Patient-derived xenograf (PDX) models, applications and challenges in cancer research. *J. Transl. Med.* **2022**, *20*, 206. [CrossRef]
36. Brock, R.M.; Beitel-White, N.; Coutermarsh-Ott, S.; Grider, D.J.; Lorenzo, M.F.; Ringel-Scaia, V.M.; Manuchehrabadi, N.; Martin R.C.G.; Davalos, R.V.; Allen, I.C. Patient Derived Xenografts Expand Human Primary Pancreatic Tumor Tissue Availability for ex vivo Irreversible Electroporation Testing. *Front. Oncol.* **2020**, *10*, 843. [CrossRef]
37. Sharma, M.; Sharma, S.; Roy, S.; Varma, S.; Bose, M. Pulmonary epithelial cells are a source of interferon-gamma in response to *Mycobacterium tuberculosis* infection. *Immunol. Cell Biol.* **2007**, *85*, 229–237. [CrossRef]
38. Jakubowska, K.; Guzinska-Ustymowicz, K.; Famulski, W.; Cepowicz, D.; Jagodzinska, D.; Pryczynicz, A. Reduced expression of caspase-8 and cleaved caspase-3 in pancreatic ductal adenocarcinoma cells. *Oncol. Lett.* **2016**, *11*, 1879–1884. [CrossRef]
39. Poruk, K.E.; Gay, D.Z.; Brown, K.; Mulvihill, J.D.; Boucher, K.M.; Scaife, C.L.; Firpo, M.A.; Mulvihill, S.J. The clinical utility of CA 19-9 in pancreatic adenocarcinoma: Diagnostic and prognostic updates. *Curr. Mol. Med.* **2013**, *13*, 340–351. [CrossRef] [PubMed]
40. Tan, Y.; Demeter, M.R.; Ruan, H.; Comb, M.J. BAD Ser-155 phosphorylation regulates BAD/Bcl-XL interaction and cell survival *J. Biol. Chem.* **2000**, *275*, 25865–25869. [CrossRef] [PubMed]
41. Cotter, T.G. Apoptosis and cancer: The genesis of a research field. *Nat. Rev. Cancer* **2009**, *9*, 501–507. [CrossRef]
42. Garcia, P.L.; Miller, A.L.; Yoon, K.J. Patient-Derived Xenograft Models of Pancreatic Cancer: Overview and Comparison with Other Types of Models. *Cancers* **2020**, *12*, 1327. [CrossRef] [PubMed]
43. Hanahan, D.; Weinberg, R.A. Hallmarks of cancer: The next generation. *Cell* **2011**, *144*, 646–674. [CrossRef] [PubMed]
44. Gillen, S.; Schuster, T.; Meyer Zum Buschenfelde, C.; Friess, H.; Kleeff, J. Preoperative/neoadjuvant therapy in pancreatic cancer A systematic review and meta-analysis of response and resection percentages. *PLoS Med.* **2010**, *7*, e1000267. [CrossRef] [PubMed]

45. Spranger, S.; Koblish, H.K.; Horton, B.; Scherle, P.A.; Newton, R.; Gajewski, T.F. Mechanism of tumor rejection with doublets of CTLA-4, PD-1/PD-L1, or IDO blockade involves restored IL-2 production and proliferation of CD8(+) T cells directly within the tumor microenvironment. *J. Immunother. Cancer* **2014**, *2*, 3. [CrossRef] [PubMed]
46. Mirlekar, B.; Pylayeva-Gupta, Y. IL-12 Family Cytokines in Cancer and Immunotherapy. *Cancers* **2021**, *13*, 167. [CrossRef]
47. Selleck, W.A.; Canfield, S.E.; Hassen, W.A.; Meseck, M.; Kuzmin, A.I.; Eisensmith, R.C.; Chen, S.H.; Hall, S.J. IFN-gamma sensitization of prostate cancer cells to Fas-mediated death: A gene therapy approach. *Mol. Ther.* **2003**, *7*, 185–192. [CrossRef]
48. Wigginton, J.M.; Gruys, E.; Geiselhart, L.; Subleski, J.; Komschlies, K.L.; Park, J.W.; Wiltrout, T.A.; Nagashima, K.; Back, T.C.; Wiltrout, R.H. IFN-gamma and Fas/FasL are required for the antitumor and antiangiogenic effects of IL-12/pulse IL-2 therapy. *J. Clin. Investig.* **2001**, *108*, 51–62. [CrossRef]
49. Barnett, D.; Liu, Y.; Partyka, K.; Huang, Y.; Tang, H.; Hostetter, G.; Brand, R.E.; Singhi, A.D.; Drake, R.R.; Haab, B.B. The CA19-9 and Sialyl-TRA Antigens Define Separate Subpopulations of Pancreatic Cancer Cells. *Sci. Rep.* **2017**, *7*, 4020. [CrossRef]
50. Azizian, A.; Ruhlmann, F.; Krause, T.; Bernhardt, M.; Jo, P.; Konig, A.; Kleiss, M.; Leha, A.; Ghadimi, M.; Gaedcke, J. CA19-9 for detecting recurrence of pancreatic cancer. *Sci. Rep.* **2020**, *10*, 1332. [CrossRef]

cancers

MDPI

Article

The Unmet Needs of Pancreatic Cancer Carers Are Associated with Anxiety and Depression in Patients and Carers

Thi N. T. Huynh [1,2], Gunter Hartel [1,2,3], Monika Janda [2], David Wyld [2,3,4], Neil Merrett [5], Helen Gooden [6], Rachel E. Neale [1,2] and Vanessa L. Beesley [1,2,3,*]

1 Population Health Department, QIMR Berghofer Medical Research Institute, Brisbane, QLD 4006, Australia; justine.huynh@qimrberghofer.edu.au (T.N.T.H.); gunter.hartel@qimrberghofer.edu.au (G.H.); rachel.neale@qimrberghofer.edu.au (R.E.N.)

2 Faculty of Medicine, The University of Queensland, Brisbane, QLD 4006, Australia; m.janda@uq.edu.au (M.J.); david.wyld@health.qld.gov.au (D.W.)

3 School of Nursing, Queensland University of Technology, Brisbane, QLD 4059, Australia

4 Cancer Care Services, Royal Brisbane and Women's Hospital, Herston, QLD 4029, Australia

5 School of Medicine, Western Sydney University, Sydney, NSW 2560, Australia; neil.merrett@health.nsw.gov.au

6 School of Nursing and Midwifery, University of Sydney, Sydney, NSW 2006, Australia; hmg@iinet.net.au

* Correspondence: vanessa.beesley@qimrberghofer.edu.au

Simple Summary: This is the first population-based study to quantitatively assess the supportive care needs of pancreatic cancer patients' carers and their associations with psychological outcomes for patient–carer dyads. We show that for this patient group, carers have exceptionally high levels of unmet needs, particularly in the healthcare and information domains, and some of these needs are strongly associated with anxiety and depression among carers and the patients they care for. The results of this study provide a strong rationale for the implementation of optimal care guidelines to promote early referrals to palliative care for pancreatic cancer patients in which the routine assessment and management of supportive care needs among family carers (and patients) occurs.

Abstract: Pancreatic cancer has one of the lowest survival rates, and patients experience debilitating symptoms. Family carers provide essential daily care. This study determined the prevalence of and risk factors for unmet supportive care needs among carers for pancreatic cancer patients and examined which carer needs were associated with anxiety and depression in carers and patients. Eighty-four pancreatic cancer patients and their carers were recruited. The carers completed a needs survey (SCNS-P&C). Both carers and patients completed the Hospital Anxiety and Depression Scale. Log binomial regression was used to identify associations between carer needs and anxiety and depression among carers and patients. The top 10 moderate-to-high unmet needs reported by $\geq$28% of carers were related to healthcare (e.g., discussing concerns with doctors) and information need domains (e.g., information about a patient's physical needs), plus one other item related to hospital parking. Being male or caring for a patient within 4 months of their diagnosis were associated with greater unmet needs. Some unmet needs, including 'accessing information about treatments' and 'being involved in patient care', were associated with both carers and patients having anxiety and depression. Carers should be involved in health care consultations and provided with information and opportunities to discuss concerns.

Keywords: pancreatic cancer; family carers; supportive care needs; anxiety; depression

1. Introduction

Pancreatic cancer it is the third most common cause of cancer death in developed countries [1]. Surgical resection is the only potentially curative treatment [2]. This cancer is typically asymptomatic early in its development, and there is no reliable screening test for early detection; thus, approximately 80% of patients present with unresectable (metastatic or locally advanced) disease [3]. During the limited time prior to death (the median survival time is 5 months [4]), patients suffer from fatigue, jaundice, abdominal or back pain, poor appetite, unintended weight loss, nausea, vomiting [5], anxiety and depression [6]. Supportive care plays an important role in managing these symptoms.

In the pancreatic cancer setting, family carers provide considerable care alongside professionally trained carers. They manage symptoms or treatment-related side effects and help with daily activities and end-of-life decision making [7]. They also provide financial, emotional, social and spiritual support [8] while facing the impending loss of their loved one. When caring demands exceed their resources, they can experience negative impacts on their mental health [8]. A systematic review found that 33% of people providing informal care to patients with pancreatic cancer have symptoms indicative of clinical anxiety and 12–32% have symptoms indicative of clinical depression [9].

Understanding and satisfying carers' explicit supportive care needs can result in cost savings for health systems [10]. There are no published quantitative studies documenting the supportive care needs of family carers for people diagnosed with pancreatic cancer [9]. The complex symptoms and the rare and rapidly progressing nature of pancreatic cancer are likely to be uniquely challenging for these carers. The aims of this work were to determine the prevalence of and risk factors for the unmet supportive care needs of this population, using quantitative methods and a validated multidimensional needs assessment tool. Additionally, we examined which specific carer needs were correlated with carers' and patients' anxiety or depression.

2. Materials and Methods

2.1. Participants and Procedures

Participants were recruited from the Queensland Pancreatic Cancer Study—Quality of Life (QPCS-QoL), which was a longitudinal, repeated-measures study of patient–carer dyads who self-reported outcomes at two, four, six and eight months after a diagnosis of pancreatic cancer. The QoL study was nested within the QPCS, a population-based case–control study examining environmental and genetic risk factors for pancreatic cancer [6]. The QPCS used a rapid ascertainment approach, recruiting patients diagnosed with pancreatic cancer between January 2007 and June 2011, as early as possible after their diagnosis, based on referral from a state-wide network of treating clinicians in hospitals and private practices.

QPCS participants recruited from July 2009 were invited to participate in the QPCS-QoL and to nominate a carer who was also invited to participate in this sub-study. Of the 351 QPCS participants recruited from July 2009, 97 were excluded due to a physical or mental inability to complete the study documents, 57 refused, 23 died shortly after receiving the questionnaire, and 38 patients did not return the questionnaire. One hundred thirty-six QPCS participants completed at least one QoL questionnaire (54% of those approached). Of these 136 patients, 21 did not nominate a carer and 31 carers declined to participate. Thus, 84 (62%) patient–carer dyads completed the questionnaire(s). We used data from the first questionnaire completed by the 84 dyads in this analysis.

2.2. Measures

2.2.1. Personal and Disease Information

We collected the age, gender and education level of the patients and carers. Carers were also asked about their relationship to patients and if they were living together. Postcodes were used to assign the remoteness of participants' residences based on the Accessibility and Remoteness Index of Australia [11].

Clinical information about the patients' date of diagnosis and disease status, defined as resectable, locally advanced or metastatic, was extracted from medical records.

2.2.2. Carers' Supportive Care Needs

The Supportive Care Needs Survey—Partners and Caregivers (SCNS-P&C) was used to assess 45 need items across four domains: healthcare service (10 items), psychological and emotional (14 items), work and social (7 items) and information (8 items) [12]. It also assesses six other items that are not classified into a domain. The SCNS-P&C asks participants to rate each need item across five response categories: '1 = no unmet need—not applicable', '2 = no unmet need—satisfied', '3 = low unmet need', '4 = moderate unmet need' and '5 = high unmet need'. In this analysis, we dichotomised each item into 'no-or-low need' versus 'moderate-to-high need'. We also calculated the number of moderate-to-high unmet needs in each domain and overall. The domains have been shown to have good internal validity; Cronbach's alpha ranged from 0.88 to 0.94 [12].

2.2.3. Carers' and Patients' Anxiety and Depression

Anxiety and depression symptoms were assessed using the Hospital Anxiety and Depression Scale (HADS) [13]. It comprises two separate 7-item subscales. The HADS-A measures symptoms of anxiety, including restlessness, nervousness and feelings of panic. The items assess emotional and cognitive aspects of anxiety, such as feeling tense or having a sense of impending doom. The HADS-D assesses symptoms of depression, including low mood, loss of interest or pleasure and a sense of hopelessness. It explores emotional and cognitive aspects of depression, like feeling sad and experiencing a lack of enjoyment in daily activities. Participants rate each symptom as '0 = absent'; '1 = occasional'; '2 = quite often'; or '3 = very often'. The total score of each subscale ranges from 0 to 21 and is classified as normal (0–7), sub-clinical (8–10) or clinical (11–21). The HADS is a reliable measure of anxiety and depression, with respective Cronbach's alpha values of 0.88 and 0.92 for internal validity [14], and has good external validity with the Depression Anxiety Stress Scales (DASS-42) (Pearson's correlation coefficient $r = 0.76$ ($p < 0.001$)) [15].

2.3. *Statistical Analysis*

To identify the carers' most prevalent unmet needs, we calculated the proportion reporting each need as moderate-to-high out of the number of participants who completed each item. The amount of missing data for each need item varied from 2 to 7 carer responses except for the need item 'reducing stress in the person with cancer's life'. This item had 60 missing responses due to being inadvertently deleted from an updated version of the questionnaire. As a consequence, this variable is not reported in this manuscript.

To identify which personal and disease risk factors were associated with carers reporting at least one moderate-to-high need, we used log-binomial regression to estimate prevalence ratios (PRs) and 95% confidence intervals (CIs). We considered PRs ≥ 2.0 to be clinically significant.

Log-binomial regression models were also used to estimate associations between (a) carers' individual need items, (b) the number of needs reported (categorised into tertiles), (c) having a need in each domain and (d) the number of domains carers had a need in (categorised as 0, 1–3 or 4) and (i) the carers' sub-clinical or clinical anxiety, (ii) the carers' sub-clinical or clinical depression, (iii) the patients' sub-clinical or clinical anxiety and (iv) the patients' sub-clinical or clinical depression. The Expectation Maximisation algorithm was applied to handle missing data. This method uses observed data to obtain maximum likelihood estimates of variables when missing values are present [16]. When the log-binomial model did not converge, we used Poisson regression models [17].

All analyses were conducted using R software version 4.1.2 (R Foundation for Statistical Computing, Vienna, Austria).

3. Results

3.1. *Sample Characteristics*

The characteristics of the 84 patient–carer dyads are shown in Table 1. In most cases, spouses or partners (81%) took on the role of informal carer, and almost all carers (94%)

lived with the patient. Nearly three-quarters of the carers were female, 62% were 60 years of age or older and for 57%, the highest level of education attained was a high school diploma or lower. The majority of patients were male (66%) and 60 years of age or older (74%), and less than half completed a high school education (44%). Thirty-six percent of patients were treated via surgical resection. Of the 54 patients who did not undergo resection, more than half (30; 56%) had metastatic disease. At the time of the questionnaire's completion, all patients were between 0and 9 months from the time of the pancreatic cancer diagnosis; 35% were within 2 months and 82% were within 4 months.

Table 1. Demographic and clinical characteristics of participants.

Characteristics	Carers (n = 84) n (%)	Patients (n = 84) n (%)
Relationship to patient		
Husband/wife/partner	68 (81.0)	
Son/daughter	10 (11.9)	
Father/mother/friend/other	6 (7.1)	
Lives with patient		
Yes	79 (94)	
No	5 (6)	
Gender		
Male	23 (27.4)	55 (65.5)
Female	61 (72.6)	29 (34.5)
Age		
≤60 years	32 (38.1)	22 (26.2)
61–70 years	31 (36.9)	33 (39.3)
≥71 years	21 (25.0)	29 (34.5)
Highest level of education		
High school or lower	48 (57.1)	37 (44.0)
College/diploma/trade certificate	21 (25)	33 (39.3)
University	15 (17.9)	14 (16.7)
Disease status		
Resection completed—curative disease		30 (35.7)
No resection—locally advanced disease		20 (23.8)
No resection—metastatic disease		30 (35.7)
Resection not attempted due to age, comorbidities or patient decline		4 (4.8)
Months post diagnosis		
≤2 months		29 (34.5)
3–4 months		40 (47.6)
5–9 months		15 (17.9)

3.2. The Top Moderate-to-High Unmet Supportive Care Needs of Carers

Overall, 63% of the carers reported having at least one moderate-to-high unmet need. The top 10 needs were from the healthcare services (five items) and information (four items) supportive care domains, plus one non-specific item (Table 2). More than a third of carers reported a moderate-to-high unmet need for information about the person with cancer's physical needs (39%), opportunities to discuss concerns with doctors (36%), accessible hospital parking (36%), help with fear about the patients' deterioration (35%) and information about the benefits and side-effects of treatments (34%). The most frequently reported psychological needs were for help with balancing the needs of the person with cancer and their own needs (26%), understanding the patient experience (23%), finding meaning (21%) and making decisions in the context of uncertainty (21%). The most frequently unmet work/social needs were for help with the impact caring has had on their working life or usual activities (24%) and adapting to changes in the patient's work or activities (23%).

Table 2. Moderate-to-high unmet needs reported by carers for pancreatic cancer patients.

Rank	Need Item	Domain	Mod–High Need	
			n	%
1	Accessing information about what the person with cancer's physical needs are	Information	31	39
2	Having opportunities to discuss your concerns with doctors	Healthcare	29	36
3	Finding more accessible hospital parking	Other	29	36
4	Addressing fears about the person with cancer's deterioration	Healthcare	28	35
5	Accessing information about the benefits and side-effects of treatments	Information	27	34
6	Being involved in the person with cancer's care, together with a medical team	Healthcare	26	32
7	Finding out about financial support and government benefits	Information	26	32
8	Accessing information about the person with cancer's prognosis	Information	24	30
9	Ensuring that there is an ongoing case manager to coordinate services	Healthcare	23	29
10	Obtaining the best medical care for the person with cancer	Healthcare	22	28
11	Balancing the needs of the person with cancer and your own needs	Psychological	22	27
12	Accessing information relevant to your needs as a carer/partner	Information	20	26
13	Feeling confident that all the doctors are talking to each other	Healthcare	21	26
14	The impact that caring for the person with cancer has had on your working life, or usual activities	Work/social	20	25
15	Accessing information about support services for carers/partners	Information	19	24
16	Adapting to changes in the person with cancer's working life or usual activities	Work/social	19	24
17	Accessing local health care services when needed	Healthcare	19	23
18	Understanding the experience of the person with cancer	Psychological	19	23
19	Making decisions about your life in the context of uncertainty	Psychological	18	23
20	Finding meaning in the person with cancer's illness	Psychological	18	23
21	Making sure that complaints regarding the person with cancer's care are properly addressed	Healthcare	18	22
22	Obtaining adequate pain control for the person with cancer	Healthcare	17	21
23	Accessing information about alternative therapies	Information	15	19
24	Working through your feelings about death and dying	Psychological	15	19
25	Dealing with others not acknowledging the impact caring has on your life	Psychological	15	19
26	Adjusting to changes in the person with cancer's body	Psychological	14	18
27	Looking after your own health, including eating and sleeping properly	Healthcare	14	17
28	Obtaining emotional support for your loved ones	Psychological	13	16
29	Communicating with family	Work/social	12	15
30	Managing concerns about the cancer returning	Psychological	12	15
31	Obtaining emotional support for yourself	Psychological	12	15
32	Coping with the person with cancer's recovery not turning out the way you expected	Psychological	12	15
33	The impact cancer has had on your relationship with the person with cancer	Psychological	11	14
34	Exploring your spiritual beliefs	Psychological	10	13
35	Having opportunities to participate in making decisions about treatment	Information	9	12
36	Communicating with the person you are caring for	Work/social	9	11
37	Receiving more support from your family	Work/social	8	10
38	Talking to other people who have cared for someone with cancer	Work/social	8	10
39	Caring for the person with cancer on a practical level, such as with bathing, changing dressings, or giving medications	Other	6	7
40	Obtaining life and/or travel insurance for the person with cancer	Other	5	6
41	Accessing legal services	Other	5	6
42	Addressing problems with your sex life	Psychological	5	6
43	Handling the topic of cancer in social situations or at work	Work/social	3	4
44	Accessing information about potential fertility problems in the person with cancer	Other	2	3

3.3. *Personal and Disease Risk Factors Associated with Carers Having at Least One Moderate-to-High Unmet Need*

While the numbers in some groups were small, bivariable analyses indicated that male carers were more likely than female carers to report a moderate-to-high unmet need (PR = 1.36; 95% CI = 1.01–1.85) and, compared to carers for patients who were 5–9 months post-diagnosis, those within 2 or 3–4 months of the diagnosis had significantly higher prevalences of moderate-to-high unmet needs (PR = 2.46; 95% CI = 1.02–5.92 and PR = 2.81; 95% CI = 1.19–6.63, respectively) (Table 3). The carer's age, relationship to the patient and level of education and the patient's disease status were not significantly associated with carers having an unmet need (Table 3).

Table 3. Personal and disease risk factors associated with carers having at least one moderate-to-high unmet supportive care need.

Personal and Disease Factors	Having at Least One Moderate-to-High Unmet Supportive Care Need		PR (95% CI)
	No n = 31 (36.9%)	Yes n = 53 (63.1%)	
	n (Column %)	n (Column %)	
Carer's gender			
Male	5 (16.1)	18 (34.0)	1.36 (1.01–1.85)
Female	26 (83.9)	35 (66.0)	1
Carer's age			
≤60 years	11 (35.5)	21 (39.6)	1.06 (0.70–1.61)
61–70 years	12 (38.7)	19 (35.8)	0.99 (0.64–1.53)
≥71 years	8 (25.8)	13 (24.5)	1
Carer's relationship with the patient			
Husband/Wife/Partner	26 (83.9)	42 (79.2)	1
Other	5 (16.1)	11 (20.8)	1.11 (0.76–1.63)
Carers' education level			
High school or less	21 (67.7)	27 (50.9)	1
College/diploma/trade certificate	5 (16.1)	16 (30.2)	1.35 (0.96–1.91)
University	5 (16.1)	10 (18.9)	1.19 (0.77–1.83)
Patient's disease status			
Resection completed—curative disease	10 (32.3)	20 (40.8)	1.33 (0.86–2.07)
No resection—locally advanced disease	6 (19.4)	14 (28.6)	1.40 (0.88–2.21)
No resection—metastatic disease	15 (48.4)	15 (30.6)	1
Resection not attempted		4	
Months after the patient's diagnosis			
≤2 months	10 (32.3)	19 (35.8)	2.46 (1.02–5.92)
3–4 months	10 (32.3)	30 (56.6)	2.81 (1.19–6.63)
5–9 months	11 (35.5)	4 (7.5)	1

3.4. Relationship between Carers' Unmet Needs and Carers' Anxiety and Depression

There was a significant association between carers reporting moderate-to-high unmet need(s) in any of the supportive care domains and also reporting subclinical or clinical anxiety and depression (Table 4, Supplementary Tables S1 and S2). The strongest associations were between depression and the healthcare (PR 5.08; 95% CI 2.12–12.20) or psychological needs domains (PR 3.85; 95% CI 1.72–8.61).

Carers reporting unmet needs in four domains were more than three times as likely to have anxiety (PR 3.57; 95% CI 1.90–6.70) and five times as likely to have depression (PR 5.10; 95% CI 1.92–13.52) compared to carers not reporting any unmet needs in any domain. Carers reporting unmet needs in 1–3 domains only showed a significant association with carer anxiety (PR 2.72; 95% CI 1.39–5.33). Compared with carers who had no moderate-to-high needs, carers with 13–35 moderate-to-high needs (the highest tertile) were significantly more likely to have anxiety and depression (PR 3.32 and 95% CI 1.67–6.60 and PR 4.43 and 95% CI 1.68–11.67, respectively).

The majority (35) of the 44 individual need items reported by carers were significantly associated with both carer anxiety and depression (Supplementary Table S3). The strongest individual needs associated with carer anxiety were needing help finding meaning in the patient's illness (PR 2.32; 95% CI 1.67–3.22), decision making in uncertainty (PR 2.22; 95% CI 1.57–3.15) and needing information about the patient's prognosis (PR 2.19; 95% CI 1.53–3.13). The strongest items associated with carer depression were needing to talk to other cancer carers (PR 4.50; 95% CI 2.92–6.93), needing help with knowing how to discuss cancer socially (PR 3.67; 95% CI 2.55–5.28) and needing help with feelings about death (PR 3.46; 95% CI 1.98–6.03).

Table 4. The association of carers' supportive care needs with carers' and patients' anxiety and depression.

	n (%)	Carers' Subclinical or Clinical Anxiety	Carers' Subclinical or Clinical Depression	Patients' Subclinical or Clinical Anxiety	Patients' Subclinical or Clinical Depression
		Unadjusted PR (95% CI)	Unadjusted PR (95% CI)	Unadjusted PR (95% CI)	Unadjusted PR (95% CI)
Individual need domains					
Having at least one moderate-to-high unmet need in the healthcare service domain					
No	46 (55)	1	1	1	1
Yes	38 (45)	2.42 (1.55–3.78)	5.08 (2.12–12.20)	2.94 (1.36–6.34)	2.06 (1.07–3.95)
Having at least one moderate-to-high unmet need in the psychological/emotional domain					
No	45 (54)	1	1	1	1
Yes	39 (46)	2.55 (1.61–4.06)	3.85 (1.72–8.61)	4.38 (1.81–10.64)	1.96 (1.02–3.77)
Having at least one moderate-to-high unmet need in the information domain					
No	39 (46)	1	1	1	1
Yes	45 (54)	2.38 (1.44–3.94)	2.89 (1.29–6.46)	3.29 (1.36–8.00)	1.47 (0.77–2.83)
Having at least one moderate-to-high unmet need in the work/social domain					
No	50 (60)	1	1	1	1
Yes	34 (40)	2.42 (1.60–3.67)	3.31 (1.63–6.73)	2.06 (1.04–4.08)	2.14 (1.14–4.02)
Number of domains with least one moderate-to-high unmet need					
0	34 (40)	1	1	1	1
1–3	25 (30)	2.72 (1.39–5.33)	2.38 (0.78–7.26)	2.38 (0.78–7.26)	1.02 (0.40–2.57)
4	25 (30)	3.57 (1.90–6.70)	5.10 (1.92–13.52)	4.42 (1.63–11.95)	2.21 (1.08–4.51)
Number of moderate-to-high unmet need items reported					
Lowest tertile (0)	31 (37)	1	1	1	1
Middle tertile (1–12)	25 (30)	3.01 (1.49–6.10)	1.86 (0.59–5.88)	3.31 (0.98–11.18)	1.65 (0.66–4.14)
Highest tertile (13–35)	28 (33)	3.32 (1.67–6.60)	4.43 (1.68–11.67)	4.80 (1.52–15.10)	2.40 (1.06–5.45)

3.5. Relationship between Carers' Unmet Needs and Patients' Anxiety and Depression

Carers who reported at least one moderate-to-high need in the healthcare, psychological or work/social domains were significantly more likely to be caring for a patient with anxiety or depression symptoms. The strongest association was between carers having at least one unmet psychological need and patient anxiety (PR 4.38; 95% CI 1.81–10.64). Carers reporting at least one moderate-to-high information need was associated with patient anxiety (PR 3.29; 95% CI 1.36–8.00) but not with patient depression.

Carers who reported moderate-to-high needs across all four domains were four times (PR 4.42; 95% CI 1.63–11.95) more likely to be caring for a patient with anxiety symptoms and two times (PR 2.21; 95% CI 1.08–4.51) more likely to be caring for a patient with depressive symptoms compared to carers who did not report any moderate-to-high needs. An increasing number of moderate-to-high unmet needs reported by carers was associated with an increased likelihood of patients experiencing anxiety or depression. Compared with patients whose carers had no moderate-to-high needs (the lowest tertile), patients whose carers reported 13–35 moderate-to-high needs (the highest tertile) were significantly more likely to have anxiety and depression (PR 4.80; 95% CI 1.52–15.10 and PR 2.40; 95% CI 1.06–5.45, respectively).

Having high supportive care needs in each of 14 of the 44 individual need items was significantly associated with patient anxiety, and 11 items were significantly associated with patient depression (Supplementary Table S3). The strongest associations with anxiety and depression in cancer patients occurred with carers having a need for help with adjusting to changes in the patient's body (PR 3.03 and 95% CI 1.65–5.56 and PR = 2.95 and 95% CI 1.72–5.06, respectively). Balancing their own and the patient's needs (PR 2.93;

95% CI 1.52–5.63) and obtaining the best medical care for patients (PR 2.59; 95% CI 1.32–5.09) were the other carer unmet needs strongly associated with patient anxiety. Carers needing help with communicating with the family (PR 2.46; 95% CI 1.41–4.28) and practical caring tasks (PR 2.27; 95% CI 1.17–4.42) were significantly more likely to be caring for a patient with depression.

There were five unmet carer needs significantly associated with all psychological outcomes for carers and patients. These included needing help with 'accessing information about the benefits and side-effects of treatments', 'obtaining the best medical care for the person with cancer', 'being involved in the person with cancer's care, together with the medical team', 'balancing the needs of the person with cancer and your own needs' and 'adjusting to changes in the person with cancer's body'.

4. Discussion

This population-based study of 84 pancreatic cancer patient–carer dyads is the first to identify that nearly two-thirds (63%) of pancreatic cancer carers reported having at least one moderate-to-high level need, the most prevalent of which were in the healthcare service and information domains. Importantly, we further identified that carers who reported more than 13 unmet needs (i.e., the highest tertile of needs vs. the lowest tertile of needs) were significantly more likely to be experiencing anxiety or depression and caring for a patient with anxiety or depression. Although the direction of the effect cannot be inferred, this nevertheless sends a strong message that we need to ensure that the basic healthcare and educational requirements of this caregiver population are met, not only to provide optimal care to carers but potentially to also reduce carers' and patients' psychological morbidity.

A systematic review quantifying unmet needs in carers for adults with cancers across eight studies found that 16–68% of carers had at least one unmet need [18]. The highest prevalence of 68% was reported by carers for patients with colorectal cancer two months after their diagnosis [19]; however this study combined low, moderate and high needs in their prevalence of unmet needs, whereas we combined only moderate and high needs. The prevalence of unmet needs in the other seven studies from this systematic review was lower than what we observed [20–26]. The variation in prevalence may be attributable to different measures and cut points used to assess unmet needs, but it also may be due to the characteristics of the patient population. Carers for people with pancreatic cancer, with which the majority of patients have an incurable disease at the outset and a significantly shorter expected survival, may respond differently to other populations in which the disease is potentially curative at diagnosis.

Similar to a recent qualitative literature review on the needs of people caring for patients with pancreatic cancer which identified key domains as 'clinical communication', 'support and briefings' and 'navigating health systems' [9], we found that the healthcare and information need domains were priorities. In particular, we found that approximately a third of carers felt inadequately informed about the benefits and side-effects of treatments, the person with cancer's prognosis and physical needs, and about financial support. We also identified that a third of carers were not feeling supported in relation to opportunities to discuss concerns with doctors, being able to be involved in care together with the medical team, help with fear about the patients' deterioration and ensuring that there is an ongoing case manager to coordinate services. Existing quantitative studies of carers for advanced cancer patients, irrespective of the type of cancer, found that information needs were the most commonly reported unmet needs, including illness and treatment information (26–100%) and care-related information (21–100%) [27]. In addition to information needs, other domains such as physical and psychological well-being, healthcare services and spiritual and social lives were also identified [27].

We show that all four need domains (healthcare, information, psychological and work/social) we measured were related to patient and carer anxiety and carer depression and that all but the information domain were also significantly associated with patient depression. Furthermore, we found that the higher the number of unmet needs reported by carers, the higher the psychological morbidity both they and their patients were experiencing. A study of cancer carers in the United States found similar associations between psychosocial and medical need domains and carers' mental health [19], and a Taiwanese study of carers for people with advanced lung cancer also found strong associations between patients' anxiety or depression and carers having healthcare, psychological and work/social needs [28]. Both studies emphasise the importance of integrating needs assessment for carers into routine clinical care to minimise the likelihood of patients and carers experiencing poor psychological health. However, the practicalities of achieving this are complicated in a hospital setting in which staff have limited time [29] and the carer is not 'a patient' and so cannot directly be provided and billed for care. Such assessments may require early referral to palliative care in which person- and family-centred care are provided.

Our finding that carers' anxiety and depression were associated with a higher number of unmet carer needs was in line with previous reports for Icelandic carers for patients with various types of cancer [30], and our finding that patients' anxiety and depression were associated with a higher number of unmet carer needs was in line with previous reports from a study of multiple myeloma [24].

Importantly, we identified the need for help with making decisions in the context of uncertainty to be the most strongly associated with carers' anxiety or depression and that needing help with 'accessing information about the benefits and side-effects of treatments', 'obtaining the best medical care for the person with cancer' and 'being involved in the person with cancer's care, together with the medical team' were significantly associated with all psychological outcomes for carers and patients. Again, this speaks to the need to actively include carers in medical consultations where possible.

Finally, we identified that being a male carer and caring for a patient in the first four months after their diagnosis were associated with greater unmet needs. Higher needs closer to the time of diagnosis might reflect increased demands immediately after the diagnosis and during initial treatment [31]. Although the difference in needs between male and female carers found in this study was relatively small, it may have implications for future interventions. In some Western societies, it is less common for men to take on a caregiving role [32]. Men may need more support to feel comfortable and confident [33–36].

Clinical practice guidelines recommend that clinicians discuss and develop supportive care plans in consultation with patients and their carers [29]. Further, the optimal care pathways for people with pancreatic cancer state that given the poor prognosis, all patients with pancreatic cancer should be offered an early referral for a palliative care assessment as an integrated aspect of their overall oncology care [37]. Many studies have shown that palliative care interventions improve health outcomes among carers, including decreased levels of psychological distress [38]. However, it is estimated that only 28% of pancreatic cancer patients see a care coordinator or have a care plan, and less than half (45%) access palliative care [39,40]. A lack of communication about palliative care may exist when healthcare professionals fear damaging patients' and carers' hope [41]. Investments in programs to improve information exchange as well as shared decision making between health professionals and family carers could be useful to better meet carers' needs [38].

A major strength of this study is the use of validated measures to quantitatively assess unmet needs and psychological outcomes in the largest cohort of pancreatic cancer carers to date. However, several limitations should be taken into account. Firstly, the analysis was cross-sectional, so temporality cannot be inferred; that is, we did not look at anxiety and depression at future time points due to significant missing repeated measures as participants died or became moribund. We also did not have information about pre-existing anxiety or depression to adjust for confounding. Thus, we do not know if having high unmet needs leads to poor psychological outcomes or if having pre-existing anxiety or depression results in high needs. Nevertheless, meeting needs remains important irrespective of the direction of the effect. Secondly, a higher proportion of patients in the study had a surgical resection than is expected in the general population. However, we found that the disease status in our patients was not associated with carers having high unmet needs and is thus likely to have had relatively little impact on the results. Thirdly, as the study used a representative cohort from Queensland, a state in Australia, it may limit the generalisability of the results to different populations across other states and territories, as well as countries. A further limitation is that the data were collected over 10 years ago, and changes in clinical practice (e.g., more access to cancer care coordinators and palliative care services) and the prevalence of unmet needs in carers may have occurred. Up-to-date data are necessary to inform service providers of current needs for intervention.

5. Conclusions

This study contributes to the understanding of the needs of people caring for patients with pancreatic cancer and the relationship between needs and anxiety and depression in both carers and patients. Although clinical practice guidelines provide evidence-based recommendations for the delivery of optimal care to cancer patients and their family members, our study found that many carers for pancreatic cancer patients report unmet needs, particularly in relation to healthcare and information. This may be due to the lack of involvement of the carer as part of the healthcare team or a lack of early referral to palliative care in which carers' needs are assessed. Failing to meet carers' expectations for information and involve them in the person with cancer's care can have significant associations with adverse psychological outcomes in patients and the carers themselves. The association of carers' needs with both carer and patient anxiety and depression provides a strong rationale for the implementation of optimal care guidelines to promote early referral to palliative care and routine assessments of supportive care needs among family carers for triage to effective interventions to manage those needs.

Supplementary Materials: The following supporting information can be downloaded at https://www.mdpi.com/article/10.3390/cancers15225307/s1, Table S1: Numbers and percentages of subclinical or clinical anxiety or depression among carers or patients; Table S2: Numbers and percentages of subclinical or clinical anxiety or depression among carers or patients by individual carer needs; Table S3: Associations between carers' unmet needs and carers' and patients' subclinical or clinical anxiety or depression.

Author Contributions: T.N.T.H. conducted the analyses and wrote the manuscript. All authors contributed to the study conception and the interpretation of data and critically reviewed the manuscript and approved the final version. All authors have read and agreed to the published version of the manuscript.

Funding: This study was funded by a National Health and Medical Research Council (NHMRC) (Australia) project grant (Project Nos. 442302 & 613654). R.E. Neale was funded by an NHMRC senior research fellowship (No. 1060183).

Institutional Review Board Statement: The study was conducted in accordance with the Declaration of Helsinki and approved by the QIMR Berghofer Medical Research Institute Human Research Ethics Committees (protocol code P1145) on 1 April 2008.

Informed Consent Statement: Written informed consent was obtained from all participants involved in the study.

Data Availability Statement: The data are available upon request and with appropriate Human Research Ethics Committee approval and data transfer agreements in place.

Acknowledgments: We acknowledge the contribution of Dianne O'Connell and David Goldstein who provided input for the conception of the study design. We also acknowledge the contribution of the study staff: Rebekah Cicero, Lea Jackman, Fran Millar, Andrea McMurtrie, Lisa Ferguson, Chris Hill, Tracey Corish, Annaka Schulte, Madeleine Payne and Therese Lawton. We are grateful for the support of clinicians in Queensland who assisted with participant recruitment, particularly Rick Abraham, Reza Adib, Mark Appleyard, John Avramovic, Andrew Barbour, Ian Baxter, Matthew Burge, Boris Chern, Michelle Cronk, Ben Devereaux, Paul Eliadis, Robert Finch, John Gibbons, David Grimes, Brendan Hanrahan, George Hopkins, Luke Hourigan, Sybil Kellner, Laurent Layani, Stephen

Lynch, Ian Martin, Judith McEniery, Lesley Nathanson, Nicholas O'Rourke, Tom O'Rourke, Harald Puhalla, Matthew Remedios, Leigh Rutherford, Sabe Sabesan, Candice Silverman, Kellee Slater, Craig Sommerville, Paul Vasey, Johannes Wittman, Louise Welch and Shinn Yeung. Finally, we thank all of the men and women who participated in the study.

Conflicts of Interest: The authors declare no conflict of interest.

References

1. Sung, H.; Ferlay, J.; Siegel, R.L.; Laversanne, M.; Soerjomataram, I.; Jemal, A.; Bray, F. Global cancer statistics 2020: GLOBOCAN estimates of incidence and mortality worldwide for 36 cancers in 185 countries. *CA Cancer J. Clin.* **2021**, *71*, 209–249. [CrossRef] [PubMed]
2. Brunner, M.; Wu, Z.; Krautz, C.; Pilarsky, C.; Grützmann, R.; Weber, G.F. Current clinical strategies of pancreatic cancer treatment and open molecular questions. *Int. J. Mol. Sci.* **2019**, *20*, 4543. [CrossRef] [PubMed]
3. Burmeister, E.A.; Waterhouse, M.; Jordan, S.J.; O'Connell, D.L.; Merrett, N.D.; Goldstein, D.; Wyld, D.; Beesley, V.; Gooden H.; Janda, M.; et al. Determinants of survival and attempted resection in patients with non-metastatic pancreatic cancer: An Australian population-based study. *Pancreatology* **2016**, *16*, 873–881. [CrossRef]
4. Dumbrava, M.I.; Burmeister, E.A.; Wyld, D.; Goldstein, D.; O'Connell, D.L.; Beesley, V.L.; Gooden, H.M.; Janda, M.; Jordan, S.J. Merrett, N.D. Chemotherapy in patients with unresected pancreatic cancer in Australia: A population-based study of uptake and survival. *Asia-Pac. J. Clin. Oncol.* **2018**, *14*, 326–336. [CrossRef] [PubMed]
5. American Cancer Society. Signs and Symptoms of Pancreatic Cancer. Available online: https://www.cancer.org/cancer/pancreatic-cancer/detection-diagnosis-staging/signs-and-symptoms.html (accessed on 5 July 2022).
6. Janda, M.; Neale, R.E.; Klein, K.; O'Connell, D.L.; Gooden, H.; Goldstein, D.; Merrett, N.D.; Wyld, D.K.; Rowlands, I.J.; Beesley V.L. Anxiety, depression and quality of life in people with pancreatic cancer and their carers. *Pancreatology* **2017**, *17*, 321–327 [CrossRef] [PubMed]
7. Roberts, K.E.; Panjwani, A.A.; Marziliano, A.; Applebaum, A.J.; Lichtenthal, W.G. End-of-life care and cancer: Psychosocial needs of patients and the bereaved. In *Quality Cancer Care: Survivorship before, during, and after Treatment*; Hopewood, P., Milroy, M.J. Eds.; Springer: Cham, Switzerland, 2018; pp. 243–268.
8. Honea, N.J. Caregiver burden. In *A Guide to Oncology Symptom Management*, 2nd ed.; Brown, C.G., Ed.; Oncology Nursing Society Pittsburgh, PA, USA, 2015; pp. 143–169.
9. Chong, E.; Crowe, L.; Mentor, K.; Pandanaboyana, S.; Sharp, L. Systematic review of caregiver burden, unmet needs and quality-of-life among informal caregivers of patients with pancreatic cancer. *Support. Care Cancer* **2023**, *31*, 74. [CrossRef]
10. Védie, A.-L.; Neuzillet, C. Best Supportive Care in Advanced Pancreatic Cancer. In *Textbook of Pancreatic Cancer*; Søreide, K. Stättner, S., Eds.; Springer: Cham, Switzerland, 2021; pp. 1293–1307.
11. Australian Bureau of Statistics. *Australian Statistical Geography Standard (ASGS): Volume 5-Remoteness Structure*; Australian Bureau of Statistics: Canberra, Australia, 2016; Volume 5.
12. Girgis, A.; Lambert, S.; Lecathelinais, C. The supportive care needs survey for partners and caregivers of cancer survivors Development and psychometric evaluation. *Psycho-Oncology* **2011**, *20*, 387–393. [CrossRef]
13. Bjelland, I.; Dahl, A.A.; Haug, T.T.; Neckelmann, D. The validity of the Hospital Anxiety and Depression Scale: An updated literature review. *J. Psychosom. Res.* **2002**, *52*, 69–77. [CrossRef]
14. Whelan-Goodinson, R.; Ponsford, J.; Schönberger, M. Validity of the Hospital Anxiety and Depression Scale to assess depression and anxiety following traumatic brain injury as compared with the Structured Clinical Interview for DSM-IV. *J. Affect. Disord* **2009**, *114*, 94–102. [CrossRef]
15. Dahm, J.; Wong, D.; Ponsford, J. Validity of the Depression Anxiety Stress Scales in assessing depression and anxiety following traumatic brain injury. *J. Affect. Disord.* **2013**, *151*, 392–396. [CrossRef]
16. Donoghoe, M.W.; Marschner, I.C. Logbin: An R package for relative risk regression using the log-binomial model. *J. Stat. Softw* **2018**, *86*, 1–22. [CrossRef]
17. Petersen, M.R.; Deddens, J.A. A comparison of two methods for estimating prevalence ratios. *BMC Med. Res. Methodol.* **2008**, *8*, 9 [CrossRef] [PubMed]
18. Lambert, S.D.; Harrison, J.D.; Smith, E.; Bonevski, B.; Carey, M.; Lawsin, C.; Paul, C.; Girgis, A. The unmet needs of partners and caregivers of adults diagnosed with cancer: A systematic review. *BMJ Support. Palliat. Care* **2012**, *2*, 224–230. [CrossRef] [PubMed]
19. Kim, Y.; Kashy, D.A.; Spillers, R.L.; Evans, T.V. Needs assessment of family caregivers of cancer survivors: Three cohorts comparison. *Psycho-Oncology* **2010**, *19*, 573–582. [CrossRef] [PubMed]
20. Girgis, A.; Lambert, S.D.; McElduff, P.; Bonevski, B.; Lecathelinais, C.; Boyes, A.; Stacey, F. Some things change, some things stay the same: A longitudinal analysis of cancer caregivers' unmet supportive care needs. *Psycho-Oncology* **2013**, *22*, 1557–1564 [CrossRef]
21. Hodgkinson, K.; Butow, P.; Hobbs, K.M.; Hunt, G.E.; Lo, S.K.; Wain, G. Assessing unmet supportive care needs in partners of cancer survivors: The development and evaluation of the Cancer Survivors' Partners Unmet Needs measure (CaSPUN) *Psycho-Oncology* **2007**, *16*, 805–813. [CrossRef]

22. Hodgkinson, K.; Butow, P.; Hunt, G.E.; Wyse, R.; Hobbs, K.M.; Wain, G. Life after cancer: Couples' and partners' psychological adjustment and supportive care needs. *Support. Care Cancer* **2007**, *15*, 405–415. [CrossRef] [PubMed]
23. Hwang, S.S.; Chang, V.T.; Alejandro, Y.; Osenenko, P.; Davis, C.; Cogswell, J.; Srinivas, S.; Kasimis, B. Caregiver unmet needs, burden, and satisfaction in symptomatic advanced cancer patients at a Veterans Affairs (VA) medical center. *Palliat. Support. Care* **2003**, *1*, 319–329. [CrossRef]
24. Molassiotis, A.; Wilson, B.; Blair, S.; Howe, T.; Cavet, J. Unmet supportive care needs, psychological well-being and quality of life in patients living with multiple myeloma and their partners. *Psycho-Oncology* **2011**, *20*, 88–97. [CrossRef]
25. Soothill, K.; Morris, S.M.; Harman, J.C.; Francis, B.; Thomas, C.; McIllmurray, M.B. Informal carers of cancer patients: What are their unmet psychosocial needs? *Health Soc. Care Community* **2001**, *9*, 464–475. [CrossRef]
26. Stafford, L.; Judd, F. Partners of long-term gynaecologic cancer survivors: Psychiatric morbidity, psychosexual outcomes and supportive care needs. *Gynecol. Oncol.* **2010**, *118*, 268–273. [CrossRef] [PubMed]
27. Wang, T.; Molassiotis, A.; Chung, B.P.M.; Tan, J.Y. Unmet care needs of advanced cancer patients and their informal caregivers: A systematic review. *BMC Palliat. Care* **2018**, *17*, 1–29. [CrossRef] [PubMed]
28. Chen, S.-C.; Chiou, S.-C.; Yu, C.-J.; Lee, Y.-H.; Liao, W.-Y.; Hsieh, P.-Y.; Jhang, S.-Y.; Lai, Y.-H. The unmet supportive care needs—What advanced lung cancer patients' caregivers need and related factors. *Support. Care Cancer* **2016**, *24*, 2999–3009. [CrossRef] [PubMed]
29. Beesley, V.L.; Staneva, A.; Nehill, C.; Milch, V.; Hughes, F.; Webb, P.M. Patterns of, and barriers to supportive care needs assessment and provision for Australian women with gynecological cancer and their caregivers: A mixed-methods study of clinical practice. *Palliat. Support. Care* **2020**, *18*, 170–177. [CrossRef] [PubMed]
30. Friðriksdóttir, N.; Sævarsdóttir, Þ.; Halfdánardóttir, S.Í.; Jónsdóttir, A.; Magnúsdóttir, H.; Ólafsdóttir, K.L.; Guðmundsdóttir, G.; Gunnarsdóttir, S. Family members of cancer patients: Needs, quality of life and symptoms of anxiety and depression. *Acta Oncol.* **2011**, *50*, 252–258. [CrossRef] [PubMed]
31. Peh, C.X.; Liu, J.; Mahendran, R. Quality of life and emotional distress among caregivers of patients newly diagnosed with cancer: Understanding trajectories across the first year post-diagnosis. *J. Psychosoc. Oncol.* **2020**, *38*, 557–572. [CrossRef] [PubMed]
32. O'Grady, H. *Woman's Relationship with Herself: Gender, Foucault and Therapy*; Routledge: New York, NY, USA, 2005.
33. Allen, S.M.; Lima, J.C.; Goldscheider, F.K.; Roy, J. Primary Caregiver Characteristics and Transitions in Community-Based Care. *J. Gerontol. Ser. B Psychol. Sci. Soc. Sci.* **2012**, *67*, 362–371. [CrossRef]
34. Baker, K.L.; Robertson, N. Coping with caring for someone with dementia: Reviewing the literature about men. *Aging Ment. Health* **2008**, *12*, 413–422. [CrossRef]
35. Daire, A.P.; Torres, J.; Edwards, N.N. Family Caregivers: Psychosocial Impacts and Clinical Needs. *Adultspan J.* **2009**, *8*, 67–80. [CrossRef]
36. Potter, A.J. Care Configurations and Unmet Care Needs in Older Men and Women. *J. Appl. Gerontol.* **2019**, *38*, 1351–1370. [CrossRef]
37. Cancer Council Victoria; Department of Health Victoria. *Optimal Care Pathway for People with Pancreatic Cancer*, 2nd ed.; Cancer Council Victoria: Melbourne, Australia, 2021.
38. Corry, M.; While, A.; Neenan, K.; Smith, V. A systematic review of systematic reviews on interventions for caregivers of people with chronic conditions. *J. Adv. Nurs.* **2015**, *71*, 718–734. [CrossRef] [PubMed]
39. Beesley, V.L.; Janda, M.; Goldstein, D.; Gooden, H.; Merrett, N.D.; O'Connell, D.L.; Rowlands, I.J.; Wyld, D.; Neale, R.E. A tsunami of unmet needs: Pancreatic and ampullary cancer patients' supportive care needs and use of community and allied health services. *Psycho-Oncology* **2016**, *25*, 150–157. [CrossRef] [PubMed]
40. Beesley, V.L.; Wockner, L.F.; O'Rourke, P.; Janda, M.; Goldstein, D.; Gooden, H.; Merrett, N.D.; O'Connell, D.L.; Rowlands, I.J.; Wyld, D.K.; et al. Risk factors for current and future unmet supportive care needs of people with pancreatic cancer. A longitudinal study. *Support. Care Cancer* **2016**, *24*, 3589–3599. [CrossRef] [PubMed]
41. Sarradon-Eck, A.; Besle, S.; Troian, J.; Capodano, G.; Mancini, J. Understanding the Barriers to Introducing Early Palliative Care for Patients with Advanced Cancer: A Qualitative Study. *J. Palliat. Med.* **2019**, *22*, 508–516. [CrossRef]

cancers

MDPI

Article

Real-Life Results of Palliative Chemotherapy in Metastatic Pancreatic Ductal Adenocarcinoma

Bianca Varzaru [1,2], Razvan A. Iacob [1,3], Adina E. Croitoru [4,5,*], Speranta M. Iacob [1,3], Cristina E. Radu [6], Stefania M. Dumitrescu [4] and Cristian Gheorghe [1,3]

1 Faculty of Medicine, Carol Davila University of Medicine and Pharmacy, 020021 Bucharest, Romania; bianca.stoica@drd.umfcd.ro (B.V.); drcgheorghe@gmail.com (C.G.)
2 Gastroenterology Department, Sanador Clinical Hospital, 010991 Bucharest, Romania
3 Digestive Diseases and Liver Transplantation Center, Fundeni Clinical Institute, 022238 Bucharest, Romania
4 Oncology Department, Fundeni Clinical Institute, 022238 Bucharest, Romania
5 Faculty of Medicine, Titu Maiorescu University, 040441 Bucharest, Romania
6 Saint Mary Clinical Hospital, 011172 Bucharest, Romania
* Correspondence: oncologie@icfundeni.ro

Simple Summary: The available chemotherapeutic regimens for metastatic pancreatic ductal adenocarcinoma (mPDAC) in Romania include FOLFIRINOX (FFX), gemcitabine-based regimens (GB), and gemcitabine monotherapy (Gem). The purpose of our study was to compare the efficacy of FFX, GB, and Gem in patients with mPDAC in real-world scenarios. Our research revealed that the overall survival (OS) of patients receiving FFX or GB was comparable, twice as long as that of patients receiving Gem, and the progression-free survival (PFS) was highest for patients receiving FFX as first-line chemotherapy (L1). Male gender, Eastern Cooperative Oncology Group Performance (ECOG-PS) 0/1, the FFX regimen, and neutrophil-to-lymphocyte ratio (NLR) > 4.15 were all independently linked to a longer OS. L1 with FFX improved both OS and PFS for second-line chemotherapy (L2).

Abstract: Purpose: To assess the efficacy of FOLFIRINOX(FFX), gemcitabine-based regimens (GB), and gemcitabine monotherapy (Gem) in patients with metastatic pancreatic ductal adenocarcinoma (mPDAC). Methods: This is a retrospective study that included 83 patients with mPDAC treated with first-line chemotherapy (L1) with either FFX, GB or Gem between 2015 and 2017. Progression-free survival (PFS) for L1 and second-line chemotherapy (L2) (PFS-L1 and PFS-L2) and overall survival (OS) were estimated using the Kaplan–Meier method. Results: Median PFS-L1 for FFX, GB and Gem groups was 9 months (95% (Confidence Interval) CI 2.76–15.24), 5 months (95%CI 3.44–6.56), and 5 months (95%CI 3.76–6.24), respectively (p = 0.04). OS was 14 months (95%CI 11.16–16.85), 12 months (95%CI: 9.44–11.56), and 7 months (95%CI: 5.7–8.3) for patients treated with FFX, GB, and Gem, respectively (p = 0.0001). ECOG-PS (0/1) (Hazard Ratio (HR) 6.74, p = 0.002), age > 70 years (HR 0.25, p = 0.04), body tumors (HR 2.8, p = 0.048), CA19–9 > 39 U/mL (HR 0.26, p = 0.02), and neutrophil-to-lymphocyte ratio (NLR) > 4.15 (HR 6.76, p = 0.001) were independent prognostic factors for PFS-L1. Male gender (HR 3.02, p = 0.026), ECOG-PS (0/1) (HR 4.21, p = 0.003), L1 with FFX (HR 0.255, p = 0.007), and NLR > 4.15 (HR 2.65, p = 0.04) were independent prognostic factors of OS. PFS-L2 (HR 6.91, p = 0.013) and OS-L2 (HR 6.95, p = 0.037) were significantly higher in patients first treated with FFX. Conclusions: The OS of patients who receive FFX or GB is comparable. The best PFS-L1 belongs to the FFX group. Male gender, ECOG-PS 0/1, the FFX regimen, and NLR > 4.15 were independent predictors of OS. PFS-L2 and OS-L2 were favorably impacted by L1 with FFX.

Keywords: metastatic pancreatic adenocarcinoma; palliative chemotherapy; overall survival; progression-free survival

1. Introduction

Pancreatic adenocarcinoma is one of the most lethal cancers in the world, with an incidence rate approximately equal to the mortality rate [1,2]. Although diagnosis accuracy has greatly improved over the past two decades [3], 28% of patients are diagnosed with locally advanced pancreatic cancer and 53% with metastatic disease [4], with median OS of approximately 12 months and 6 months, respectively [5]. The optimal treatment for pancreatic cancer remains controversial. Resection is the only curative therapy for patients with localized pancreatic cancer; however, management is mainly limited to chemotherapy, sometimes combined with radiotherapy for loco-regional diseases [6].

Gem was the usual chemotherapy regimen until 2011, when FFX was presented as a novel, more efficient L1 regimen for advanced pancreatic cancer. In 2011, Conroy et al. (PRODIGE trial) showed that the median OS for chemotherapy-naive patients treated with FFX was approximately 11 months, compared to 6.8 months for patients treated with Gem, with median PFS of 6.4 months and 3.3 months, respectively (HR, 0.47, 95% CI 0.37 to 0.59; $p = 0.001$) [7]. Patients with mPDAC who received gemcitabine combined with nanoparticle albumin-bound (nab)-paclitaxel (nab-paclitaxel) had a significantly better OS (8.5 vs. 6.7 months) as compared to those who received Gem, according to Von Hoff et al. [8].

When recommending L2 to patients with mPDAC, the L1 regimen should be taken into account. [7,9]. FFX is often administered first when patients are in relatively good general condition [8]. Less than half of patients with advanced or mPDAC who experienced L1 treatment failure remain in good general condition and may receive subsequent L2 regimens [10]. Combinations of 5-fluorouracil (FU) with oxaliplatin [11] or nanoliposomal irinotecan [9] can be suggested as L2 after Gem fails.

Even though FFX and gemcitabine plus nab-paclitaxel are both considered standard L1 [7,8] for patients with PDAC, nab-paclitaxel is not currently covered by insurance in our country. At this moment, the palliative chemotherapy regimens available in our country are based on FFX, GB (gemcitabine combined with capecitabine, cisplatin, or oxaliplatin), or Gem. The choice of L1 takes into account the patient's characteristics: age, ECOG-PS, bilirubin levels, nutritional status, and comorbidities.

The aim of this study was to compare the efficacy of the chemotherapy regimens available in our country (FFX, GB, and Gem) and identify the prognostic factors of OS and PFS in a real-world setting.

2. Materials and Methods

We analyzed data from 83 consecutive patients diagnosed with mPDAC between 2015–2017 in the Oncology Department of Fundeni Clinical Institute (Bucharest, Romania). In this research, only patients who received FFX, GB or Gem were considered. Pathological confirmation was provided for each patient. Since this group of patients was retrospectively reviewed, there were no ethical issues.

Medical record variables were gathered and entered into a database. Baseline characteristics (age, gender, tumor location, ECOG-PS, presence of diabetes mellitus, CA 19-9 levels), as well as NLR and L1 and L2 regimens, were analyzed with respect to their prognostic significance. OS was defined as the period from the time of diagnosis until death (from complications related to pancreatic cancer or other causes) or the end of follow-up. PFS-L1 was calculated from the first chemotherapy dosage to either the first sign of tumor progression or the patient's death, whichever came first. For patients who received L2 therapy, the OS-L2 and PFS-L2 were computed. The OS-L2 was calculated starting with the date of progression under L1 (or the date of initial administration of L2 if no progression was observed under L1) and ending with the date of death from any cause. PFS-L2 was computed from the date of progression under L1 (or the date of first administration of L2 if no progression was recorded under L1) until the date of progression, death from any cause, or the end of follow-up. Survival data were censored at the last follow-up. The cut-off date for follow-up was 30 June 2019.

SPSS statistical software (IBM SPSS Statistics 20.0) was used for all analyses. According to the Kaplan–Meier method, a survival analysis was conducted, and survival curves were compared using the log rank test, considering $p < 0.05$ for statistical significance. The optimal cut-off value for baseline NLR was determined using a time-dependent receiver operating characteristic (ROC) analysis, considering 6-month survival as the reference time point.

The multivariate survival analysis was further conducted using the Cox regression model, submitting into analysis variables that were found to be significant ($p < 0.05$) in univariate analysis and adjusting for age and ECOG-PS.

The study's goals were to assess the effectiveness of the chemotherapy regimens that are used in our nation and to pinpoint the variables that affect OS and PFS in the real world.

3. Results

3.1. Patients' Characteristics

Between January 2015 and December 2017, 83 consecutive patients diagnosed with mPDAC and treated with chemotherapy regimens in the oncology department were included in this analysis. Clinical parameters, information on the L1 and L2 regimens, PFS, and OS were recorded.

Table 1 displays demographic information and disease features at the beginning of the L1 regimens. The male-to-female ratio was 48:35, and the median age was 63 years (interquartile range (IQR), 57–71). The median age of the patients in the Gem group was 67 years (IQR: 58.5–73), compared to 61 years (IQR: 54–66) for the GB group and 60 years (IQR: 54–65) for the FFX group. In about 54% of patients, the tumor was located in the head or uncinate process of the pancreas; in 27% of patients, it was found in the pancreatic corpus, and in 19% of patients, it was found in the tail of the pancreas. The patients in the analyzed group had an ECOG-PS of 0/1 or 2 (51.8% and 48.19%, respectively), and 37.4% of them suffered from type 2 diabetes. The majority of patients (almost 81%) had elevated baseline levels of CA 19-9 (>39 UI/mL), and the median NLR was 3.35 (IQR: 2.14–4.75). Gem was used as the L1 regimen in 53.01% of cases, GB in 24.09% of cases, and FFX in 22.9% of cases. Almost 29% of patients ($n = 24$) underwent L2 regimens. Patients treated with L2 regimens received 5-FU plus leucovorin, irinotecan, and/or oxaliplatin ($n = 11$, 45.83%), Gem ($n = 5$, 20.83%), GB ($n = 5$, 20.83%), and other chemotherapy, such as oxaliplatin, irinotecan, or capecitabine ($n = 3$, 12.5%).

3.2. Statistical Analysis

The median PFS-L1 and median OS were 5 months (95% CI 3.88–6.12) and 10 months (95% CI 7.77–12.23), respectively, with variation regarding the chemotherapy regimens. Patients in the FFX group had a median PFS-L1 of 9 months (95% CI 2.76–15.24), whereas the GB group and Gem group had median PFS-L1 of 5 months (95% CI 3.44–6.56) and 5 months (95% CI 3.76–6.24), respectively ($p = 0.044$) (Figure 1). OS for patients treated with FFX was 14 months (95% CI 11.16–16.85), for patients treated with GB, it was 12 months (95% CI 9.44–14.56), and for patients treated with Gem, it was 7 months (95% CI 5.7–8.3), $p < 0.0001$ (Figure 2).

At 6, 12, 18, and 24 months, the OS rates in the Gem group were 71.11%, 24.44%, 2.22%, and 0%, compared to 94.74%, 57.9%, 26.32%, and 0% in the GB group and 84.21%, 68.42%, 31.58%, and 10.52%, respectively, in the FFX group.

The median PFS-L2 and OS-L2 for patients who received L2 were 4 months (95% CI 2.16–5.84) and 6 months (95% CI 4.97–7.03), respectively. PFS-L2 was longer in patients initially treated with FFX followed by Gem (PFS-L2 = 6 months, 95% CI 4.83–7.17) or GB (PFS-L2 = 6 months, 95% CI 1.2–10.8), as well as in patients receiving in L1 GB followed in L2 by 5-FU-based regimens (PFS-L2 = 5 months, 95% CI 3.61–6.38), $p = 0.014$ (Figure 3). The longest OS-L2 was recorded in patients treated with the sequence FFX → GB (13 months, 95% CI 11.4–14.6), followed by those treated with FFX → Gem (6 months, 95% CI 2.77–9.22) and GB → 5-FU-based regimens (6 months, 95% CI 4.54–7.46), $p < 0.0001$ (Figure 4).

Table 1. Baseline characteristics of patients treated with palliative chemotherapy.

Variable	All (n = 83)	Gem (n = 44)	GB (n = 20)	FFX (n = 19)
Age (years)	63 (57–71)	67 (58.5–73)	61 (54–66)	60 (54–65)
Age ≥ 70 years, n (%)	23 (27.71)	19 (43.18)	2 (10)	2 (10.53)
Sex, male, n (%)	48 (57.83)	20 (45.45)	13 (65)	14 (73.86)
ECOG-PS				
0/1, n (%)	43 (51.8)	14 (31.81)	12 (60)	17 (89.47)
2, n (%)	40 (48.19)	30 (68.18)	8 (40)	2 (10.53)
Primary tumor location				
head/uncinate process, n (%)	45 (54.22)	26 (59.09)	9 (45)	10 (52.63)
body, n (%)	22 (26.5)	12 (27.27)	5 (25)	5 (26.32)
tail, n (%)	16 (19.28)	6 (13.63)	6 (30)	4 (21.05)
Diabetes Mellitus, n (%)	31 (37.35)	18 (40.90)	4 (20)	9 (47.37)
CA 19-9				
>39 UI/mL	67 (80.72)	36 (81.82)	15 (75)	16 (84.21)
≤39 UI/mL	16 (19.28)	9 (18.18)	5 (25)	3 (15.79)
NLR	3.35 (2.14–4.52)	3.9 (2.55–4.75)	3.28 (2.17–3.95)	2.72 (1.61–4.19)

All variables are provided as median (IQR) or number (percentage). Abbreviations: Gem: Gemcitabine monotherapy, GB: gemcitabine-based regimens, FFX: FOLFIRINOX, ECOG-PS: Eastern Cooperative Oncology Group Performance Status, NLR: neutrophil-to-lymphocyte ratio.

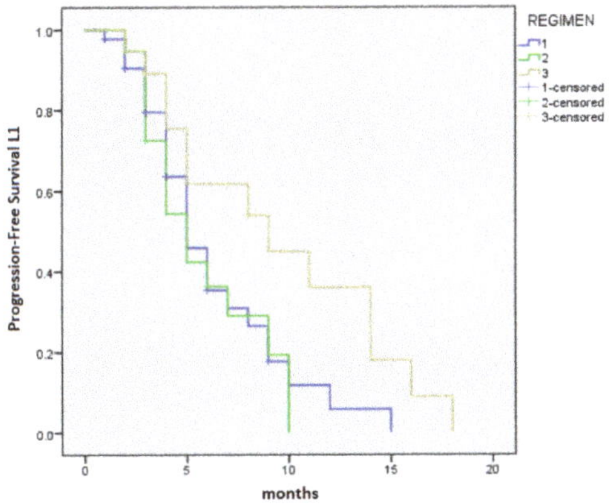

Figure 1. Median progression-free survival for first-line chemotherapy: 1—Gemcitabine monotherapy: 5 months, 2—Gemcitabine-based regimens: 5 months, 3—FOLFIRINOX: 9 months (p = 0.044).

A Cox regression model was used to assess the relationship between patients' characteristics and survival. This analysis took into account factors like age, gender, tumor location, diabetes, ECOG-PS, L1 and L2 regimens, CA 19-9, and NLR at diagnosis. A time-dependent receiver operating characteristic (ROC) analysis was conducted using 6-month survival as the reference time point in order to determine the cut-off value for baseline NLR. The optimal cut-off value for baseline NLR was 4.15, with an area under the curve (AUC) of 0.754 (95% CI 0.594–0.913, p = 0.003).

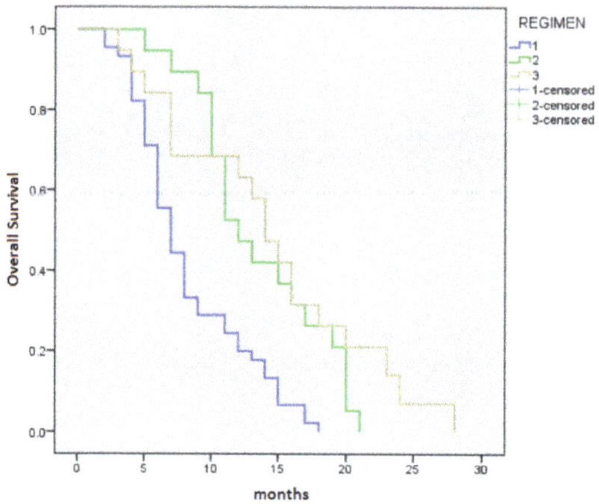

Figure 2. Median overall survival: 1—Gemcitabine: 7 months, 2—Gemcitabine-based regiments: 12 months 3—FOLFIRINOX: 14 months ($p < 0.0001$).

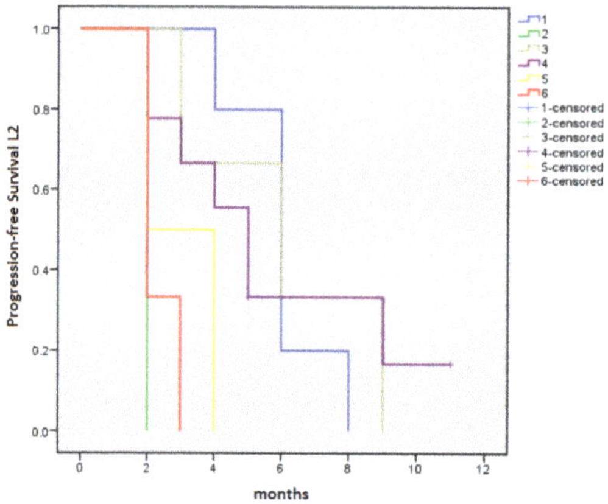

Figure 3. Median progression-free survival for second-line chemotherapy: 1—FOLFIRINOX → Gemcitabine monotherapy (6 months), 2—Gemcitabine monotherapy → 5-FU-based regimens (2 months), 3—FOLFIRINOX → Gemcitabine-based regimens (6 months), 4—Gemcitabine-based regimens → 5—FU-based regimens (5 months), 5—Gemcitabine monotherapy → Gemcitabine-based regimens (2 months), 6—others (2 months), $p = 0.014$.

The multivariate survival analysis was further conducted using the Cox regression model. Multivariate survival analyses were performed by submitting into analysis variables that were found to be significant ($p < 0.05$) or near significant in univariate analysis and by adjusting for age and ECOG-PS.

In univariate analyses, CA 19-9 > 39 UI/mL (HR 2.46, 95% CI 1.18–5.14, $p < 0.016$), NLR > 4.15 (HR 0.52, 95% CI 0.29–0.92, $p = 0.024$), L1 with FFX vs. Gem (HR 2.42, 95% CI 1.06–5.49, $p = 0.035$), and L1 with GB vs. Gem (HR 2.13, 95% CI 1.03–4.39, $p = 0.041$) were prognostic factors of the PFS-L1. In the multivariate Cox regression model, age > 70 years (HR 0.25, 95% CI 0.07–0.95, $p = 0.04$), ECOG-PS (0/1 vs. 2) (HR 6.74, 95% CI 1.99–22.87, $p = 0.002$), tumor location (corpus vs. head) (HR 2.8, 95% CI 1.01–7.73, $p = 0.048$), increased CA 19-9 (>39 UI/mL) at diagnosis (HR 0.26, 95% CI 0.08–0.83, $p = 0.02$), and NLR > 4.15 at diagnosis (HR 6.76, 95% CI 2.24–20.37, $p = 0.001$) were all independent predictors of PFS-L1. ECOG-PS 0/1 was associated with a longer PFS-L1, while age > 70, elevated CA 19-9 levels,

NLR > 4.15, and tumor in the pancreatic body were linked with a shorter PFS-L1 (Table 2). There was no statistically significant correlation between PFS-L1 and gender, diabetes, or chemotherapy treatment.

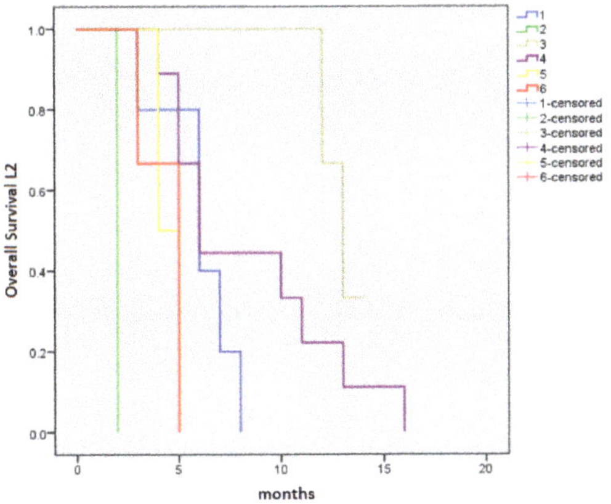

Figure 4. Median overall survival for second-line chemotherapy: 1—FOLFIRINOX → Gemcitabine monotherapy (6 months), 2—Gemcitabine monotherapy → 5-FU-based regimens (2 months), 3—FOLFIRINOX → Gemcitabine-based regimens (13 months), 4—Gemcitabine-based regimens → 5-FU-based regimens (6 months), 5—Gemcitabine monotherapy → Gemcitabine-based regimens (4 months), 6—others (5 months), $p < 0.0001$.

Table 2. Prognostic factors of the progression-free survival for first-line chemotherapy.

Prognostic Factor	Univariate Analyses		Multivariate Analyses	
	p	HR (95% CI)	p	HR (95% CI)
Age (years)	0.68	0.99 (0.97–1.02)		
Age > 70 years	0.65	1.16 (0.62–2.14)	0.04	0.25 (0.07–0.95)
Sex: male vs. female	0.58	1.16 (0.67–2.02)	0.21	0.52 (0.18–1.44)
Diabetes	0.55	1.18 (0.68–2.05)		
Baseline ECOG-PS (0/1 vs. 2)	0.063	0.58 (0.33–1.03)	0.002	6.74 (1.99–22.87)
Tumor location				
head vs. body	0.22	2.02 (1.11–3.69)	0.048	2.8 (1.01–7.73)
head vs. tail	0.73	1.13 (0.54–2.37)	0.142	2.75 (0.71–10.6)
CA 19-9 > 39 UI/mL vs. ≤ 39 UI/mL	0.016	2.46 (1.18–5.14)	0.02	0.26 (0.08–0.83)
NLR > 4.15 vs. NLR ≤ 4.15	0.024	0.52 (0.29–0.92)	0.001	6.76 (2.24–20.37)
First-line chemotherapy				
FFX vs. Gem	0.035	2.42 (1.06–5.49)	0.37	0.47 (0.08–2.5)
GB vs. Gem	0.041	2.13 (1.03–4.39)	0.97	0.98 (0.32–2.96)

Abbreviations: ECOG-PS: Eastern Cooperative Oncology Group Performance Status, FFX: FOLFIRINOX, Gem: Gemcitabine monotherapy, GB: gemcitabine-based regimens, NLR: neutrophil-to-lymphocyte ratio.

In univariate analysis, baseline ECOG-PS 0/1 vs. 2 (HR 2.49, 95% CI 1.56–3.98, $p < 0.0001$), NLR > 4.15 (HR 0.6, 95% CI 0.37–0.97, $p = 0.036$), L1 with FFX vs. Gem (HR 0.29, 95% CI 0.16–0.56, $p < 0.0001$), and L1 with GB vs. Gem (HR 0.41, 95% CI 0.23–0.72, $p = 0.002$) were independent prognostic factors of OS. In the multivariate analysis, male gender (HR 3.02, 95% CI 1.14–7.98, $p = 0.026$), ECOG-PS (0/1 vs. 2) (HR 4.21, 95% CI 1.61–11, $p = 0.003$), palliative chemotherapy FFX (HR 0.255, 95% CI 0.09–0.69, $p = 0.007$), and baseline NLR > 4.15 (HR 2.65, 95% CI 1.04–6.75, $p = 0.04$) were the independent prognostic factors of OS. Male gender, ECOG-PS 0/1, and L1 with FFX (vs. Gem) were linked to improved OS, whereas higher NLR was linked to lower OS. A worse OS was also indicated by increased CA 19-9 at diagnosis, although the association lacked statistical significance (HR 0.41, 95% CI 0.17–1, p = 0.05) (Table 3). In the multivariate analysis, L1 with FFX (vs. Gem) was an independent predictor for PFS-L2 (HR 6.91, 95% CI 1.5–31.9, p = 0.013) and OS-L2 (HR 6.95, 95% CI 1.12–43.07, p = 0.037). OS-L2 and PFS-L2 did not correlate statistically significantly with gender, age at the start of L2, or the L2 regimen.

Table 3. Prognostic factors of overall survival.

Prognostic Factor	Univariate Analyses		Multivariate Analyses	
	p	HR (95% CI)	p	HR (95% CI)
Age (years)	0.879	1.01 (0.98–1.02)		
Age > 70 years	0.279	0.76 (0.47–1.24)	0.33	0.62 (0.24–1.61)
Sex: male vs. female	0.685	1.1 (0.70–1.71)	0.026	3.02 (1.14–7.98)
Diabetes	0.571	1.14 (0.72–1.79)		
Baseline ECOG-PS (0/1 vs. 2)	0.0001	2.49 (1.56–3.98)	0.003	4.21 (1.61–11)
Tumor location				
head vs. body	0.881	1.04 (0.62–1.75)		
head vs. tail	0.756	0.91 (0.50–1.64)		
CA 19-9 > 39 UI/mL vs. ≤ 39 UI/mL	0.460	1.23 (0.71–2.14)	0.05	0.41 (0.17–1)
NLR > 4.15 vs. NLR ≤ 4.15	0.036	0.60 (0.37–0.97)	0.04	2.65 (1.04–6.75)
First-line chemotherapy				
FFX vs. Gem	0.0001	0.29 (0.16–0.56)	0.007	0.26 (0.09–0.69)
GB vs. Gem	0.002	0.41 (0.23–0.72)	0.253	0.49 (0.14–1.68)

Abbreviations: ECOG-PS: Eastern Cooperative Oncology Group Performance Status, FFX: FOLFIRINOX, Gem: Gemcitabine monotherapy, GB: gemcitabine-based regimens, NLR: neutrophil-to-lymphocyte ratio.

4. Discussion

In this study, we retrospectively analyzed the clinical outcomes of patients with mPDAC. The patient characteristics included in our study were similar to those published in previous epidemiological studies in terms of gender, age, and tumor location [5,7,12,13]. Consistent with the results of previous studies [7,12], we noticed significant improvement in OS in patients treated with FFX or GB regimens [14] compared to patients receiving Gem (12 months and 14 months, respectively, vs. 8 months).

A retrospective multinational study, which included 1089 patients from the UK, Sweden, Germany, Italy, and Hungary with mPDAC undergoing palliative chemotherapy between 2012 and 2015, analyzed the efficacy of FFX and gemcitabine plus nab-paclitaxel versus Gem and GB regimens like gemcitabine plus oxaliplatin, gemcitabine plus cisplatin, and gemcitabine plus capecitabine. The median OS was 9 months for the FFX group (95% CI 7.1–10.9), 7 months for gemcitabine plus nab-paclitaxel (95% CI 5.8–8.2), 7 months for GB regimens (95% CI 6.0–8.0), and 5 months for the Gem group (95% CI 4.3–5.7) [15].

It is interesting to note that a recent systematic review comparing the safety and efficacy of FFX to gemcitabine plus nab-paclitaxel and gemcitabine plus capecitabine in the treatment of pancreatic cancer revealed that FFX was linked to significantly longer survival than gemcitabine plus nab-paclitaxel and gemcitabine plus capecitabine. In the adjuvant pancreatic cancer setting, combination regimens (FFX, gemcitabine plus capecitabine, and gemcitabine plus nab-paclitaxel) had statistically significant differences for OS (HR 0.78, 95% CI: 0.69–0.89) and relapse-free survival/disease-free survival (HR 0.77, 95% CI 0.60–0.98) compared to Gem. Also, in advanced/metastatic pancreatic cancer, FFX showed significantly better OS (HR 0.71, 95% CI 0.60–0.85) and PFS (HR 0.65, 95% CI 0.57–0.74) compared to gemcitabine plus capecitabine [16].

In our retrospective cohort, the proportion of patients receiving L2 was ~29%, which is consistent with reports from other studies [17,18]. A retrospective study on real-world unselected patients with pancreatic cancer reported a median OS-L2 of 5.2 months (95% CI 4.7–5.7) [17]. In another retrospective study on 366 patients with advanced pancreatic cancer who had received palliative chemotherapy, 28.4% underwent L2, the median OS-L2 was 6.4 months (95% CI 4.5–8.6), and the median PFS-L2 was 4.5 months (95% CI 2.7–6.3) [18]. Despite the lack of statistical significance, Gränsmark et al. noticed a better OS-L2 in patients receiving gemcitabine plus nab-paclitaxel as L1 compared to the Gem subgroup (HR = 0.70, 95% CI 0.48–1.03, $p = 0.067$) [17].

A Cox regression model was used to assess the relationship between patients' characteristics and survival. In our cohort study, the multivariate analysis showed that ECOG-PS 0/1 was associated with prolonged PFS-L1, while age over 70, increased levels of CA 19-9, NLR > 4.15, and tumors located in the pancreatic body negatively influenced PFS-L1. Greater OS was linked to male gender, ECOG-PS 0/1, and the L1 regimen with FFX (vs. Gem), while lower survival was linked to higher NLR. A worse survival was also predicted by higher CA 19-9 levels at diagnosis, although this prediction was not statistically significant (HR 0.41, 95% CI 0.17–1, $p = 0.05$). Furthermore, L1 with FFX (vs. Gem) was an independent predictor for PFS-L2 (HR 6.91, 95% CI 1.5–31.9, $p = 0.013$) and OS-L2 (HR 6.95, 95% CI 1.12–43.07, $p = 0.037$).

Artinyan et al. examined the relationship between tumor location and survival. In multivariate analysis, body and tail locations were significant prognostic factors for decreased survival (HR 1.11, 95% CI 1.00–1.23, $p = 0.05$) [19]. Further, in a systematic review and meta-analysis of 93 studies, studying the outcome of head compared to body and tail pancreatic cancer, multivariate analysis showed that the head site was an independent prognostic factor for survival (HR 0.95, 95% CI 0.92–0.99, $p = 0.02$), and tumors of the head were associated with a similar PFS to tail cancers (HR 0.99, 95% CI 0.84–1.16, $p = 0.91$) [20]. In another study, normal baseline albumin (HR 0.63, 95% CI 0.41–0.97), male sex (HR 0.65, 95% CI 0.43–0.97), and L2 therapy (HR 0.50, 95% CI 0.28–0.86) were correlated with better survival [21].

In a multivariate analysis of 154 patients with inoperable pancreatic cancer treated with Gem and/or 5-FU-based therapy, the baseline CA 19-9 above or below the median value (958 U/mL) was an independent prognostic factor for OS (HR 1.8, 95% CI 1.3–2.5, $p = 0.0004$) [22]. In a retrospective analysis, patients with increased levels of the biomarkers CA 19-9 and CEA, or the location of cancer in the pancreatic tail, were associated with a worse prognosis.

Based on our cohort data and according to the ROC curve, the cut-off value of the NLR was 4.15, which is consistent with that in previous studies [23–26]. In several studies, multivariate analysis revealed that elevated NLR (cut-off values ranged from 2 to 5) indicated a worse prognosis than in patients with lower NLR [27,28].

A systematic review published in 2013 [29], analyzing the relationship between the NLR and cancer outcome (OS/cancer-specific survival/disease recurrence, or response to treatment), demonstrated that the NLR had prognostic value in a variety of tumor types, and in cancer patients receiving chemo/radiotherapy, elevated baseline NLR was associated with poor OS.

Several retrospective studies analyzing patients with locally advanced or metastatic pancreatic cancer treated with palliative chemotherapy assessed the prognostic value of NLR. For example, Luo et al. retrospectively reviewed 403 patients undergoing chemotherapy for advanced pancreatic adenocarcinoma and showed that both baseline NLR (NLR > 3.1, HR = 1.42; $p = 0.001$) and post-treatment NLR (NLR > 3.1, HR = 2.39; $p > 0.0001$) were independent prognostic factors of OS [25]. An et al. demonstrated that elevated pre-treatment NLR (> 5) was a predictor of shorter survival in patients with advanced pancreatic cancer ($p = 0.001$) [30]. Also, in another retrospective study, a multivariate analysis revealed that a high NLR > 3.74 (HR 2.430; 95% CI 1.484–3.977; $p < 0.001$) was independently associated with OS [24].

5. Conclusions

Oncologists continue to face difficulties in the management of mPDAC. In this study, FFX was an effective L1 option for patients with ECOG-PS 0/1.

The patients with the best PFS-L1 (9 months) in our real-life mPDAC cohort scenario are those who received FFX as an L1 regimen. Patients who underwent either the FFX or GB regimens had similar OS (14 months and 12 months, respectively).

Our results demonstrate that age over 70 years, increased levels of CA 19-9, NLR > 4.15, and tumors located in the pancreatic body negatively influenced PFS-L1, while ECOG-PS 0/1 was associated with prolonged PFS-L1. None of the following factors were statistically significantly linked with PFS-L1: gender, diabetes, or chemotherapy regimen. Male gender, ECOG-PS 0/1, and L1 with FFX (vs. Gem) were associated with better OS, while increased NLR was correlated with decreased OS. At the same time, patients with elevated CA 19-9 values at diagnosis had lower OS. In this study, around one-third of the patients received L2, and regardless of the L2 regimen, those who received FFX first had significantly greater PFS-L2 and OS-L2 than those who did not. There is very limited information available regarding the treatment strategies for pancreatic cancer in Eastern Europe. As far as we are aware, this is the first study comparing the effectiveness of mPDAC palliative chemotherapeutic options currently available in Romania. We believe that our research's conclusions may be helpful in assisting oncologists in making decisions regarding their choice of chemotherapy regimens given the difficulties they experience in controlling mPDAC.

There are some limitations in this research, as it is a retrospective study performed in a single center with a small number of patients. Additionally, due to the study's retrospective character, no information on the patients' psychosocial or emotional effects could be gathered, despite the fact that an increasing amount of research suggests a connection between psychological stress and site-specific cancer mortality. To confirm our findings, we think a multicenter, nationwide prospective validation is required.

Author Contributions: B.V.: conceptualization, methodology, investigation, formal analysis, writing—original draft, visualization; R.A.I.: conceptualization; supervision; writing—review & editing, methodology; A.E.C.: methodology, investigation, data curation, writing—review & editing, supervision; S.M.I.: conceptualization, methodology, writing—review & editing, C.E.R.: conceptualization, investigation, data curation, methodology, writing—review & editing; S.M.D.: methodology, writing—review & editing; C.G.: conceptualization, supervision, writing—review & editing. All authors have read and agreed to the published version of the manuscript.

Funding: This research received no external funding.

Institutional Review Board Statement: This retrospective study was approved by the Internal Review Board of Fundeni Clinical Institute, Bucharest, Romania—IRB:26717/24.05.2023.

Informed Consent Statement: For retrospective studies, informed consent is not required.

Data Availability Statement: Data are available upon reasonable request and with the permission of the corresponding author.

Conflicts of Interest: The authors declare that there is no conflict of interest. The authors are solely responsible for the content and writing of the paper.

References

1. GLOBOCAN 2020. *Estimated Number of Cases Worldwide, Both Sexes;* The International Agency for Research on Cancer: Geneva, Switzerland, 2020; Volume 144.
2. Lu, Y.; Gentiluomo, M.; Macauda, A.; Gioffreda, D.; Gazouli, M.; Petrone, M.C.; Kelemen, D.; Ginocchi, L.; Morelli, L.; Papiris, K.; et al. Identification of Recessively Inherited Genetic Variants Potentially Linked to Pancreatic Cancer Risk. *Front. Oncol.* **2021**, *11*, 771312. [CrossRef] [PubMed]
3. Winter, K.; Talar-Wojnarowska, R.; Dąbrowski, A.; Degowska, M.; Durlik, M.; Gąsiorowska, A.; Głuszek, S.; Jurkowska, G.; Kaczka, A.; Lampe, P.; et al. Diagnostic and Therapeutic Recommendations in Pancreatic Ductal Adenocarcinoma. Recommendations of the Working Group of the Polish Pancreatic Club. *Prz. Gastroenterol.* **2019**, *14*, 1–18. [CrossRef]
4. Sheahan, A.V.; Biankin, A.V.; Parish, C.R.; Khachigian, L.M. Targeted Therapies in the Management of Locally Advanced and Metastatic Pancreatic Cancer: A Systematic Review. *Oncotarget* **2019**, *9*, 21613–21627. [CrossRef]

5. Peixoto, R.D.A.; Speers, C.; Mcgahan, C.E.; Renouf, D.J.; Schaeffer, D.F.; Kennecke, H.F. Prognostic Factors and Sites of Metastasis in Unresectable Locally Advanced Pancreatic Cancer. *Cancer Med.* **2015**, *4*, 1171–1177. [CrossRef]
6. Chen, J.; Chen, L.; Yu, J.; Xu, Y.; Wang, X.; Zeng, Z.; Liu, N.; Xu, F.; Yang, S. Meta-Analysis of Current Chemotherapy Regimens in Advanced Pancreatic Cancer to Prolong Survival and Reduce Treatment-Associated Toxicities. *Mol. Med. Rep.* **2019**, *19*, 477–489. [CrossRef] [PubMed]
7. Conroy, T.; Ychou, M.; Bouché, O.; Guimbaud, R.; Bécouarn, Y.; Adenis, A.; Raoul, J.-L.; Gourgou-Bourgade, S.; De La Fouchardière, C.; Bennouna, J.; et al. FOLFIRINOX versus Gemcitabine for Metastatic Pancreatic Cancer. *N. Engl. J. Med.* **2011**, *364*, 1817–1825. [CrossRef]
8. Von Hoff, D.D.; Ervin, T.; Arena, F.P.; Chiorean, E.G.; Infante, J.; Moore, M.; Seay, T.; Tjulandin, S.A.; Ma, W.W.; Saleh, M.N.; et al. Increased Survival in Pancreatic Cancer with Nab-Paclitaxel plus Gemcitabine. *N. Engl. J. Med.* **2013**, *369*, 1691–1703. [CrossRef]
9. Ducreux, M.; Cuhna, A.S.; Caramella, C.; Hollebecque, A.; Burtin, P.; Goéré, D.; Seufferlein, T.; Haustermans, K.; Van Laethem, J.L.; Conroy, T.; et al. Cancer of the Pancreas: ESMO Clinical Practice Guidelines for Diagnosis, Treatment and Follow-Up. *Ann. Oncol.* **2015**, *26* (Suppl. 5), v56–v68. [CrossRef]
10. Walker, E.J.; Ko, A.H. Beyond First-Line Chemotherapy for Advanced Pancreatic Cancer: An Expanding Array of Therapeutic Options? *World J. Gastroenterol.* **2014**, *20*, 2224–2236. [CrossRef]
11. Oettle, H.; Riess, H.; Stieler, J.M.; Heil, G.; Schwaner, I.; Seraphin, J.; Görner, M.; Mölle, M.; Greten, T.F.; Lakner, V.; et al. Second-Line Oxaliplatin, Folinic Acid, and Fluorouracil versus Folinic Acid and Fluorouracil Alone for Gemcitabine-Refractory Pancreatic Cancer: Outcomes from the CONKO-003 Trial. *J. Clin. Oncol.* **2014**, *32*, 2423–2429. [CrossRef] [PubMed]
12. Ergun, Y.; Numune, A.; Yildirim Ozdemir, N.; Karci Guner, E.; Esin, E.; Ali Sendur, M.; Berna Koksoy, E.; Serkan Demirci, N.; Eren, T.; Dede, I.; et al. Comparison of Gemcitabine Monotherapy with Gemcitabine and Cisplatin Combination in Metastatic Pancreatic Cancer: A Retrospective Analysis. *JBUON* **2018**, *23*, 116–121.
13. Ozaka, M.; Nakachi, K.; Kobayashi, S.; Ohba, A.; Imaoka, H.; Terashima, T.; Ishii, H.; Mizusawa, J.; Katayama, H.; Kataoka, T.; et al. A Randomised Phase II Study of Modified FOLFIRINOX versus Gemcitabine plus Nab-Paclitaxel for Locally Advanced Pancreatic Cancer (JCOG1407). *Eur. J. Cancer* **2023**, *181*, 135–144. [CrossRef]
14. Williet, N.; Saint, A.; Pointet, A.L.; Tougeron, D.; Pernot, S.; Pozet, A.; Bechade, D.; Trouilloud, I.; Lourenco, N.; Hautefeuille, V.; et al. Folfirinox versus Gemcitabine/Nab-Paclitaxel as First-Line Therapy in Patients with Metastatic Pancreatic Cancer: A Comparative Propensity Score Study. *Therap. Adv. Gastroenterol.* **2019**, *12*, 1756284819878660. [CrossRef]
15. Javed, M.A.; Beyer, G.; Le, N.; Vinci, A.; Wong, H.; Palmer, D.; Morgan, R.D.; Lamarca, A.; Hubner, R.A.; Valle, J.W.; et al. Impact of Intensified Chemotherapy in Metastatic Pancreatic Ductal Adenocarcinoma (PDAC) in Clinical Routine in Europe. *Pancreatology* **2019**, *19*, 97–104. [CrossRef] [PubMed]
16. Kharat, A.; Brendle, M.; Chhibber, A.; Chaiyakunapruk, N.; Biskupiak, J. Comparative Safety and Efficacy of Therapeutic Options in Resectable and Advanced/Metastatic Pancreatic Cancer: A Systematic Review and Indirect Comparison. *Oncol. Res. Treat.* **2021**, *44*, 476–484. [CrossRef] [PubMed]
17. Gränsmark, E.; Bågenholm Bylin, N.; Blomstrand, H.; Fredrikson, M.; Åvall-Lundqvist, E.; Elander, N.O. Real World Evidence on Second-Line Palliative Chemotherapy in Advanced Pancreatic Cancer. *Front. Oncol.* **2020**, *10*, 1176. [CrossRef]
18. Jung, H.; Lee, E.M. The Clinical Outcomes of Second-Line Chemotherapy in Patients with Advanced Pancreatic Cancer: A Retrospective Study. *J. Yeungnam Med. Sci.* **2022**, *39*, 124–132. [CrossRef] [PubMed]
19. Artinyan, A.; Soriano, P.A.; Prendergast, C.; Low, T.; Ellenhorn, J.D.I.; Kim, J. The Anatomic Location of Pancreatic Cancer Is a Prognostic Factor for Survival. *HPB* **2008**, *10*, 371–376. [CrossRef]
20. Tomasello, G.; Ghidini, M.; Costanzo, A.; Ghidini, A.; Russo, A.; Barni, S.; Passalacqua, R.; Petrelli, F. Outcome of Head Compared to Body and Tail Pancreatic Cancer: A Systematic Review and Meta-Analysis of 93 Studies. *J. Gastrointest. Oncol.* **2019**, *10*, 259–269. [CrossRef]
21. Papneja, N.; Zaidi, A.; Chalchal, H.; Moser, M.; Tan, K.; Olson, C.; Haider, K.; Shaw, J.; Ahmed, S. Comparisons of Outcomes of Real-World Patients with Advanced Pancreatic Cancer Treated with FOLFIRINOX Versus Gemcitabine and Nab-Paclitaxel: A Population-Based Cohort Study. *Pancreas* **2019**, *48*, 920–926. [CrossRef]
22. Maisey, N.R.; Norman, A.R.; Hill, A.; Massey, A.; Oates, J.; Cunningham, D. CA19-9 as a Prognostic Factor in Inoperable Pancreatic Cancer: The Implication for Clinical Trials. *Br. J. Cancer* **2005**, *93*, 740–743. [CrossRef] [PubMed]
23. Chen, Y.; Yan, H.; Wang, Y.; Shi, Y.; Dai, G. Significance of Baseline and Change in Neutrophil-to-Lymphocyte Ratio in Predicting Prognosis: A Retrospective Analysis in Advanced Pancreatic Ductal Adenocarcinoma. *Sci. Rep.* **2017**, *7*, 753. [CrossRef] [PubMed]
24. Iwai, N.; Okuda, T.; Sakagami, J.; Harada, T.; Ohara, T.; Taniguchi, M.; Sakai, H.; Oka, K.; Hara, T.; Tsuji, T.; et al. Neutrophil to Lymphocyte Ratio Predicts Prognosis in Unresectable Pancreatic Cancer. *Sci. Rep.* **2020**, *10*, 65. [CrossRef]
25. Luo, G.; Guo, M.; Liu, Z.; Xiao, Z.; Jin, K.; Long, J.; Liu, L.; Liu, C.; Xu, J.; Ni, Q.; et al. Blood Neutrophil–Lymphocyte Ratio Predicts Survival in Patients with Advanced Pancreatic Cancer Treated with Chemotherapy. *Ann. Surg. Oncol.* **2015**, *22*, 670–676. [CrossRef]
26. Stotz, M.; Gerger, A.; Eisner, F.; Szkandera, J.; Loibner, H.; Ress, A.L.; Kornprat, P.; Zoughbi, W.A.; Seggewies, F.S.; Lackner, C.; et al. Increased Neutrophil-Lymphocyte Ratio Is a Poor Prognostic Factor in Patients with Primary Operable and Inoperable Pancreatic Cancer. *Br. J. Cancer* **2013**, *109*, 416–421. [CrossRef]

27. Mowbray, N.G.; Griffith, D.; Hammoda, M.; Shingler, G.; Kambal, A.; Al-Sarireh, B. A Meta-Analysis of the Utility of the Neutrophil-to-Lymphocyte Ratio in Predicting Survival after Pancreatic Cancer Resection. *HPB* **2018**, *20*, 379–384. [CrossRef] [PubMed]
28. Kadokura, M.; Ishida, Y.; Tatsumi, A.; Takahashi, E.; Shindo, H.; Amemiya, F.; Takano, S.; Fukasawa, M.; Sato, T.; Enomoto, N. Performance Status and Neutrophil-Lymphocyte Ratio Are Important Prognostic Factors in Elderly Patients with Unresectable Pancreatic Cancer. *J. Gastrointest. Oncol.* **2016**, *7*, 982–988. [CrossRef]
29. Guthrie, G.J.K.; Charles, K.A.; Roxburgh, C.S.D.; Horgan, P.G.; McMillan, D.C.; Clarke, S.J. The Systemic Inflammation-Based Neutrophil-Lymphocyte Ratio: Experience in Patients with Cancer. *Crit. Rev. Oncol. Hematol.* **2013**, *88*, 218–230. [CrossRef]
30. An, X.; Ding, P.R.; Li, Y.H.; Wang, F.H.; Shi, Y.X.; Wang, Z.Q.; He, Y.J.; Xu, R.H.; Jiang, W.Q. Elevated Neutrophil to Lymphocyte Ratio Predicts Survival in Advanced Pancreatic Cancer. *Biomarkers* **2010**, *15*, 516–522. [CrossRef] [PubMed]

cancers

MDPI

Review

Advancing Precision Medicine in PDAC: An Ethical Scoping Review and Call to Action for IHC Implementation

Lyanne A. Delgado-Coka [1,2,*], Lucia Roa-Peña [3], Andrew Flescher [2,†], Luisa F. Escobar-Hoyos [1,4,5,6,†] and Kenneth R. Shroyer [1,†]

1 Department of Pathology, Renaissance School of Medicine, Stony Brook University, Stony Brook, NY 11794, USA; luisa.escobar-hoyos@yale.edu (L.F.E.-H.)
2 Program of Public Health and Department of Preventative Medicine, Renaissance School of Medicine, Stony Brook University, Stony Brook, NY 11794, USA; andrew.flescher@stonybrook.edu
3 Department of Pathology, School of Medicine, Universidad Nacional de Colombia, Bogotá 110110, Colombia
4 Department of Therapeutic Radiology, Yale University, New Haven, CT 06510, USA
5 Department of Molecular Biophysics and Biochemistry, Yale University, New Haven, CT 06520, USA
6 Division of Oncology-Medicine-Oncology, Yale University, New Haven, CT 06510, USA
* Correspondence: lyanne.delgadocoka@stonybrookmedicine.edu
† Co-senior authors.

Simple Summary: Pancreatic cancer is among the deadliest cancers, with few patients qualifying for surgery, the only potential cure. For everyone else, treatments remain limited, and survival rates are disturbingly low. While expensive genetic tests only help a small fraction of patients, this review examines how a widely available and affordable laboratory test—immunohistochemistry (IHC)—could transform cancer care by matching patients with the most effective treatments. Instead of relying on a one-size-fits-all treatment approach for pancreatic cancer, using IHC to detect specific biomarkers can help guide clinicians in tailoring therapies to each patient's unique tumor, potentially improving outcomes while minimizing side effects. We analyze the ethical imperative to expand clinical trials of IHC-based testing, ensuring this life-saving technology reaches all communities, regardless of their resources or location. By implementing this cost-effective approach in hospitals worldwide, we could dramatically improve how we treat pancreatic cancer, saving lives and reducing healthcare expenditure while offering hope to patients and families facing this aggressive disease. This practical solution could become a model for delivering more equitable and effective cancer care across the healthcare system.

Abstract: Pancreatic ductal adenocarcinoma (PDAC) presents significant challenges in diagnosis, prevention, and treatment. Predictive biomarkers offer the potential to revolutionize clinical management, particularly in the preoperative setting, but their implementation requires careful consideration of ethical implications. This scoping review analyzes the ethical landscape of using immunohistochemistry (IHC) for molecular subtyping in PDAC, focusing on its utility, accessibility, and potential impact on patient care. We conducted a systematic literature search in the PubMed, Scopus and Google Scholar databases (2015–2025) using COVIDENCE, which identified 130 references. Of these, 79 were reviewed in a full-text format, and 9 ultimately met the inclusion criteria for our analysis. IHC offers several advantages as a companion diagnostic tool. It is relatively inexpensive, widely available in most pathology laboratories, and can be readily integrated into existing clinical workflows. This contrasts with more complex molecular subtyping methods, such as gene expression profiling, which can be costly, require specialized equipment and expertise, and may not be readily accessible in all clinical settings. Furthermore, accurate analysis of gene expression requires the localized targeting of individual cells; therefore, digesting the sample for bulk analysis would be less informative than using spatial localization techniques such as

IHC. Because biomarker regulation can occur at the level of transcription or translation, protein-level assessment via IHC is often more accurate than mRNA analysis. Standardized IHC protocols for biomarker assessment are therefore essential for translating the molecular subtyping of PDAC into clinically actionable treatment strategies, especially for aggressive subtypes like basal-like tumors. This readily deployable IHC-based approach can optimize therapy selection, maximizing patient benefits and minimizing exposure to ineffective and potentially toxic treatments. This review critically analyzes the ethical dimensions of this method, grounded in the principles of autonomy, beneficence, non-maleficence, and justice. The review urges the medical community to fully utilize the potential of IHC-driven molecular subtyping to improve outcomes in PDAC, while ensuring equitable and responsible access to the benefits of precision oncology for all patients.

Keywords: pancreatic ductal adenocarcinoma; PDAC; immunohistochemistry; IHC; molecular subtyping; ethical considerations; scoping review; autonomy; beneficence; non-maleficence; justice

1. Introduction

1.1. Highlighting the Persistent Challenge of Pancreatic Cancer

Pancreatic ductal adenocarcinoma (PDAC) remains a formidable challenge in oncology, characterized by a dismal prognosis and limited treatment options. Notably, despite advances in cancer care, only a minority (approximately 20%) of PDAC patients present with resectable disease, the only potentially curative intervention [1]. In contrast, for the remaining majority, systemic therapies offer limited long-term survival benefit [2]. This stark reality underscores the urgent need for innovative diagnostic and therapeutic strategies to improve outcomes for all PDAC patients, regardless of resectability. The aggressive nature of PDAC [3,4] and its projected rise as a leading cause of cancer-related death worldwide further underscore the pressing need for innovative approaches to treatment and patient management.

The current clinical management of PDAC heavily relies on the detection of incidental lesions via imaging studies, typically performed using computed tomography (CT) or magnetic resonance imaging (MRI conducted for unrelated medical issues). This is invariably followed by tissue biopsy [5] for histopathological confirmation and the assessment of tumor resectability (Figure 1) [6].

However, while often combined with neoadjuvant chemotherapy, this standard approach yields disappointingly low long-term survival [7]. This limitation stems from the fact that routine histopathology does not fully capture the complex biological behavior of PDAC, including its aggressiveness, chemoresistance, and metastatic potential. Additionally, the inherent chemoresistance of PDAC, coupled with significant genetic heterogeneity and a dense stromal microenvironment [8], further complicates effective treatment. As highlighted by Hilmi et al., PDAC exhibits both inter- and intratumoral heterogeneity, encompassing variations between patients and within individual tumors [9]. This heterogeneity manifests histologically, with diverse architectures like squamous/non-gland-forming (associated with the basal-like subtype) and glandular/gland-forming (associated with the classical subtype) varieties coexisting within the same tumor. Existing interventions, including surgery, radiation, chemotherapy, immunotherapy, and targeted therapies, often only provide marginal improvements in overall survival. This underscores the critical need to identify and validate novel biomarkers to enhance personalized treatment strategies.

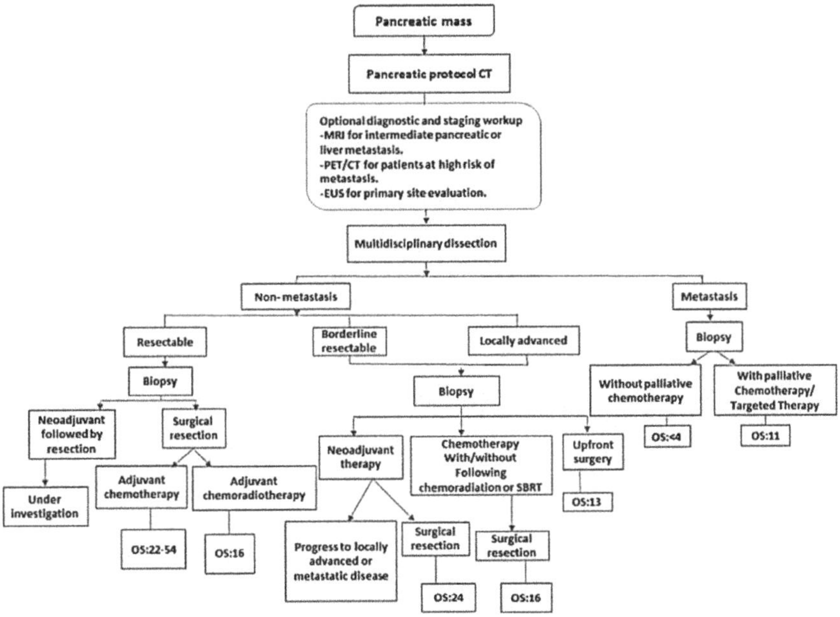

Figure 1. Current diagnostic and therapeutic pathways for staging, tumor response evaluation, and management of borderline or resectable PDAC. CT, computed tomography; EUS, endoscopic ultrasound; MRI, magnetic resonance imaging; PET, positron emission tomography; SBRT, stereotactic body radiation therapy. NCCN guidelines recommend that biopsy is not required for proof of malignancy prior to surgical resection and should not delay surgical resection in patients with high clinical suspicion of pancreatic cancer. Reprinted from Bugazia, Doaa et al. [5].

Transcriptomic subtyping has emerged as a valuable tool for predicting treatment response and tailoring therapy based on individual tumor biology [10,11]. Specifically, some studies demonstrate that basal-like PDAC carries a poorer prognosis and greater chemoresistance compared to the classical subtype, highlighting the importance of subtype-specific treatment strategies [12–15]. However, bulk transcriptomic analyses, while informative, are costly, difficult to implement clinically, and struggle to fully capture the complexities of intratumoral heterogeneity due to their inherent averaging effect across diverse cell populations. This averaging effect obscures critical information about the spatial distribution and interactions of different cell types within the tumor. As a result, the limitations of bulk transcriptomics have led to the proposal of continuous molecular gradients to better represent tumor characteristics, but these still lack information on intratumoral heterogeneity [9]. While single-cell studies offer higher resolution and have revealed the co-occurrence of classical and basal-like subtypes within individual tumors (hybrid/mixed tumors), including an intermediate phenotype with the co-expression of both classical and basal markers [16], their widespread clinical application remains limited by cost, complexity, and the need for specialized expertise. The application of deep learning models to H&E staining to identify intermediate tumors—where cells cannot be clearly assigned to either subtype—further emphasizes the complexity of PDAC heterogeneity and the need for more robust and accessible methods to characterize it [17,18]. Biomarker-driven testing is thus becoming a cornerstone of personalized medicine in PDAC [19]. By identifying specific tumor characteristics, such as basal subtype, clinicians can move away from a one-size-fits-all approach towards tailored therapies, maximizing efficacy and minimizing treatment-related toxicity [20]. Additionally, trials like SWOG S1505 reveal the difficulty of assessing chemotherapy efficacy in unselected populations, thus reinforcing the need for genomically driven precision and patient stratification. Consequently, integrating biomarker-enriched designs into neoadjuvant settings is therefore crucial for advancing precision medicine in PDAC [21].

1.2. The Promise of IHC in the Era of Advanced Molecular Technologies

While next-generation sequencing (NGS), artificial intelligence, and multi-omics have revolutionized our understanding of tumor biology, their complexity and cost limit widespread clinical application [22]. Although NGS accessibility and affordability are increasing, barriers to broader adoption persist, including investment costs, limited reimbursement, infrastructure limitations, centralization in specialized centers, and the lack of standardized guidelines. While the further research and development of targeted therapies, based on actionable mutations identified by NGS, remain crucial, immunohistochemistry (IHC) offers a pragmatic solution. As emphasized by Hilmi et al. (2025), IHC provides a cost-effective and readily accessible method for analyzing individual tumor cells while preserving their spatial context, enabling the more precise assessment of intratumoral heterogeneity compared to bulk transcriptomics or H&E staining alone [9]. This spatial resolution, which allows for the analysis of individual cells and their localization, is critical for understanding the complex interplay between different cell populations within the tumor microenvironment and for developing more accurate diagnostic and prognostic tools [23,24]. Furthermore, IHC avoids the averaging effect of bulk transcriptomics and the complexities of single-cell analysis, providing a practical and efficient approach to characterizing tumor heterogeneity, particularly when applied on a larger scale, where current methods are lacking [9]. To translate these theoretical advantages into clinical practice, IHC provides a readily available, cost-effective, and easily integrated method for biomarker detection in routine clinical practice, particularly benefiting those patients deemed unresectable, whose treatment goal is palliative care. Developing an IHC-based biomarker assay to guide neoadjuvant and adjuvant chemotherapy selection is critical. However, despite IHC's practical advantages, one key challenge remains, namely, identifying robust panels of IHC biomarkers that accurately predict treatment benefits and comprehensively capture the complexities of intratumoral heterogeneity.

To address these challenges and develop a robust IHC-based tool for predicting treatment response in PDAC, careful biomarker selection is essential, particularly given the limitations of traditional RNA-based approaches in distinguishing tumor-specific markers from stromal signatures. Building on established molecular knowledge, when selecting appropriate biomarkers for IHC analysis, ideal biomarkers should (i) be expressed by tumor cells only and not by stromal cells, (ii) have available antibodies that produce staining compatible with routine clinical use (considering intensity, ease of interpretation, and robustness), and (iii) be informative of treatment response independently of other tumor characteristics. Bulk transcriptomic analysis can misrepresent gene expression differences in PDAC subtypes. For instance, while *KRT6A* is associated with the epithelial component in both basal-like and classical tumors, its expression appears higher in basal-like tumors, simply due to their increased cellularity. This difficulty in interpreting true subtype-specific expression limits the clinical utility of bulk transcriptomics in PDAC [9]. Previous studies, along with our own findings, support the need for a panel of markers rather than single markers to address PDAC heterogeneity [12]. For example, Ragavhan et al. (2021) recently proposed a multiplex immunofluorescence panel including six markers (CLDN18.2, TFF1, GATA6, KRT17, KRT5, and S100A2) [16]. Several clinical trials like the PRODIGE-104 (NeoPREDICT) phase II trial aim to personalize neoadjuvant chemotherapy according to transcriptomic signatures in borderline resectable PDAC. To enhance the clinical utility of this trial, the IHC staining of a classical marker (e.g., CLDN18) and two specific basal markers (S100A2 and MUC16) were incorporated into the ancillary studies. This combined approach promises to refine patient prognosis and facilitate the implementation of these markers in routine clinical practice. Similarly, the ongoing NeoPANCOne phase II trial (NCT04472910) is evaluating the value of GATA6 (assessed by FISH and IHC) in predicting chemotherapy resistance in resectable PDAC [25]. Facilitating the assessment of tumor heterogeneity through IHC could also prove valuable in evaluating treatment response in trials of novel therapies that modulate PDAC phenotypes, such as epigenetic therapies [26,27].

In resectable PDAC, the indiscriminate administration of neoadjuvant chemotherapy can be detrimental, potentially leading to disease progression or toxicity that precludes curative surgery. Given the limited progress in developing robust predictive biomarkers, current patient selection for neoadjuvant chemotherapy relies on high-risk clinical and radiographic features, such as the detection of suspicious lymphadenopathy/metastases via imaging and elevated CA19-9 levels. IHC offers a practical approach to detecting prognostic and predictive biomarkers, holding immense potential for advancing personalized medicine in diverse healthcare settings. Leveraging IHC-based biomarkers in preoperative clinical trials allows for refined risk stratification and informs decisions regarding primary systemic therapy by identifying markers of therapy resistance or sensitivity. This personalized approach not only improves patient outcomes but also minimizes treatment-related toxicity and improves quality of life for patients and their families. Given the limitations of current PDAC management and the potential of IHC, this scoping review systematically evaluates the existing literature on IHC-based biomarkers in PDAC. This review will perform the following tasks:

- Delineate the current landscape of predictive IHC biomarkers in PDAC, highlighting successes and challenges.
- Analyze the ethical implications of using IHC to guide treatment decisions, focusing on the principles of autonomy, beneficence, non-maleficence, and justice.
- Assess how IHC-based approaches align with clinical needs and patient welfare.

By providing a comprehensive overview of the evidence, this review aims to inform future public health policies and clinical practices, ultimately promoting the effective integration of IHC into personalized medicine strategies for combating pancreatic cancer.

2. Methods

A scoping review was conducted between November 2024 and February 2025 using the PRISMA-ScR (Preferred Reporting Items for Systematic reviews and Meta-Analyses extension for Scoping Reviews) guidelines. A protocol was developed for the scoping review. This consisted of the following steps: exploratory investigation of the literature; the identification of research aims; the formulation of eligibility criteria; database searches; the screening and identification of studies; and extraction and charting of data.

Initial Search: To gain insight into the topic area, an exploratory investigation of the literature was undertaken, employing broad criteria across multiple databases. This investigation informed the selection of keywords for the searches and formulation of the eligibility criteria.

Search Strategy and Screening: The following electronic databases were searched: PubMed, Google Scholar, and Scopus. The most recent search was undertaken on 26 March 2025. Searches were conducted for each database from 2015 to the present. Keywords and Medical Subject Heading (MeSH) terms encompassed "Pancreatic Ductal Adenocarcinoma", "PDAC", "Transcriptomics", "Gene Expression Profiling", "Immunohistochemistry", "Molecular Subtyping", "Precision Medicine", "Biomarkers", "Predictive",

"Treatment Outcome", and "Clinical Utility". A total of 79 articles were identified from the search. The references of the articles were scanned to identify any additional relevant articles; no additional studies were included. Duplicates were removed.

Eligibility Criteria: Studies meeting the following criteria were included: the population criterion referred to patients diagnosed with PDAC; the concept criterion referred to studies investigating the ethical implications of IHC-based molecular subtyping in PDAC. This includes evaluations of IHC utility, accessibility, cost-effectiveness, and the impact on treatment decisions and patient outcomes. Studies were excluded if they were not related to PDAC; did not employ IHC-based molecular subtyping in PDAC; lacked sufficient clinical outcome data related to identified subtypes; or were reviews offering no novel insights (with some flexibility for context-providing narrative reviews). Studies on adults with all stages of PDAC were included. Studies in which biomarkers were not assessed as an outcome were excluded. All types of clinical trials were included to maximize the comprehensive nature of the search.

Study Selection: Two reviewers (L.A.D.-C, L.R.-P) conducted an initial screening of article titles and abstracts, followed by full-text assessments based on predefined inclusion and exclusion criteria. The selection process was documented using a PRISMA flow diagram, ultimately yielding nine publications for inclusion in this review.

Data Extraction: A standardized form was used to capture essential information from each study, incorporating both publication and scientific details. To assess the credibility and academic reach of the articles, we carefully documented several journal-related attributes like journal name, whether it was indexed (e.g., in PubMed, Web of Science, or Scopus), and its standard (two-year) impact factor. We noted whether the journal employed single-blind, double-blind, or open peer review, or if any indication of peer-review rigor was provided. This offered insight into the quality control measures taken before publication. Disclosures about conflicts of interest were documented. We also extracted the article title, study ID, and the country in which the study was conducted. In terms of scientific content, we noted the biomarkers analyzed, the methods used, the aim of the study, and the overall design (including the total number of participants and any comparisons made).

Data Synthesis and Analysis: A narrative synthesis summarized and analyzed the extracted data. Studies were grouped thematically (e.g., prognostic value, predictive value, technical challenges). Different subtyping approaches and their clinical implications were described and critically appraised. Finally, knowledge gaps and the future research directions were identified.

3. Results

Seventy-nine studies were identified through our search strategy. Following deduplication, 75 studies remained and were screened by title, abstract, and full text, resulting in the inclusion of 9 retrospective studies. Figure 2 presents a flow diagram, adapted from the PRISMA flow chart, of the literature retrieval process.

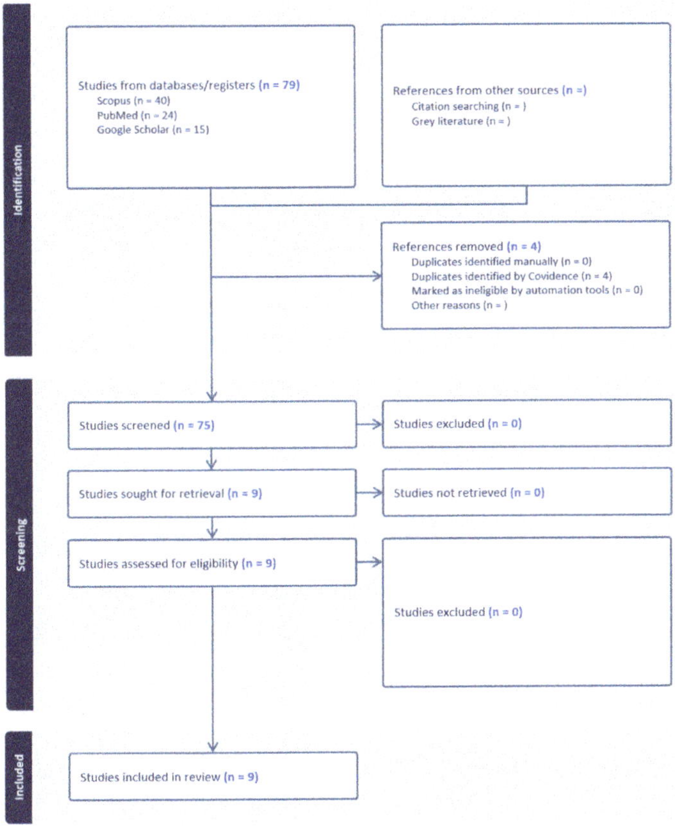

Figure 2. Flow diagram illustrates process of study identification, screening, and identification of studies for inclusion. Adapted from PRISMA flow diagram.

Table 1 presents the biomarkers measured in the studies selected. The most frequently evaluated biomarker was GATA6, measured in four of the studies, followed by Keratin17 (KRT17) and Keratin81 (KRT81), which were included in two studies, respectively. Several studies investigated the potential of various biomarkers, including CREB3L1, GATA6, KRT81, HNF1A, and KRT17, to predict treatment response and prognosis. For instance, Xu et al. (2025) found that CREB3L1 expression was lower in patients who responded well to immunotherapy, suggesting its potential as a biomarker for treatment selection [28]. Similarly, studies exploring GATA6 as a prognostic marker indicated its association with enhanced immune surveillance and improved outcomes in certain PDAC subtypes. Other studies explored combinations of markers, such as KRT81 and HNF1A, to refine subtyping and predict responses to specific therapies like erlotinib and FOLFIRINOX. These findings highlight the potential of IHC-based molecular subtyping to personalize PDAC treatment.

Table 1. Characteristics and outcomes of published studies.

Journal Name	Journal Indexed	Impact Factor	Journal Peer Review Process	Conflict of Interest	Author	Title	Study ID	Country in Which the Study Conducted	Biomarker(s)	Methods	Aim of Study	Study Design	Total Number of Participants	Comparison	Outcome	Conclusion
Journal for ImmunoTherapy of Cancer	Yes	10.3	Single anonymized	None	Xu, 2025 [28]	CREB3L1 facilitates pancreatic tumor progression and reprograms intratumoral tumor-associated macrophages to shape an immunotherapy-resistance microenvironment	https://doi.org/10.1136/jitc-2024-010029	China	CREB3L1	IHC	Explore CREB3L1's role in PDAC and its correlation with clinical features	Cohort study	94	Responders (ORR) vs. non- ORR; IHC-based CREB3L1 expression	Lower CREB3L1 expression found in those responding well to immunotherapy	CREB3L1 expression predicts immunotherapy response and outcome in PDAC
Cell Reports Medicine	Yes	11.7	Single anonymized	None	Van Eijck, 2024 [29]	GATA6 identifies an immune-enriched phenotype linked to favorable outcomes in patients with pancreatic cancer undergoing upfront surgery	https://doi.org/10.1016/j.xcrm.2024.101557	Other: the Netherlands	GATA6	Transcriptomic profiling/IHC	Investigate prognostic value of GATA6 IHC in treatment-naive vs. gemcitabine-based nCRT-treated PDAC patients	Cohort study	88	GATA6 expression, immune cell infiltration, and survival in treatment-naive vs. chemotherapy-treated patients	Strongly treatment-naive GATA6 tumors exhibit enhanced immunological features and immunostimulatory mechanisms	GATA6 expression correlates with distinct immune landscapes and better outcomes, underscoring its prognostic significance
The Journal of Pathology: Clinical Research	Yes	3.4	Single anonymized	None	Rao, 2024 [27]	KRT81 and HNF1A expression in pancreatic ductal adenocarcinoma: investigation of predictive and prognostic value of immunohistochemistry-based subtyping	https://doi.org/10.1002/2056-4538.12377	Other: Germany	KRT81 and HNF1A	IHC	Validate revised subtyping in a controlled phase III trial (CONKO-005) assessing erlotinib + gemcitabine vs. gemcitabine	Cohort study	269	Gemcitabine–erlotinib combination vs. gemcitabine only	HNF1A-positive subtype benefited more from gemcitabine–erlotinib compared with KRT81-positive or double-negative subtypes	KRT81/HNF1A IHC serves as a partial surrogate for RNA-defined PDAC subtypes and informs potential treatment choices
Clinical Cancer Research	Yes	10.4	double-blind review	A. Stenzinger reports receiving speaker's bureau honoraria from AstraZeneca, Illumina, Novartis, and Thermo Fisher Scientific and is a consultant/advisory board member for AstraZeneca, Bristol-Myers Squibb, Illumina, Novartis, and Thermo Fisher Scientific. M.R. Sprick is listed as a co-inventor on a pending patent application on the use of KRT81 and HNF1A for the stratification of PDAC patients. This is owned by HI-STEM gGmbH. No potential conflicts of interest were disclosed by the other authors.	Muckenhuber, 2018 [30]	Pancreatic Ductal Adenocarcinoma Subtyping Using the Biomarkers Hepatocyte Nuclear Factor-1A and Cytokeratin-81 Correlates with Outcome and Treatment Response	https://doi.org/10.1158/1078-0432.CCR-17-2180	Other: Germany	HNF1A and KRT81	IHC	Validate HNF1A/KRT81 subtypes in resectable and unresectable PDAC, and assess their predictive value for chemotherapy	Cohort study	204	Survival and treatment response (FOLFIRINOX vs. gemcitabine) by HNF1A/KRT81 IHC subtypes	KRT81-positive patients derived less benefit from FOLFIRINOX; HNF1A-positive patients had a significantly better initial response to FOLFIRINOX compared with gemcitabine	An IHC-based HNF1A/KRT81 classification reliably identifies PDAC subtypes, aiding pre-therapeutic stratification and personalized therapy

Table 1. *Cont.*

Journal Name	Journal Indexed	Impact Factor	Journal Peer Review Process	Conflict of Interest	Author	Title	Study ID	Country in Which the Study Conducted	Biomarker(s)	Methods	Aim of Study	Study Design	Total Number of Participants	Comparison	Outcome	Conclusion
Translational Research	Yes	6.4	Single anonymized	MFB has received research funding from Celgene, Frame Therapeutics, and Lead Pharma, and has acted as a consultant to Servier and Olympus. HWML Consultant or advisory role: BMS, Daiichy, Dragonfly, Eli Lilly, MSD, Nordic Pharma, Servier. Research funding and/or medication supply: Bayer, BMS, Celgene, Janssen, Incyte, Eli Lilly, MSD, Nordic Pharma, Philips, Roche, Servier. Speaker role: Astellas, Daiichy, Novartis. JPM has acted as a consultant to AbbVie. JWW Consultant or advisory role: MSD, Servier, Astra Zeneca, Research funding: MSD, Nordic, Servier. Speaker role: MSD, Servier. None of these parties were involved in the design of this study or drafting of the manuscript. All other authors declare no conflicts of interest.	Lansbergen, 2024 [31]	Transcriptome-based classification to predict FOLFIRINOX response in a real-world metastatic pancreatic cancer cohort	https://doi.org/10.1016/j.trsl.2024.08.002	Other: the Netherlands	GATA6 and keratin-17 (KRT17)	IHC	Assess predictive value of molecular subtypes for FOLFIRINOX response in advanced PDAC	Cohort study	86	IHC-based stratification into good vs. poor responders to FOLFIRINOX	GATA6 H-score reliably predicts response to FOLFIRINOX	GATA6 (±KRT17) IHC can be integrated into diagnostic routines to guide chemotherapy choice and inform patient prognosis
Scientific Reports	Yes	3.8	Single anonymized	The authors declare no competing interests.	Duan, 2021 [25]	The value of GATA6 immunohistochemistry and computer-assisted diagnosis to predict clinical outcome in advanced pancreatic cancer	https://doi.org/10.1038/s41598-021-94544-3	Canada	GATA6	IHC	Evaluate GATA6 IHC as a single biomarker for advanced PDAC and examine computer-assisted analysis	Cohort study	110	Response to chemotherapy according to GATA6 IHC	Among mFFX-treated patients, disease progression was 39% in GATA6-low vs. 12% in GATA6-high PDAC	GATA6 IHC can serve as a single predictive biomarker for mFFX response in advanced PDAC; warrants prospective validation
American Journal of Clinical Pathology	Yes	5.4	double-blind review	K.R.S. and L.F.E.-H. are consultants for KDx Diagnostics. E.M.B. is an employee of Perthera and owns stocks in the company. He also has consulted for Theralink Technologies and received compensation as chair of the Science Advisory Board and owns stock in the company. The additional authors have nothing to disclose.	Delgado-Coka, 2024 [12]	Keratin 17 is a prognostic and predictive biomarker in pancreatic ductal adenocarcinoma	https://doi.org/10.1093/AJCP/AQAE038	United States	Keratin 17	IHC	Define K17 IHC thresholds for chemotherapy response to optimize therapeutic interventions in PDAC	Cohort study	305	K17 expression in the context of survival after adjuvant chemotherapy	High K17 marks resistance to gemcitabine-based therapies and predicts better response to 5-FU-based regimens	K17 IHC testing serves as a rapid predictive marker to guide the best chemotherapy choice based on tumor expression profiles
Scientific Reports	Yes	3.8	Single anonymized	CI-D receives research support from BMS. All other authors (TS, AH, MT, K-Ki, YJH, K-Ka, TY, SK, Ko-K, KO, KG, NO, JM, YS, TH, JS) declare that they have no conflicts of interest in relation to this work.	Shibayama, 2024 [26]	Combination immunohistochemistry for CK5/6, p63, GATA6, and HNF4a predicts clinical outcome in treatment-naive pancreatic ductal adenocarcinoma	https://doi.org/10.1038/s41598-024-65900-w	Other: Japan	CK5/6, p63, GATA6, and HNF4a	Immunohistochemistry (IHC) on endoscopic ultrasound-guided fine-needle aspiration biopsy (EUS-FNAB) samples	Determine surrogate biomarkers (K5/6, p63, GATA6, HNF4a) for molecular signatures in advanced PDAC	Cohort study	190	IHC-based subtypes (Classical, Transitional, Basal-like)	Basal-like pattern correlated with squamous differentiation and worst survival; (Transitional/Basal vs. Classical) = poor prognosis	IHC expression patterns identify Basal-like PDAC, aiding in prognostic assessment and therapeutic decision-making.

Table 1. *Cont.*

Journal Name	Journal Indexed	Impact Factor	Journal Peer Review Process	Conflict of Interest	Author	Title	Study ID	Country in Which the Study Conducted	Biomarker(s)	Methods	Aim of Study	Study Design	Total Number of Participants	Comparison	Outcome	Conclusion
Cancers	Yes	5.2	Single anonymized	Authors declare no conflict of interest	Okada, 2021 [32]	Identification of LAMC2 as a prognostic and predictive biomarker for determining response to gemcitabine-based therapy in pancreatic ductal adenocarcinoma	https://doi.org/10.1016/j.ejca.2020.12.031	Japan	LAMC2 (Laminin γ2)	IHC on EUS-FNAB samples.	Identify and validate biomarkers for gemcitabine-based therapy response in PDAC	Retrospective analysis of datasets and clinical cohorts	423	LAMC2 expression compared with overall survival, relapse-free survival, and gemcitabine response	High LAMC2 correlates with poor prognosis and reduced response to gemcitabine	LAMC2 serves as a prognostic and predictive biomarker for gemcitabine-based therapies in PDAC

Our scoping review identified several key predictive immunohistochemical (IHC) biomarkers for pancreatic ductal adenocarcinoma (PDAC). The review of studies highlights the critical role of predictive biomarkers in pancreatic ductal adenocarcinoma (PDAC) and their potential to enhance clinical outcomes. PDAC is characterized by its aggressive nature and poor prognosis, with a median overall survival (OS) of approximately 10–12 months for advanced stages and up to 28 months for resected cases with optimal adjuvant chemotherapy [33]. Recent research has identified various molecular subtypes of PDAC, with classifications based on gene expression patterns correlating with treatment responses and prognostic outcomes. These subtypes, such as the classical and basal-like groups defined by Moffitt et al. [34] and the quasimesenchymal and squamous subtypes identified by Collisson [15] and Bailey [35], offer potential for personalized therapy. For instance, the basal-like subtype is associated with poorer prognosis and chemoresistance. While promising, molecular subtyping has limitations. Gene expression can vary within a tumor, and the chosen technology may not capture all relevant molecular features, potentially leading to misclassification and hindering clinical translation [13,36,37].

Specific biomarkers such as KRT17 [12,38,39], GATA6 [26], HNF1A, and KRT81 [27] have emerged as significant predictors of clinical outcomes. GATA6, for example, has been shown to correlate positively with classical phenotype markers and negatively with basal-like markers in treatment-naive tumor [25]. The expression of KRT81 and HNF1A has also been linked to patient stratification, with implications for treatment response to therapies like erlotinib [27]. Briefly, IHC subtyping based on KRT81 and HNF1A effectively stratified PDAC into clinically relevant subgroups, with HNF1A expression correlating with superior overall and disease-free survival compared to KRT81. These results underscore the importance of identifying molecular subtypes and biomarkers to optimize patient stratification and guide individualized treatment strategies. Moreover, the role of KRT17 as a prognostic and predictive biomarker in pancreatic ductal adenocarcinoma (PDAC) sheds significant light on its potential utility in clinical settings. The identification of KRT17 as not only a marker of prognosis but also a predictive factor for treatment response represents a pivotal advancement in our understanding of PDAC pathology [12]. This research supports the implementation of KRT17 as a companion diagnostic marker, providing critical therapeutic insights that could guide more personalized treatment plans [12]. By incorporating KRT17 into routine diagnostic assessments, clinicians could better predict disease course, tailor treatment modalities to individual patients, and ultimately improve clinical outcomes in PDAC. Such findings reinforce the necessity of integrating robust molecular markers in the management of complex cancers, highlighting a step forward in the evolution of personalized oncology.

Overall, these studies suggest that the integration of these biomarkers into clinical practice is crucial for enhancing patient management. The development of immunohistochemistry (IHC) assays for these biomarkers could facilitate their implementation in routine diagnostics, allowing for more personalized treatment approaches. However, these studies promptly reported that the retrospective nature of the analyses represented a limitation, suggesting that further prospective multi-center studies with larger patient populations and that the ongoing clinical trials evaluating the utility of these biomarkers in guiding treatment decisions in randomized controlled trials are needed [31,40]. The potential for these biomarkers to refine treatment selection and improve outcomes in PDAC is promising, but further studies are needed to establish their clinical applicability and effectiveness in diverse patient populations. In conclusion, the identification and validation of prognostic and predictive biomarkers in PDAC represent significant advancements in the quest for improved clinical outcomes. By enabling more precise patient stratification and personalized treatment strategies, these biomarkers have the potential to transform the management of this challenging malignancy (Figure 3).

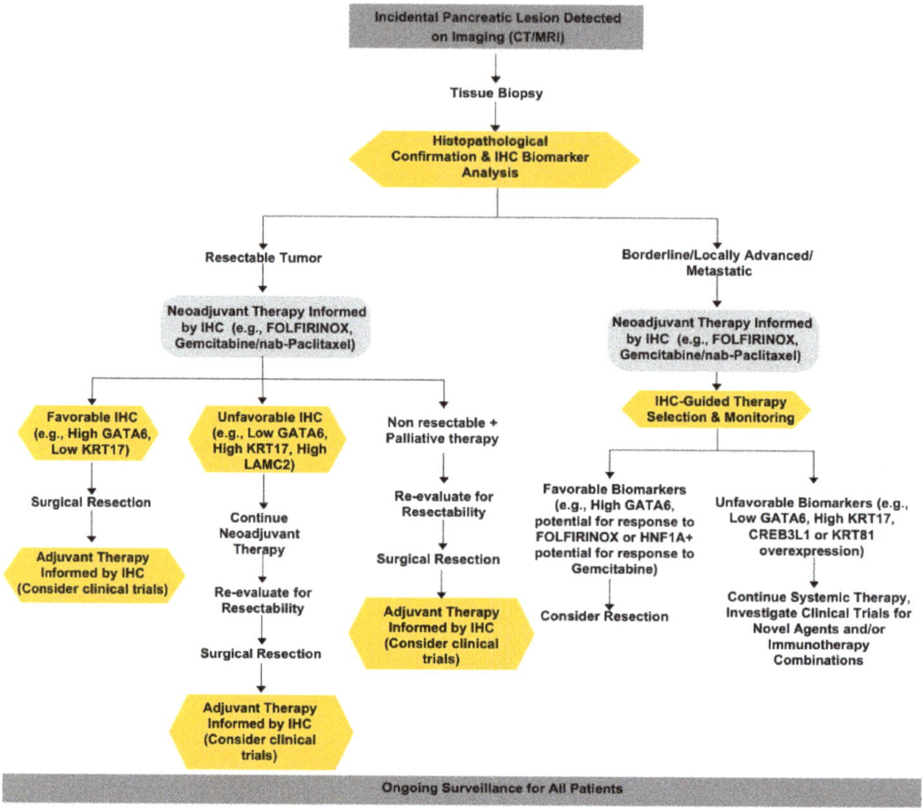

Figure 3. Proposed clinical management of pancreatic cancer patients.

3.1. The Utility and Clinical Imperative of IHC Biomarkers in PDAC

Mosele et al. (2024) highlight a crucial point: despite the theoretical promise of next-generation sequencing (NGS), its clinical utility in advanced PDAC remains limited in routine practice [41]. While NGS can identify a wide range of genomic alterations, only germline BRCA1/2 alterations currently hold ESCAT level I status (strong evidence of clinical actionability) in this setting. Although KRAS G12C mutations, detectable by PCR, provide a readily actionable target, they represent a small minority (1.5%) of PDAC cases [41,42]. This disparity between identifying molecular alterations and demonstrating improved patient outcomes underscores the central challenge—the "utility dilemma". In contrast, immunohistochemistry (IHC), a technique used to visualize the presence and localization of specific proteins within a tissue sample, offers a pragmatic and readily implementable approach for assessing biomarker expression for several key reasons. IHC involves using labeled antibodies that bind specifically to the target protein. These antibodies are then detected through various methods, allowing for the visualization of the protein's distribution within the tissue. Firstly, IHC is more cost-effective than more complex molecular techniques (e.g., gene expression profiling), making it a practical option for broader clinical use. Secondly, IHC is widely available in most pathology laboratories, requiring standard equipment and readily accessible reagents and thus eliminating the need for specialized infrastructure or highly trained personnel. This widespread availability facilitates easier integration into existing clinical workflows and diagnostic pathways. This is particularly important in developing countries, where the infrastructure for advanced molecular techniques is limited and expensive. Thirdly, IHC provides spatial context crucial for accurate interpretation, allowing for the visualization and assessment of protein expression within the tissue microenvironment and at the single-cell level. This is particularly important in heterogeneous tumors, where bulk molecular analyses may mask critical differences in expression patterns across distinct cell populations. Finally, for biomarkers whose regulation occurs predominantly at the translational rather than transcriptional level, IHC offers a more accurate representation of protein activity and functional status, directly measuring the protein product rather than the intermediary mRNA transcript. These combined advantages position IHC as a highly practical and readily deployable method that can be used for evaluating target biomarkers in routine clinical practice [43]. This rapid, readily available approach can inform timely treatment decisions, particularly crucial given the often-indiscriminate and potentially toxic "one-size-fits-all" approach to chemotherapy employed when treating metastatic PDAC [19]. By identifying patients most likely to benefit from specific treatments, based on IHC-detectable biomarkers, we can move towards a more personalized and effective approach to PDAC management, ultimately improving patient outcomes and minimizing harm.

3.2. The Utility Dilemma: Balancing Cost, Actionability, and Patient Benefit

The utility dilemma in PDAC centers on the challenge of balancing the potential benefits of advanced molecular diagnostics with the realities of cost, turnaround time, and clinical actionability. While the European Society for Medical Oncology (ESMO) guidelines recommend the use of tumor NGS within clinical genomics programs and trials, particularly for accessing PARP and NRG1 inhibitors [41], this recommendation is contingent on access to targeted therapies and local cost-effectiveness assessments. This highlights the inherent tension within the utility dilemma: the desire to provide cutting-edge diagnostics versus the responsible stewardship of healthcare resources. NGS, while offering a comprehensive genomic profile, is expensive, requires specialized infrastructure, and has long turnaround times, making it often incompatible with the rapid progression of PDAC. Furthermore, many identified alterations lack clear clinical actionability in the absence of readily available targeted therapies, diminishing the immediate patient benefit despite the high cost of testing. This raises the crucial ethical question: is it justifiable to expend significant resources on testing that yields limited actionable information, especially in a resource-constrained environment?

3.3. IHC: A Value-Based Solution to the Utility Dilemma

Immunohistochemistry (IHC) presents a strategically and fiscally responsible alternative to patient stratification in pancreatic ductal adenocarcinoma (PDAC) treatment. IHC is a technique that uses antibodies to detect specific proteins in tissue samples, allowing for the identification of biomarkers that can guide treatment decisions. In the US healthcare system, which is grappling with a trillion-dollar debt, the indiscriminate use of costly systemic chemotherapies, with often-limited efficacy in advanced PDAC [37], further exacerbates this financial burden. By using IHC to stratify patients based on their tumor biology, clinicians can select targeted therapies that are more likely to be effective, potentially minimizing the use of ineffective treatments and their associated costs and toxicities.

Compared to more expensive molecular profiling techniques like next-generation sequencing (NGS), IHC is cost-effective and widely available, making it a readily deployable solution for refining treatment selection. Its fiscal advantage is particularly relevant in the context of value-based healthcare, where the goal is to optimize patient outcomes while managing cost [36,44]. By directing resources towards targeted therapies that are more likely to benefit specific patient subgroups, IHC-guided treatment stratification can potentially improve the cost-effectiveness of PDAC care. In addition to its financial benefits, IHC also offers rapid results, often within 24 h with automated systems. This is a critical advantage given the aggressive nature of PDAC, where timely treatment initiation is crucial. The rapid turnaround time of IHC allows for prompt treatment decisions, maximizing the opportunity for intervention and aligning with the ethical imperative to avoid delays in care. In contrast, NGS results may take several weeks, potentially delaying treatment and compromising patient outcomes.

The current "one-size-fits-all" approach, particularly using FOLFIRINOX or gemcitabine/nab-paclitaxel without biomarker guidance, carries significant ethical baggage [21,45]. Subjecting patients to potentially unnecessary toxicity without a commensurate survival benefit raises serious ethical concerns. IHC-guided treatment selection has the potential to minimize these harmful effects, improving patient quality of life and reducing the burden on patients, caregivers, and families.

IHC has already demonstrated its value in guiding treatment decisions in other cancers. For example, in breast cancer, IHC is routinely used to assess estrogen receptor (ER), progesterone receptor (PR), and HER2 status [46]. Patients with ER/PR-positive tumors benefit from endocrine therapy [47], while those with HER2-positive tumors are candidates for targeted therapies like trastuzumab [48]. Similarly, in non-small-cell lung cancer, IHC is used to detect PD-L1 expression, which predicts the response to immune checkpoint inhibitors [49,50]. By tailoring treatment to the biology of each individual tumor, IHC has improved the outcomes and quality of life for patients with these cancers.

While NGS can identify alterations in 12–25% of PDAC cases [51,52], many lack immediate clinical utility [17]. IHC offers a pragmatic approach that can be used to address the utility dilemma by providing actionable information linked to established therapeutic strategies (31). Prioritizing IHC, therefore, not only aligns with financial responsibility but also upholds the ethical principles of beneficence and non-maleficence. A concerted effort to assess biomarkers with cost-effective methods like IHC is essential for realizing the tangible clinical benefits of precision oncology and ensuring equitable access to potentially life-saving diagnostic information [44].

3.4. Ethical Principles Guiding the Implementation of IHC Predictive Biomarkers

The ethical imperatives underlying pancreatic cancer care extend far beyond mere utility or efficiency. The current state of PDAC care, characterized by high mortality and limited treatment options, represents a significant challenge. This applies not just clinically, but ethically. The slow translation of research into clinical tools constitutes an ethical crisis demanding immediate action.

3.5. Autonomy

Patient autonomy requires individuals to make informed decisions about their medical care, which includes a comprehensive understanding of the purpose, implications, and limitations of, as well as alternatives to, IHC testing. This informed decision-making process is best achieved through shared decision-making, where clinicians and patients collaborate to make treatment choices aligned with the patient's values and preferences [53]. IHC can facilitate this process by providing relatively easy-to-understand information compared to complex genomic data. However, clinicians must carefully present this information to ensure patient comprehension without causing information overload [54], particularly considering the difficult prognosis associated with PDAC and the emotional vulnerability of patients and their families. Maintaining patient trust is paramount, which necessitates transparency regarding the rationale for using IHC and interpreting its results [55]. Relying exclusively on "physician preference" to guide treatment decisions is unacceptable. Instead, physicians have a responsibility to engage in open communication with patients, actively discussing preferences and values, to ensure treatment recommendations reflect a genuinely shared decision-making process. [56]. Despite the benefits of IHC and shared decision-making, the application of patient autonomy in the context of novel diagnostics like IHC raises several important questions.

(1) The Right to the "Best" vs. the Right to Choose: Patient autonomy does not guarantee a right to the newest treatments or diagnostic tools simply because they exist. While patients have the right to make informed choices about their care, this right applies to available and appropriate options, considering factors such as cost, availability, and proven benefit. The principle of justice requires prioritizing interventions with established clinical utility over those with uncertain benefits or limited access, ensuring equitable resource allocation.

(2) Autonomy, Privilege, and the Zero-Sum Game: A "right" to the newest interventions for one patient might limit resources for others that are less privileged, highlighting the potential for privilege to influence autonomous decision-making. Prioritizing cost-effective, readily available tools like IHC becomes an ethical imperative to ensure equitable access to essential diagnostic information. Transparent communication about the benefits and limitations of different companion diagnostic approaches is crucial for empowering all patients to make informed decisions, regardless of socioeconomic status.

(3) Shared Decision-Making—Balancing Patient Input and Physician Expertise: Effective shared decision-making necessitates open communication and mutual respect. Physicians should provide clear information about available options, while patients share their values and preferences. In PDAC subtyping, this involves discussing the trade-offs between IHC and more complex molecular testing, considering factors such as cost, turnaround time, and clinical impact. While patient preferences are paramount, physicians have a responsibility to guide patients toward medically and ethically appropriate decisions based on the best available evidence [57]. The physician's role extends beyond merely presenting options; it includes contextualizing those options within the framework of evidence-based medicine and ethical principles. This collaborative, evidence-based approach ensures personalized care while mitigating potential therapeutic misconceptions and upholding responsible resource allocation. It fosters trust by demonstrating transparency and a commitment to compassionate care and scientifically rigorous practice. The goal is to arrive at a decision that respects the patient's autonomy while adhering to the physician's responsibility to provide the best possible care based on the strongest available evidence.

3.6. Beneficence

The principle of beneficence dictates that healthcare providers should act in the best interests of their patients, maximizing benefits and minimizing potential harm [54]. IHC-based predictive biomarkers can promote beneficence by identifying the patients most likely to respond to specific therapies, improving treatment success rates, guiding the selection of less toxic therapies when appropriate, and potentially leading to earlier intervention. Furthermore, IHC can contribute to the development of more effective treatment strategies overall by facilitating the identification and validation of new therapeutic targets. However, the pursuit of beneficence must be tempered by a realistic assessment of the limitations of IHC and the potential for false-positive or false-negative results. Moreover, the scientific community must be vigilant against the unequal advancement and inclusion of biomarkers, a practice that can skew the landscape of available diagnostic and therapeutic options. This inequality often arises not purely from scientific need or clinical urgency but from a milieu influenced by publication pressures, funding opportunities, and the pursuit of prestige. These dynamics can cultivate an environment where certain biomarkers are disproportionately highlighted, not for their clinical utility but for their novelty and the academic currency they provide. This brings to light the concern of "self-promoted experts" who, perhaps driven by the need for career advancement, might disproportionately endorse specific biomarkers. Such endorsements can perpetuate a cycle where biomarkers are pursued aggressively at the expense of others, potentially sidelining equal or more effective alternatives that lack similar scientific or commercial backing. To navigate this complex landscape, it is essential for the medical community to foster a robust framework for validation and replication, emphasizing transparency and integrity in research. Further, engagement in multidisciplinary discourse and critique should be encouraged, ensuring that decisions around the adoption of specific IHC markers in PDAC are grounded in a broad consensus rather than the narrow interests of a few. It is only through rigorous scholarly examination and strict adherence to ethical standards that we can ensure the pursuit of beneficence in medical practice is genuinely fulfilled, thereby advancing patient care in both effective and morally responsible ways [58].

3.7. Non-Maleficence

This principle, often summarized as "do no harm", requires healthcare providers to avoid causing unnecessary harm to patients. Given the known complexity and heterogeneity of PDAC, we and others have advocated for the inclusion of companion diagnostic markers that add predictive value in the clinical management of patients from the time of PDAC diagnosis (Figure 2) [12,59]. For example, the high expression of the transcription factor GATA6 and low expression of KRT17 have been associated with better responses to FOLFIRINOX chemotherapy in PDAC patients. In contrast, low GATA6 expression has been linked to a poor response to FOLFIRINOX but potentially better outcomes with gemcitabine-based regimens [25]. By incorporating these IHC biomarkers into treatment decision-making, clinicians can select therapies that are more likely to be effective based on the molecular profile of each patient's tumor. This approach not only maximizes the potential for therapeutic benefit but also minimizes the risk of exposing patients to ineffective and potentially harmful treatments. It is important to note that while IHC itself is a minimally invasive procedure with minimal direct risks to patients, the potential harm lies in the misinterpretation or misapplication of IHC results, which could lead to suboptimal treatment choices. Therefore, it is crucial that IHC biomarker testing is performed in accredited laboratories with rigorous quality control measures and interpreted by experienced pathologists to ensure accurate and reliable results are obtained [45]. As our understanding of PDAC biology continues to evolve, the use of IHC biomarkers to guide treatment selection will become increasingly important in upholding the principle of non-maleficence and providing the best possible care for PDAC patients.

3.8. Justice

The principle of justice demands the fair and equitable distribution of healthcare resources. This is particularly relevant to the implementation of IHC biomarkers in PDAC, given the existing disparities in access to advanced cancer care [60]. IHC's lower cost and wider accessibility, including in resource-limited settings, ensure that more patients can benefit from personalized treatment strategies. This is crucial in PDAC, where socioeconomic factors significantly influence access to care and outcomes. In contrast, expensive molecular tests like NGS may only be available in specialized centers or to patients with comprehensive insurance coverage or financial resources [61]. This disparity can create a two-tiered system, where some patients have access to cutting-edge molecular profiling while others are left with a one-size-fits-all approach. Prioritizing IHC as a cost-effective tool for patient stratification can help to close the treatment disparity gap and ensure that all patients, regardless of financial status or location, have the opportunity to receive tailored therapies based on their tumor's molecular profile.

Moreover, IHC's technical simplicity compared to NGS allows for more widespread adoption across different healthcare settings, including community hospitals and clinics. This decentralization of diagnostic capabilities can bridge the access gap between academic medical centers and local healthcare providers, enabling more patients to receive personalized care closer to home [62]. This is especially relevant for PDAC patients, who may face challenges related to transportation, time off work, and caregiver responsibilities when seeking care at distant, specialized centers. While IHC may serve as an interim solution, it facilitates more widespread treatment as we continue to progress towards discovering a definitive cure—something every patient rightfully deserves. However, the centralization of advanced molecular technologies in specialized centers and the lack of sociodemographic diversity among cancer clinical trial participants represent major barriers to advancing cancer care for the entire patient population [63]. Health systems often lack the specialized bioinformatics capacity required to analyze and interpret the complex data generated by tumor sequencing [64]. Despite evidence demonstrating improved outcomes in high-volume centers, a significant proportion of PDAC patients are diagnosed and treated in community hospitals with limited access to advanced molecular technologies and/or resources to use the information, highlighting the disparity in access related to the location of treatment [65]. To truly honor the spirit of medical innovation and ethical integrity, we must foster strategies that embrace the diversity of our society and advance equity within clinical trials, meticulously balancing the fine line between individual care and collective advancements in health sciences [66]. This commitment will ensure that our pursuit of knowledge remains just, transparent, and fundamentally aligned with the enduring welfare of humanity. By leveraging the equity-promoting characteristics of IHC, we can work towards a more just and inclusive approach to precision medicine in PDAC, ensuring that all patients have access to the diagnostic tools and tailored therapies that can improve their outcomes and quality of life. This commitment to reducing access disparities aligns with the ethical principle of justice, which calls for the fair distribution of healthcare resources and the elimination of unjust barriers to care.

4. Discussion

The pursuit of improved outcomes in pancreatic ductal adenocarcinoma (PDAC) necessitates a multi-faceted approach, and transcriptomic subtyping holds significant promise in this endeavor. As outlined in the preceding sections, large-scale, multi-center, and interdisciplinary efforts are crucial. Initiatives like COMPASS, PREDICT-PACA, Precision Promise, and others represent critical steps toward developing more effective, personalized treatment regimens. The PRIMUS-002 trial, performed as part of the PRECISION-Panc platform, exemplifies a prospective approach, integrating genomic and transcriptomic data with circulating biomarkers and clinical outcomes. This holistic approach, incorporating preoperative biopsies and resection specimens, is essential for understanding the dynamic interplay between molecular subtypes, therapeutic responses, and tumor heterogeneity. Critically, biomarker-based preoperative trials are paramount for validating predictive factors, moving beyond retrospective analyses to directly inform clinical decision-making.

However, the situation is further complicated by the scarcity of biomarker-driven clinical trials for PDAC patients, the inherent difficulties in conducting adequately powered trials in small molecular subgroups, and the practical considerations of turnaround time, cost-effectiveness, and reimbursement for molecular analyses. Innovative platforms like PRECISION-Panc, EPPIC, and Precision Promise represent potential solutions, integrating discovery, preclinical development, and innovative clinical trial design. The PRECISION-Panc Master Protocol, with its focus on EUS-guided biopsies and peripheral blood sampling, demonstrates a pragmatic approach to real-world personalized clinical trials, achieving a high success rate in molecular profiling.

5. Ethical Considerations: Utility, Equity, and Transparency

The advancement of transcriptomic subtyping and biomarker-driven approaches in PDAC is not solely a scientific endeavor; it is deeply intertwined with ethical considerations. Several key tensions emerge when analyzing this progress through the lens of ethical principles:

Utility vs. Equity: The principle of utility, aiming for the greatest good for the greatest number, is central to the pursuit of precision medicine. While sophisticated molecular profiling offers the potential for significant benefit, its high cost, complexity, and limited availability creates disparities in access. This aligns with the observation that the high cost, complexity, and limited availability of advanced technologies create significant disparities in access, as not all patients or healthcare systems have the resources to implement them. Patients treated in specialized centers with access to cutting-edge technologies and clinical trials are more likely to benefit from these developments than those treated in resource-constrained settings. This disparity raises fundamental questions of justice and fairness. A truly ethical approach demands a commitment to ensuring that the benefits of precision medicine are accessible to all patients, regardless of their geographic location, socioeconomic status, or race/ethnicity. This necessitates the prioritization of more equitable solutions like IHC, which can provide similar benefits at a lower cost and with wider accessibility. Therefore, ongoing efforts are needed to address these underlying disparities such as geographic location and socioeconomic status and ensure fair access to healthcare resources. This requires innovative strategies to reduce costs, decentralize expertise, and expand access to clinical trials. For instance, implementing reimbursement policies that cover the cost of molecular profiling and providing funding for research and development to improve the efficiency and affordability of these technologies are essential steps. Additionally, establishing guidelines and standards for use in clinical practice can also help streamline access. As Varkey et al. point out, even when treating physicians act with knowledge, skill, and empathy, treatment selection may be made without absolute certainty about effectiveness, highlighting the need for therapies established on a rigorous scientific foundation that is accessible to all [54].

Utility vs. Transparency: The principle of utility is intrinsically linked to transparency in research, demanding openness in data, protocols, and processes to ensure the validation of findings and foster scientific advancement. Transparency's absence, characterized by data hoarding and replication difficulties, obstructs progress and compromises research ethics. A shift towards open science, emphasizing rigorous hypothesis testing over mere confirmation, is paramount. This requires the use of freely accessible methodologies, protocols, raw data, software, and code. Critically, procedural justice necessitates the careful examination of who defines utility, access, and associated trade-offs. The meaningful engagement of key stakeholders, representing the diverse voices of the public, is vital. Such inclusive dialogue ensures that the pursuit of utility does not disproportionately favor some at the expense of others. Deliberate efforts to incorporate diverse perspectives into scientific governance and decision-making are essential. Neglecting these considerations risks inequitable outcomes, undermining the very utility that transparency aims to promote. This highlights the need for greater equity within the realm of open science itself.

Internal Tensions within Utility (Cost–Benefit Analysis): Tensions even arise within the principle of utility itself. The pursuit of precision medicine involves significant costs—financial, technological, and human. A rigorous cost–benefit analysis is essential, weighing the potential benefits of improved outcomes against the resources required. This analysis must consider not only the direct costs of molecular profiling and targeted therapies but also the indirect costs associated with infrastructure, training, and data management. A purely utilitarian perspective would suggest that the most cost-effective strategies that benefit the most patients should be prioritized. That could mean prioritizing basic research and widely applicable, less expensive screening methods (like IHC) instead of more complex and individualized molecular tests.

Biomarker-Based vs. Biomarker-Agnostic Strategies: Navigating the future of PDAC care requires careful consideration of both biomarker-based and biomarker-agnostic approaches. While targeted therapies based on specific mutations can be highly effective, many patients either lack access to comprehensive molecular profiling or do not present with actionable mutations. In these instances, readily available approaches such as IHC (immunohistochemistry) become vital. Moving forward, a comprehensive strategy that integrates both biomarker-based and biomarker-agnostic treatments will help ensure that all PDAC patients receive appropriately tailored care. Previously, next-generation sequencing (NGS) was employed to pinpoint the "needle in the haystack"—roughly 5% of patients with microsatellite instability or DNA damage response mutations. This was the group that could benefit from immunotherapy or PARP inhibitors [67]. Although the cost–benefit ratio justified NGS for this select group, emerging evidence suggests that broader sequencing may be less crucial for most patients. For example, results from clinical trials of RevMed's RAS-ON inhibitors (RMC-6236 and RMC-7977)—which targets both mutant and wild-type KRAS—hold exceptional promise and could revolutionize PDAC therapy if approved. In contrast, mutant-specific KRAS inhibitors (e.g., MRTX1133 G12Di) have not shown similarly positive outcomes, leaving NGS screening relevant primarily for that small subgroup with actionable mutations [68,69]. Looking ahead, the critical question is determining who stands to gain the most from RAS-ON inhibitors once standard-of-care chemotherapy (e.g., gemcitabine/nab-paclitaxel or FOLFIRINOX) loses effectiveness. Recent findings by Dilly et al. suggest that basal like tumors—easily identified through the IHC detection of surrogate markers such as KRT17—are especially responsive to these agents [70]. This highlights the pivotal role of IHC-based testing in guiding both first-line therapy and second-line decisions regarding RAS-ON inhibitors. As a result, expanding IHC use has the potential to enhance clinical decision-making, ensuring that emerging treatments are deployed for those most likely to benefit.

By examining these aspects, we can identify the best practices and develop strategies to accelerate the translation of research findings into clinical benefit for all PDAC patients.

6. Conclusions

In line with prior research, our study underscores the vital necessity of advanced, ethically informed strategies for managing pancreatic ductal adenocarcinoma (PDAC). By integrating early molecular classification into treatment protocols, we can enhance patient outcomes, reflecting the critical importance of timely and strategic interventions. To fulfill this promise, it is imperative that we foster broad-based collaboration among diverse stakeholders—ranging from policymakers to academicians and industry experts—to universally advance access to predictive biomarkers and precision medicine. This concerted effort aims to bridge clinical and socioeconomic gaps but also to propel society into a new era of cancer treatment. Embracing such a holistic approach, underscored by a commitment to ethical principles and fueled by robust interdisciplinary cooperation, holds the key to transformative advances in PDAC therapy, ensuring that these innovations benefit patients globally and culminate in a future where the devastating impact of this disease is markedly diminished.

Author Contributions: Conceptualization, K.R.S., L.F.E.-H., L.A.D.-C. and A.F.; methodology, L.A.D.-C.; data curation, L.R.-P. and L.A.D.-C.; writing—original draft preparation, L.A.D.-C.; writing—review and editing, L.A.D.-C., L.R.-P. and A.F.; visualization, L.A.D.-C.; supervision, K.R.S. and L.F.E.-H.; project administration, K.R.S.; funding acquisition, K.R.S. All authors have read and agreed to the published version of the manuscript.

Funding: This work was supported by academic enrichment funds of the Department of Pathology at the Renaissance School of Medicine, the Marvin Kuschner endowed professorship (K.R.S.) of Stony Brook University.

Conflicts of Interest: K.R.S. and L.F.E.-H. are consultants for KDx Diagnostics. The additional authors declare no conflict of interest.

References

1. Schepis, T.; De Lucia, S.S.; Pellegrino, A.; Del Gaudio, A.; Maresca, R.; Coppola, G.; Chiappetta, M.F.; Gasbarrini, A.; Franceschi, F. Candelli, M.; et al. State-of-the-Art and Upcoming Innovations in Pancreatic Cancer Care: A Step Forward to Precision Medicine *Cancers* **2023**, *15*, 3423. [CrossRef] [PubMed]
2. Li, B.; Zhang, Q.; Castaneda, C.; Cook, S. Targeted Therapies in Pancreatic Cancer: A New Era of Precision Medicine. *Biomedicines* **2024**, *12*, 2175. [CrossRef] [PubMed]
3. Blackford, A.L.; Canto, M.I.; Dbouk, M.; Hruban, R.H.; Katona, B.W.; Chak, A.; Brand, R.E.; Syngal, S.; Farrell, J.; Kastrinos F.; et al. Pancreatic Cancer Surveillance and Survival of High-Risk Individuals. *JAMA Oncol.* **2024**, *10*, 1087–1096. [CrossRef] [PubMed]
4. Prades, J.; Arnold, D.; Brunner, T.; Cardone, A.; Carrato, A.; Coll-Ortega, C.; De Luze, S.; Garel, P.; Goossens, M.E.; Grilli, R. et al. Bratislava Statement: Consensus recommendations for improving pancreatic cancer care. *ESMO Open* **2020**, *5*, e001051 [CrossRef]
5. Bugazia, D.; Al-Najjar, E.; Esmail, A.; Abdelrahim, S.; Abboud, K.; Abdelrahim, A.; Umoru, G.; Rayyan, H.A.; Abudayyeh, A.; Al Moustafa, A.E.; et al. Pancreatic ductal adenocarcinoma: The latest on diagnosis, molecular profiling, and systemic treatments *Front. Oncol.* **2024**, *14*, 1386699. [CrossRef]
6. Garajova, I.; Peroni, M.; Gelsomino, F.; Leonardi, F. A Simple Overview of Pancreatic Cancer Treatment for Clinical Oncologists *Curr. Oncol.* **2023**, *30*, 9587–9601. [CrossRef]
7. Tirpe, A.; Streianu, C.; Isachesku, E.; Simon, I.; Berindan-Neagoe, I. The road to overcome pancreatic cancer: Where are we? *Heliyon* **2024**, *10*, e38196. [CrossRef]
8. de la Fouchardiere, C.; Adham, M.; Marion-Audibert, A.M.; Duclos, A.; Darcha, C.; Berthelet, O.; Hervieu, V.; Artru, P.; Labrosse H.; Fayet, Y.; et al. Management of Patients with Pancreatic Ductal Adenocarcinoma in the Real-Life Setting: Lessons from the French National Hospital Database. *Cancers* **2021**, *13*, 3515. [CrossRef]
9. Hilmi, M.; Delecourt, F.; Raffenne, J.; Bourega, T.; Dusetti, N.; Iovanna, J.; Blum, Y.; Richard, M.; Neuzillet, C.; Couvelard, A.; et al Redefining phenotypic intratumor heterogeneity of pancreatic ductal adenocarcinoma: A bottom-up approach. *J. Pathol.* **2025** *265*, 448–461. [CrossRef]
10. Yu, B.; Shao, S.; Ma, W. Frontiers in pancreatic cancer on biomarkers, microenvironment, and immunotherapy. *Cancer Lett.* **2025** *610*, 217350. [CrossRef]
11. Robertson, F.P.; Cameron, A.; Spiers, H.V.M.; Joseph, N.; Taylor, E.; Ratnayake, B.; Jamieson, N.B.; Pandanaboyana, S. Evidence for molecular subtyping in pancreatic ductal adenocarcinoma: A systematic review. *HPB* **2024**, *26*, 609–617. [CrossRef] [PubMed]
12. Delgado-Coka, L.A.; Roa-Pena, L.; Babu, S.; Horowitz, M.; Petricoin, E.F., III; Matrisian, L.M.; Blais, E.M.; Marchenko, N.; Allard, F.D.; Akalin, A.; et al. Keratin 17 is a prognostic and predictive biomarker in pancreatic ductal adenocarcinoma. *Am. J. Clin. Pathol.* **2024**, *162*, 314–326. [CrossRef] [PubMed]
13. Juiz, N.; Elkaoutari, A.; Bigonnet, M.; Gayet, O.; Roques, J.; Nicolle, R.; Iovanna, J.; Dusetti, N. Basal-like and classical cells coexist in pancreatic cancer revealed by single-cell analysis on biopsy-derived pancreatic cancer organoids from the classical subtype *FASEB J.* **2020**, *34*, 12214–12228. [CrossRef] [PubMed]

14. Kokumai, T.; Omori, Y.; Ishida, M.; Ohtsuka, H.; Mizuma, M.; Nakagawa, K.; Maeda, C.; Ono, Y.; Mizukami, Y.; Miura, S.; et al. *GATA6* and *CK5* Stratify the Survival of Patients with Pancreatic Cancer Undergoing Neoadjuvant Chemotherapy. *Mod. Pathol.* **2023**, *36*, 100102. [CrossRef]
15. Collisson, E.A.; Sadanandam, A.; Olson, P.; Gibb, W.J.; Truitt, M.; Gu, S.; Cooc, J.; Weinkle, J.; Kim, G.E.; Jakkula, L.; et al. Subtypes of pancreatic ductal adenocarcinoma and their differing responses to therapy. *Nat. Med.* **2011**, *17*, 500–503. [CrossRef]
16. Raghavan, S.; Winter, P.S.; Navia, A.W.; Williams, H.L.; DenAdel, A.; Lowder, K.E.; Galvez-Reyes, J.; Kalekar, R.L.; Mulugeta, N.; Kapner, K.S.; et al. Microenvironment drives cell state, plasticity, and drug response in pancreatic cancer. *Cell* **2021**, *184*, 6119–6137.e26. [CrossRef]
17. Hayashi, H.; Higashi, T.; Miyata, T.; Yamashita, Y.I.; Baba, H. Recent advances in precision medicine for pancreatic ductal adenocarcinoma. *Ann. Gastroenterol. Surg.* **2021**, *5*, 457–466. [CrossRef] [PubMed]
18. Ahmadvand, P.; Farahani, H.; Farnell, D.; Darbandsari, A.; Topham, J.; Karasinska, J.; Nelson, J.; Naso, J.; Jones, S.J.M.; Renouf, D.; et al. A Deep Learning Approach for the Identification of the Molecular Subtypes of Pancreatic Ductal Adenocarcinoma Based on Whole Slide Pathology Images. *Am. J. Pathol.* **2024**, *194*, 2302–2312. [CrossRef]
19. Passaro, A.; Al Bakir, M.; Hamilton, E.G.; Diehn, M.; Andre, F.; Roy-Chowdhuri, S.; Mountzios, G.; Wistuba, I.I.; Swanton, C.; Peters, S. Cancer biomarkers: Emerging trends and clinical implications for personalized treatment. *Cell* **2024**, *187*, 1617–1635. [CrossRef]
20. Giannis, D.; Moris, D.; Barbas, A.S. Diagnostic, Predictive and Prognostic Molecular Biomarkers in Pancreatic Cancer: An Overview for Clinicians. *Cancers* **2021**, *13*, 1071. [CrossRef]
21. Lyu, J.; Jiang, M.; Zhu, Z.; Wu, H.; Kang, H.; Hao, X.; Cheng, S.; Guo, H.; Shen, X.; Wu, T.; et al. Identification of biomarkers and potential therapeutic targets for pancreatic cancer by proteomic analysis in two prospective cohorts. *Cell Genom.* **2024**, *4*, 100561. [CrossRef] [PubMed]
22. Mirza, M.; Goerke, L.; Anderson, A.; Wilsdon, T. Assessing the Cost-Effectiveness of Next-Generation Sequencing as a Biomarker Testing Approach in Oncology and Policy Implications: A Literature Review. *Value Health* **2024**, *27*, 1300–1309. [CrossRef] [PubMed]
23. Li, Y.; Ding, Z.; Cheng, T.; Hu, Y.; Zhong, F.; Ren, S.; Wang, S. Single-cell transcriptomics analysis reveals dynamic changes and prognostic signature in tumor microenvironment of PDAC. *Sci. Rep.* **2025**, *15*, 4025.
24. Pompella, L.; Tirino, G.; Pappalardo, A.; Caterino, M.; Ventriglia, A.; Nacca, V.; Orditura, M.; Ciardiello, F.; De Vita, F. Pancreatic Cancer Molecular Classifications: From Bulk Genomics to Single Cell Analysis. *Int. J. Mol. Sci.* **2020**, *21*, 2814. [CrossRef]
25. Duan, K.; Jang, G.H.; Grant, R.C.; Wilson, J.M.; Notta, F.; O'Kane, G.M.; Knox, J.J.; Gallinger, S.; Fischer, S. The value of *GATA6* immunohistochemistry and computer-assisted diagnosis to predict clinical outcome in advanced pancreatic cancer. *Sci. Rep.* **2021**, *11*, 14951. [CrossRef] [PubMed]
26. Shibayama, T.; Hayashi, A.; Toki, M.; Kitahama, K.; Ho, Y.J.; Kato, K.; Yamada, T.; Kawamoto, S.; Kambayashi, K.; Ochiai, K.; et al. Combination immunohistochemistry for *CK5/6, p63, GATA6*, and *HNF4a* predicts clinical outcome in treatment-naive pancreatic ductal adenocarcinoma. *Sci. Rep.* **2024**, *14*, 15598. [CrossRef]
27. Rao, J.; Sinn, M.; Pelzer, U.; Riess, H.; Oettle, H.; Demir, I.E.; Friess, H.; Jager, C.; Steiger, K.; Muckenhuber, A. *KRT81* and *HNF1A* expression in pancreatic ductal adenocarcinoma: Investigation of predictive and prognostic value of immunohistochemistry-based subtyping. *J. Pathol. Clin. Res.* **2024**, *10*, e12377. [CrossRef]
28. Xu, H.; Xue, S.; Sun, Y.; Ma, J.; Li, S.; Wang, Y.; Mao, T.; Ge, W.; Yue, M.; Shentu, D.; et al. *CREB3L1* facilitates pancreatic tumor progression and reprograms intratumoral tumor-associated macrophages to shape an immunotherapy-resistance microenvironment. *J. Immunother. Cancer* **2025**, *13*, e010029. [CrossRef]
29. van Eijck, C.W.; Real, F.X.; Malats, N.; Vadgama, D.; van den Bosch, T.P.; Doukas, M.; van Eijck, C.H.; Mustafa, D.A. GATA6 identifies an im-mune-enriched phenotype linked to favorable outcomes in patients with pancreatic cancer undergoing upfront surgery. *Cell Rep. Med.* **2024**, *5*, 101557. [CrossRef] [PubMed]
30. Muckenhuber, A.; Berger, A.K.; Schlitter, A.M.; Steiger, K.; Konukiewitz, B.; Trumpp, A.; Eils, R.; Werner, J.; Friess, H.; Esposito, I.; Klöppel, G. Pancreatic Ductal Adenocar-cinoma Subtyping Using the Biomarkers Hepatocyte Nuclear Factor-1A and Cytokeratin-81 Correlates with Outcome and Treatment Response. *Clin. Cancer Res.* **2018**, *24*, 351–359. [CrossRef]
31. Lansbergen, M.F.; Dings, M.P.G.; Manoukian, P.; Farina, A.; Waasdorp, C.; Hooijer, G.K.J.; Verheij, J.; Koster, J.; Zwijnenburg, D.A.; Wilmink, J.W.; et al. Transcriptome-based classification to predict FOLFIRINOX response in a real-world metastatic pancreatic cancer cohort. *Transl. Res.* **2024**, *273*, 137–147. [CrossRef]
32. Okada, Y.; Nishiwada, S.; Yamamura, K.; Sho, M.; Baba, H.; Takayama, T.; Goel, A. Identification of laminin $\gamma 2$ as a prognostic and predictive biomarker for determining response to gemcitabine-based therapy in pancreatic ductal adenocarcinoma. *Eur. J. Cancer* **2021**, *146*, 125–134. [CrossRef]
33. Dreyer, S.B.; Rae, S.; Bisset, K.; Upstill-Goddard, R.; Gemenetzis, G.; Johns, A.L.; Dickson, E.J.; Mittal, A.; Gill, A.J.; Duthie, F.; et al. The Impact of Molecular Subtyping on Pathological Staging of Pancreatic Cancer. *Ann. Surg.* **2023**, *277*, e396–e405. [CrossRef]

34. Moffitt, R.A.; Marayati, R.; Flate, E.L.; Volmar, K.E.; Loeza, S.G.; Hoadley, K.A.; Rashid, N.U.; Williams, L.A.; Eaton, S.C.; Chung, A.H.; et al. Virtual microdissection identifies distinct tumor- and stroma-specific subtypes of pancreatic ductal adenocarcinoma. *Nat. Genet.* **2015**, *47*, 1168–1178. [CrossRef]
35. Bailey, P.; Chang, D.K.; Nones, K.; Johns, A.L.; Patch, A.M.; Gingras, M.C.; Miller, D.K.; Christ, A.N.; Bruxner, T.J.; Quinn, M.C.; et al. Genomic analyses identify molecular subtypes of pancreatic cancer. *Nature* **2016**, *531*, 47–52. [CrossRef] [PubMed]
36. Zhou, X.; Hu, K.; Bailey, P.; Springfeld, C.; Roth, S.; Kurilov, R.; Brors, B.; Gress, T.; Buchholz, M.; An, J.; et al. Clinical Impact of Molecular Subtyping of Pancreatic Cancer. *Front. Cell Dev. Biol.* **2021**, *9*, 743908. [CrossRef] [PubMed]
37. Christofyllakis, K.; Bittenbring, J.T.; Thurner, L.; Ahlgrimm, M.; Stilgenbauer, S.; Bewarder, M.; Kaddu-Mulindwa, D. Cost-effectiveness of precision cancer medicine-current challenges in the use of next generation sequencing for comprehensive tumour genomic profiling and the role of clinical utility frameworks (Review). *Mol. Clin. Oncol.* **2022**, *16*, 21. [CrossRef] [PubMed]
38. Roa-Pena, L.; Leiton, C.V.; Babu, S.; Pan, C.H.; Vanner, E.A.; Akalin, A.; Bandovic, J.; Moffitt, R.A.; Shroyer, K.R.; Escobar-Hoyos, L.F. Keratin 17 identifies the most lethal molecular subtype of pancreatic cancer. *Sci. Rep.* **2019**, *9*, 11239. [CrossRef]
39. Roa-Pena, L.; Babu, S.; Leiton, C.V.; Wu, M.; Taboada, S.; Akalin, A.; Buscaglia, J.; Escobar-Hoyos, L.F.; Shroyer, K.R. Keratin 17 testing in pancreatic cancer needle aspiration biopsies predicts survival. *Cancer Cytopathol.* **2021**, *129*, 865–873. [CrossRef]
40. Rashid, N.U.; Peng, X.L.; Jin, C.; Moffitt, R.A.; Volmar, K.E.; Belt, B.A.; Panni, R.Z.; Nywening, T.M.; Herrera, S.G.; Moore, K.J.; et al. Purity Independent Subtyping of Tumors (PurIST), A Clinically Robust, Single-sample Classifier for Tumor Subtyping in Pancreatic Cancer. *Clin. Cancer Res.* **2020**, *26*, 82–92. [CrossRef]
41. Mosele, M.F.; Westphalen, C.B.; Stenzinger, A.; Barlesi, F.; Bayle, A.; Bieche, I.; Bonastre, J.; Castro, E.; Dienstmann, R.; Kramer, A.; et al. Recommendations for the use of next-generation sequencing (NGS) for patients with advanced cancer in 2024: A report from the ESMO Precision Medicine Working Group. *Ann. Oncol.* **2024**, *35*, 588–606. [CrossRef]
42. Racu, M.L.; Schiavo, A.A.; Van Campenhout, C.; De Neve, N.; Masuy, T.; Maris, C.; Decaestecker, C.; Remmelink, M.; Salmon, I.; D'Haene, N. Validation of a targeted next-generation sequencing panel for pancreatic ductal adenocarcinomas. *Exp. Mol. Pathol.* **2024**, *139*, 104920. [CrossRef]
43. Torres, C.; Grippo, P.J. Pancreatic cancer subtypes: A roadmap for precision medicine. *Ann. Med.* **2018**, *50*, 277–287. [CrossRef]
44. Zhou, Y.; Tao, L.; Qiu, J.; Xu, J.; Yang, X.; Zhang, Y.; Tian, X.; Guan, X.; Cen, X.; Zhao, Y. Tumor biomarkers for diagnosis, prognosis and targeted therapy. *Signal Transduct. Target. Ther.* **2024**, *9*, 132. [PubMed]
45. Frank, T.S.; Sun, X.; Zhang, Y.; Yang, J.; Fisher, W.E.; Gingras, M.C.; Li, M. Genomic profiling guides the choice of molecular targeted therapy of pancreatic cancer. *Cancer Lett.* **2015**, *363*, 1–6. [CrossRef] [PubMed]
46. Turner, B.M.; Katerji, H.; Zhang, H.; Hicks, D.G. Biomarker and multigene assay testing in ER positive, HER-2 negative breast carcinomas: An international guidelines-based approach. *Hum. Pathol. Rep.* **2021**, *26*, 300574. [CrossRef]
47. Zaha, D.C. Significance of immunohistochemistry in breast cancer. *World J. Clin. Oncol.* **2014**, *5*, 382–392. [CrossRef]
48. Wang, J.; Xu, B. Targeted therapeutic options and future perspectives for HER2-positive breast cancer. *Signal Transduct. Target. Ther.* **2019**, *4*, 34. [CrossRef]
49. Sholl, L.M. Biomarkers of response to checkpoint inhibitors beyond PD-L1 in lung cancer. *Mod. Pathol.* **2022**, *35* (Suppl. S1), 66–74. [CrossRef] [PubMed]
50. Kim, H.; Chung, J.H. PD-L1 Testing in Non-small Cell Lung Cancer: Past, Present, and Future. *J. Pathol. Transl. Med.* **2019**, *53*, 199–206. [CrossRef]
51. Horgan, D.; Hamdi, Y.; Lal, J.A.; Nyawira, T.; Meyer, S.; Kondji, D.; Francisco, N.M.; De Guzman, R.; Paul, A.; Bernard, B.; et al. Framework for Adoption of Next-Generation Sequencing (NGS) Globally in the Oncology Area. *Healthcare* **2023**, *11*, 431. [CrossRef]
52. Herbst, B.; Zheng, L. Precision medicine in pancreatic cancer: Treating every patient as an exception. *Lancet Gastroenterol. Hepatol.* **2019**, *4*, 805–810. [CrossRef]
53. Ubel, P.A.; Scherr, K.A.; Fagerlin, A. Autonomy: What's Shared Decision Making Have to Do with It? *Am. J. Bioeth.* **2018**, *18*, W11–W12. [CrossRef]
54. Varkey, B. Principles of Clinical Ethics and Their Application to Practice. *Med. Princ. Pract.* **2021**, *30*, 17–28. [CrossRef] [PubMed]
55. Schildmann, J.; Ritter, P.; Salloch, S.; Uhl, W.; Vollmann, J. 'One also needs a bit of trust in the doctor . . .': A qualitative interview study with pancreatic cancer patients about their perceptions and views on information and treatment decision-making. *Ann. Oncol.* **2013**, *24*, 2444–2449. [CrossRef] [PubMed]
56. Byrne, M.; Mattison, R.; Bercovitz, R.; Lottenberg, R.; Rezende, S.M.; Silverstein, R.; Terrell, D.; Kunkle, R.; Smith, D.; Bollard, C.; et al. Identifying experts for clinical practice guidelines: Perspectives from the ASH Guideline Oversight Subcommittee. *Blood Adv.* **2023**, *7*, 4323–4326. [CrossRef]
57. Entwistle, V.A.; Carter, S.M.; Cribb, A.; McCaffery, K. Supporting patient autonomy: The importance of clinician-patient relationships. *J. Gen. Intern. Med.* **2010**, *25*, 741–745. [CrossRef] [PubMed]

58. Baliga, M.S.; Marakala, V.; Madathil, L.P.; George, T.; D'Souza, R.F.; Palatty, P.L. Ethical and moral principles for oncology healthcare workers: A brief report from a Bioethics consortium emphasizing on need for education. *J. Educ. Health Promot.* **2024**, *13*, 145. [CrossRef]
59. Casolino, R.; Braconi, C.; Malleo, G.; Paiella, S.; Bassi, C.; Milella, M.; Dreyer, S.B.; Froeling, F.E.M.; Chang, D.K.; Biankin, A.V.; et al. Reshaping preoperative treatment of pancreatic cancer in the era of precision medicine. *Ann. Oncol.* **2021**, *32*, 183–196. [CrossRef]
60. Marron, J.M.; Charlot, M.; Gaddy, J.; Rosenberg, A.R. The Ethical Imperative of Equity in Oncology: Lessons Learned From 2020 and a Path Forward. *Am. Soc. Clin. Oncol. Educ. Book* **2021**, *41*, e13–e19. [CrossRef]
61. Zakout, G.A. Practicing equitable principles in cancer clinical research: Has the EU got it right? *J. Cancer Policy* **2023**, *37*, 100435. [CrossRef]
62. Kirkwood, M.K.; Schenkel, C.; Hinshaw, D.C.; Bruinooge, S.S.; Waterhouse, D.M.; Peppercorn, J.M.; Subbiah, I.M.; Levit, L.A. State of Geographic Access to Cancer Treatment Trials in the United States: Are Studies Located Where Patients Live? *JCO Oncol. Pract.* **2025**, *21*, 427–437. [CrossRef]
63. Villamar, D.M.P.; Blasé, N. The Promise of Cancer Health Justice: How Stakeholders and the Community Can Build a Sustained and Equitable System of Cancer Care Through the Lens of Colorectal Cancer Interventions. *Cancer J.* **2023**, *29*, 338–342. [CrossRef]
64. Zalis, M.; Viana Veloso, G.G.; Aguiar, P.N., Jr.; Gimenes, N.; Reis, M.X.; Matsas, S.; Ferreira, C.G. Next-generation sequencing impact on cancer care: Applications, challenges, and future directions. *Front. Genet.* **2024**, *15*, 1420190. [CrossRef] [PubMed]
65. Qadir, R.; Umair, M.B.; Tariq, U.B.; Ahmad, A.; Kiran, W.; Shahid, M.H. Unraveling Pancreatic Cancer: Epidemiology, Risk Factors, and Global Trends. *Cureus* **2024**, *16*, e72816. [CrossRef]
66. Vidal, L.; Dlamini, Z.; Qian, S.; Rishi, P.; Karmo, M.; Joglekar, N.; Abedin, S.; Previs, R.A.; Orbegoso, C.; Joshi, C.; et al. Equitable inclusion of diverse populations in oncology clinical trials: Deterrents and drivers. *ESMO Open* **2024**, *9*, 103373. [CrossRef]
67. Singh, R.R.; Goldberg, J.; Varghese, A.M.; Yu, K.H.; Park, W.; O'Reilly, E.M. Genomic profiling in pancreatic ductal adenocarcinoma and a pathway towards therapy individualization: A scoping review. *Cancer Treat. Rev.* **2019**, *75*, 27–38. [CrossRef] [PubMed]
68. Holderfield, M.; Lee, B.J.; Jiang, J.; Tomlinson, A.; Seamon, K.J.; Mira, A.; Patrucco, E.; Goodhart, G.; Dilly, J.; Gindin, Y.; et al. Concurrent inhibition of oncogenic and wild-type RAS-GTP for cancer therapy. *Nature* **2024**, *629*, 919–926. [CrossRef]
69. Wasko, U.N.; Jiang, J.; Dalton, T.C.; Curiel-Garcia, A.; Edwards, A.C.; Wang, Y.; Lee, B.; Orlen, M.; Tian, S.; Stalnecker, C.A.; et al. Tumour-selective activity of RAS-GTP inhibition in pancreatic cancer. *Nature* **2024**, *629*, 927–936. [CrossRef]
70. Dilly, J.; Hoffman, M.T.; Abbassi, L.; Li, Z.; Paradiso, F.; Parent, B.D.; Hennessey, C.J.; Jordan, A.C.; Morgado, M.; Dasgupta, S.; et al. Mechanisms of Resistance to Oncogenic KRAS Inhibition in Pancreatic Cancer. *Cancer Discov.* **2024**, *14*, 2135–2161. [CrossRef]

cancers

MDPI

Review

The Role of Nanoparticles in Therapy of Real-World Patients with Pancreatic Cancer: A Scoping Review

Ioannis Konstantinidis [1,*], Sophia Tsokkou [1,2,*], Dimitrios Katsikeros [3], Paraskevi Chatzikomnitsa [2], Menelaos Papakonstantinou [2], Eftychia Liampou [2], Evdokia Toutziari [2], Dimitrios Giakoustidis [2], Petros Bageas [2], Vasileios Papadopoulos [2], Alexandros Giakoustidis [2] and Theodora Papamitsou [4]

1 Department of Medicine, Faculty of Health Sciences, Aristotle University of Thessaloniki, 54124 Thessaloniki, Greece

2 First Department of Surgery, General Hospital Papageorgiou, Aristotle University of Thessaloniki, 56429 Thessaloniki, Greece; voula.hatzikomnitsa@yahoo.gr (P.C.); menelaospap.md@gmail.com (M.P.); liampouef7@yahoo.gr (E.L.); evdo-t@hotmail.com (E.T.); dgiak@auth.gr (D.G.); pbangeas@gmail.com (P.B.); papadvas@auth.gr (V.P.); algiak@auth.gr (A.G.)

3 Faculty of Medicine, School of Health Sciences, University of Thessaly, 41334 Larissa, Greece; dkatsikeros@uth.gr

4 Laboratory of Histology-Embryology, Department of Medicine, Faculty of Health Sciences, Aristotle University of Thessaloniki, 54124 Thessaloniki, Greece; thpapami@auth.gr

* Correspondence: ikonsc@auth.gr (I.K.); stsokkou@auth.gr (S.T.)

Simple Summary: Pancreatic cancer remains one of the deadliest malignancies, largely due to its aggressive biology, late diagnosis, and the presence of a dense tumor stroma that hampers effective drug delivery. Nanoparticle-based therapies offer a promising solution by enabling targeted delivery, enhancing chemotherapy's bioavailability, and modulating the tumor microenvironment to reduce systemic toxicity. This review evaluated real-world clinical evidence on nanoparticle-based therapies in pancreatic cancer through a scoping review approach guided by the PRISMA Extension for Scoping Reviews. A systematic search was conducted across PubMed, MEDLINE, the Cochrane Library, and Embase on 2 April 2025, which identified 2144 records. Utilizing the PICOTS framework and the pre-set eligibility criteria, studies were independently screened by two reviewers, ultimately including 19 studies published between 2006 and 2023. Clinical evidence indicates that nanoparticle-based therapies, particularly with agents such as nanoparticle albumin-bound paclitaxel and nanoliposomal irinotecan, can improve survival outcomes and reduce toxicity compared with conventional treatments. Nonetheless, challenges remain in dosing optimization, biomarker-driven patient selection, and ensuring long-term safety. Overall, nanoparticle-based approaches show promising potential to be integrated into standard treatment regimens within the coming decade, warranting further clinical investigation to ultimately benefit broader patient populations worldwide.

Abstract: Background: Pancreatic cancer, one of the most aggressive malignancies, poses significant treatment challenges due to its aggressive nature, late detection, and dense tumor stroma that not only impedes drug delivery but also promotes tumor progression and immune evasion. Nanoparticle-based therapies offer a promising solution by enabling targeted drug delivery, enhancing chemotherapeutic bioavailability, and modulating the tumor microenvironment to reduce systemic toxicity. **Objectives:** This scoping review systematically evaluates real-world clinical evidence to elucidate the translational potential of nanoparticle technologies and identify future directions for integrating these approaches into effective clinical treatment paradigms for pancreatic cancer. **Methods:** A scoping review was conducted following the PRISMA Extension for Scoping Reviews to comprehensively map research on nanoparticle-based therapies in pancreatic cancer over the past

https://doi.org/10.3390/cancers17101726

20 years. The research question was identified using the PICOTS framework. A systematic search was performed across PubMed, MEDLINE, Cochrane Library, and Embase on 2 April 2025, using a predefined query: "((pancreatic cancer) OR (pancreatic carcinoma) OR (pancreatic adenocarcinoma) OR (pancreatic neoplasm)) AND (nanoparticles)". Eligible full-text studies were independently screened by two reviewers, and key study variables were extracted and descriptively synthesized. **Results:** From 2144 initial records, 19 studies were included after screening and eligibility assessment. These studies, published between 2006 and 2023, comprised 14 clinical trials, 2 retrospective cohorts, and 3 case reports, with the majority evaluating nanoparticle albumin-bound paclitaxel, followed by nanoliposomal irinotecan. **Conclusions:** NP-based therapies have emerged as a promising strategy to enhance drug delivery, improve survival outcomes, and reduce toxicity in pancreatic cancer. Clinical evidence, particularly with agents such as nab-PTX and nal-IRI, underscores their potential to overcome the delivery challenges posed by the tumor microenvironment. However, optimizing dosing, biomarker-driven patient selection, and ensuring long-term safety remain critical hurdles. In the coming decade, the integration of nanoparticle therapies into standard-of-care regimens is anticipated to transform pancreatic cancer's management, contingent upon further rigorous clinical investigations and refined translational strategies.

Keywords: pancreatic cancer; pancreatic carcinoma; pancreatic adenocarcinoma; pancreatic neoplasm; nanoparticles; nanomedicine; nanoliposomal irinotecan; nanoparticle albumin-bound paclitaxel; nal-IRI; nab-PTX

1. Introduction

Pancreatic cancer (PC) is one of the most aggressive and fatal malignancies worldwide, posing a significant global health challenge due to its high mortality rates, late-stage diagnosis, and limited therapeutic efficacy. In the United States, PC ranks as the tenth most common malignancy and the third leading cause of cancer-related mortality, with an estimated 67,440 new diagnoses and approximately 51,980 deaths reported annually as of 2025 [1,2]. In Europe, mortality rates reached 17 per 100,000 among women and 22.3 per 100,000 among men in 2022, indicating a higher prevalence in the male population [3,4]. On a global scale, according to data from the Global Cancer Observatory 2022 (GLOBOCAN), PC was ranked twelfth in incidence, with 510,992 diagnosed cases, and sixth in mortality, with 467,409 recorded deaths [5,6]. The incidence of PC increases with age, with a median age at diagnosis of 71 years based on data from 2018 to 2022, a median age at death of 73 years based on data from 2019 to 2023, and approximately 90% of cases occurring in individuals over 55 years, particularly among those over 70. Moreover, nearly 1.6% of both men and women are diagnosed with PC during their lifetime [1]. Histopathologically, pancreatic ductal adenocarcinoma (PDAC) is the predominant subtype, accounting for over 90% of cases, while additional types such as cystadenocarcinoma and acinar cell carcinoma are also observed [7]. The elevated mortality associated with PC is largely attributable to its asymptomatic early stages, leading to delayed diagnosis and the limited efficacy of current therapeutic interventions [7].

1.1. Pancreatic Cancer—Risk Factors

PC is influenced by both modifiable and non-modifiable risk factors. According to the American Cancer Society, tobacco use, obesity, type 2 diabetes (T2DM), chronic pancreatitis, and occupational exposure to carcinogens significantly increase the risk of developing PC. Specifically, smoking is associated with a 25% increased risk, while cessation is linked to a decline in incidence. Additionally, excess body weight, particularly central adiposity and chronic pancreatitis, often consequent to prolonged alcohol consumption, can further increase susceptibility [8,9].

Non-modifiable risk factors include advanced age, male gender, and race, with African Americans being more predisposed than Caucasians. Familial predisposition also demonstrates a key role; individuals with a family history of PC or those with inherited genetic syndromes, such as mutations in BRCA, KRAS, TP53, or CDKN2A, as well as Lynch syndrome and hereditary pancreatitis, face a higher risk. Moreover, emerging studies suggest that dietary factors, physical inactivity, certain infections (including *Helicobacter pylori* and hepatitis B virus), heavy alcohol consumption, and gestational diabetes mellitus may contribute to PC risk, although further research is necessary to substantiate these associations (Figure 1) [8,9].

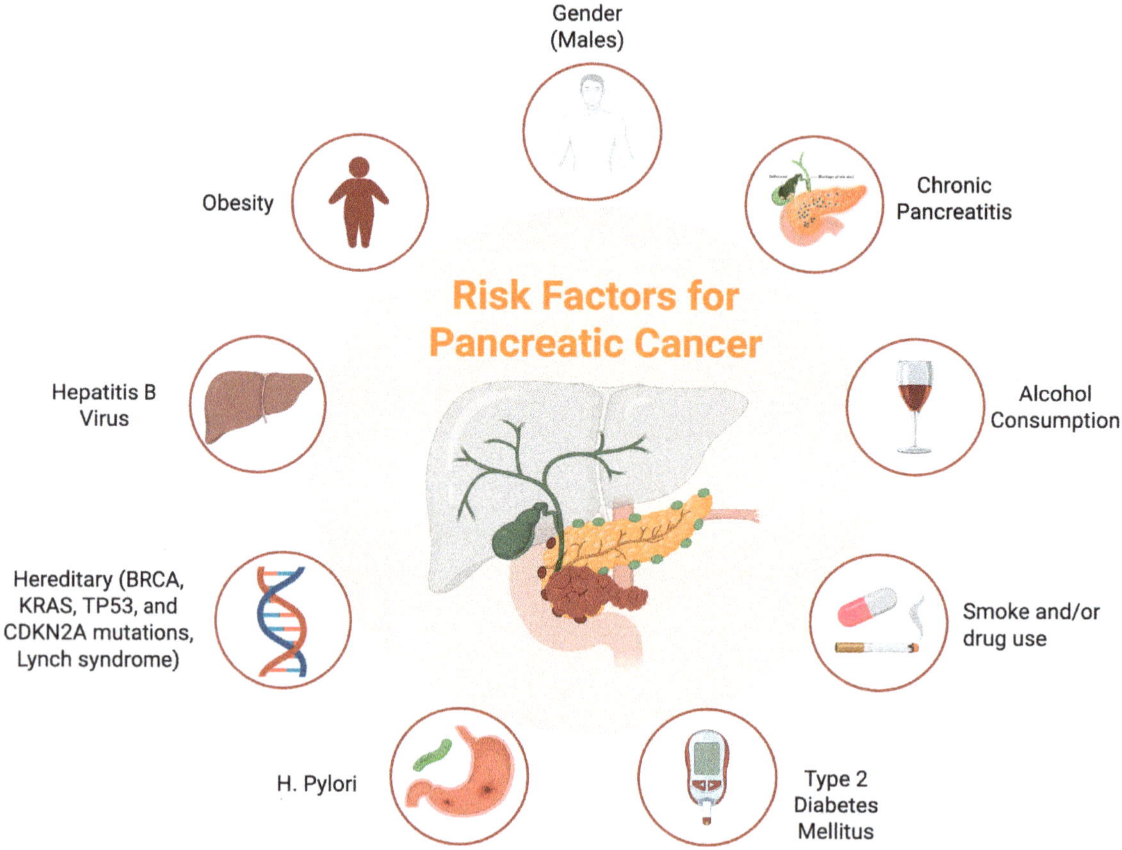

Figure 1. Risk factors for pancreatic cancer development.

1.2. Molecular and Cellular Alterations–Pancreatic Ductal Adenocarcinoma

PDAC is predominantly driven by somatic mutations in both oncogenes and tumor suppressor genes. In particular, activating mutations in the oncogene *KRAS* and loss-of-function mutations in the tumor suppressor genes *CDKN2A*, *TP53*, and *SMAD4* are among the most frequently observed genetic alterations in *PDAC* patients (Figure 2) [10]. Moreover, *PDACs* exhibit significant alterations in the composition of immune cell subpopulations, contributing to an immunosuppressive or "cold" tumor microenvironment. Notably, there is an enrichment of regulatory T cells and myeloid-derived suppressor cells, which impede the effective immune-mediated targeting of cancer cells [10]. Also, tumor-associated macrophages promote the progression of precancerous lesions by the secretion of interleukin-6 (IL-6). Immune alterations in *PDAC* negatively impact disease progression by contributing to the lack of responsiveness to immunotherapeutic strategies, including checkpoint inhibition. Elucidating the molecular signals that drive the formation of this immunosuppressive microenvironment may uncover novel therapeutic targets to enhance treatment efficacy [10].

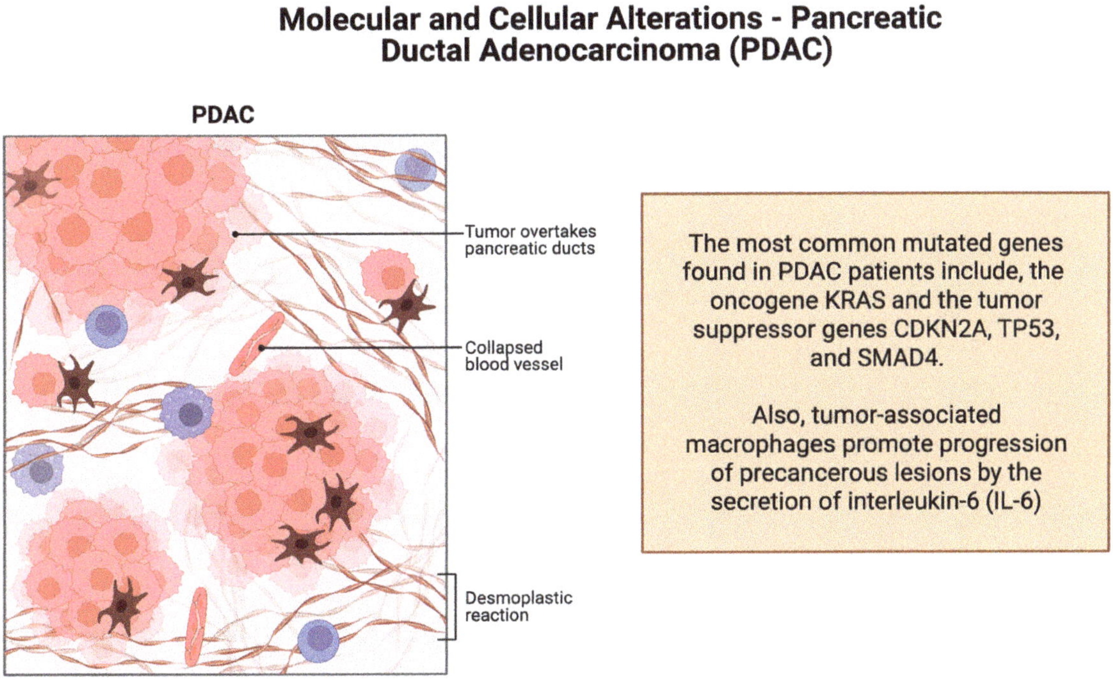

Figure 2. Molecular and cellular alterations—pancreatic ductal adenocarcinoma.

1.3. Pancreatic Cancer Therapy

The aggressive nature of PC and its frequent late-stage diagnosis make it one of the most challenging malignancies to treat. Current treatment strategies depend on the patient's health status, tumor resectability, and the stage of the disease. For tumors confined to the pancreas, without vascular invasion, the Whipple procedure (pancreaticoduodenectomy) is the standard approach, with surgical resection representing the only curative option [11–13]. However, only approximately 20% of patients are eligible for surgery at the time of diagnosis. Neoadjuvant therapy, which encompasses both chemotherapy and radiation, is increasingly employed to reduce the tumor burden and improve surgical outcomes in cases of borderline resectability [11–13].

Chemotherapy is the first-line treatment for locally advanced and metastatic pancreatic cancer. The FOLFIRINOX regimen, comprising fluorouracil, leucovorin, irinotecan, and oxaliplatin, has demonstrated superior efficacy compared to gemcitabine monotherapy, resulting in a significant increase in survival rates. For patients unable to tolerate FOLFIRINOX, gemcitabine combined with nab-paclitaxel serves as a more tolerable and widely utilized alternative [11–13]. Furthermore, emerging personalized treatment approaches include targeted therapies, such as PARP inhibitors (e.g., olaparib) for patients with BRCA mutations, as well as tyrosine kinase inhibitors. Additionally, immunotherapy—which includes immune checkpoint inhibitors—has demonstrated potential in other malignancies; however, its application in pancreatic cancer remains under investigation due to the immunosuppressive tumor microenvironment [11–13]. In advanced cases, radiation therapy is frequently employed in conjunction with chemotherapy to alleviate symptoms and achieve local tumor control [11–13].

Recently, the U.S. Food and Drug Administration (FDA) approved NALIRIFOX, a novel chemotherapy regimen that integrates liposomal irinotecan (nal-IRI), fluorouracil, leucovorin, and oxaliplatin [11–13]. Preliminary evidence indicates that NALIRIFOX exhibits enhanced efficacy in the treatment of metastatic pancreatic cancer. This advancement reflects ongoing efforts to improve patient outcomes and treatment efficacy. Concurrently, current research is focusing on biomarker-driven therapies, modulation of the tumor microenvironment, and innovative drug delivery systems [11–13].

1.4. Nanoparticles in Pancreatic Cancer Therapy

Nanoparticles (NPs) have revolutionized cancer treatment by offering innovative solutions to overcome the limitations of conventional therapies. These nanoscale particles, ranging from 1 to 100 nanometers in size, are meticulously engineered to enhance drug delivery, optimize therapeutic efficacy, and minimize systemic toxicity. NPs can be selectively designed to target only tumor cells by exploiting the enhanced permeability and retention (EPR) effect, or through active targeting approaches using ligands that bind to cancer-specific biomarkers. This targeted delivery facilitates the accumulation of therapeutic agents at the tumor site while reducing off-target effects, thereby potentially improving clinical outcomes [14–26].

Various types of NPs, including liposomes, polymeric NPs, metallic NPs and lipid-based NPs (LBNPs), as well as novel mRNA-lipoplex vaccines targeting somatic mutation-derived neoantigens, have been implemented in cancer therapy. These nanoscale carriers can encapsulate chemotherapeutic agents, thus facilitating controlled and programmed release at the target site while enhancing drug stability in systemic circulation and minimizing off-target complications [9–20]. Additionally, multifunctional NPs are engineered to combine therapeutic and diagnostic capabilities, thereby enabling real-time imaging and treatment monitoring. NPs also play a crucial role in overcoming drug resistance by delivering combination therapies or modulating the tumor microenvironment. For instance, lipid–polymeric hybrid NPs have demonstrated enhanced radiosensitivity and radiation-triggered drug delivery, providing synergistic effects in cancer treatment. Despite this promise, challenges such as scalability, biocompatibility, and regulatory approval continue to represent critical areas of ongoing research [16–27].

PC remains one of the most formidable challenges in oncology due to its aggressive biology, late-stage diagnosis, and intrinsic resistance to conventional therapies such as chemotherapy and radiotherapy. The complex and dense tumor stroma, which is characteristic of PC, not only serves as a physical barrier that hinders the effective penetration of therapeutic agents but also fosters a microenvironment that promotes tumor growth and immune evasion. NPs have emerged as a promising means to overcome these impediments, owing to their ability to enhance targeted drug delivery, improve the bioavailability of chemotherapeutic agents, and modulate both the tumor microenvironment and immune responses. These engineered nanoplatforms enable the precise delivery of drugs directly to tumor sites, thereby potentially increasing therapeutic efficacy while minimizing systemic toxicity. Given these innovative capabilities, the present scoping review aims to systematically explore and critically appraise the application of NP-based therapies in the management of PC, with a specific focus on evidence derived from real-world clinical settings. By synthesizing the current research on NP-mediated drug delivery systems, stromal barrier modulation, and immune microenvironment alteration, this review seeks to elucidate the translational potential of NP technologies and identify future directions for integrating these approaches into effective clinical treatment paradigms for PC.

2. Materials and Methods

A scoping review approach was adopted for this project in lieu of a formal systematic review, due to the diverse approaches encountered in studies addressing NP applications in PC therapy. This methodological choice was made to comprehensively map the extent of the research, including variability in study designs, implementation strategies, and outcome measures, rather than attempting to synthesize data from highly disparate sources into a single analysis. By using a scoping review framework, we aimed to delineate critical gaps in the current literature, particularly regarding the effectiveness of novel NP strategies in overcoming the unique challenges of PC in real-world clinical settings, and identify key advancements. This approach not only facilitates the characterization of existing evidence on therapeutic effectiveness, it also provides a foundational understanding of implementation strategies across diverse patient populations and elucidates the practical challenges associated with translating NP technologies from experimental models to routine clinical practice, thereby informing future systematic reviews and guiding translational research efforts in this evolving field. A detailed protocol for this scoping review was systematically developed, and all results were documented following the Preferred Reporting Items for Systematic Reviews and Meta-Analyses (PRISMA) checklist adapted for scoping reviews, as detailed in Supplementary Table S1.

2.1. Identifying Research Questions

To clarify the research query, a PICOTS (Population, Intervention, Comparator, Outcome, Time, Study design) framework was employed, as detailed in Table 1. Thus, the following review question was developed: "Among adult (≥18 years) patients with PC, what is the evidence regarding the efficacy of NP-based pharmacological approaches in improving overall survival (OS), progression-free disease (PFS), disease control rate (DCR), partial remission (PR), complete remission (CR), stable disease (SD) and treatment-emergent adverse events (TEAEs), compared with conventional pharmacological regimens over the past twenty years?".

Table 1. Population, Intervention, Comparator, Outcome, Time and Study design (PICOTS) table.

P (Population)	Adult (≥18 years) patients with pancreatic cancer
I (Intervention)	Nanoparticle-based pharmacotherapy
C (Comparator)	Conventional pharmacological regimens
O (Outcome)	OS, PFS, DCR, PR, CR, SD, and TEAEs
T (Time)	20 Years (2005–2025)
S (Study design)	Clinical trials, cohorts (retrospective or prospective), case reports

2.2. Identifying Relevant Studies

A comprehensive search was conducted on 2 April 2025, across multiple biomedical databases, including PubMed, MEDLINE, Cochrane Library, and Embase, using the following query string: "((pancreatic cancer) OR (pancreatic carcinoma) OR (pancreatic adenocarcinoma) OR (pancreatic neoplasm)) AND (nanoparticles)". References were reviewed for the identification of any additional relevant articles.

2.3. Study Selection—Eligibility and Screening

The review was restricted to full-text research studies published in peer-reviewed journals in the English language. Eligible studies had to meet the following criteria: the study must include adult (≥18 years) patients with PC of any histopathological type or clinical stage; the study design must be a clinical trial, prospective or retrospective cohort, or case report; the study should focus primarily on the effectiveness of NP-based regimens for treatment of PC and, when available, a direct comparison with conventional pharmacotherapy; the study must have been published during the past twenty years, i.e., between 2005 and 2025. Duplicate records, review articles, systematic reviews and meta-analyses, protocols and guidelines, animal studies, conference abstracts and presentations, preprints, clinical trials under patient recruitment or without published results, ongoing clinical trials, and studies deemed irrelevant were excluded.

After the exclusion of articles based on the above criteria by both the automated tools and the researchers, the final set of articles was retrieved. To ensure accuracy and objectivity, two independent reviewers (I.K. and S.T.) initially screened the titles and abstracts in a double-blinded process. For studies that passed this initial screening, the full texts were obtained and further evaluated to determine their final eligibility. Any discrepancies during the screening process were resolved by a third reviewer (T.P.).

2.4. Data Charting

Key variables were systematically extracted from all included studies by the primary researchers (I.K. and S.T.), comprising the first author, publication year, study design, number of participants, NP-based regimen discussed, pharmacological regimens assessed, mean age of participants in years, median overall survival in months, median progression-free disease in months, disease control rates, partial remission rate, complete remission rate, stable disease rate, treatment-emergent adverse events reported, and finally, the key findings as a conclusion.

2.5. Collating, Summarizing, and Reporting Results

The extracted data were synthesized into results tables. Given the scoping nature of this review, a meta-analysis was not conducted; instead, a descriptive synthesis of the principal findings was performed to explore and evaluate the application of NP-based therapies in the management of PC, particularly within real-world clinical settings.

3. Results

The PRISMA flow diagram (Figure 3) outlines the review selection and exclusion process. Initially, a total of 2144 records were retrieved from the aforementioned databases. Automated screening excluded 2063 records, leaving 81 records for further consideration. Of these, 11 duplicate records were removed manually. Subsequently, 45 studies were excluded based on ineligible study design, as determined through title and abstract screening. After a full-text review of the remaining 25 articles, a total of 19 studies met the inclusion criteria and, thus, were included in the review.

The included studies were published between 2006 and 2023 (Tables 2 and 3). Most of the studies (n = 14) were clinical trials, whereas two were retrospective cohorts and three were case reports. Most of the studies (n = 10) assessed nanoparticle albumin-bound paclitaxel, whereas four evaluated nanoliposomal irinotecan, two weighed both of the aforementioned regimens, one considered CYT-6091, one NK105, and finally, one reviewed nanoliposomal cisplatin.

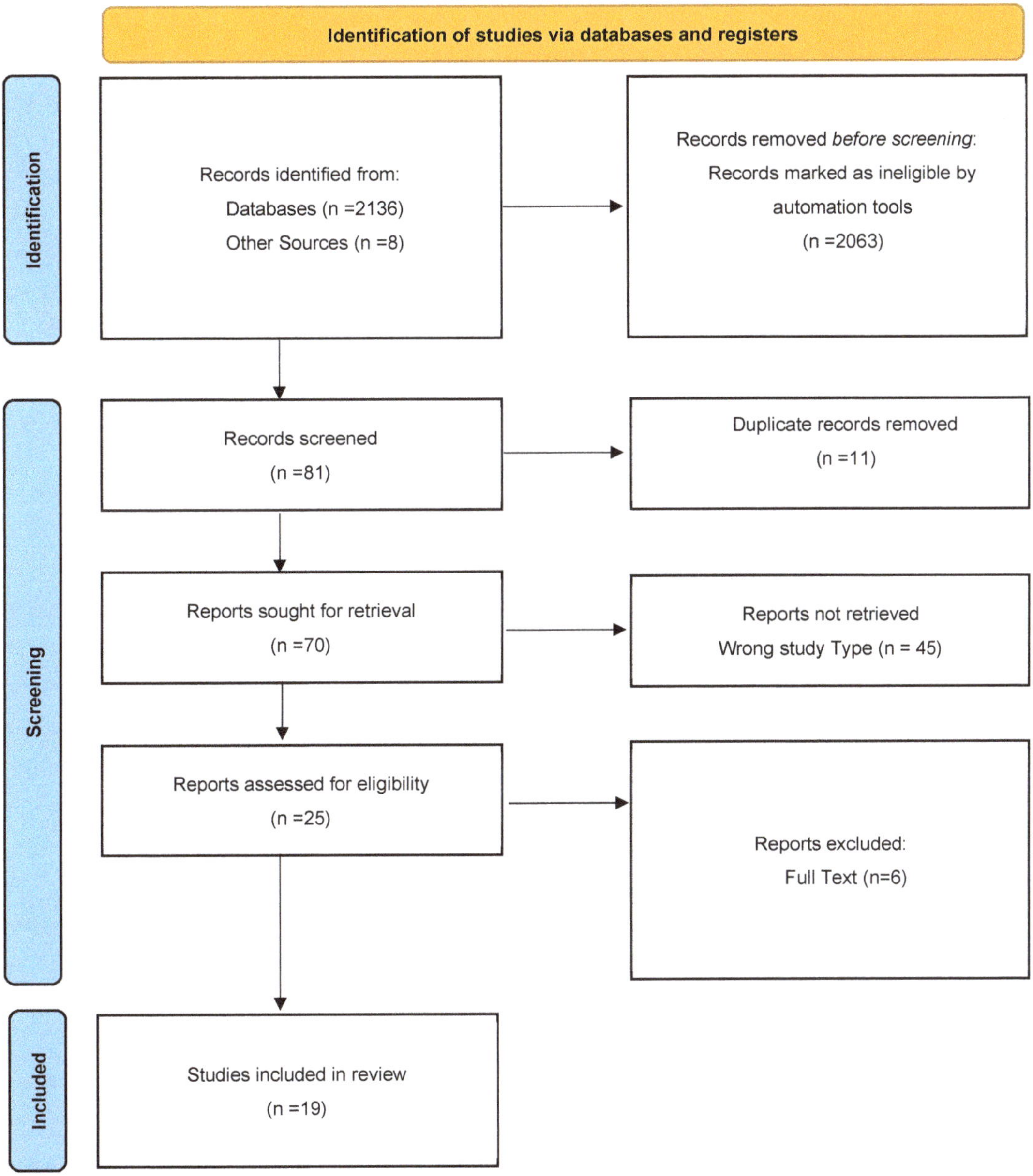

Figure 3. PRISMA flow diagram.

Table 2. Comparative summary table of clinical trials and retrospective studies. N: number of participants; NPs: nanoparticles; mOS: median overall survival; mo: months; CI: confidence interval; mPFS: median progression-free survival; DCR: disease control rate; PR: partial remission; CR: complete remission; SD: stable disease; TEAEs: treatment-emergent adverse events; nab-PTX: nanoparticle albumin-bound paclitaxel; nal-IRI: nanoliposomal irinotecan: mPDAC: metastatic pancreatic ductal adenocarcinoma; 5-FU: 5-fluorouracile; LV: leucovorin; NALIRIFOX: nal-IRI, oxaliplatin, 5-FU, LV; FOLFIRINOX: irinotecan, oxaliplatin, 5-FU, LV; mFOLFIRINOX: modified FOLFIRINOX; ECOG PS: Eastern Cooperative Oncology Group Performance Status.

Author, Year	Type of Study	N	Patients	NPs	Regimens	Age (Years)	mOS (mo; 95% CI)	mPFS (mo; 95% CI)	DCR (%, 95% CI)	PR (%, 95% CI)	CR (%, 95% CI)	SD (%, 95% CI)	TEAEs	Conclusions
Nanoliposomal Irinotecan and Nanoparticle Albumin-Bound Paclitaxel														
Wainberg ZA et al., 2023 [28]	Phase III randomized clinical trial (NAPOLI 3; NCT04083235)	770	Previously untreated mPDAC	Nanoliposomal irinotecan and nanoparticle albumin-bound paclitaxel	NALIRIFOX (N = 383) vs. nab-PTX + gemcitabine (N = 387)	64 (20–85) vs. 65 (36–82)	11.1 (10.0–12.1) vs. 9.2 (8.3–10.6)	7.4 (6.0–7.7) vs. 5.6 (5.3–5.8)	41.8 (36.8–46.9) vs. 36.2 (21.4–41.2)	42 vs. 36	<1 vs. <1	26 vs. 26	Grade 3–4: neutropenia; diarrhea; hypokalemia in the NALIRIFOX group Grade 3–4: neutropenia; anemia; peripheral neuropathy in the nab-PTX + gemcitabine group	NALIRIFOX promising treatment for mPDAC; improved survival and tolerability; fewer hematological TEAEs
Nanoliposomal Irinotecan														
Bockorny B et al., 2021 [29]	Phase IIa clinical trial (COMBAT/ KEYNOTE-202; NCT02826486)	43	De novo mPDAC with documented radiographic progression after treatment with first-line gemcitabine-based chemotherapy	Nanoliposomal irinotecan	Motixafortide + pembrolizumab + nal-IRI + 5-FU + LV	68 (40–85)	6.6 (4.5–8.7)	3.8 (1.6–5.1)	63.2 (47.8–78.5)	N/A	N/A	42.1 (26.4–57.8)	Grade 3–4: nausea and vomiting (18.6%); asthenia (16.3%); diarrhea (14%); serious neutropenia (7%); febrile neutropenia (2.3%); reactions at the injection site (4.7%)	Safe; well tolerated; promising efficacy; lower-than-expected rates of neutropenia and infections
Park SJ et al., 2021 [30]	Retrospective cohort study	51	mPDAC previously treated with gemcitabine-based therapy	Nanoliposomal irinotecan	nal-IRI + 5-FU + LV	67 (50–78)	7.0 (6.0–7.9)	2.8 (1.8–3.7)	60.8	5.9	0	54.9	Anemia (84.3%); neutropenia (84.3%; Grade 3–4: 58.8%); nausea (43.1%); diarrhea (23.5%); fatigue (21.6%); febrile neutropenia (7.8%)	Clinical benefits; gemcitabine plus nab-PTX remains a viable first-line treatment option for a significant portion of patients with mPDAC
Glassman DC et al., 2018 [31]	Retrospective study	56	mPDAC previously treated with gemcitabine-based therapy	Nanoliposomal irinotecan	FOLFIRINOX or FOLFOX, followed by nab-PTX + gemcitabine and nal-IRI + 5-FU + LV (Sequence 1) vs. gemcitabine alone or nab-PTX + gemcitabine followed by nal-IRI + 5-FU + LV (Sequence 2)	68 (42–88)	4.1 vs. 9.0	2.2 vs. 4.8	N/A	5	0	41	GI toxicities (nausea and vomiting; diarrhea); fatigue; anorexia; neutropenia; anemia (Grade 3/4)	Confirmed safety and efficacy of nal-IRI + 5-FU/LV for advanced PDAC after gemcitabine-based therapy; earlier use in treatment and absence of irinotecan-refractory disease correlated with improved progression-free survival; dose reductions did not compromise outcomes; genetic predictors of response require further validation; promising OS with sequential integration into combination chemotherapy

Table 2. *Cont.*

Author, Year	Type of Study	N	Patients	NPs	Regimens	Age (Years)	mOS (mo; 95% CI)	mPFS (mo; 95% CI)	DCR (%, 95% CI)	PR (%, 95% CI)	CR (%, 95% CI)	SD (%, 95% CI)	TEAEs	Conclusions
Wang-Gillam A et al., 2016 [32]	Phase III randomized clinical trial (NAPOLI-1; NCT01494506)	417	mPDAC previously treated with gemcitabine-based therapy	Nanoliposomal irinotecan	nal-IRI + 5-FU + LV (N = 117) vs. 5-FU + LV (N = 149) vs. nal-IRI monotherapy (N = 151)	63 (57–70) vs. 65 (58–70) vs. 63 (55–69)	6.1 (4.8–8.9) vs. 4.2 (3.3–5.3) vs. 4.9 (4.2–5.6)	3.1 (2.7–4.2) vs. 1.5 (1.4–1.8) vs. 2.7 (2.1–2.9)	N/A	N/A	N/A	N/A	Grade 3–4 neutropenic sepsis and febrile neutropenia (3% vs. 0 vs. 4%); Grade 4 (10% vs. 7% vs. 16%); resulting in death: gastrointestinal toxicity, infectious enterocolitis, septic shock, and disseminated intravascular coagulation with pulmonary embolism	Improves survival and other key efficacy measures in metastatic PC patients previously treated with gemcitabine-based therapy; manageable and mostly reversible safety profile; new treatment option, although its applicability to patients with low performance status remains uncertain
Nanoparticle albumin-bound paclitaxel														
Ceelen W et al., 2022 [33]	Phase I clinical trial (NCT03304210)	20	Peritoneal metastases from ovarian, breast, gastric, hepatobiliary, or pancreatic origin	Nanoparticle albumin-bound paclitaxel	Pressurized intraperitoneal aerosol chemotherapy (PIPAC) nab-PTX	57 (49–65)	N/A	N/A	N/A	N/A	N/A	N/A	Hematological toxicity (moderate); Grade 3 neutropenia	Safety and potential effectiveness for advanced, unresectable peritoneal metastases; well-tolerated dosing; stable patient quality of life; promising anticancer activity
Sohal DPS et al., 2021 [34]	Phase II randomized clinical trial (NCT02562716)	102	Treatment-naïve PDAC with no metastases	Nanoparticle albumin-bound paclitaxel	mFOLFIRINOX (N = 55) vs. nab-PTX + gemcitabine (N = 47)	66 (44–76) vs. 64 (46–75)	23.2 (17.6–45.9) vs. 23.6 (17.8–31.7)	N/A	N/A	N/A	N/A	N/A	Neoadjuvant: neutropenia (19% vs 27%); (11% vs 4%)	Safety and efficacy; no improved OS compared to historical adjuvant trials
Azmi AS et al., 2020 [35]	Phase Ib study (NCT02178436)	5	mPDAC not treated with chemotherapy	Nanoparticle albumin-bound paclitaxel	Selinexor + gemcitabine + nab-PTX	N/A	N/A	N/A	N/A	N/A	N/A	N/A	N/A	Synergy between selinexor and GEM-nab-PTX in PDAC models, including stem cells and patient-derived xenografts
Hasegawa R et al., 2019 [36]	Clinical trial (UMIN000018907)	27	Unresectable advanced PC + age ≥ 75 years	Nanoparticle albumin-bound paclitaxel	nab-PTX + gemcitabine	77 (75–85)	10.3 (8.2–12.5)	7.0 (6.0–8.1)	N/A	44.4	N/A	48.1	Grade 3–4: hemotoxic (51.9%); non-hemotoxic (59.3%): peripheral nerve disorder (22.2%)	Improved progression-free survival in elderly patients; favorable disease control even in stage IV cases; feasible with proper dose management; elderly patients more susceptible to non-hemotoxic TEAEs
Macarulla T et al., 2019 [37]	Phase I trial	24	Locally advanced or advanced PDAC; ECOG PS of 2	Nanoparticle albumin-bound paclitaxel	nab-PTX at 150 mg/m^2 (arm A) or 125 mg/m^2 (arm C) + gemcitabine; nab-PTX at 100 mg/m^2 (arm B) or 125 mg/m^2 (arm D) + gemcitabine	N/A	N/A	N/A	N/A	N/A	N/A	N/A	N/A	Not designed for direct comparison; both arms showed similar efficacy and toxicity; potential treatment option in clinical practice
	Phase II randomized trial (NCT02382263)	221	Locally advanced or advanced PDAC; ECOG PS of 2		nab-PTX at 100 mg/m^2 (arm B; N = 111) or 125 mg/m^2 (arm D; N = 110) + gemcitabine	71 (43–89) vs. 68 (35–84)	7.7 (6.3–9.1) vs. 9.8 (7.5–11.8)	5.4 (4–6.9) vs. 6.6 (5.6–7.6)	64.9 (56–73.7) vs. 71.8 (63.4–80.2)	20.7 vs. 21.8	0 vs. 0.9	N/A	Hematological toxicity (neutropenia); fatigue; peripheral neuropathy	

Table 2. *Cont.*

Author, Year	Type of Study	N	Patients	NPs	Regimens	Age (Years)	mOS (mo; 95% CI)	mPFS (mo; 95% CI)	DCR (%, 95% CI)	PR (%, 95% CI)	CR (%, 95% CI)	SD (%, 95% CI)	TEAEs	Conclusions
Von Hoff DD et al., 2013 [38]	Phase III Randomized control trial (MPACT; NCT00844649)	861	mPDAC not treated with chemotherapy	Nanoparticle albumin-bound paclitaxel	nab-PTX + gemcitabine (N = 431) vs. gemcitabine monotherapy (N = 430)	63 (27–88)	8.5 (7.89–9.53) vs. 6.7 (6.01–7.23)	5.5 (4.5–5.9) vs. 3.7 (3.6–4.0)	48 (43–53) vs. 33 (28–37)	23 vs. 7	<1 vs. 0	20 vs. 26	Grade 3–4: neutropenia; leukopenia; fatigue; peripheral neuropathy (mostly in nab-PTX cohort)	Significantly improved survival; benefits observed across multiple time points and subgroups; increased myelosuppression and peripheral neuropathy, reversible; potential as an effective treatment option
Hosein PJ et al., 2013 [39]	Phase II clinical trial (NCT00691054)	19	Advanced PC that progressed on gemcitabine-based therapy with unresectable locally advanced or metastatic disease	Nanoparticle albumin-bound paclitaxel	nab-PTX monotherapy	61 (24–80)	7.3 (2.8–15.8)	1.7 (1.5–3.5)	5	5	0	32	Grades 3–4 neutropenia (26%); Grades 3–4 anemia (11%); neutropenic fever (11%); hypocalcemia	The nab-PTX monotherapy demonstrated preliminary activity in a subset of patients and was well tolerated
Von Hoff DD et al., 2011 [40]	Phase I/II clinical trial (NCT00398086.)	67	Previously untreated advanced PC	Nanoparticle albumin-bound paclitaxel	100 (N = 20), 125 (N = 44; Results), or 150 (N = 3) mg/m^2 nab-PTX + gemcitabine	62 (30–86) vs. 61 (28–78) vs. 69 (53–72)	12.2 (8.9–17.9)	7.9 (5.8–11.0)	68	48	0	20	Grade 3–4 fatigue (21%); sensory neuropathy (15%); neutropenia (67%); leukopenia (44%); thrombocytopenia (23%)	Favorable safety and encouraging antitumor activity; patient selection may influence outcomes
Other Nanoparticle-Based Targeted Therapies														
Libutti SK et al., 2010 [41]	Phase I clinical trial	3	Advanced-stage PC patients	CYT-6091	PEGylated colloidal gold nanoparticle carrying rhTNF-a	N/A	N/A	N/A	N/A	N/A	N/A	N/A	Grade 3–4 lymphopenia (89%); hypoalbuminemia (17%); hypokalemia (17%); hypophosphatemia (17%); hyperbilirubinemia (17%), increased AST (17%)	Promising tumor targeting; potential benefits when administered systemically before chemotherapy or surgery, particularly for solid tumors
Hamaguchi T et al., 2007 [42]	Phase I clinical trial	11	PC refractory to conventional chemotherapy	NK105	Polymeric micellar nanoparticle paclitaxel	57 (43–72)	N/A	N/A	N/A	N/A	N/A	N/A	Grade 3–4: neutropenia; Grade 1–2: fever; nausea; fatigue; stomatitis; rash; alopecia	Reduction in the size of metastatic lesions; minimal severity of adverse events; favorable therapeutic response and manageable safety profile
Stathopoulos GP et al., 2006 [43]	Phase I/II clinical trial	24	Advanced PDAC after chemotherapy pretreatment and recurrent or non-responsive disease	Nanoliposomal cisplatin	Lipoplatin + gemcitabine	66 (47–80)	4 (2–8)	N/A	N/A	8.3	N/A	58.3	Grade 3 myelotoxicity (50%)	Well tolerated in advanced pretreated PC patients; promising efficacy with symptom relief and disease stability

Table 3. Comparative summary of case reports. NPs: nanoparticles; nab-PTX: nanoparticle albumin-bound paclitaxel; nal-IRI: nanoliposomal irinotecan; SCC: squamous-cell carcinoma; mPDAC: metastatic pancreatic ductal adenocarcinoma; 5-FU: 5-fluorouracile; LV: leucovorin.

Author, Year	Type	Disease	Gender	Age	NPs	Regimen	Conclusions
Huang X et al., 2021 [44]	Case report	Stage IV primary SCC of the pancreas harboring a deleterious BRCA2 somatic mutation	F	52	NP albumin-bound paclitaxel	nab-PTX + cisplatin	Significant tumor reduction; prolonged survival; improved tumor resectability; the longest reported survival for metastatic pancreatic SCC to date
Otsubo M et al., 2021 [45]	Case report	Stage IV PC with hepatic and lymph node metastases	M	70	NP albumin-bound paclitaxel	nab-PTX + gemcitabine	Taxane-related cystoid macular edema (CME) as a rare but notable side effect of nab-PTX, affecting bilateral central vision; CME resolved after stopping nab-PTX, with no intervention other than topical dorzolamide
Assi HA et al., 2020 [46]	Case report	T4, N1, and M1 primary pancreatic adenocarcinoma	F	57	Nanoliposomal irinotecan and NP albumin-bound paclitaxel	nab-PTX + gemcitabine followed by nal-IRI + 5-FU + LV	Rare instance of long-term survival in an mPDAC patient treated with nal-IRI + 5-FU/LV; despite initial disease progression, sustained response for over two years, receiving 58 cycles without dose adjustments; PFS and OS reached 31 and 40 months, respectively; potential clinical benefits

4. Discussion

Pancreatic cancer, most commonly presenting as PDAC, remains one of the most dreadful malignancies due to its limited therapeutic options and dismal survival outcomes. The integration of NP-based technologies into PC treatment has yielded significant advancements, notably in enhancing drug delivery, improving therapeutic efficacy, and reducing systemic adverse effects and toxicities. By modifying pharmacokinetics, increasing tumor penetration, and refining second-line treatment strategies, nanomedicine has fundamentally transformed treatment paradigms for PC.

4.1. Nanoparticle Albumin-Bound Paclitaxel (nab-PTX) in Pancreatic Cancer

Nanoparticle albumin-bound paclitaxel (nab-PTX) accounts for a major advancement in PC treatment by enhancing drug delivery and tumor penetration while diminishing treatment-emergent adverse events (TEAEs) and toxicities correlated with conventional paclitaxel. This formulation leverages albumin as a carrier to accelerate active transport through gp60 receptors and the caveolin-1-SPARC pathway, permitting more efficient intratumoral drug accumulation [40]. This mechanism of action results in significant clinical benefits, comprising improved OS and PFS, superior tumor response rates, and enhanced chemotherapy delivery to neoplastic tissues (Figure 4) [40].

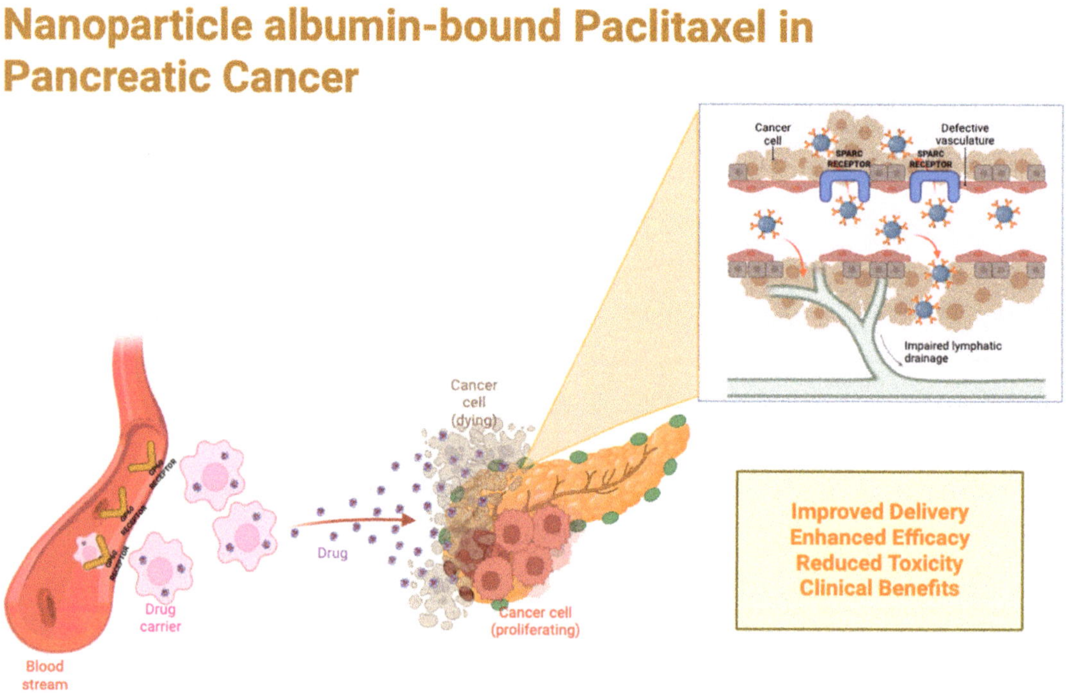

Figure 4. Nanoparticle albumin-bound paclitaxel in pancreatic cancer: mechanisms of action and advantages compared to conventional chemotherapy regimens.

Regarding the mechanism of action and tumor microenvironment modulation, nab-PTX demonstrates a dual function as both a cytotoxic agent and a tumor stroma modifier.

In a phase I/II clinical trial by Von Hoff DD et al. in 2011, critical preclinical evidence demonstrated that nab-PTX depletes the tumor stroma, thereby enhancing intratumoral gemcitabine concentrations through increased vascular perfusion [40]. This stromal depletion is significant, as the dense fibrotic stroma characteristic of pancreatic tumors frequently inhibits effective drug delivery and, therefore, nab-PTX facilitates chemotherapy penetration, improving drug accumulation and enhancing tumor cell death [40]. Additionally, the study demonstrated that elevated expression of Secreted Protein Acidic and Rich in Cysteine (SPARC) in the tumor stroma is associated with improved survival rates, supporting the hypothesis that targeting stromal components is essential for maximizing treatment efficacy. These findings underline the significance of integrating stromal-depleting therapies with standard chemotherapy regimens to optimize drug penetration and overall therapeutic outcomes [40]. Furthermore, an alternative nab-PTX formulation—NK105, a polymeric micelle formulation of paclitaxel—was evaluated by Hamaguchi T et al. in 2007 for its pharmacokinetic advantages. NK105 exhibited a plasma area under the curve (AUC) 15 to 20 times higher than that of conventional paclitaxel, thereby augmenting the drug stability and improving tumor targeting [42]. The study further demonstrated that lower tissue distribution of NK105 resulted in reduced toxicity in normal tissues, particularly neurotoxicity, suggesting that it may offer an alternative paclitaxel delivery system with a more favorable adverse event profile [42].

Concerning clinical efficacy and survival benefits, the pivotal MPACT randomized control trial by Von Hoff DD et al. (2013) verified that nab-PTX in combination with gemcitabine significantly enhanced survival outcomes compared with gemcitabine monotherapy in patients with mPDAC who had not received prior chemotherapy [38]. The mOS improved by 1.8–8.5 (95% CI 7.89–9.53) months versus 6.7 (95% CI 6.01–7.23) months in the gemcitabine-only arm, with long-term survival rates similarly favoring the combination therapy (35% vs. 22% at one year and 9% vs. 4% at two years). Similarly, the mPFS increased by 31%, with values of 5.5 (95% CI 4.5–5.9) months in the control arm compared to 3.7 (95% CI 3.6–4.0) months in the control group, thereby reducing the risk of disease progression or death [38]. Moreover, the study indicated that declining serum CA19–9 levels were strongly correlated with improved survival, reaffirming the prognostic significance of this biomarker, and that nab-PTX was shown to enhance chemotherapy delivery by modulating the tumor stroma to facilitate increased drug penetration [38]. Furthermore, a subsequent phase II randomized trial by Macarulla T et al. (2019) evaluated nab-PTX in patients with locally advanced or advanced PDAC and an Eastern Cooperative Oncology Group (ECOG) performance status of 2. The findings confirmed that the regimen was both efficacious and tolerable in this more vulnerable patient population, with mOS and mPFS sustained at 8.5 and 5.5 months, respectively, values comparable to the results of the MPACT trial [37]. However, baseline patient heterogeneity within the study cohort may have influenced tolerability and outcomes, underscoring the need for more robust patient stratification tools. Moreover, the incorporation of objective biomarkers, such as albumin levels, inflammatory markers, and body composition, could aid in refining patient selection and optimizing treatment strategies [37].

In this context, Hasegawa et al. (2019) conducted a clinical trial in patients with unresectable advanced pancreatic adenocarcinoma or adenosquamous carcinoma aged over 75 years. Despite lower-than-expected chemotherapy completion rates, the combination of nab-PTX and gemcitabine improved mOS and mPFS in elderly patients compared to gemcitabine monotherapy, as confirmed by an mOS of 10.3 (95% CI 8.2–12.5) months and an mPFS of 7.0 (95% CI 6.0–8.1) months, with favorable disease control observed even in stage IV cases [36]. While this regimen remains feasible with appropriate dose management, elderly patients, particularly those with sarcopenia, appear more susceptible to non-hemotoxic adverse events, highlighting the need for further large-scale studies and improved patient selection criteria [36]. Furthermore, a phase II clinical trial by Hosein PJ et al. (2013) investigated nab-PTX monotherapy in patients with unresectable locally advanced or metastatic PC who had progressed on gemcitabine-based therapy, reporting an mOS of 7.3 (95% CI 2.8–15.8) months and an mPFS of 1.7 (95% CI 1.5–3.5) months, with 37% of patients surviving beyond thirteen weeks. Notably, one patient remained on nab-PTX therapy for nearly two years, establishing the feasibility of prolonged administration of nab-PTX in selected individuals [39].

In the context of peritoneal metastases associated with advanced PC, patients confront unique therapeutic challenges due to inadequate drug penetration into the tumor core. In this setting, pressurized intraperitoneal aerosol chemotherapy (PIPAC) has emerged as an innovative drug delivery technique to overcome these impediments. In a phase I clinical trial, Ceelen W et al. (2022) evaluated aerosolized nab-PTX and established that the regimen was well tolerated while achieving enhanced tumor uptake over multiple treatment cycles. Importantly, systemic exposure remained significantly lower compared to intravenous administration, thereby diminishing the risk of adverse events [33]. The study reported a histological response rate of 35% among patients receiving two or more PIPAC cycles, with the survival data indicating that more than half of the patients survived beyond one year. These promising findings warrant further clinical investigation, particularly to refine dose selection and sequencing strategies for this modality [33].

In a phase II randomized clinical trial by Sohal DPS et al. (2021), nab-PTX was evaluated in the neoadjuvant setting as part of a perioperative chemotherapy regimen for treatment-naïve pancreatic adenocarcinoma without metastases. The study reported a slightly higher mOS in the nab-PTX plus gemcitabine cohort, at 23.6 (95% CI 17.8–31.7) months, compared to 23.2 (95% CI 17.6–45.9) months in the modified FOLFIRINOX arm. However, this difference did not represent an improvement in OS when compared with historical perioperative chemotherapy trials [34]. Additionally, while a modestly higher incidence of neutropenia was observed in the nab-PTX cohort (27% versus 19%), severe diarrhea was more common in the mFOLFIRINOX arm (11% versus 4%), although neither of these differences was statistically significant [34].

With reference to toxicity and other safety considerations, nab-PTX necessitates meticulous management, particularly concerning neurotoxicity and myelosuppression. The MPACT trial by Von Hoff DD et al., in 2013, identified peripheral neuropathy as a noteworthy adverse effect, although these symptoms were reversible with treatment suspension and dose modifications [38]. Additionally, sepsis and pneumonitis risks were effectively managed through protocol adjustments, and myelosuppression was manageable with appropriate supportive care [38]. Comparative safety analyses by Hosein PJ et al. (2013) established improved tolerability with nab-PTX monotherapy, characterized by minimal non-hematological toxicities and an absence of Grade 3–4 peripheral neuropathy [39]. Moreover, Macarulla T et al. (2019) noted that a lower dose maintained survival benefits while reducing toxicity and enhancing tolerability, particularly among more fragile patients with an ECOG performance status of 2 [37]. Similarly, Otsubo M et al. (2021) reported taxane-related cystoid macular edema (CME) as a rare yet noteworthy adverse event affecting bilateral central vision in a patient with stage IV PC undergoing a nab-PTX plus gemcitabine regimen [45]. Encouragingly, CME resolved after the suspension of nab-PTX and treatment with local dorzolamide, suggesting a potential management strategy for similar cases [45].

As treatment regimens for mPDAC continue to advance, integrating nab-PTX with emerging therapies demonstrates considerable promise. For instance, Azmi AS et al., in 2020, assessed the combination of nab-PTX with selinexor, a nuclear export inhibitor targeting XPO1. By retaining tumor suppressor proteins within the nucleus of the tumor cells, selinexor enhances cancer cell apoptosis and suppresses PDAC proliferation [35]. Preclinical evidence from this study established that the combination was particularly effective in PDAC stem cells and patient-derived xenograft models, indicating that targeting multiple cancer cell survival pathways could overcome chemotherapy resistance mechanisms and further improve treatment outcomes [35]. Additionally, Huang X et al. (2021) reported a case of a patient with stage IV primary squamous-cell carcinoma of the pancreas harboring a deleterious BRCA2 somatic mutation. The combination of cisplatin and nab-PTX in this patient resulted in significant tumor reduction and prolonged survival, along with improved tumor resectability, and represented the longest reported survival for metastatic pancreatic squamous-cell carcinoma to date. These findings underscore the potential clinical impact of such combination therapies [44].

4.2. Nanoliposomal Irinotecan (nal-IRI) in Pancreatic Cancer

Nanoliposomal irinotecan (nal-IRI) represents a significant advancement in the treatment of mPDAC, markedly altering the disease's prognosis. By encapsulating irinotecan within liposomes, nal-IRI enhances drug stability, improves tumor penetration and minimizes systemic toxicities compared to conventional irinotecan formulations (Figure 5). Multiple clinical trials have demonstrated its efficacy, establishing nal-IRI as an essential component of second-line treatment regimens following gemcitabine-based therapies.

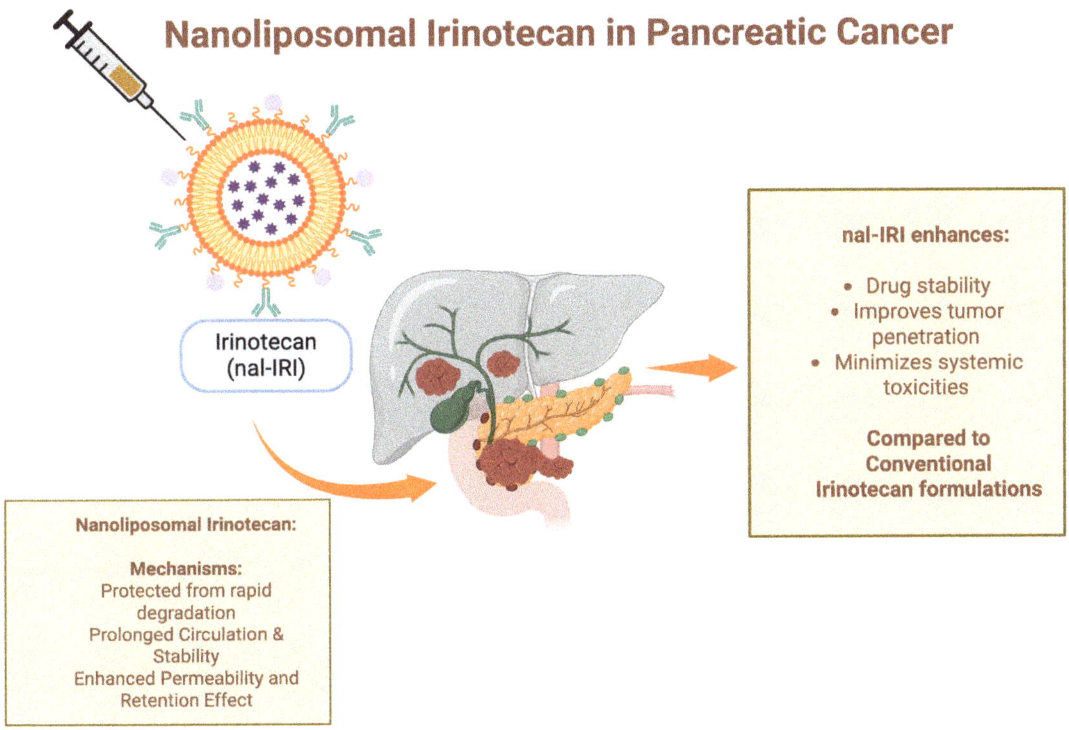

Figure 5. Nanoliposomal irinotecan in pancreatic cancer: mechanism of action and advantages compared to conventional irinotecan-based regimens.

With respect to the clinical efficacy and survival benefits of nal-IRI, the NAPOLI-1 trial by Wang-Gillam A et al. (2016) demonstrated that the combination of nal-IRI with 5-fluorouracil (5-FU) and folinic acid/leucovorin (LV) is superior to fluorouracil monotherapy for patients with metastatic PC previously treated with gemcitabine-based regimens [32]. Specifically, the trial reported a significant improvement in mOS and mPFS to 6.1 (95% CI 4.8–8.9) and 3.1 (95% CI 2.7–4.2) months, respectively, compared to 4.2 (95% CI 3.3–5.3) and 1.5 (95% CI 1.4–1.8) months in the monotherapy cohort, respectively. In addition to these survival benefits, the combination regimen enhanced objective tumor response rates and significantly reduced CA19–9 levels, thereby reaffirming its viability as a treatment option [32]. Further evidence supporting the value of nal-IRI in second-line treatment came from a retrospective cohort study by Park SJ et al. in 2021, which evaluated nal-IRI plus 5-FU/LV in patients with progressed or recurrent mPDAC previously treated with gemcitabine-based therapy. This study reported survival outcomes consistent with the NAPOLI-1 trial, with an mOS of 7.0 (95% CI 6.0–7.9) months and an mPFS of 2.8 (95% CI 1.8–3.7) months, along with manageable toxicities [30]. However, a higher incidence of Grade 3–4 neutropenia was noted compared to the NAPOLI-1 findings, emphasizing the necessity for vigilant hematological monitoring. Notably, nal-IRI remains a first-line treatment in only 20–40% of patients with metastatic PC, underscoring the importance of patient selection and individualized dosing strategies [30].

Another retrospective study by Glassman DC et al. (2018) further elucidated the role of nal-IRI in sequencing treatment strategies. Patients who received nab-PTX with gemcitabine, followed by nal-IRI plus 5-FU/LV as a second-line therapy, without prior irinotecan exposure, achieved an mOS of 9.0 months and an mPFS of 4.8 months. In contrast, patients who had undergone prior treatment with the FOLFIRINOX regimen (and consequently received nal-IRI as a third-line treatment) exhibited an mOS of 4.1 months and an mPFS of 2.2 months. These findings advocate for the strategic integration of nal-IRI into the treatment algorithm to prolong survival [31]. Complementing these data, a case report by Assi HA et al. (2020) described a rare instance of long-term survival in a patient with mPDAC under nal-IRI + 5-FU/LV therapy following disease progression on a nab-PTX plus gemcitabine regimen [46]. The patient exhibited a sustained response for over two years, receiving 58 cycles without dose adjustments. Remarkably, the reported PFS and OS were 31 and 40 months, respectively, underscoring the potential benefits of this regimen and the need for further refinement of sequential regimen therapies [46]. Further evidence was derived from the NAPOLI-3 phase III randomized clinical trial by Wainberg ZA et al. (2023), which compared a quadruplet regimen of NALIRIFOX (incorporating nal-IRI) with FOLFIRINOX, as evaluated in the PRODIGE 4/ACCORD 11 phase III clinical trial by Conroy T et al. (2011). In NAPOLI-3, the mPFS was 7.4 (95% CI 6.0–7.7) months for NALIRIFOX, compared to 6.4 (95% CI 5.5–7.2) months for FOLFIRINOX in PRODIGE, insinuating that nal-IRI confers advantages over conventional irinotecan-based regimens [28]. Importantly, nal-IRI was correlated with a lower incidence of neutropenia and neuropathy relative to FOLFIRINOX, positioning it as a more tolerable alternative for patients with compromised performance status and those at risk of TEAEs [28,30,47]. Moreover, in the context of sequential combination chemotherapy regimens, Bockorny B et al. (2021) conducted a phase IIa clinical trial (COMBAT/KEYNOTE-202) investigating the incorporation of motixafortide to potentiate immune responses by increasing circulating lymphocytes and neutrophils, in combination with pembrolizumab and nal-IRI plus 5-FU/LV, in patients with de novo mPDAC who had documented radiographic progression after first-line gemcitabine-based therapy. This regimen demonstrated clinical benefit, with durable responses, reflected in an mOS of 6.6 (95% CI 4.5–8.7) months, an mPFS of 3.8 (95%

CI 1.6–5.1), and a notably lower rate of severe neutropenia (7%, compared to 27% in the NAPOLI-1 trial), likely attributable to CXCR4 inhibition by motixafortide [29].

Regarding toxicity and safety considerations, despite its established efficacy, nal-IRI is correlated with specific toxicity concerns, predominantly hematological toxicity. In the NAPOLI-1 trial, higher rates of Grade 3–4 neutropenia were reported, an effect mainly attributed to the fluorouracil and folinic acid components of the regimen [32]. Notably, incidents of neutropenic sepsis were rare, indicating that these risks are manageable with appropriate supportive care [32]. Consistent with these observations, Park SJ et al. (2021) documented an increased incidence of neutropenia (58.8% versus 27% in NAPOLI-1), while severe diarrhea was observed less frequently (5.9% versus 13% in NAPOLI-1). This underscores the necessity for proactive management and suggests that treatment modifications may significantly influence the tolerability profile [30]. Moreover, Wainberg ZA et al. (2023) attested that nal-IRI exhibited lower rates of Grade 3–4 peripheral neuropathy and hematological adverse events compared to the nab-PTX plus gemcitabine regimen [28].

Furthermore, emerging evidence suggests that biomarker-driven approaches may enhance the application of nal-IRI in personalized oncology. Glassman DC et al., in 2018, investigated the association between TP53 mutation status and mPFS in patients treated with the nal-IRI plus 5-FU/LV regimen. The study demonstrated that patients harboring wild-type TP53 experienced significantly improved treatment efficacy, with an mPFS of 6.0 months, compared to only 2.2 months in those with TP53 mutations [31]. The underlying biological rationale for these observations likely involves the crucial role of p53 in orchestrating cellular responses to DNA damage. In tumors with an intact *TP53* gene, nal-IRI-induced DNA damage, primarily through the active metabolite of irinotecan, triggers p53 activation, which subsequently upregulates downstream effectors, such as $p21^{WAF1/CIP1}$ [48]. This cascade enforces a robust cell-cycle arrest, ultimately leading to apoptosis when the damage is irreparable. Conversely, in tumors harboring TP53 mutations, the disruption of this critical checkpoint mechanism results in an attenuated p53 response, permitting continued cell-cycle progression, and thereby diminishing the cytotoxic efficacy of nal-IRI [48]. Although definitive conclusions cannot be drawn from studies with limited sample sizes, this preliminary evidence highlights the potential of TP53 status as a predictive biomarker and underscores the critical need for further genomic profiling in larger, controlled patient cohorts to optimize patient stratification and to enhance therapeutic outcomes [31,48]. Similarly, Wainberg ZA et al., in 2023, recommended that future research should seek insight into integrating genomic biomarkers into treatment algorithms to ensure that nal-IRI is administered to patients most likely to derive clinical benefit [28].

4.3. Other Nanoparticle-Based Targeted Therapies

The advancement of NP-based targeted therapies has introduced innovative strategies to enhance chemotherapy delivery while diminishing systemic toxicity. In a phase I/II trial, Stathopoulos GP et al. (2006) demonstrated that a nanoliposomal formulation of cisplatin, known as lipoplatin, when combined with gemcitabine, is well tolerated in advanced pretreated PC patients. The study reported promising efficacy, with symptom relief observed in one-third and disease stability achieved in more than half of patients [47]. Moreover, incorporating lipoplatin into the gemcitabine regimen was shown to minimize nephrotoxicity and exhibit manageable myelotoxicity, all while maintaining robust antitumor efficacy [43].

Additionally, Libutti SK et al. (2010) introduced a novel PEGylated colloidal gold NP, CYT-6091, engineered by concurrently conjugating recombinant human tumor necrosis factor alpha (rhTNF-a) and thiolated polyethylene glycol to the surface of 27 nm colloidal gold particles [41]. Evaluated in a phase I dose-escalation clinical trial involving advanced

PC patients, CYT-6091 demonstrated selective accumulation in tumor tissues via the enhanced permeability and retention effect. Electron microscopy confirmed intratumoral NP accumulation, thereby supporting its potential role in vascular disruption therapy. The preliminary clinical findings, which revealed partial responses in metastatic ocular melanoma, further underscore the need for additional trials to assess the integration of CYT-6091 with standard chemotherapy protocols [41].

4.4. Limitations, Challenges, and Prospective Views

NP-based therapies have emerged as promising candidates for the management of PC; however, several limitations and challenges must be acknowledged when considering their clinical application in real-world patients. A significant concern is biocompatibility, as the materials used in NP formulations may elicit unexpected toxicities or compromise cellular integrity, necessitating a delicate balance between therapeutic efficacy and safety. Additionally, the intricate interactions between NPs and the immune system raise the potential for immunogenic responses that could undermine treatment outcomes and adversely affect patient tolerance. Tumor heterogeneity further complicates the therapeutic landscape, as variations in tumor microenvironment, genetic profile, and phenotypic expression can significantly impact NPs' delivery, penetration, and overall efficacy. Finally, clinical translation is hampered by regulatory complexities, scalability challenges in manufacturing processes, and the absence of standardized evaluation protocols, all of which underscore the need for rigorous, multidisciplinary research to bridge the gap between preclinical promise and effective clinical implementation.

This scoping review synthesizes the existing literature on NP-based therapeutics for PC; however, several limitations compromise the interpretability and generalizability of its conclusions. One major limitation is the absence of rigorous statistical analyses that would facilitate the evaluation of significant differences among the various NP therapies. This gap limits the ability to discern whether the observed therapeutic effects are truly attributable to the NP interventions or are instead a product of underlying variability. Furthermore, the heterogeneity inherent in clinical trial populations represents a critical challenge. Variations in baseline performance status, differences in previous lines of therapy, and other patient-specific factors can markedly influence treatment outcomes. For instance, patients with a higher baseline performance status or fewer prior treatments might respond differently to NP-based therapies compared to those with more advanced disease or multiple prior therapies. Such discrepancies could raise concerns about the applicability of these findings to real-world clinical settings, where patient populations are diverse. Another concern is the lack of a systematic quality assessment within the review. Without a robust methodological appraisal of the included studies, potential biases stemming from variations in study design, data collection, and outcome reporting may remain unaddressed, further complicating the interpretation of the aggregated data. To address these limitations, we propose a prospective systematic review complemented by a meta-analysis that specifically incorporates subgroup analyses based on patient-level characteristics, such as performance status and treatment history. By employing advanced statistical methods, this approach will enable us to unravel the complex interplay between patient heterogeneity and treatment efficacy. Ultimately, this strategy aims to yield a more nuanced and clinically relevant understanding of how NP therapies impact quality of care and health outcomes in PC, thereby informing clinical decision-making and guiding future research directions.

5. Conclusions

Nanoparticle-based therapeutics has emerged as a transformative paradigm in the management of pancreatic cancer. Evidence from multiple clinical trials demonstrates that formulations such as nanoparticle albumin-bound paclitaxel and nanoliposomal irinotecan markedly enhance intratumoral drug delivery, improve overall and progression-free survival, and reduce systemic toxicity compared with conventional chemotherapy. These innovative agents achieve more effective cytotoxicity through enhanced tumor penetration and modulation of the tumor microenvironment, thereby offering promise in overcoming the inherent challenges posed by a dense, fibrotic stroma that traditionally impedes drug efficacy. Furthermore, modifications in dosing strategies have rendered these therapies feasible across diverse patient populations, including elderly patients and those with compromised performance status.

Despite these promising advances, several challenges remain. Unresolved questions include optimizing dosing regimens, identifying and validating predictive biomarkers (such as TP53 status), and ensuring long-term biocompatibility and safety. Moreover, issues related to regulatory approval pathways and manufacturing scalability must be rigorously addressed to bridge the gap between preclinical promise and real-world clinical application.

Over the next decade, nanoparticle-based therapies are expected to become integral to the standard of care for pancreatic cancer. These modalities are poised to serve as critical components in multimodal treatment strategies, working synergistically with chemotherapy, immunotherapy, and targeted agents to reshape therapeutic approaches. Future research must prioritize large-scale, rigorously designed clinical trials and comprehensive meta-analyses that incorporate patient-level subgroup analyses. Such efforts are essential not only for optimizing dosing and sequencing strategies but also for establishing precise patient selection criteria to maximize clinical benefit and improve survival outcomes. This integrative approach heralds a transformative era in personalized oncology, where the strategic deployment of nanoparticle platforms could ultimately redefine the prognosis of one of the most challenging malignancies.

Supplementary Materials: The following supporting information can be downloaded at https://www.mdpi.com/article/10.3390/cancers17101726/s1, Table S1: Preferred Reporting Items for Systematic reviews and Meta-Analyses Extension for Scoping Reviews (PRISMA-ScR) checklist.

Author Contributions: Conceptualization, I.K., S.T., A.G. and T.P.; methodology, I.K. and S.T.; software, I.K., S.T. and E.L.; validation, I.K., S.T., P.C. and D.K.; formal analysis, I.K. and S.T.; investigation, I.K. and S.T.; resources, I.K., S.T. and E.L.; data curation, I.K. and S.T.; writing—original draft preparation, I.K. and S.T.; writing—review and editing, I.K., S.T., M.P., E.T., D.G., P.B., V.P., A.G. and T.P.; visualization, I.K. and S.T.; supervision, D.G., P.B., V.P., A.G. and T.P.; project administration, T.P.; funding acquisition, I.K. and S.T. All authors have read and agreed to the published version of the manuscript.

Funding: This research received no external funding.

Conflicts of Interest: The authors declare no conflicts of interest.

References

1. Stoffel, E.M.; Brand, R.E.; Goggins, M. Pancreatic Cancer: Changing Epidemiology and New Approaches to Risk Assessment, Early Detection, and Prevention. *Gastroenterology* **2023**, *164*, 752–765. [CrossRef] [PubMed]
2. Pancreatic Cancer—Cancer Stat Facts. Available online: https://seer.cancer.gov/statfacts/html/pancreas.html (accessed on 2 May 2025).

3. Gagliardi, J. *Mortality Rate of Pancreatic Cancer in Europe in 2022, by Country and Gender*; Health Pharma Medtech: Washington DC, USA, 2024. Available online: https://www.statista.com/statistics/1452352/pancreatic-cancer-mortality-rate-in-europe-by-country-and-gender/ (accessed on 2 May 2025).
4. Partyka, O.; Pajewska, M.; Kwaśniewska, D.; Czerw, A.; Deptała, A.; Budzik, M.; Cipora, E.; Gąska, I.; Gazdowicz, L.; Mielnik, A. et al. Overview of Pancreatic Cancer Epidemiology in Europe and Recommendations for Screening in High-Risk Populations. *Cancers* **2023**, *15*, 3634. [CrossRef]
5. Cancer Site Ranking. Available online: https://gco.iarc.who.int/media/globocan/factsheets/cancers/13-pancreas-fact-sheet.pdf (accessed on 11 April 2025).
6. Rawla, P.; Sunkara, T.; Gaduputi, V. Epidemiology of Pancreatic Cancer: Global Trends, Etiology and Risk Factors. *World J. Oncol* **2019**, *10*, 10–27. [CrossRef] [PubMed]
7. Puckett, Y.; Garfield, K. Pancreatic Cancer. In *StatPearls*; StatsPearls Publishing: Treasure Island, FL, USA, 2025. Available online https://www.ncbi.nlm.nih.gov/books/NBK518996/ (accessed on 11 April 2025).
8. Rock, C.L.; Thomson, C.; Gansler, T.; Gapstur, S.M.; McCullough, M.L.; Patel, A.V.; Bandrews, K.S.; Bandera, E.V.; Spees, C.K. Robien, K.; et al. American Cancer Society guideline for diet and physical activity for cancer prevention. *CA Cancer J. Clin.* **2020** *70*, 245–271. [CrossRef]
9. Tsokkou, S.; Konstantinidis, I.; Georgaki, M.N.; Kavvadas, D.; Papadopoulou, K.; Keramas, A.; Sioga, A.; Papamitsou, T. Karachrysafi, S. Gestational Diabetes Mellitus and Its Correlation in the Development of Pancreatic Cancer: A 10-Year Systematic Review. *Cancers* **2024**, *16*, 1840. [CrossRef]
10. Wood, L.D.; Canto, M.I.; Jaffee, E.M.; Simeone, D.M. Pancreatic Cancer: Pathogenesis, Screening, Diagnosis, and Treatment *Gastroenterology* **2022**, *163*, 386. [CrossRef]
11. Hayat, U.; Croce, P.S.; Saadeh, A.; Desai, K.; Appiah, J.; Khan, S.; Khan, Y.I.; Kumar, K.; Hanif, A. Current and Emerging Treatment Options for Pancreatic Cancer: A Comprehensive Review. *J. Clin. Med.* **2025**, *14*, 1129. [CrossRef]
12. Dallavalle, S.; Campagnoli, G.; Pastena, P.; Martinino, A.; Schiliró, D.; Giovinazzo, F. New Frontiers in Pancreatic Cancer Management: Current Treatment Options and the Emerging Role of Neoadjuvant Therapy. *Medicina* **2024**, *60*, 1070. [CrossRef]
13. Gall, T.M.H.; Tsakok, M.; Wasan, H.; Jiao, L.R. Pancreatic cancer: Current management and treatment strategies. *Postgrad. Med. J* **2015**, *91*, 601–607. [CrossRef]
14. Nanotechnology Cancer Therapy Treatment—NCI. Available online: https://www.cancer.gov/nano/cancer-nanotechnology/treatment (accessed on 11 April 2025).
15. Gavas, S.; Quazi, S.; Karpiński, T.M. Nanoparticles for Cancer Therapy: Current Progress and Challenges. *Nanoscale Res. Lett* **2021**, *16*, 173. [CrossRef]
16. Au, M.; Emeto, T.I.; Power, J.; Vangaveti, V.N.; Lai, H.C. Emerging Therapeutic Potential of Nanoparticles in Pancreatic Cancer: A Systematic Review of Clinical Trials. *Biomedicines* **2016**, *4*, 20. [CrossRef] [PubMed]
17. Rojas, L.A.; Sethna, Z.; Soares, K.C.; Olcese, C.; Pang, N.; Patterson, E.; Lihm, J.; Ceglia, N.; Guasp, P.; Chu, A.; et al. Personalized RNA neoantigen vaccines stimulate T cells in pancreatic cancer. *Nature* **2023**, *618*, 144–150. [CrossRef]
18. Sethna, Z.; Guasp, P.; Reiche, C.; Milighetti, M.; Ceglia, N.; Patterson, E.; Lihm, J.; Payne, G.; Lyudovyk, O.; Rojas, L.A.; et al. RNA neoantigen vaccines prime long-lived CD8+ T cells in pancreatic cancer. *Nature* **2025**, *639*, 1042–1051. [CrossRef]
19. Yang, Y.; Bteich, J.; Li, S.D. Current Update of a Carboxymethylcellulose-PEG Conjugate Platform for Delivery of Insoluble Cytotoxic Agents to Tumors. *AAPS J.* **2017**, *19*, 386–396. [CrossRef] [PubMed]
20. Stainthorpe, A.; Greenhalgh, J.; Bagust, A.; Richardson, M.; Boland, A.; Beale, S.; Duarte, R.; Kotas, E.; Banks, L.; Palmer, D Paclitaxel as Albumin-Bound Nanoparticles with Gemcitabine for Untreated Metastatic Pancreatic Cancer: An Evidence Review Group Perspective of a NICE Single Technology Appraisal. *Pharmacoeconomics* **2018**, *36*, 1153–1163. [CrossRef]
21. Roy, H.; Nayak, B.S.; Nandi, S. Chitosan Anchored Nanoparticles in Current Drug Development Utilizing Computer-Aided Pharmacokinetic Modeling: Case Studies for Target Specific Cancer Treatment and Future Prospective. *Curr. Pharm. Des.* **2020**, *26*, 1666–1675. [CrossRef]
22. Song, S.Y.; Kim, K.P.; Jeong, S.Y.; Park, J.; Park, J.; Jung, J.; Chung, H.K.; Lee, S.-W.; Seo, M.H.; Lee, J.-S.; et al. Polymeric nanoparticle-docetaxel for the treatment of advanced solid tumors: Phase I clinical trial and preclinical data from an orthotopic pancreatic cancer model. *Oncotarget* **2016**, *7*, 77348–77357. [CrossRef]
23. Sloat, B.R.; Sandoval, M.A.; Li, D.; Chung, W.-G.; Lansakara-P, D.S.; Proteau, P.J.; Kiguchi, K.; DiGiovanni, J.; Cui, Z. In vitro and in vivo anti-tumor activities of a gemcitabine derivative carried by nanoparticles. *Int. J. Pharm.* **2011**, *409*, 278–288. [CrossRef]
24. Bagley, A.F.; Ludmir, E.B.; Maitra, A.; Minsky, B.D.; Smith, G.L.; Das, P.; Koong, A.C.; Holliday, E.B.; Taniguchi, C.M.; Katz, M.H., et al. NBTXR3, a first-in-class radioenhancer for pancreatic ductal adenocarcinoma: Report of first patient experience. *Clin. Transl. Radiat. Oncol.* **2022**, *33*, 66–69. [CrossRef]
25. Chen, N.; Brachmann, C.; Liu, X.; Pierce, D.W.; Dey, J.; Kerwin, W.S.; Li, Y.; Zhou, S.; Hou, S.; Carleton, M.; et al. Albumin-bound nanoparticle (nab) paclitaxel exhibits enhanced paclitaxel tissue distribution and tumor penetration. *Cancer Chemother. Pharmacol.* **2015**, *76*, 699–712. [CrossRef]

26. Daman, Z.; Ostad, S.; Amini, M.; Gilani, K. Preparation, optimization and in vitro characterization of stearoyl-gemcitabine polymeric micelles: A comparison with its self-assembled nanoparticles. *Int. J. Pharm.* **2014**, *468*, 142–151. [CrossRef] [PubMed]
27. Appidi, T.; China, D.; Ştefan, G.R.; Moreau, M.; Mao, S.; Velarde, E.; Toyang, N.; Lowe, H.; Rengan, A.K.; Ding, K.; et al. Engineered multifunctional nanoparticles for enhanced radiation therapy: Three-in-one approach for cancer treatment. *Mol. Cancer* **2025**, *24*, 68. [CrossRef]
28. Wainberg, Z.A.; Melisi, D.; Macarulla, T.; Cid, R.P.; Chandana, S.R.; De La Fouchardière, C.; Dean, A.; Kiss, I.; Lee, W.J.; Goetze, T.O.; et al. NALIRIFOX versus nab-paclitaxel and gemcitabine in treatment-naive patients with metastatic pancreatic ductal adenocarcinoma (NAPOLI 3): A randomised, open-label, phase 3 trial. *Lancet* **2023**, *402*, 1272–1281. [CrossRef]
29. Bockorny, B.; Macarulla, T.; Semenisty, V.; Borazanci, E.; Feliu, J.; Ponz-Sarvise, M.; Abad, D.G.; Oberstein, P.; Alistar, A.; Muñoz, A.; et al. Motixafortide and Pembrolizumab Combined to Nanoliposomal Irinotecan, Fluorouracil, and Folinic Acid in Metastatic Pancreatic Cancer: The COMBAT/KEYNOTE-202 Trial. *Clin. Cancer Res.* **2021**, *27*, 5020–5027. [CrossRef]
30. Park, S.J.; Kim, H.; Shin, K.; Hong, T.H.; Suh, J.H.; Lee, M.A. Nanoliposomal irinotecan plus fluorouracil and folinic acid as a second-line treatment option in patients with metastatic pancreatic ductal adenocarcinoma: A retrospective cohort study. *BMC Cancer* **2021**, *21*, 1176. [CrossRef]
31. Glassman, D.C.; Palmaira, R.L.; Covington, C.M.; Desai, A.M.; Ku, G.Y.; Li, J.; Harding, J.J.; Varghese, A.M.; O'reilly, E.M.; Yu, K.H. Nanoliposomal irinotecan with fluorouracil for the treatment of advanced pancreatic cancer, a single institution experience. *BMC Cancer* **2018**, *18*, 693. [CrossRef]
32. Wang-Gillam, A.; Li, C.P.; Bodoky, G.; Dean, A.; Shan, Y.-S.; Jameson, G.; Macarulla, T.; Lee, K.-H.; Cunningham, D.; Blanc, J.F.; et al. Nanoliposomal irinotecan with fluorouracil and folinic acid in metastatic pancreatic cancer after previous gemcitabine-based therapy (NAPOLI-1): A global, randomised, open-label, phase 3 trial. *Lancet* **2016**, *387*, 545–557. [CrossRef]
33. Ceelen, W.; Sandra, L.; Van de Sande, L.; Graversen, M.; Mortensen, M.B.; Vermeulen, A.; Gasthuys, E.; Reynders, D.; Cosyns, S.; Hoorens, A.; et al. Phase I study of intraperitoneal aerosolized nanoparticle albumin based paclitaxel (NAB-PTX) for unresectable peritoneal metastases. *EBioMedicine* **2022**, *82*, 104151. [CrossRef]
34. Sohal, D.P.S.; Duong, M.; Ahmad, S.A.; Gandhi, N.S.; Beg, M.S.; Wang-Gillam, A.; Wade, J.L.; Chiorean, E.G.; Guthrie, K.A.; Lowy, A.M.; et al. Efficacy of Perioperative Chemotherapy for Resectable Pancreatic Adenocarcinoma. *JAMA Oncol.* **2021**, *7*, 421. [CrossRef]
35. Azmi, A.S.; Khan, H.Y.; Muqbil, I.; Aboukameel, A.; Neggers, J.E.; Daelemans, D.; Mahipal, A.; Dyson, G.; Kamgar, M.; Al-Hallak, M.N.; et al. Preclinical Assessment with Clinical Validation of Selinexor with Gemcitabine and Nab-Paclitaxel for the Treatment of Pancreatic Ductal Adenocarcinoma. *Clin. Cancer Res.* **2020**, *26*, 1338–1348. [CrossRef]
36. Hasegawa, R.; Okuwaki, K.; Kida, M.; Yamauchi, H.; Kawaguchi, Y.; Matsumoto, T.; Kaneko, T.; Miyata, E.; Uehara, K.; Iwai, T.; et al. A clinical trial to assess the feasibility and efficacy of nab-paclitaxel plus gemcitabine for elderly patients with unresectable advanced pancreatic cancer. *Int. J. Clin. Oncol.* **2019**, *24*, 1574–1581. [CrossRef] [PubMed]
37. Macarulla, T.; Pazo-Cid, R.; Guillén-Ponce, C.; López, R.; Vera, R.; Reboredo, M.; Martin, A.M.; Rivera, F.; Beveridge, R.D.; La Casta, A.; et al. Phase I/II Trial to Evaluate the Efficacy and Safety of Nanoparticle Albumin-Bound Paclitaxel in Combination with Gemcitabine in Patients with Pancreatic Cancer and an ECOG Performance Status of 2. *J. Clin. Oncol.* **2019**, *37*, 230–238. [CrossRef]
38. Von Hoff, D.D.; Ervin, T.; Arena, F.P.; Chiorean, E.G.; Infante, J.; Moore, M.; Seay, T.; Tjulandin, S.A.; Ma, W.W.; Saleh, M.N.; et al. Increased Survival in Pancreatic Cancer with nab-Paclitaxel plus Gemcitabine. *N. Engl. J. Med.* **2013**, *369*, 1691–1703. [CrossRef]
39. Hosein, P.J.; de Lima Lopes, G.; Pastorini, V.H.; Gomez, C.; Macintyre, J.A.; Zayas, G.C.; Reis, I.; Montero, A.J.; Merchan, J.R.; Lima, C.M.R. A Phase II Trial of nab-Paclitaxel as Second-line Therapy in Patients with Advanced Pancreatic Cancer. *Am. J. Clin. Oncol.* **2013**, *36*, 151–156. [CrossRef]
40. Von Hoff, D.D.; Ramanathan, R.K.; Borad, M.J.; Laheru, D.A.; Smith, L.S.; Wood, T.E.; Korn, R.L.; Desai, N.; Trieu, V.; Iglesias, J.L.; et al. Gemcitabine Plus *nab*-Paclitaxel Is an Active Regimen in Patients with Advanced Pancreatic Cancer: A Phase I/II Trial. *J. Clin. Oncol.* **2011**, *29*, 4548–4554. [CrossRef]
41. Libutti, S.K.; Paciotti, G.F.; Byrnes, A.A.; Alexander, H.R.; Gannon, W.E.; Walker, M.; Seidel, G.D.; Yuldasheva, N.; Tamarkin, L. Phase I and Pharmacokinetic Studies of CYT-6091, a Novel PEGylated Colloidal Gold-rhTNF Nanomedicine. *Clin. Cancer Res.* **2010**, *16*, 6139–6149. [CrossRef]
42. Hamaguchi, T.; Kato, K.; Yasui, H.; Morizane, C.; Ikeda, M.; Ueno, H.; Muro, K.; Yamada, Y.; Okusaka, T.; Shirao, K.; et al. A phase I and pharmacokinetic study of NK105, a paclitaxel-incorporating micellar nanoparticle formulation. *Br. J. Cancer* **2007**, *97*, 170–176. [CrossRef]
43. Stathopoulos, G.; Boulikas, T.; Vougiouka, M.; Rigatos, S.; Stathopoulos, J. Liposomal cisplatin combined with gemcitabine in pretreated advanced pancreatic cancer patients: A phase I-II study. *Oncol. Rep.* **2006**, *15*, 1201–1204. [CrossRef]
44. Huang, X.; Wang, C.; Ma, T.; Huang, Z.; Zhou, H.; Xu, L.; Zhang, R.; Zhao, J.; Zhang, Y.; Huang, Z.; et al. The Efficacy of Combined Cisplatin and Nanoparticle Albumin-Bound Paclitaxel in a Stage IV Pancreatic Squamous Cell Carcinoma Patient with a Somatic BRCA2 Mutation: A Case Report. *Front. Oncol.* **2021**, *11*, 585983. [CrossRef]

45. Otsubo, M.; Kinouchi, R.; Kamiya, T.; Yoshida, A. Regression of taxane-related cystoid macular edema after topical dorzolamide treatment: Two case reports. *J. Med. Case Rep.* **2021**, *15*, 355. [CrossRef]
46. Assi, H.A.; Shikdar, S.; Alhyari, L.; Aljumaily, R. Long-Term Survival with Nanoliposomal Irinotecan in Pancreatic Cancer. *Pancreas* **2020**, *49*, e95–e96. [CrossRef] [PubMed]
47. Conroy, T.; Desseigne, F.; Ychou, M.; Bouché, O.; Guimbaud, R.; Bécouarn, Y.; Adenis, A.; Raoul, J.-L.; Gourgou-Bourgade, S.; De La Fouchardière, C.; et al. FOLFIRINOX versus Gemcitabine for Metastatic Pancreatic Cancer. *N. Engl. J. Med.* **2011**, *364*, 1817–1825. [CrossRef] [PubMed]
48. Abal, M.; Bras-Goncalves, R.; Judde, J.G.; Fsihi, H.; de Cremoux, P.; Louvard, D.; Magdelenat, H.; Robine, S.; Poupon, M.-F. Enhanced sensitivity to irinotecan by Cdk1 inhibition in the p53-deficient HT29 human colon cancer cell line. *Oncogene* **2004**, *23*, 1737–1744. [CrossRef] [PubMed]

cancers

MDPI

Review

Innate Immunity and Platelets: Unveiling Their Role in Chronic Pancreatitis and Pancreatic Cancer

Juliane Blümke [1,†], Moritz Schameitat [2,†], Atul Verma [3], Celina Limbecker [2], Elise Arlt [2], Sonja M. Kessler [4], Heike Kielstein [2], Sebastian Krug [3,5], Ivonne Bazwinsky-Wutschke [2,‡] and Monika Haemmerle [1,*,‡]

1 Institute of Pathology, Section of Experimental Pathology, Medical Faculty, Martin Luther University Halle-Wittenberg, 06112 Halle (Saale), Germany; juliane.bluemke@uk-halle.de
2 Institute of Anatomy and Cell Biology, Medical Faculty, Martin Luther University Halle-Wittenberg, 06108 Halle (Saale), Germany; moritz.schameitat@uk-halle.de (M.S.); celina.limbecker@uk-halle.de (C.L.); heike.kielstein@uk-halle.de (H.K.); ivonne.bazwinsky@uk-halle.de (I.B.-W.)
3 Department of Internal Medicine I, Medical Faculty, Martin Luther University Halle-Wittenberg, 06120 Halle (Saale), Germany; atul.verma@uk-halle.de (A.V.); sebastian.krug@med.uni-heidelberg.de (S.K.)
4 Institute of Pharmacy, Experimental Pharmacology for Natural Sciences, Faculty of Natural Sciences, Martin Luther University Halle-Wittenberg, 06120 Halle (Saale), Germany; sonja.kessler@pharmazie.uni-halle.de
5 Department of Internal Medicine IV, University Hospital Heidelberg, 69120 Heidelberg, Germany
* Correspondence: monika.haemmerle@uk-halle.de
† These authors contributed equally to this work.
‡ These authors also contributed equally to this work.

Simple Summary: Chronic pancreatitis (CP) is a common risk factor for pancreatic ductal adenocarcinoma (PDAC), which is a highly aggressive cancer. The development of PDAC is influenced by interactions between tumor cells and their surrounding microenvironment, including immune cells as well as platelets. Immune cells can either help or hinder tumor growth, while platelets play a major role in supporting tumor growth and metastasis. Understanding these interactions is key to developing treatments that impact the immune and coagulation systems to fight PDAC and improve patient outcomes.

Abstract: Pancreatic ductal adenocarcinoma (PDAC) is one of the most aggressive and lethal forms of cancer, characterized by a highly desmoplastic tumor microenvironment. One main risk factor is chronic pancreatitis (CP). Progression of CP to PDAC is greatly influenced by persistent inflammation promoting genomic instability, acinar–ductal metaplasia, and pancreatic intraepithelial neoplasia (PanIN) formation. Components of the extracellular matrix, including immune cells, can modulate this progression phase. This includes cells of the innate immune system, such as natural killer (NK) cells, macrophages, dendritic cells, mast cells, neutrophils, and myeloid-derived suppressor cells (MDSCs), either promoting or inhibiting tumor growth. On one hand, innate immune cells can trigger inflammatory responses that support tumor progression by releasing cytokines and growth factors, fostering tumor cell proliferation, invasion, and metastasis. On the other hand, they can also activate immune surveillance mechanisms, which can limit tumor development. For example, NK cells are cytotoxic innate lymphoid cells that are able to kill tumor cells, and active dendritic cells are crucial for a functioning anti-tumor immune response. In contrast, mast cells and MDSCs rather support a pro-tumorigenic tumor microenvironment that is additionally sustained by platelets. Once thought to play a role in hemostasis only, platelets are now recognized as key players in inflammation and cancer progression. By releasing cytokines, growth factors, and pro-angiogenic mediators, platelets help shape an immunosuppressive microenvironment that promotes fibrotic remodeling, tumor initiation, progression, metastasis, and immune evasion. Neutrophils and macrophages exist in different functional subtypes that can both act pro- and anti-tumorigenic. Understanding

 https://doi.org/10.3390/cancers17101689

the complex interactions between innate immune cells, platelets, and early precursor lesions, as well as PDAC cells, is crucial for developing new therapeutic approaches that can harness the immune and potentially also the coagulation system to target and eliminate tumors, offering hope for improved patient outcomes.

Keywords: innate immune cells; immune microenvironment; platelets; pancreatitis; PDAC

1. Introduction

Chronic pancreatitis (CP) is a major cause of morbidity and a global burden for healthcare systems [1]. It is a chronic inflammatory condition of the pancreas leading to progressive scarring of pancreatic tissue, endocrine and exocrine tissue dysfunction, and increased risk for pancreatic cancer development [2–4]. Persistent tissue damage of the pancreas is caused primarily by prolonged alcohol abuse or smoking, and more rarely by hereditary genetic disorders [5–7]. This leads to direct or indirect cellular damages that result in an inflammatory reaction, activation of pancreatic stellate cells, and ultimately replacement of orthotopic pancreatic tissue with fibrotic tissue. The key histological features (Figure 1a–c) are intralobular, interlobular and periductal fibrosis, atrophy of acinar parenchyma and acinar–ductal metaplasia (ADM), ductal changes including ductal dilation and distortion with protein plugs and calcifications and associated interstitial inflammation [8,9], that ultimately persist after progression to pancreatic ductal adenocarcinoma (PDAC, Figure 1a,d,e).

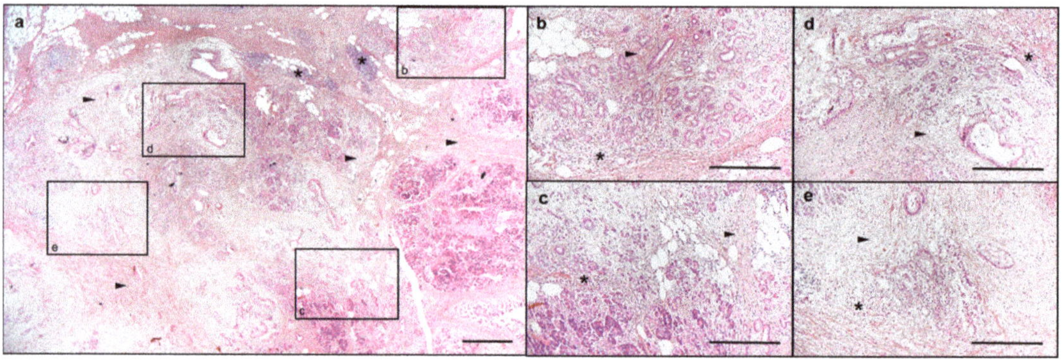

Figure 1. Histology of PDAC with associated features of chronic pancreatitis. Overview of an HE-stained section of a pancreatic resection specimen (**a**) of a patient with PDAC (**d**,**e**) with associated parenchyma atrophy and extensive inter- and intralobular fibrosis with interstitial inflammation and ADM lesions of surrounding peritumoral pancreatic tissue characterizing chronic pancreatitis (**b**,**c**). Arrowheads mark areas with fibrosis and/or desmoplasia, asterisks show areas of inflammation. Scale bar for (**a**) 1000 μm, scale bar for (**b**–**e**) 500 μm.

It is well-recognized that CP is a risk factor for PDAC development. A large multicenter retrospective study found that subjects with chronic pancreatitis had a 14-fold increased risk of developing PDAC [4]. Other studies estimate the risk of PDAC development in patients with CP to be even higher [10]. Mechanistically, both genetic as well as epigenetic mechanisms, subsequent inflammatory processes, and oxidative stress resulting in DNA damage have been implicated in the progressive development of PDAC from CP [11]. A recent study aimed to identify hub genes in the development of CP and PDAC by analyzing transcriptomic data of various publicly available datasets. This study identified the gene *CEL* (carboxyl ester lipase), a glycoprotein secreted from the pancreas, as particularly important for CP and PDAC, and its expression correlated with the pancreatic immune cell landscape [12]. Others identified genes related to cell cycle and DNA replication to be key for the development of CP and pancreatic cancer [13]. In general, chronic inflammation, as seen in CP, is known to cause DNA damage, endoplasmic reticulum (ER) stress and autophagy. Tumor-promoting inflammation is one of the prerequisites for sustaining proliferative activity and promoting angiogenesis [14–16]. Finally, the accumulation of mutations in acinar or ductal cells of the pancreas can lead to dysplasia and the development of PDAC [17]. Based on the most recent global cancer statistics, PDAC is the third leading cause of cancer-related death worldwide [18]. The molecular pathology of PDAC is dominated by activating mutations in codon 12 of the proto-oncogene *KRAS* that occur in >90% of PDACs [19,20]. In the course of the disease, additional mutations arise, including inactivating mutations in tumor suppressor genes like *TP53*, *CDKN2A*, or *SMAD4*. It is well accepted that *KRAS* mutations occur very early in disease development and are already detected in preneoplastic lesions, including ADM and pancreatic intraepithelial neoplasia (PanIN) [21–23]. In mice, a *KRAS* G12D mutation is able to promote ADM and PanIN formation and spontaneously induce invasive cancer [24], accelerated by an additional inflammatory trigger [25,26]. Interestingly, *KRAS* mutations not only regulate intrinsic signaling pathways to sustain cellular proliferation and inhibit apoptosis in mutated cells. They are also able to regulate the tumor microenvironment (TME) by supporting a tumor-promoting inflammatory milieu that eventually contributes to immune escape [27]. In general, it is believed that KRAS induces several inflammatory cytokines and chemokines as well as signaling pathways, which promote tumorigenesis. For example, *KRAS* mutations have been shown to promote the progression of PanIN lesions and PDAC, which depended on the secretion of IL-6 (interleukin-6) by myeloid cells, activation of STAT3 (signal transducer and activator of transcription 3) and, SOCS3 (suppressor of cytokine signaling 3) [28]. In addition, KRAS and IL-6 synergism caused activation of the mitogen-activated protein kinase (MAPK) signaling pathway that was responsible for the initiation of pancreatic cancer precursor lesions [29]. Similarly to IL-6, the CXCR2 (C-X-C motif chemokine receptor 2)/IL-8 axis induced by KRAS was shown to be crucial for promoting phenotype alterations of CAFs (cancer-associated fibroblasts) and increased secretion of pro-tumoral cytokines that eventually promoted the development of PDAC [30]. Moreover, STAT5 activation downstream of oncogenic KRAS signaling can trigger inflammation-mediated ADM formation and PDAC growth [31]. Interestingly, oncogenic $KRAS^{G12D}$ can be transferred to tumor cells via platelet-like particles leading to a growth advantage in *KRAS* wildtype cells [32]. In addition, it was shown that *KRAS*-mutated cancer cells induce platelet aggregation [33], a phenomenon called TCIPA (tumor cell-induced platelet aggregation) that is associated with metastasis formation and might be an emerging therapeutic target in cancer therapy [34]. Once activated by tumor cells, platelets can secrete a plethora of inflammatory cytokines that lead to the recruitment and activation of immune cells, which then secrete chemotactic factors to regulate other immune cells [35]. Various classes of regulatory and cytotoxic immune cells were frequently identified within the microenvironment of the pancreas and pancreatic cancer tissue [36–38], showing differences in diverse tumor areas as well as changes upon disease progression and neoadjuvant therapy. During early cancer progression, immune cells are still able to eliminate precancerous cells. However, tumor cytotoxicity or anti-tumor immunity are mainly suppressed in PDAC, suggesting increasing dysfunction of the immune response, which is likely mediated by the PDAC cells themselves [35,39]. Moreover, tumor-associated immune cells can be divided into tumor-antagonizing and tumor-promoting immune cells, playing various roles in the different stages of tumor progression [40]. PDAC cells can influence the metabolic reprogramming of immune cells [41]. In addition, the interaction of immune cells with platelets, both in the circulation and within the TME, appears to play a critical role in modulating immune cell infiltration, differentiation, and activity, thereby regulating tumor growth and immune evasion [42–44]. Altogether, this suggests that both genetic and non-genetic factors regulate microenvironmental changes in pancreatic tissue that impact tumorigenesis and cancer dissemination. Moreover, persistent organ injury and chronic inflammation induce DNA damage in preneoplastic lesions, ultimately resulting in the breaching of basement membranes and invasive cancer.

In this review, we focus on the role of innate immune effector cells and platelets in chronic pancreatitis and pancreatic cancer, given their involvement in tissue injury and repair, fibrosis, stromal remodeling, tumor growth, and metastasis. We focused on the main key signaling pathways that drive the reorganization of the tumor immune microenvironment in PDAC, highlighting their potential as therapeutic targets. Additionally, we emphasize the emerging role of platelets as orchestrators of innate immunity and potential facilitators of immune evasion in cancer.

2. Innate Immune Cells in Chronic Pancreatitis and PDAC

Innate immune cells are active players in the pathogenesis of both CP and PDAC. They perpetuate chronic inflammation, shape the tumor microenvironment, promote or inhibit tumor progression, and influence immune evasion. In addition, they are altered in their function, maturation, or number which might have clinical implications. Crucial functions and intercellular interactions of innate immune cells and tumor cells and their impact on T cells within the TME are summarized in Figures 2 and 3 and described in more detail in the following paragraphs.

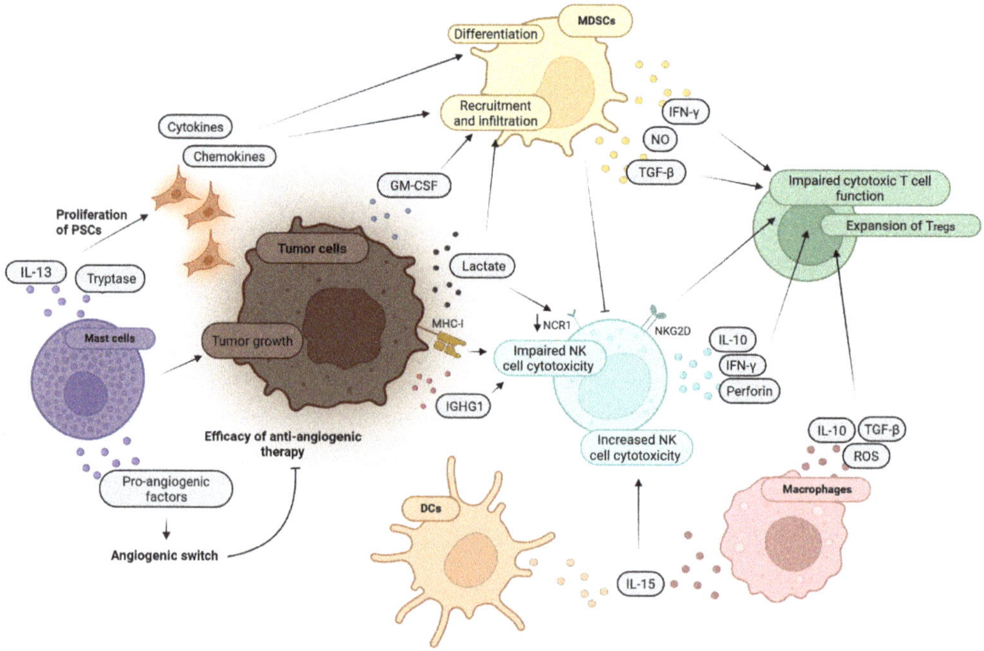

Figure 2. Interplay of tumor cells with NK (natural killer) cells, MDSCs (myeloid-derived suppressor cells) and mast cells. Tumor cell secretion of lactate and IGHG1 (Igγ-1 chain C region) leads to an impaired NK cell cytotoxicity, e.g., via downregulation of the surface receptor NCR1. Additionally,

MHC (major histocompatibility complex) class I molecules on the tumor cell surface similarly suppress NK cell cytotoxicity. Increased NK cell cytotoxicity is mediated via IL-15 (interleukin-15), secreted by DCs (dendritic cells) or macrophages. Active NK cells can reduce cytotoxic T cell function and regulate the expansion of Tregs either directly by engaging NKG2D or indirectly by the secretion of IFN-γ (interferon gamma), IL-10 or perforin. Other mechanisms that can limit adaptive immune responses include secretion of cytokines by MDSCs or macrophages, including TGF-β (transforming growth factor beta) among others. MDSCs are recruited via tumor cell-derived lactate or GM-CSF (granulocyte-macrophage colony-stimulating factor). In addition, PSCs (pancreatic stellate stells) support the recruitment and infiltration as well as differentiation of MDSCs via the STAT3 (signal transducer and activator of transcription 3) pathway. Proliferation of PSCs is induced via mast cell-derived IL-13 and tryptase. In addition, mast cells are considered tumor-promoting in PDAC and secrete pro-angiogenic factors that induce an angiogenic switch and limit the efficacy of anti-angiogenic therapy. The figure was created with BioRender.com.

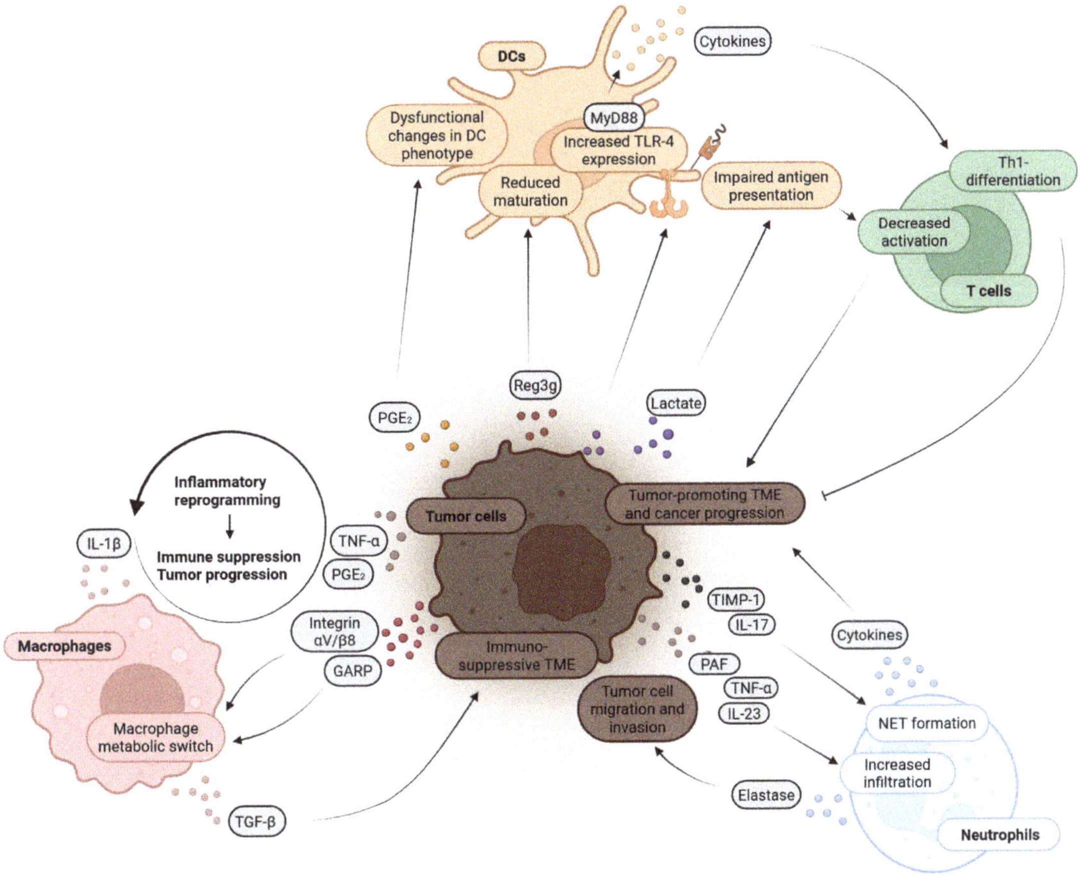

Figure 3. Interplay of tumor cells with macrophages, DCs and neutrophils. Integrin $\alpha V/\beta 8$ and GARP (glycoprotein a repetitions predominant) secreted by tumor cells lead to a metabolic switch in macrophages promoting the secreting of TGF-β that supports an immunosuppressive and tumor-promoting TME (tumor microenvironment). In addition, tumor cells secreted TNF-α (tumor necrosis factor alpha) and PGE_2 (prostaglandin E_2) are part of a positive feedback loop, which triggers IL-1β secretion by macrophages. This sustains a tumor-promoting inflammatory response, facilitating immune

suppression and tumor progression. Tumor cell-derived PGE_2, Reg3g (regenerating islet-derived protein 3 gamma) and lactate induced dysfunctional phenotypic changes in DCs, reduced DC maturation and impaired antigen presentation by DCs, respectively. In addition, tumor cells increase TLR4 (toll-like-receptor 4) expression in DCs which leads to a secretion of cytokines via the MyD88 pathways that favor Th1 cell differentiation. In summary, tumor cells can influence DCs in ways that induce both anti-tumorigenic and pro-tumorigenic effects in the T cell compartment. A close interaction also exists between tumor cells and neutrophils. Tumor-derived cytokines induce infiltration of neutrophils into tumor tissue and induce NET formation. On the other hand, neutrophils secrete cytokines that support a tumor-promoting TME and induce tumor cell migration and invasion. The figure was created with BioRender.com.

2.1. *Natural Killer (NK) Cells*

2.1.1. Key Physiological Functions

Natural killer (NK) cells have been the focus of fundamental research for quite some time, as they represent an efficient endogenous first-line defense against cancer [45,46]. As part of the innate immune system, NK cells are "naturally" cytotoxic, which means they are able to identify virus-infected [45] or malignant cells and eliminate them via induction of apoptosis without prior antigen exposure. The activity of NK cells is balanced by activating and inhibitory receptors on their surface [47–51], which in turn are affected by activating and inhibitory signals. NK cells recognize if a proximal cell expresses a ligand profile associated with oncogenic transformation. The joint activating and inhibitory signals decide whether a cell is targeted for killing [52]. Activating NK cell receptors recognize stress-induced ligands on the target cells, as well as other alert molecules and toll-like-receptor ligands. Additionally, NK cells are able to exert ADCC (antibody-dependent cell cytotoxicity) by recognizing antibody-coated target cells with the Fc receptor CD16 [53]. Inhibitory receptors recognize constitutively expressed self-molecules on potentially altered target cells and induce NK cell tolerance, especially the MHC-I (major histocompatibility complex class I molecule) [54]. According to the "missing self"-hypothesis, NK cells contribute to T cell-mediated killing by eliminating cells that lack MHC-I [50]. However, other inhibitory ways exist that are independent of MHC-I molecules. In this context, the inhibition of NK cells via the 2B4 receptor is one of the best-characterized mechanisms. Other NK-cell inhibitory receptors that have non-MHC-molecule ligands include, for example, the NK-cell-receptor protein 1 family, the carcinoembryonic antigen family, the sialic-acid-binding immunoglobulin-like lectins [55].

2.1.2. Pathophysiology in PDAC

NK cells should kill single tumor cells before they develop into solid tumors. Also, they should contribute to preventing metastasis by eliminating circulating tumor cells [56]. Previous studies have shown that the pathophysiology and progression of pancreatic cancer are strongly affected by the interaction of cancer cells with the TME, and are closely associated with dysfunctional NK cells [57–61]. Impairment of NK cells is associated with a reduced ability of the organism to target tumor cells and thus promotes cancer spread [62]. PDAC cells are able to develop mechanisms to inhibit NK cell function and thus protect themselves from the host immune system [63–65]. NK cells in the TME markedly downregulate activating receptors in response to immune evasion factors produced by tumor cells [66]. For example, tumor-derived lactate causes a downregulation of NCR1 (NKp46), therefore, inhibiting NK cell cytotoxicity [67]. Tumor cells can also secrete the protein IGHG1 (Igγ-1 chain C region), which attenuates the cytotoxic activity of NK cells by inhibiting ADCC [68]. He et al. discovered that PDAC cells actively consume vitamin B6, which NK cells need as a critical energy source for activation via glycogen metabolism [69]. Besides the direct influence of tumor cells, NK cells are indirectly affected by other immune cells and platelets found in the TME. For example, lactate increases the amount of MDSCs (myeloid-derived suppressor cells) in the tumor tissue and, therefore, leads to NK cell suppression indirectly [67]. It could be shown that natural killer T (NKT) cells have a beneficial effect on NK cell activity [70]. IL-15 (interleukin-15) produced by dendritic cells, monocytes, and macrophages increases NK cell cytotoxicity [71]. In contrast to that, platelets have a suppressive effect on NK cell function, as described in detail below [72,73].

2.1.3. Clinical Implications in PDAC

Despite the limited functionality of NK cells as mentioned above, the amount of circulating NK cells in the peripheral blood of PDAC patients is a positive prognostic biomarker for resectable pancreatic cancer [74]. NK cells in the peripheral blood of PDAC patients display a reduced cytotoxic function and adopt a regulatory, IL-10-producing phenotype [66]. PDAC patients with high NK cell infiltration in the tumor displayed improved survival [69]. Interferon type I and II, produced by NK cells, are enriched in tumors with later recurrence [74]. As NK cells are able to kill tumor cells without prior sensitization, they have become a key focus of cell-mediated cancer immunotherapy. It could be shown that less differentiated tumor cells were more sensitive to NK cell-mediated killing, as higher differentiated tumors could re-increase their expression of MHC-I [75]. Highly differentiated cells were, in turn, more sensitive to chemotherapy. This suggests that a combination of surgical resection, chemotherapy, and immunotherapy might be a promising tool for the treatment of pancreatic cancer treatment. Especially after tumor resection and adjuvant treatment, NK cells play a crucial role in the control of recurrence [75]. Brooks et al. showed that the activation of $CD8^+$ T cells and NK cells after surgery increased perioperative survival. Additionally, neoadjuvant anti-PD-1 and gemcitabine treatment, followed by tumor resection, and adjuvant anti-CD96 therapy, stimulated NK cell activation and led to significantly improved survival [76].

2.1.4. Therapeutic Strategies

Various approaches exist to NK cell immunotherapy. One is to block NK cell MHC-I specific inhibitory receptors to increase NK cell effector function against tumor cells. This was successfully tested in mice with leukemia [77]. It is also possible to upregulate the expression of NKG2D, which is the strongest NK cell activator [52]. Another approach would be to isolate NK cells from the patient's peripheral blood, followed by in vitro stimulation with IL-2 and/or co-culture with K562 tumor cells, resulting in proliferation and activation. NK cells are then released back into the patient's bloodstream [52,78]. It is also possible to produce CAR-NK cells that bind to specific surface molecules of the tumor [52]. For example, CD70-targeting CAR NK cells were able to eliminate both PDAC cells and CAFs (cancer-associated fibroblasts) in vitro and in vivo when stimulated with IL-15 [79]. In conclusion, NK cells play a crucial role in tumor development, especially in the early stages, and are a promising target for immunotherapies.

2.2. *Macrophages*

2.2.1. Key Physiological Functions

Macrophages play a wide role in tissue maintenance and pathological conditions, and their divergent role depends on several factors like origin, residence, and micro-environmental conditions [80]. Macrophages play a dynamic role in the immune system and are traditionally classified into two polarization states. While M1 macrophages are considered pro-inflammatory cells with anti-tumor properties, M2 macrophages have anti-inflammatory and pro-tumor properties [81]. Recent studies have revealed that macrophages can have mixed origins. In pancreatic cancer, both tissue-resident macrophages as well as inflammatory monocytes can be the source of TAMs (tumor-associated macrophages), exhibiting distinct functions depending on their source [82]. Macrophages are phenotypically highly plastic by nature, and polarization depends on external stimuli. In PDAC, macrophages are more prone to a pro-tumorigenic, or M2 polarization state. M2 macrophages can promote tumor angiogenesis, immune evasion, chemotherapy resistance, metabolic rewiring, and metastasis [37]. The phenotypic properties of macrophages highly depend on TME factors like hypoxia, cachexia, fibrosis, and immune-mediated secreted factors [80].

2.2.2. Pathophysiology in Chronic Pancreatitis or PDAC

TAMs are the most abundant inflammatory cells in chronic pancreatitis and pancreatic cancer. TAMs are present and increase in number with disease progression from the early stage of PanIN to the metastatic stage of PDAC [83]. A detailed multi-institutional study of more than 300 patients by Väyrynen et al. reported that a higher density of macrophages in PDAC is associated with a worse prognosis and DFS (disease-free survival). While M2 macrophages were associated with worse prognosis and DFS, M1 macrophages did not show any specific correlation with prognosis [84]. However, macrophages might not only have disease-promoting functions but are also necessary for maintaining tissue homeostasis during pancreatic inflammation. Baer et al. identified a subset of TRMs (tissue-resident macrophages) showing high levels of LYVE1 and expression of genes important for tissue homeostasis. TRMs were necessary for tissue fibrosis and mediated a protective effect in cerulean-induced acute pancreatitis. In contrast, LYVE1+ TRMs supported pancreatitis-accelerated PDAC progression [85]. Another recent publication demonstrated the role of IL-1β^+ TAMs in pancreatic cancer. This study highlighted that this subset of TAMs interacted with PDAC cells expressing an IL-1β response signature, leading to worse prognosis and survival of patients. Upon exposure to TNF (tumor necrosis factor) and PGE_2 (prostaglandin E_2) secreted by PDAC cells infiltrating monocytes differentiated to IL-1β^+ TAMs and facilitated inflammatory reprogramming of cancer cells to potentiate the release of TNF, PGE_2, and other factors for maintenance of an IL-1β^+ TAM state. This positive feedback loop helped to mediate the inflammatory reprogramming leading to tumor-promoting inflammation, facilitating immune suppression and tissue repair in the tumor, and establishing the PGE_2–IL-1β axis as a key driver of the inflammation-induced tumor progression [86]. Macrophages also play important roles in cachexia in pancreatic cancer. A current study highlighted the role of TWEAK (TNF-related weak inducer of apoptosis), a pro-inflammatory cytokine belonging to the TNF family, which led to muscle wasting. Specifically, tumor cells induced secretion of CCL2 (C-C motif chemokine ligand 2), leading to macrophage activation and subsequent TWEAK secretion by tumor cells via the CCL5/TRAF6 (TNF receptor-associated factor 6)/NF-κB signaling axis, which stimulated muscular atrophy [87]. Macrophage function and phenotypic switch largely depend on changes in their metabolic state [88,89]. M1 macrophage mediate their metabolism through glycolysis by increased glucose consumption, whilst M2 macrophages show an increase in oxidative phosphorylation [90]. A study performed by Zhang et al. using a co-culture model to understand the metabolic crosstalk between cancer cells and macrophages described the capability of PDAC cells to metabolically alter M1 macrophages to release the M2-specific cytokine IL-10. The results from the study suggested that the metabolic switch of M1 macrophages happens via direct interaction with PDAC cells, mediated by GARP (glycoprotein a repetitions predominant) and integrin αV/β8, and ultimately leads to TGF-β (transforming growth factor beta) secretion. Interestingly, selective reprogramming induced by PDAC cell interaction was only possible in M1 macrophages, whereas M2-like macrophages retained their phenotype upon tumor cell interaction. The same study highlighted that PDAC cells induced DNA methylation of genes related to glucose metabolism and oxidative phosphorylation (OXPHOS), including quinone oxidoreductase (NQO-1) and aldehyde dehydrogenase 1A3 (ALDH1A3), in M1 macrophages. This led to metabolic dysregulation. In M2 macrophages, these metabolism-related genes were upregulated [91]. Metabolic changes in macrophages might also influence chemoresistance. Halbrook et al. generated tumor-educated macrophages (TEMs) by growing bone marrow-derived macrophages in conditioned media from PDAC cells and performing metabolomics profiling. They identified an increased release of pyrimidine nucleosides and nucleobases in TEMs compared to control macrophages that impeded gemcitabine cytotoxic activity through molecular competition [92].

2.2.3. Clinical Implications and Therapeutic Strategies

A deeper and better understanding of signaling pathways involved in tumor-associated macrophage recruitment and functional properties has led to the development of several macrophage-targeted therapies in various cancers. For example, trabectedin and its analog lurbinectedin selectively depleted monocytes and TAMs in patients and mice through the TNFRSF10 (tumor necrosis factor receptor superfamily member 10, also known as TRAIL)-dependent apoptosis pathway [93]. CD40, which is a key component of both the innate and adaptive immune system, remains an attractive target for cancer immunotherapy. CD40 receptor agonists are used to facilitate the production of TNF, reactive oxygen, and nitrogen species, which mediate the bactericidal and tumoricidal activity of macrophages. CD40 agonist administration caused an increased influx of $CD4^+$ T cells into the TME. The safety of APX005M (CD40 agonistic antibody) was assessed in a phase I study in patients with metastatic pancreatic cancer. However, promising results demand further investigation in phase II/III clinical trials [94,95]. Altogether, this suggests that macrophages are an integral part of the pancreatic TME. The opportunity to understand TAM diversity at a single cell level and within a spatial context will enable a better characterization of pro- and anti-tumor behaviors of macrophages in PDAC [93].

2.3. *Dendritic Cells*

2.3.1. Key Physiological Functions

Dendritic cells (DCs) are characterized as professional antigen-presenting cells [96] that bridge the innate and adaptive immune system [96]. DCs can differentiate in various ways to fulfill their tasks [96]. All DC subsets originate from HSCs (hematopoietic stem cells) within the bone marrow [97,98]. HSCs develop into CMPs (common myeloid progenitors) and CLPs (common lymphoid progenitors). CMPs generate imDCs (immature DCs) and monocytes, which can differentiate into cDCs (conventional DCs) or moDCs (monocyte-derived DCs) [98]. cDCs are further classified into cDC1s, which become interstitial DCs, and cDC2s, which differentiate into Langerhans cells in the epidermis [96,99–101]. The only DC subtype that develops from CLPs is the pDC (plasmacytoid DC) subtype, which can produce high amounts of type I IFN (interferon) to actively participate in antiviral immunity [100,102]. In PDAC, several DC subtypes can be affected. However, cDC1 dendritic cells are particularly important because of their ability to present antigens to T cells. Although this classification is simplified, recent studies have defined multiple new DC types with unique functional properties [103].

2.3.2. Pathophysiology in PDAC

Disturbed maturation and a reduced number of DCs are fundamental problems in PDAC. The maturation of DCs can also be influenced by Reg3g (regenerating islet-derived protein 3 gamma) expression in PDAC cells. Reg3g promoted pancreatic cancer carcinogenesis via a STAT3 signaling pathway in a murine model of chronic pancreatitis [104]. Regarding an intratumoral immune response, Reg3g triggered an immunosuppressive microenvironment, including suppression of DC maturation, upregulation of EGFR (epidermal growth factor receptor) expression, and increase in Th2 cytokines in DCs while suppressing and inactivating $CD8^+$ T cell responses [105]. Ochi et al. showed that MyD88 (myeloid differentiation primary response 88 innate immune signal transduction adaptor) inhibition exacerbated pancreatic inflammation and progression to invasive cancer [106]. TLR4 (toll-like-receptor 4) activation on DCs usually triggers either a MyD88-dependent or -independent pathway [107]. The MyD88-dependent pathway is the predominant one in DCs and leads to the production of pro-inflammatory cytokines, favoring Th1-differentiation. This, in turn, can activate anti-tumor immunity and suppress pancreatic tumor growth. Blocking the MyD88-dependent-pathway induces pancreatic antigen-restricted, Th2-deviated $CD4^+$ T cells, leading to a transition from pancreatitis to pancreatic carcinoma [106]. A similar report by Lin and colleagues showed that cDC1 abundance and maturation declined progressively during pancreatic carcinogenesis. They remained in a semi-mature state associated with the upregulation of inflammation-related genes but impaired production of T-cell polarizing cytokines. Consequently, cDC1-mediated $CD8^+$ T cell priming was compromised [108]. The TME, featuring hypoxia, dense stroma, a high presence of immunosuppressive cells like MDSCs and Tregs (regulatory T cells), and low pH due to the glycolytic metabolism of tumor cells can also affect DC function [109,110]. Elevated glycolytic activity in PDAC cells led to decreased DC infiltration and impaired antigen-presenting functions due to low glucose and high lactate concentrations, which were detrimental to DC mitochondrial and antigen-presenting capabilities [111]. Additionally, Treg infiltration suppressed the immunogenicity of DCs, contributing to a disturbed T cell activation [112]. Kenkel et al. described an immunosuppressive subset of DCs that promoted Treg expansion, thus leading to a higher risk of tumor metastasis [113].

2.3.3. Clinical Implications in PDAC

Disturbed maturation and a reduced number of DCs are associated with poor prognosis and low survival rates in PDAC patients [114–116]. In addition, DCs play a crucial role in immunotherapy against various cancers, including PDAC [117–120]. PDAC patients exhibited decreased levels and enhanced apoptosis of cDCs and pDCs in comparison to control patients. Additionally, patients who have undergone tumor resection had lower DC counts even 12 weeks after surgery. Moreover, the authors found that high blood DC levels positively correlated with prolonged patient survival [120] and were usually associated with a better prognosis [121]. This is consistent with the data of Plesca et al., which showed that higher frequencies of tumor-infiltrating cDC1s and pDCs correlated with improved survival outcomes in PDAC patients, suggesting that the presence and functionality of DCs could serve as prognostic markers [122]. The same group claimed that the blood of PDAC patients accommodates more DCs with disturbed maturation in comparison to healthy patients. This includes both cDCs and pDCs. They showed an increased expression of CD83, CD40, B7H3 (also known as CD276), PD-L1 (also known as CD274), CCR6 (C-C chemokine receptor type 6), and CCR7 and a lowered expression of ICOSL (inducible T cell costimulator ligand), and DCIR, also known as CLEC4A (C-type lectin domain family 4 member A) [123]. Mechanistically, inflammatory factors, including elevated levels of PGE_2 in PDAC patients' plasma, were related to dysfunctional changes in DC phenotype [123]. Before pancreatic cancer development, particularly at the (IPMN) (intraductal papillary mucinous neoplasm) stage, increased secretion of CXCL17 and ICAM2 (intercellular adhesion molecule 2) led to the infiltration of cDCs, followed by T-cell-mediated cytolysis of tumor cells. Secretion of CXCL17 and ICAM2 was significantly decreased when IPMA progressed to pancreatic cancer, contributing to immune tolerance [124].

2.3.4. Therapeutic Strategies

DCs are a fundamental component of immunotherapeutic approaches in numerous cancers, including PDAC [98,116,117]. One possibility is given by pulsing DCs with tumor-specific antigens, e.g., using cell lysates, KRAS G12D$^{1-23}$ peptide, or alpha-enolase. As an example, in mice treated with alpha-enolase-pulsed DCs, T cell proliferation is stimulated. As a result, these cells secreted IFN-γ, which subsequently led to PDAC cell lysis [100,118]. Alternatively, DC vaccination might be combined with other treatments. Mahadevan et al. reported that using engineered cancer-specific cDC1s along with immunotherapy might be an approach for the treatment of pancreatitis-associated PDAC. They showed that ex vivo-engineered cDC1s stimulated with tumor antigens sensitized resistant PDAC tumors to immune checkpoint blockade [98]. A recent study showed that IL-2 promoted the expansion and intratumoral accretion of tumor-infiltrating DCs in PDAC [118]. Further approaches pursue the creation of a more favorable immune landscape to improve both DC infiltration and T cell activation and infiltration by inhibiting TNFR1 signaling or hypoxia-driven immune checkpoints [119,120]. Although DC-based therapy is promising in PDAC, further research is necessary to understand the fundamental biology and functionality of tumor-associated DCs to be able to improve or combine existing immunotherapeutic approaches.

2.4. Mast Cells

2.4.1. Key Physiological Functions

Mast cells belong to the group of granulocytes and derive from myeloid progenitor cells [125]. During mast cell differentiation and maturation, mast cell progenitor cells typically migrate to areas of the body that are in direct contact with the environment, e.g., the skin, mucosa of the conjunctiva, and the respiratory and gastrointestinal tract [126]. Therefore, they are only found as immature precursor cells in the peripheral blood [101]. Fully differentiated mast cells are traditionally classified into three categories based on the dominant serine protease secreted: MC_T (tryptase-producing mast cells), MC_C (chymase-producing mast cells), and MC_{TC}, which produce both [127]. Further classification is based on the location of the mast cell: CMCs (connective tissue mast cells) can be distinguished from MMCs (mucosal mast cells) [128]. Mast cells play a vital role in allergic reactions, especially type 1 allergic reactions. Physiologically, mast cells bind IgE antibodies, which are produced by B-lymphocytes after first antigen contact. At the time of a second antigen contact, the antigen binds to IgE on the mast cell's surface, causing its degranulation. Regulation of mast cells is mediated by the KIT receptor (CD117) [129]. Mast cell granules comprise, for instance, histamine, heparin, proteases (tryptase, chymase), and cytokines like interleukin (IL-1, -3, -4, -5, -8, -10), as well as PDGF (platelet-derived growth factor), TNF-α, TGF-β, and MMP9 (matrix metalloproteinase-9) [130].

2.4.2. Pathophysiology and Clinical Implications in PDAC

The role of mast cells in cancer is multifaceted [131–133]. In some cancer types, mast cell infiltration of the TME is associated with better outcomes [134–136]. In other tumor entities, it has a negative impact on patient prognosis [137], e.g., for melanoma [138,139], breast cancer [140,141], and gastric cancer [142,143]. In PDAC, they are considered one of the tumor-promoting cell types [144], and mast cell infiltration is associated with a lower survival rate [145–147]. Tumor-infiltrating mast cells often accumulate at the edges of the tumor, which is also observed in PDAC [148,149]. Analyses of the mast cell count in pancreatic tissue from PDAC patients after curative partial pancreas resection showed a correlation between high mast cell count and TNM stage. Remarkably, only mast cell infiltration of the intratumoral border zone could be identified as an independent prognostic factor for overall survival, whereas survival did not correlate with the mast cell count in the intratumoral central zone or in the peritumoral zone [145]. A similar effect was also described for *K-ras*^{G12V} mice, where mast cells accumulated at the tumor edge [146]. Therefore, they contributed significantly to the angiogenic switch during tumor progression [150,151]. Mast cells secrete several pro-angiogenic factors, such as VEGF (vascular endothelial growth factor), TNF-α, TGF-β, FGF-2 (fibroblast growth factor-2), and angiopoietin-1 [152–156]. Consistent with these findings, mast cell inhibition promoted the efficiency of anti-angiogenic therapy [157]. Other factors secreted by mast cells are IL-13 and tryptase, which directly induce the proliferation of pancreatic stellate cells (PSCs) [158,159]. On the other hand, tumor growth was suppressed significantly in mast cell-deficient mice [146,151]. In conclusion, mast cells infiltrate the TME of PDAC, promoting tumor progression by activating PSCs and facilitating angiogenesis.

2.4.3. Therapeutic Strategies

Mast cells can be useful targets in cancer therapy. So far, three different approaches have evolved: mast cell inhibition, decreasing the mast cell count, or altering the effects of secreted mediators [160]. Although previous findings suggested that mast cell inhibition might be a promising approach, data for PDAC therapy are scarce [144]. Decreasing their chemotaxis by pharmacological inhibition of CXCR4 resulted in reduced mast cell migration in mice, and thus improved survival [158]. The tyrosine kinase inhibitor masitinib, which selectively targets the c-Kit receptor, increased overall survival in PDAC patients when combined with gemcitabine [161–163]. However, it is not yet known to what extent the effect of masitinib on mast cells contributes to these findings. Thus, further research is needed to elucidate the potential of mast cell inhibition in PDAC therapy.

2.5. *Neutrophils*

2.5.1. Key Physiological Functions

Neutrophils are the most abundant innate immune cells in the blood and bone marrow [164,165]. They are the first cells being recruited to the site of inflammation and play a crucial role in host defense mechanisms, having antibacterial [166], antifungal [167], and antiviral [168] functions. Also, they perform phagocytosis of cell debris, an essential process for tissue regeneration and angiogenesis [169]. Some studies have proposed that two groups of tumor-associated neutrophils exist that differ according to their polarization state: tumor-suppressing N1 neutrophils and tumor-promoting N2 neutrophils [170].

2.5.2. Pathophysiology and Clinical Implications in PDAC

Since neutrophils are considered major initiators of inflammation, they play a role in both acute and chronic pancreatitis as well as PDAC. Normal pancreatic tissue is not infiltrated by neutrophils, however, infiltration is significantly increased after cerulein-mediated tissue damage and release of PAF (platelet-activating factor) [171]. Neutrophils are recruited by the secretion of pro-inflammatory factors, such as TNF-α and IL-23. On the other hand, infiltrated neutrophils secrete a number of chemokines that further attract other immune cells of the innate and adaptive immune system [60]. In addition, the secretion of cytokines, including CXCL10 and CCL-21, can promote the migration of pancreatic cancer cells towards sensory neurons [172]. Moreover, neutrophil-derived elastase has been shown to mediate the dyshesion of tumor cells and degradation of E-cadherin, contributing to enhanced migration and invasion [173]. Another important function of neutrophils is the capability of forming NETs (neutrophil extracellular traps). NETs are large, web-like structures that contain neutrophil DNA as well as cytosolic and granule proteins [174] and are considered a defense mechanism for bacterial killing. Across several cancer types, NETs may promote tumor progression and metastasis (reviewed in [175]). Pancreatic cancer cells were able to induce NET formation [176] and the serum of

PDAC patients has a higher NET-forming potential mediated by IL-17 [177]. In addition, tumor-derived TIMP-1 (tissue inhibitor of metalloproteinase-1) triggered NET formation upon interaction with its receptor CD63 and activation of ERK signaling. Inhibition of TIMP-1 or inhibition of NETosis prolonged survival in a murine PDAC model. Likewise, TIMP-1 levels correlated with local and systemic NET-formation in PDAC patients and negatively affected survival [178]. Furthermore, additional studies have shown that NETs induce migration, invasion, and EMT (epithelial–mesenchymal transition) of pancreatic cancer cells in an IL-1b/EGFR/ERK-dependent manner, which could potentially be utilized for therapy [179]. Interestingly, inhibition of PAD4 (protein arginine deiminase 4), which is critical for NET release, reduced NET formation and suppressed pancreatic tumor growth in a xenograft model [180]. NETs not only entrap pathogens but also bind platelets and contribute to cancer-associated thrombosis [181], which is associated with reduced survival in pancreatic cancer patients [182].

2.6. Myeloid-Derived Suppressor Cells (MDSCs)

2.6.1. Key Physiological Functions

MDSCs are a heterogeneous cell population of pathologically activated neutrophils (granulocytic/polymorphonuclear MDSCs; PMN-MDSCs) and monocytes (monocytic MDSCs; M-MDSCs) that show strong immune suppressive capabilities and have been implicated in multiple malignancies [183]. While M-MDSCs are mainly responsible for T cell suppression in an antigen-specific and non-specific manner, associated with the production of nitric oxide and cytokines [184], PMN-MDSCs suppress T cells primarily in an antigen-specific manner [185]. The pathological activation and recruitment of MDSCs are mediated by a large variety of mostly pro-inflammatory cytokines, indicating the increasing importance of these cells in malignancies associated with chronic inflammation, such as chronic pancreatitis with associated pancreatic adenocarcinoma.

2.6.2. Pathophysiology and Clinical Implications in PDAC

Monitoring infiltration of immune cells during disease progression in an LSL-$Kras^{G12D/+}$;$p48^{Cre}$ mouse model showed an early influx of leukocytes into pancreatic tissue. Macrophage infiltration began very early in preinvasive disease, followed by an infiltration of MDSCs. MDSCs persisted after progression to PDAC and were found to be highly immunosuppressive in vitro [83]. Several studies have revealed that the homing of MDSCs to the pancreas in preinvasive and invasive diseases is mediated by cytokines directly produced within the pancreas. For example, PDAC cells were found to be able to produce high levels of GM-CSF (granulocyte-macrophage colony-stimulating factor) in mice. GM-CSF was capable of inducing splenocyte differentiation into MDSCs that suppressed T cell responses in vitro [186]. Likewise, human PDAC prominently expressed GM-CSF as well. Neutralizing GM-CSF blocked the recruitment of MDSCs and reduced tumor growth in mice that were dependent on $CD8^+$ T cells [186]. In mice, data showed that the upregulation of GM-CSF was specifically dependent on oncogenic $Kras^{G12D}$ [187]. Furthermore, other factors including IL-1β, VEGF, CXCL1, and IL-6 can influence MDSC number in the tumor microenvironment, some of which are produced by PSCs. Mace et al. showed that PSCs secreted MDSC-promoting cytokines and chemokines and led to MDSC differentiation in a STAT3-dependent manner [188]. STAT3 signaling is suggested to be a crucial pathway regulating immunosuppressive activity in MDSCs. In head and neck squamous cell carcinoma patients, STAT3 signaling was responsible for arginase-I expression in MDSCs, which was crucial for MDSCs' suppressive function [189]. Arginase-I has been shown to be a key driver of the immunosuppressive tumor microenvironment in PDAC [190]. In addition, the transformation of monocytes to M-MDSCs was dependent on STAT3 activation contributing to stemness and increased mesenchymal properties in pancreatic cancer [191]. Porembka et al. showed that C57BL/6 mice inoculated with Panc02 pancreatic cancer cells have increased numbers of MDSCs in their bone marrow and peripheral blood, which were recruited to the tumor site and were able to decrease T cell responses. Similar results were found in PDAC patients. Recruitment of MDSCs and tumor growth could be inhibited by zoledronic acid treatment in vivo [192]. Unfortunately, translating these findings to PDAC patients was not successful as zoledronic acid did not impact overall or progression-free survival [193]. Besides inhibition of $CD8^+$ T cell function directly, MDSCs can also stimulate the expansion of immunosuppressive Tregs via TGF-β and IFN-γ [194,195], which contributes to impaired $CD8^+$ T cell function as well. In addition, the influence on NK cells as well as macrophages can also attenuate anti-tumor immunity [196–198].

2.6.3. Therapeutic Strategies

As MDSCs are key drivers of immune suppression in pancreatic cancer, targeting MDSCs might represent a potential tool to promote anti-tumor response. Interestingly, gemcitabine is known to decrease the quantity of MDSCs, thereby promoting antitumor response [199]. Another approach includes targeting mediators that promote their proliferation and recruitment, e.g., GM-CSF, as mentioned above. In addition, inhibitors of the JAK2/STAT3 signaling pathway might limit MDSC stimulation and infiltration. This was tested in immunocompetent PDAC mouse models, where the authors used CXCR4-modified Claudin 18.2-directed CAR-T cells that suppressed recruitment of MDSCs via a STAT3/NF-κB/SDF-1α axis. CXCR4 not only led to a better infiltration of CAR-T cells into tumor sites but also increased the efficacy of CAR-T cell therapy by reducing the production of STAT3-mediated cytokines [200].

While current and novel therapeutic approaches might reduce MDSC function and infiltration, it is known that chemotherapy in PDAC leads to the release of inflammatory factors, including GM-CSF, that contribute to increased numbers of intratumoral MDSCs [201,202]. In conclusion, MDSCs play a crucial role in shaping the tumor immune microenvironment in PDAC, thereby affecting initiation, disease progression, and therapy response. Understanding their function and regulation might further help to design innovative therapeutic strategies that impact the PDAC TME.

3. Platelets as Regulators of Tumor Growth and Immunity

Platelets are increasingly recognized as active contributors to tumor growth, immunity, and immune evasion beyond their traditional role in hemostasis. Interaction with immune or cancer cells happens either directly via receptor–ligand interactions or indirectly via the secretion of cytokines or growth factors. Thus, platelets are positioned at the intersection of inflammation, tumor immunity, and cancer progression.

3.1. *Key Physiological Functions*

Platelets or thrombocytes are blood components that, although not categorized as immune cells, can have considerable roles in inflammation and immune response. Megakaryocytes are the precursors of platelets and reside in the bone marrow, where platelet formation primarily occurs [203]. After their release from megakaryocytes into the blood vessels, platelets have a lifespan of 5–7 days [204]. Being highly abundant in circulation, platelets play a key role in regulating hemostasis. They are able to sense damage to blood vessels within seconds as they recognize glycosylated structures of the extracellular matrix, like collagen, von Willebrand factor, laminin, or fibronectin, that become exposed when the vessel is injured. Subsequently, platelets become activated [205]. In the past years, accumulating evidence suggests that platelets become activated by tumor cells as well and that they are not merely bystander cells but play active roles in several steps of tumorigenesis [206]. For example, platelets were shown to regulate tumor growth and therapy response [207,208]. Moreover, platelets interact with circulating tumor cells and protect them from anoikis, thereby promoting metastasis formation [209]. In addition, several studies have highlighted platelets as orchestrators of immunity and regulators of the cancer immune microenvironment with potential roles in immune evasion. It is well known that platelets store and release chemokines and cytokines upon activation that can regulate the recruitment, activation, and differentiation of immune cells [210]. In addition, platelets interact with immune cells of innate and adaptive immunity via receptor–ligand interactions, e.g., PSGL-1 (P-selectin-P-selectin glycoprotein ligand-1 interaction) that mediates rolling and adhesion of neutrophils [211]. Similarly to innate immune cells, they express PRRs (pattern recognition receptors) like TLRs, NLRs (NOD-like receptors), and CLR (C-type lectin receptors) on their surface [212] that recognize damage- or pathogen-associated molecular patterns, and they communicate with or present antigens to T cells [213].

3.2. Impact of Platelets on Immune Cells of the Innate Immune System

In several murine models of inflammation, platelets have been key in regulating the extravasation of immune cells [214,215]. When platelet numbers were low, host defense in bacterial pneumonia was impaired [216,217]. Likewise, in cancer, immune cell infiltration and activity can be regulated by platelets. This is the result of direct platelet-immune cell interactions or cytokine secretion after platelet activation (Figure 4a–c). Subsequently, this can impact tumor growth and metastasis.

It has long been recognized that NK cell-mediated tumor lysis is impaired by platelets forming a platelet coat around circulating tumor cells [218]. Mechanistically, it has been shown that platelet coating led to a transfer of MHC class I molecules onto the tumor cell surface that disrupted NK cell recognition and impaired cytotoxicity [73]. Alternatively, platelet coating reduced surface expression of NKG2D ligands, in particular, MHC class I chain-related sequence A (MICA) and MICB, on tumor cells and thereby diminished NKG2D-dependent lysis of tumor cells [219]. NKG2D expression can also be downregulated by platelet-derived TGF-β [72]. Moreover, platelet RANKL (receptor activator of nF-κB ligand) reduced IFN-γ production by NK cells and inhibited NK cell cytotoxicity [220].

Platelets can also regulate the differentiation of innate immune cells. This has been shown for DCs, where platelets reduced DC differentiation and altered production of proinflammatory and immunoregulatory cytokines [221]. In contrast to these findings, another study reported that platelets enhanced DC maturation, infiltration, and their capacity to stimulate lymphocyte proliferation [222]. Similarly, the polarisation of macrophages can be regulated by platelet interaction. Here, studies show that platelets can promote both a polarisation towards an M1- and an M2-phenotype, likely depending on the model used. In a murine sepsis model, platelets promoted macrophage polarization towards a pro-inflammatory M1 phenotype in a cell contact-dependent manner involving the glycoprotein Ib (GPIb)-CD11b axis [223]. In cancer, platelet aggregation increased hematogenous metastasis formation by triggering macrophage recruitment and promoting an M2 phenotype [224]. Other results showed that platelet-derived CXCL4 induced a unique phenotype in macrophages, showing characteristics of both M1 and M2 macrophages. The authors called these M4-macrophages [225]. A strong functional interplay between macrophages and platelets is also demonstrated for cancer-associated thrombosis driven by a pro-thrombotic niche that was induced by CXCL13-reprogrammed macrophages. This promoted metastasis across multiple cancer types including a murine PDAC model [226].

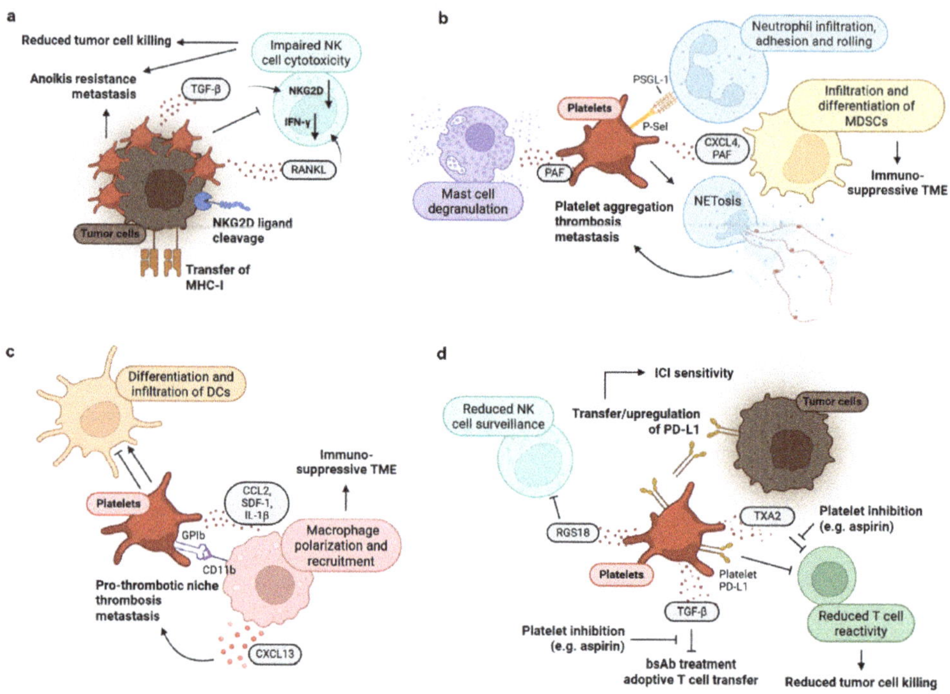

Figure 4. Platelet collaboration with innate immune cells, their role in cancer, and in immune evasion. (**a**) Tumor cell coating protects CTCs from anoikis, supports their dissemination, and shields them from NK cell cytotoxicity by secreting TGF-β or RANKL (receptor activator of nF-κB ligand). This reduces NKG2D expression or IFN-γ secretion. In addition, platelets mediate cleavage of NKG2D ligands or transfer MHC class I molecules onto the tumor cell surface. (**b**) Platelets mediate infiltration and differentiation of MDSCs, and ultimately support an immunosuppressive TME, via CXCL4 and PAF (platelet-activating factor), adhesion and rolling of neutrophils by receptor–ligand interactions, e.g., P-Sel (P-Selectin)-PSGL-1 (P-selectin glycoprotein ligand-1) among others, and induce the formation of neutrophil extracellular traps (NETosis). NET formation contributes to platelet aggregation, thrombosis and metastasis. Furthermore, platelets can induce the degranulation of perivascular mast cells via PAF. (**c**) Platelets induce macrophage polarization and recruitment via direct and indirect mechanisms and regulate differentiation and infiltration of DCs. Polarization to an M2-phenotype in tumors drives an immunosuppressive TME. Moreover, macrophages can induce a pro-thrombotic niche via CXCL13 secretion that stimulates thrombosis and metastasis. (**d**) Platelets may transfer to or upregulate PD-L1 expression in tumor cells that predicts ICI treatment sensitivity. In addition, platelet PD-L1, as well as, secretion of TXA2 (thromboxane A2) or TGF-β, reduces T cell reactivity and efficacy of T cell-based immunotherapy that can be alleviated by platelet inhibitory agents, including aspirin. Immune evasion from NK cell surveillance is induced by platelet RGS18 (regulator of G protein signaling 18). The figure was created using BioRender.com.

Due to their rapid response after vessel injury, platelets are ideally positioned between the damaged endothelium and infiltrating neutrophils. Indeed, direct interactions of platelets and neutrophils seem to be crucial for inflammatory processes, NETosis, thrombosis, and cancer. Interaction between neutrophils and platelets is mediated via multiple receptor–ligand pairs, including P-Selectin-PSGL1, ICAM2-LFA1 (lymphocyte function-associated antigen 1), JAM-3 (junctional adhesion molecule 3), Mac-1 (macrophage-1 antigen), and CD40-CD40L [211,227–229]. Platelets foster transmigration and extravasation of neutrophils after vessel injury, which is required for subsequent effective immune responses and tissue repair [230]. On the other hand, neutrophils trigger platelet activation and thrombosis during systemic infections, which suppresses pathogen dissemination [231]. It has been shown that neutrophil recruitment in the early phase of thrombus formation is indispensable for deep venous thrombosis (DVT), partly driven by tissue factor secretion. In turn, DVT propagation is supported by platelets via stimulation of NETs [232]. NET formation can be induced by cytokines secreted via tumor cells [233] or is dependent on platelet proteins, receptors, or adhesion molecules [234–236].

The impact of platelets on MDSCs is relevant for local immunosuppression. It has been shown that platelets increase the differentiation of monocytes into MDSCs, which inhibit $CD8^+$ T cell function [237]. A similar report by Servais et al. showed that platelets enhanced immunosuppression, MDSC infiltration into tumors and MDSC-mediated inhibition of T cell proliferation [238].

While the interactions between platelets and above mentioned innate immune cells are well characterized, the significance of platelet–mast cell crosstalk remains largely unexplored. It has been shown that platelets trigger perivascular mast cell degranulation via PAF [239]. In addition, platelets and mast cells might work together to promote the recruitment of eosinophils during fungal infections [240]. However, their interaction in the context of cancer has not been studied so far.

In summary, platelets play a pivotal role in modulating innate immune responses during cancer and inflammation. Platelet–immune cell interactions can trigger pro-inflammatory and pro-thrombotic pathways that link hemostasis, immunity, and oncogenesis.

3.3. *Role of Platelets in Immune Evasion*

A meta-analysis of 12 studies with 1340 cancer patients showed that the platelet–lymphocyte ratio (PLR) is a negative predictor of survival under immune checkpoint inhibitor therapy (ICI) [241]. This raised the question of whether PLR is a simple biomarker or if platelets, either alone or through interactions with immune cells in the tumor microenvironment, actively influence response to ICI, immune evasion, and disease outcome. Indeed, it has been shown that platelets can increase PD-L1 expression in cancer cells [242,243], a well-accepted and long-standing marker of immune evasion in several types of cancer [244]. Similarly, a report showed that platelet PD-L1 was able to protect PD-L1 negative tumor cells from elimination by T cells [245]. Platelets are also capable of transferring PD-L1 to tumor cells. This was shown for lung cancer cells and was dependent on fibronectin 1, integrin $\alpha5\beta1$, and GPIbα. Platelet PD-L1 inhibited $CD4^+$ and $CD8^+$ T cells and predicted response towards ICI [246]. Other T cell-based immunotherapies, e.g., T cell-recruiting bsAb (bispecific antibody) treatment, can be modulated by platelets as well. A study showed that platelets significantly reduced bsAb-mediated $CD4^+$ and $CD8^+$ T cell reactivity mediated by platelet TGF-β, providing a rationale for modulation of platelet function to reinforce the effectiveness of bsAb treatment [247]. Platelet effects are not limited to bsAb treatment but have been shown to be useful for adoptive T cell transfer as well. Platelet TGF-β reduced the efficacy of adoptive T cell transfer in murine melanoma, which could be mitigated by platelet inhibitory drugs, including aspirin and clopidogrel [248]. In general, platelet inhibitory drugs might hold great promise to overcome immune evasion. In a murine ovarian cancer model, aspirin in combination with adoptive T cell transfer led to a markedly increased infiltration of tumor-reactive $CD8^+$ T cells [249]. Similar results have been demonstrated recently, showing that aspirin prevented metastasis formation by releasing T cells from suppression of platelet thromboxane A2 [250]. NK cell-based treatments may also be affected by platelets, as numerous in vitro and vitro studies have demonstrated that platelets suppress NK cell cytotoxic activity, as highlighted above. A recent study in PDAC demonstrated that immune evasion of CTCs from NK cell surveillance, engaging the HLA-E:CD94-NKG2A immune checkpoint, is promoted by platelet-derived RGS18 (regulator of G protein signaling 18). RGS18 significantly increased hepatic metastasis, which was inhibited by the blockade of NKG2A or the knockdown of HLA-E [251].

Overall, these findings underscore the role of platelets as key contributors to immune evasion and the effectiveness of immunotherapy (summarized in Figure 4d), thereby supporting the rationale for incorporating anti-platelet therapy into certain treatment strategies.

3.4. Pathophysiology and Clinical Implications in PDAC

Pancreatic cancer cells were shown to induce platelet aggregation and activation [252]. This is associated with a release of bioactive molecules from platelet granules. Moreover, pancreatic cancer cell-derived tissue factor (TF) can lead to activation of coagulation and thrombus formation [253,254]. In fact, pancreatic cancer patients are especially prone to venous thrombosis [255], and paraneoplastic thrombocytosis is associated with worse survival in PDAC [256,257]. In line with this, the relative risk for the subsequent diagnosis of an occult pancreatic carcinoma after the occurrence of a thromboembolic event is six-fold higher [258]. In addition, high platelet-to-albumin ratios as well as high platelet-lymphocyte ratios are negative predictors of PDAC patient survival [259,260]. This suggests that platelets might be used as diagnostic and prognostic biomarkers. Indeed, the use of the RNA content of tumor-educated platelets as a source for liquid biopsy has been proposed [261]. Platelets might also be important for pancreatitis and PDAC development. Upon platelet activation, TGF-β can be released from platelet granules [262], which is a critical immunomodulatory cytokine and highly abundant in chronic pancreatitis and pancreatic cancer (reviewed in [263]). Activation of the TGF-β signaling pathway was found to be a driving force for fibrosis in chronic pancreatitis, acinar-to-ductal metaplasia, and pancreatic tumor initiation [264,265]. Furthermore, platelets actively release IL-1β [266,267], which is associated with acute and chronic pancreatitis as well as PDAC promotion [268,269]. Indeed, pannexin 1 led to increased IL-1β secretion in $CD41^+/CD62^+$ platelets that promoted migration and invasion of PDAC cells in vitro. Inhibition of pannexin 1 using a small molecule inhibitor proved its relevance also in vivo by inhibition of primary tumor growth, metastasis, and survival [270]. In addition, analyzing TCGA pancreatic cancer transcriptomics data showed an inverse correlation between platelet and $CD8^+$ T cell RNA signatures but a positive correlation with MDSC RNA signatures [237], indicating that platelets are crucial for regulating the infiltration of respective immune cells into pancreatic tumor tissue. Likewise, the expression of platelet-related genes in PDAC has been associated with immune cell infiltration and immune checkpoint expression [271]. Moreover, evasion of human PDAC CTCs from NK cell surveillance has been mediated by platelets [251].

Although several indirect associations exist, the question of whether platelets directly influence early pancreatic carcinogenesis and PDAC progression still requires more detailed investigations and is the subject of ongoing research.

3.5. Therapeutic Strategies

Platelets might not only be important for cancer development but also for cancer treatment. For example, inhibiting platelet activity by combining aspirin and the P2Y12 inhibitor clopidogrel was able to reduce progression to hepatocellular carcinoma [272]. Aspirin may hold global significance, especially regarding the prevention of pancreatic cancer [273]. In addition, the homing capabilities of platelets have been harnessed in systems where platelet mimics were loaded with a cytotoxic payload to restrict the localization of the drug to the tumor site [274–276]. The most interesting application of this methodology includes perforin/granzyme-loaded platelets that are able to kill tumor cells upon activation and subsequent alpha granule release directly at the tumor site [277]. Platelets and platelet inhibitory drugs might also regulate the efficacy of immunotherapy, as highlighted above [246–250]. Very recently, combining immunotherapy with antithrombotic therapy has been reported to improve survival of advanced melanoma patients [278]. Although PDAC is an immunologically cold tumor with low T cell infiltration and restricted efficacy of immunotherapeutic agents, adding platelet-based therapies might be a novel approach to handling this deadly disease. However, whether such a therapeutic strategy is effective in PDAC remains to be determined.

4. Future Directions and Perspectives

Intricate crosstalk exists between the innate immune system, tumor cells, and platelets that drive intratumoral inflammation, fibrosis, tumor growth, metastasis, and therapy response. However, innate immune cells and platelets also critically shape responses of the adaptive immune system. In particular, the role of platelets in regulating T cell responses and immune evasion was described in detail above. In addition, dysregulation of the innate immune system can profoundly impair adaptive immune responses, particularly in the context of cancer. Uptake and presentation of tumor antigens is a prerequisite for subsequent priming and activation of naïve T cells. Here, dendritic cells play a central role in generating specific T cell-mediated antitumor responses (see also Figure 3) to control tumor growth and dissemination [279]. However, the phenotype and function of DCs are altered by inflammatory mediators generated in the TME, which impairs their antigen-presenting capacity [280]. In addition, NK cells influence adaptive immunity and can both stimulate and inhibit T cell responses (see also Figure 2). Regulation of T cell responses can be direct or indirect. Direct mechanisms include the secretion of cytokines, e.g., IFN-γ or IL-10 that mediate T cell differentiation or T cell inhibition, respectively. Alternatively, they are able to kill $CD4^+$ and $CD8^+$ T cells in an NKG2D- and perforin-dependent manner. Effects on T cells can also be indirect via governing DC maturation and elimination or antigen cross-presentation [281]. The recruitment of immunosuppressive cells, including MDSCs and TAMs, is an additional mechanism to reduce anti-tumor T cell responses and the efficacy of immunotherapy. Similar to NK cells, both direct and indirect regulatory mechanisms exist. They inhibit T cell functions through the production of reactive oxygen species, arginase-1, IL-10, and nitric oxide. In addition, they can restrain the intratumoral localization of cytotoxic T cells while promoting the recruitment of regulatory T cells. Moreover, their presence in the tumor microenvironment can limit the effectiveness of ICI [80,183]. In summary, an effectively regulated innate immune system is crucial for orchestrating robust and functional adaptive immune responses that can also be limited by platelets. This interplay is particularly relevant for PDAC, where a dominant immunosuppressive environment hinders effective antitumor immunity. Therefore, targeting innate immune cells or platelets, alongside T cell-based therapies such as immune checkpoint blockade, represents a promising therapeutic strategy. Indeed, several currently ongoing and recently completed approaches are used in PDAC that target these cellular compartments and are summarized in Table 1.

Furthermore, emerging technologies such as single-cell RNA sequencing (scRNA-seq), spatial transcriptomics, and high-dimensional immune profiling are transforming our understanding of the tumor microenvironment. This is critical, particularly in PDAC, which is characterized by extensive cellular heterogeneity and a dense stromal compartment. This cellular heterogeneity could be uncovered using single-cell transcriptomics, e.g., in primary PDAC, metastatic lesions, as well as PDAC-derived organoids [282,283]. To further differentiate the cellular subtypes, scRNA-seq enabled the high-resolution characterization of rare or previously unrecognized subpopulations of immune cells [284–286], fibroblasts [287,288], and malignant epithelial cells. Spatial transcriptomics complements scRNA-seq by preserving the spatial architecture of the tumor, allowing researchers to map specific gene expression patterns to discrete regions within the tumor and stroma. This is crucial for understanding how cell–cell interactions and gradients of signaling molecules influence tumor progression, immune evasion or metastasis. Immune profiling, including high-dimensional flow cytometry and multiplexed imaging, adds another layer by quantifying immune cell subsets, their activation states, and interactions with other cell types such as platelets, cancer-associated fibroblasts, and endothelial cells [289]. Together, these approaches offer a powerful toolkit for dissecting the immunological landscape of PDAC, identifying novel biomarkers and causes for interindividual differences in drug responses as well as developing strategies for precision immunotherapy [36,290]. Integrating these insights with functional and translational studies will be pivotal for identifying new therapeutic targets and guiding the development of more effective, personalized immunotherapies for PDAC.

Table 1. Summary of ongoing and recently completed clinical trials targeting innate immune cells or platelets in PDAC. 5-FU: 5-Fluorouracil; ACT: Adoptive cellular therapy; CAR: chimeric antigen receptor; CCR: CC motif chemokine receptors; CD: Cluster of differentiation; CSF1R: Colony-stimulating factor 1 receptor; mTOR: Mammalian target of rapamycin; PI3K: Phosphatidylinositol 3-kinase; SIRPα: Signal-regulatory protein α; STING: Stimulator of interferon genes; CXCR: CXC motif chemokine receptor; TKI: tyrosine kinase inhibitor; ILRAP: Interleukin-1 receptor accessory protein.

NK Cells			
Compound	**Clinical Study Phase**	**Trial Number**	**Combination Drugs/Treatment**
CAR-NK Cells (CL-NK-001)	Phase 1	NCT06816823	-
Allogeneic Magicell-NK infusion	Phases 1/2	NCT06730009	SLOG chemotherapy
CAR-T/CAR-NK cells	Phase 1	NCT06572956	-
Chemotherapy Sequential NKG2D CAR-NK Cell	Phase 1	NCT06503497	Second-line chemotherapy (not specified)
Intratumoral Injection and intravenous infusion of NKG2D CAR-NK cells	Phase 1	NCT06478459	-
CAR-NK cells (CB CAR-NK182) targeting Claudin18.2	Phase 1	NCT06464965	-
TROP2-CAR/IL15-transduced CB-NK cells	Phases 1/2	NCT05922930	Cyclophosphamide, Fludarabine
NK cell infusion	Phases 1/2	NCT02718859	Irreversible electroporation (IRE)
Cytokine-induced Killer Cells	Phases 1/2	NCT01868490	-
Dendritic cell-activated Cytokine-induced killer treatment (DC-CIK)	Phases 1/2	NCT01781520	S-1
Interleukin-2	Phase 2	NCT05810792	Histamine Dihydrochloride (HDC)
FT500	Phase 1	NCT03841110	Cyclophosphamide, Fludarabine, Nivolumab, Pembrolizumab, Atezolizumab, IL-2
FATE-NK100	Phase 1	NCT03319459	Cetuximab, Trastuzumab

Table 1. *Cont.*

Macrophages			
Compound	**Preclinical/clinical study**	**Trial Number**	**Combination drug**
BMS-813160 (CCR2/CCR5 antagonist)	Phases 1/2	NCT03184870	Nivolumab, nab-paclitaxel, gemcitabine, 5-FU, leucovorin, irinotecan
BMS-813160	Phases 1/2	NCT03767582	Nivolumab, GVAX
TAK-500 (CCR2 and STING agonist)	Phase 1	NCT05070247	Pembrolizumab
PLX3397 (CSF1R inhibitors)	Phase 1	NCT02777710	Durvalumab
LY3022855 (anti-CSF1R antibody)	Phase 1	NCT03153410	Cyclophosphamide, GVAX, pembrolizumab
Cabiralizumab (anti-CSF1R antibody)	Phase 1	NCT02526017	Nivolumab
Lurbinectedin	Phase 2	NCT05229588	-
BI 754,091 (anti-CD47/SIRPα antibody)	Phase 1	NCT04752215	Ezabenlimab
CP-870, 893 (CD40 agonist antibody)	Phase 1	NCT01456585	Gemcitabine
APX005M (CD40 agonist antibody)	Phase 1	NCT02600949	Pembrolizumab, sotigalimab
APX005M	Phases 1/2	NCT05419479	Zimberelimab, domvanalimab
RO7009789 (CD40 agonist antibody)	Phase 1	NCT02588443	Nab-paclitaxel, gemcitabine
Gedatolisib (PI3K/mTOR inhibitor)	Phase 1	NCT03065062	Palbociclib
Metformin	Phase 1	NCT02336087	Gemcitabine, paclitaxel albumin-stabilized nanoparticle formulation
Metformin	Phase 2	NCT01666730	Oxaliplatin, leucovorin calcium, fluorouracil
Metformin	Phase 2	NCT04033107	Vitamin C
CT-0508 (CAR macrophages)	Phase 1	NCT04660929	Pembrolizumab
Dendritic cells			
Compound	**Preclinical/clinical study**	**Trial Number**	**Combination drug**
Metformin	Phase 2	PREOPANC trial EudraCT: 2012-003181-40	-
Toripalimab	Phases 1b/2	ChiCTR2000032293	chemotherapy
Ibrutinib	Phase 1/2	NCT02562898	Paclitaxel, gemcitabine
Wilms' tumor 1 (WT1) peptides	Phase 2	jRCTc030190195	multiagent chemotherapy
Mast cells			
Compound	**Preclinical/clinical study**	**Trial Number**	**Combination drug**
Masitinib (TKI targeting KIT)	Phase 3	NCT00789633	Gemcitabine
Neutrophils			
Compound	**Preclinical/clinical study**	**Trial Number**	**Combination drug**
Nadunolimab (IL1RAP inhibition)	Phases 1/2	NCT03267316	Cisplatin, gemcitabine, nab-paclitaxel, carboplatin, pemetrexed

Table 1. *Cont.*

MDSCs			
Compound	**Preclinical/clinical study**	**Trial Number**	**Combination drug**
Entinostat	Phase 2	NCT03250273	Nivolumab
SX-682 (CXCR1/2 Inhibitor)	Phase 1	NCT04477343	Nivolumab
Platelets			
Compound	**Preclinical/clinical study**	**Trial Number**	**Combination drug**
Avatrombopag	Phase 1	NCT06182072	Gemcitabine, nab-Paclitaxel

5. Conclusions

Chronic pancreatitis is a global health problem and an important risk factor for PDAC, which remains one of the most lethal malignancies worldwide. The innate immune system and platelets play multifaceted and often context-dependent roles in the pathogenesis and progression of chronic pancreatitis and PDAC. Persistent inflammation, partly driven by innate immune cells and platelets, contributes to tissue remodeling and fibrosis, setting the stage for malignant transformation. In PDAC, these same cells often adopt tumor-promoting phenotypes that support immune evasion, angiogenesis, and metastasis. Clinically, the complex crosstalk between innate immune cells, platelets, and tumor cells underscores the limitations of monotherapies in PDAC. A more effective approach will likely involve combination strategies that target both the tumor and its immunosuppressive microenvironment. Integrating innate immune modulators with T cell-based therapies holds promise for overcoming resistance and improving patient outcomes. In conclusion, understanding the diverse roles of innate immune cells and platelets in pancreatic inflammation and malignancy offers critical insights into disease mechanisms and reveals novel opportunities for therapeutic intervention in PDAC. Continued research into the dynamic interactions within the pancreatic tumor microenvironment is essential to translate these insights into effective clinical strategies.

Author Contributions: Conceptualization, M.H. and I.B.-W.; writing—original draft preparation, J.B., M.S., A.V., C.L., E.A., S.K., I.B.-W. and M.H.; writing—review and editing, J.B., M.S., A.V., C.L., E.A., S.K., S.M.K., H.K., I.B.-W. and M.H.; visualization, M.S. and M.H.; supervision, M.H. and I.B.-W.; funding acquisition, H.K., M.H., I.B.-W., S.K. and S.M.K. All authors have read and agreed to the published version of the manuscript.

Funding: The work was conducted within the Research Training Group InCuPanc (GRK 2751/1-2022 Project number: 449501615) funded by the DFG.

Institutional Review Board Statement: Pictures for Figure 1 were taken from a 5 μm HE section of a PDAC patient after approval from the local ethics committee of the Medical Faculty, Martin-Luther-University Halle-Wittenberg (no. 2015-16, no. 2017-81).

Acknowledgments: We thank Sina Krehahn and Nico Hesselbarth for their scientific and administrative assistance.

Conflicts of Interest: The authors declare no conflicts of interest.

References

1. Xiao, A.Y.; Tan, M.L.Y.; Wu, L.M.; Asrani, V.M.; Windsor, J.A.; Yadav, D.; Petrov, M.S. Global incidence and mortality of pancreatic diseases: A systematic review, meta-analysis, and meta-regression of population-based cohort studies. *Lancet Gastroenterol. Hepatol.* **2016**, *1*, 45–55. [CrossRef]
2. Malka, D.; Hammel, P.; Maire, F.; Rufat, P.; Madeira, I.; Pessione, F.; Lévy, P.; Ruszniewski, P. Risk of pancreatic adenocarcinoma in chronic pancreatitis. *Gut* **2002**, *51*, 849–852. [CrossRef] [PubMed]
3. Zheng, Z.; Chen, Y.; Tan, C.; Ke, N.; Du, B.; Liu, X. Risk of pancreatic cancer in patients undergoing surgery for chronic pancreatitis. *BMC Surg.* **2019**, *19*, 83. [CrossRef] [PubMed]
4. Lowenfels, A.B.; Maisonneuve, P.; Cavallini, G.; Ammann, R.W.; Lankisch, P.G.; Andersen, J.R.; Dimagno, E.P.; Andrén-Sandberg, A.; Domellöf, L. Pancreatitis and the risk of pancreatic cancer. International Pancreatitis Study Group. *N. Engl. J. Med.* **1993**, *328*, 1433–1437. [CrossRef] [PubMed]
5. Coté, G.A.; Yadav, D.; Slivka, A.; Hawes, R.H.; Anderson, M.A.; Burton, F.R.; Brand, R.E.; Banks, P.A.; Lewis, M.D.; Disario, J.A.; et al. Alcohol and smoking as risk factors in an epidemiology study of patients with chronic pancreatitis. *Clin. Gastroenterol. Hepatol.* **2011**, *9*, 266–273.e27. [CrossRef]
6. Lin, Y.; Tamakoshi, A.; Hayakawa, T.; Ogawa, M.; Ohno, Y. Associations of alcohol drinking and nutrient intake with chronic pancreatitis: Findings from a case-control study in Japan. *Am. J. Gastroenterol.* **2001**, *96*, 2622–2627. [CrossRef]
7. Rosendahl, J.; Bödeker, H.; Mössner, J.; Teich, N. Hereditary chronic pancreatitis. *Orphanet J. Rare Dis.* **2007**, *2*, 1. [CrossRef]
8. Klöppel, G. Chronic pancreatitis, pseudotumors and other tumor-like lesions. *Mod. Pathol.* **2007**, *20* (Suppl. 1), S113–S131. [CrossRef]
9. Shrikhande, S.V.; Martignoni, M.E.; Shrikhande, M.; Kappeler, A.; Ramesh, H.; Zimmermann, A.; Büchler, M.W.; Friess, H. Comparison of histological features and inflammatory cell reaction in alcoholic, idiopathic and tropical chronic pancreatitis. *Br. J. Surg.* **2003**, *90*, 1565–1572. [CrossRef]
10. Gandhi, S.; de la Fuente, J.; Murad, M.H.; Majumder, S. Chronic Pancreatitis Is a Risk Factor for Pancreatic Cancer, and Incidence Increases With Duration of Disease: A Systematic Review and Meta-analysis. *Clin. Transl. Gastroenterol.* **2022**, *13*, e00463. [CrossRef]
11. Le Cosquer, G.; Maulat, C.; Bournet, B.; Cordelier, P.; Buscail, E.; Buscail, L. Pancreatic Cancer in Chronic Pancreatitis: Pathogenesis and Diagnostic Approach. *Cancers* **2023**, *15*, 761. [CrossRef] [PubMed]
12. Guo, K.; Zhao, Y.; Cao, Y.; Li, Y.; Yang, M.; Tian, Y.; Dai, J.; Song, L.; Ren, S.; Wang, Z. Exploring the key genetic association between chronic pancreatitis and pancreatic ductal adenocarcinoma through integrated bioinformatics. *Front. Genet.* **2023**, *14*, 1115660. [CrossRef]
13. Li, H.; Hao, C.; Yang, Q.; Gao, W.; Ma, B.; Xue, D. Identification of hub genes in chronic pancreatitis and analysis of association with pancreatic cancer via bioinformatic analysis. *Gen. Physiol. Biophys.* **2022**, *41*, 15–30. [CrossRef] [PubMed]
14. Coussens, L.M.; Werb, Z. Inflammation and cancer. *Nature* **2002**, *420*, 860–867. [CrossRef] [PubMed]
15. Hanahan, D.; Weinberg, R.A. Hallmarks of cancer: The next generation. *Cell* **2011**, *144*, 646–674. [CrossRef]
16. Wang, S.; Chao, X.; Jiang, X.; Wang, T.; Rodriguez, Y.; Yang, L.; Pacher, P.; Ni, H.-M.; Ding, W.-X. Loss of acinar cell VMP1 triggers spontaneous pancreatitis in mice. *Autophagy* **2022**, *18*, 1572–1582. [CrossRef]
17. Morris, J.P.; Wang, S.C.; Hebrok, M. KRAS, Hedgehog, Wnt and the twisted developmental biology of pancreatic ductal adenocarcinoma. *Nat. Rev. Cancer* **2010**, *10*, 683–695. [CrossRef] [PubMed]
18. Siegel, R.L.; Giaquinto, A.N.; Jemal, A. Cancer statistics, 2024. *CA Cancer J. Clin.* **2024**, *74*, 12–49. [CrossRef]
19. The Cancer Genome Atlas Research Network; Raphael, B.J. Integrated Genomic Characterization of Pancreatic Ductal Adenocarcinoma. *Cancer Cell* **2017**, *32*, 185–203.e13. [CrossRef]
20. Bailey, P.; Chang, D.K.; Nones, K.; Johns, A.L.; Patch, A.-M.; Gingras, M.-C.; Miller, D.K.; Christ, A.N.; Bruxner, T.J.C.; Quinn, M.C.; et al. Genomic analyses identify molecular subtypes of pancreatic cancer. *Nature* **2016**, *531*, 47–52. [CrossRef]
21. Shi, C.; Hong, S.-M.; Lim, P.; Kamiyama, H.; Khan, M.; Anders, R.A.; Goggins, M.; Hruban, R.H.; Eshleman, J.R. KRAS2 mutations in human pancreatic acinar-ductal metaplastic lesions are limited to those with PanIN: Implications for the human pancreatic cancer cell of origin. *Mol. Cancer Res.* **2009**, *7*, 230–236. [CrossRef] [PubMed]
22. Kanda, M.; Matthaei, H.; Wu, J.; Hong, S.-M.; Yu, J.; Borges, M.; Hruban, R.H.; Maitra, A.; Kinzler, K.; Vogelstein, B.; et al. Presence of somatic mutations in most early-stage pancreatic intraepithelial neoplasia. *Gastroenterology* **2012**, *142*, 730–733.e9. [CrossRef] [PubMed]
23. Braxton, A.M.; Kiemen, A.L.; Grahn, M.P.; Forjaz, A.; Parksong, J.; Mahesh Babu, J.; Lai, J.; Zheng, L.; Niknafs, N.; Jiang, L.; et al. 3D genomic mapping reveals multifocality of human pancreatic precancers. *Nature* **2024**, *629*, 679–687. [CrossRef]
24. Hingorani, S.R.; Petricoin, E.F.; Maitra, A.; Rajapakse, V.; King, C.; Jacobetz, M.A.; Ross, S.; Conrads, T.P.; Veenstra, T.D.; Hitt, B.A.; et al. Preinvasive and invasive ductal pancreatic cancer and its early detection in the mouse. *Cancer Cell* **2003**, *4*, 437–450. [CrossRef]

25. Guerra, C.; Schuhmacher, A.J.; Cañamero, M.; Grippo, P.J.; Verdaguer, L.; Pérez-Gallego, L.; Dubus, P.; Sandgren, E.P.; Barbacid, M. Chronic pancreatitis is essential for induction of pancreatic ductal adenocarcinoma by K-Ras oncogenes in adult mice. *Cancer Cell* **2007**, *11*, 291–302. [CrossRef]
26. Guerra, C.; Collado, M.; Navas, C.; Schuhmacher, A.J.; Hernández-Porras, I.; Cañamero, M.; Rodriguez-Justo, M.; Serrano, M.; Barbacid, M. Pancreatitis-induced inflammation contributes to pancreatic cancer by inhibiting oncogene-induced senescence. *Cancer Cell* **2011**, *19*, 728–739. [CrossRef]
27. Hamarsheh, S.; Groß, O.; Brummer, T.; Zeiser, R. Immune modulatory effects of oncogenic KRAS in cancer. *Nat. Commun.* **2020**, *11*, 5439. [CrossRef] [PubMed]
28. Lesina, M.; Kurkowski, M.U.; Ludes, K.; Rose-John, S.; Treiber, M.; Klöppel, G.; Yoshimura, A.; Reindl, W.; Sipos, B.; Akira, S.; et al. Stat3/Socs3 activation by IL-6 transsignaling promotes progression of pancreatic intraepithelial neoplasia and development of pancreatic cancer. *Cancer Cell* **2011**, *19*, 456–469. [CrossRef]
29. Zhang, Y.; Yan, W.; Collins, M.A.; Bednar, F.; Rakshit, S.; Zetter, B.R.; Stanger, B.Z.; Chung, I.; Rhim, A.D.; Di Magliano, M.P. Interleukin-6 is required for pancreatic cancer progression by promoting MAPK signaling activation and oxidative stress resistance. *Cancer Res.* **2013**, *73*, 6359–6374. [CrossRef]
30. Awaji, M.; Saxena, S.; Wu, L.; Prajapati, D.R.; Purohit, A.; Varney, M.L.; Kumar, S.; Rachagani, S.; Ly, Q.P.; Jain, M.; et al. CXCR2 signaling promotes secretory cancer-associated fibroblasts in pancreatic ductal adenocarcinoma. *FASEB J.* **2020**, *34*, 9405–9418. [CrossRef]
31. Lin, Y.; Pu, S.; Wang, J.; Wan, Y.; Wu, Z.; Guo, Y.; Feng, W.; Ying, Y.; Ma, S.; Meng, X.J.; et al. Pancreatic STAT5 activation promotes KrasG12D-induced and inflammation-induced acinar-to-ductal metaplasia and pancreatic cancer. *Gut* **2024**, *73*, 1831–1843. [CrossRef] [PubMed]
32. Ceron-Hernandez, J.; Martinez-Navajas, G.; Sanchez-Manas, J.M.; Molina, M.P.; Xie, J.; Aznar-Peralta, I.; Garcia-Diaz, A.; Perales, S.; Torres, C.; Serrano, M.J.; et al. Oncogenic KRASG12D Transfer from Platelet-like Particles Enhances Proliferation and Survival in Non-Small Cell Lung Cancer Cells. *Int. J. Mol. Sci.* **2025**, *26*, 3264. [CrossRef] [PubMed]
33. Xu, D.; Liao, C.; Tan, J. KRAS-mutant colorectal cancer cell lines cause a prothrombotic state through the upregulation of thrombin: Experimental study. *Ann. Med. Surg.* **2024**, *86*, 850–855. [CrossRef]
34. Strasenburg, W.; Jóźwicki, J.; Durślewicz, J.; Kuffel, B.; Kulczyk, M.P.; Kowalewski, A.; Grzanka, D.; Drewa, T.; Adamowicz, J. Tumor Cell-Induced Platelet Aggregation as an Emerging Therapeutic Target for Cancer Therapy. *Front. Oncol.* **2022**, *12*, 909767. [CrossRef]
35. Inman, K.S.; Francis, A.A.; Murray, N.R. Complex role for the immune system in initiation and progression of pancreatic cancer. *World J. Gastroenterol.* **2014**, *20*, 11160–11181. [CrossRef]
36. Yousuf, S.; Qiu, M.; von Voith Voithenberg, L.; Hulkkonen, J.; Macinkovic, I.; Schulz, A.R.; Hartmann, D.; Mueller, F.; Mijatovic, M.; Ibberson, D.; et al. Spatially Resolved Multi-Omics Single-Cell Analyses Inform Mechanisms of Immune Dysfunction in Pancreatic Cancer. *Gastroenterology* **2023**, *165*, 891–908.e14. [CrossRef] [PubMed]
37. Yang, J.; Zhang, Q.; Wang, J.; Lou, Y.; Hong, Z.; Wei, S.; Sun, K.; Wang, J.; Chen, Y.; Sheng, J.; et al. Dynamic profiling of immune microenvironment during pancreatic cancer development suggests early intervention and combination strategy of immunotherapy. *EBioMedicine* **2022**, *78*, 103958. [CrossRef]
38. Zwart, E.S.; van Ee, T.; Affandi, A.J.; Boyd, L.N.C.; Rodriguez, E.; den Haan, J.M.M.; Farina, A.; van Grieken, N.C.T.; Meijer, L.L.; van Kooyk, Y.; et al. Spatial immune composition of tumor microenvironment in patients with pancreatic cancer. *Cancer Immunol. Immunother.* **2023**, *72*, 4385–4397. [CrossRef]
39. Wang, J.; He, P.; Gaida, M.; Yang, S.; Schetter, A.J.; Gaedcke, J.; Ghadimi, B.M.; Ried, T.; Yfantis, H.; Lee, D.; et al. Inducible nitric oxide synthase enhances disease aggressiveness in pancreatic cancer. *Oncotarget* **2016**, *7*, 52993–53004. [CrossRef]
40. Lei, X.; Lei, Y.; Li, J.-K.; Du, W.-X.; Li, R.-G.; Yang, J.; Li, J.; Li, F.; Tan, H.-B. Immune cells within the tumor microenvironment: Biological functions and roles in cancer immunotherapy. *Cancer Lett.* **2020**, *470*, 126–133. [CrossRef]
41. Xiang, H.; Yang, R.; Tu, J.; Xi, Y.; Yang, S.; Lv, L.; Zhai, X.; Zhu, Y.; Dong, D.; Tao, X. Metabolic reprogramming of immune cells in pancreatic cancer progression. *Biomed. Pharmacother.* **2023**, *157*, 113992. [CrossRef] [PubMed]
42. Schmied, L.; Höglund, P.; Meinke, S. Platelet-Mediated Protection of Cancer Cells From Immune Surveillance—Possible Implications for Cancer Immunotherapy. *Front. Immunol.* **2021**, *12*, 640578. [CrossRef] [PubMed]
43. Tuerhong, N.; Yang, Y.; Wang, C.; Huang, P.; Li, Q. Interactions between platelets and the cancer immune microenvironment. *Crit. Rev. Oncol. Hematol.* **2024**, *199*, 104380. [CrossRef]
44. Ward, M.P.; Kane, L.E.; Norris, L.A.; Mohamed, B.M.; Kelly, T.; Bates, M.; Clarke, A.; Brady, N.; Martin, C.M.; Brooks, R.D.; et al. Platelets, immune cells and the coagulation cascade; friend or foe of the circulating tumour cell? *Mol. Cancer* **2021**, *20*, 59. [CrossRef]
45. Abel, A.M.; Yang, C.; Thakar, M.S.; Malarkannan, S. Natural Killer Cells: Development, Maturation, and Clinical Utilization. *Front. Immunol.* **2018**, *9*, 1869. [CrossRef]
46. Guillerey, C. NK Cells in the Tumor Microenvironment. *Adv. Exp. Med. Biol.* **2020**, *1273*, 69–90. [CrossRef]

47. Pegram, H.J.; Andrews, D.M.; Smyth, M.J.; Darcy, P.K.; Kershaw, M.H. Activating and inhibitory receptors of natural killer cells. Immunol. *Cell Biol.* **2011**, *89*, 216–224. [CrossRef]
48. Reschner, A.; Hubert, P.; Delvenne, P.; Boniver, J.; Jacobs, N. Innate lymphocyte and dendritic cell cross-talk: A key factor in the regulation of the immune response. *Clin. Exp. Immunol.* **2008**, *152*, 219–226. [CrossRef]
49. Koehl, U.; Toubert, A.; Pittari, G. Editorial: Tailoring NK Cell Receptor-Ligand Interactions: An Art in Evolution. *Front. Immunol.* **2018**, *9*, 351. [CrossRef]
50. Kärre, K. NK cells, MHC class I molecules and the missing self. *Scand. J. Immunol.* **2002**, *55*, 221–228. [CrossRef]
51. Ljunggren, H.G.; Kärre, K. In search of the 'missing self': MHC molecules and NK cell recognition. *Immunol. Today* **1990**, *11*, 237–244. [CrossRef] [PubMed]
52. Shimasaki, N.; Jain, A.; Campana, D. NK cells for cancer immunotherapy. *Nat. Rev. Drug Discov.* **2020**, *19*, 200–218. [CrossRef] [PubMed]
53. Vivier, E.; Tomasello, E.; Baratin, M.; Walzer, T.; Ugolini, S. Functions of natural killer cells. *Nat. Immunol.* **2008**, *9*, 503–510. [CrossRef]
54. Parham, P. MHC class I molecules and KIRs in human history, health and survival. *Nat. Rev. Immunol.* **2005**, *5*, 201–214. [CrossRef]
55. Kumar, V.; McNerney, M.E. A new self: MHC-class-I-independent natural-killer-cell self-tolerance. *Nat. Rev. Immunol.* **2005**, *5*, 363–374. [CrossRef] [PubMed]
56. López-Soto, A.; Gonzalez, S.; Smyth, M.J.; Galluzzi, L. Control of Metastasis by NK Cells. *Cancer Cell* **2017**, *32*, 135–154. [CrossRef]
57. Ferretti, E.; Carlomagno, S.; Pesce, S.; Muccio, L.; Obino, V.; Greppi, M.; Solari, A.; Setti, C.; Marcenaro, E.; Della Chiesa, M.; et al. Role of the Main Non HLA-Specific Activating NK Receptors in Pancreatic, Colorectal and Gastric Tumors Surveillance. *Cancers* **2020**, *12*, 3705. [CrossRef] [PubMed]
58. Peng, Y.-P.; Zhu, Y.; Zhang, J.-J.; Xu, Z.-K.; Qian, Z.-Y.; Dai, C.-C.; Jiang, K.-R.; Wu, J.-L.; Gao, W.-T.; Li, Q.; et al. Comprehensive analysis of the percentage of surface receptors and cytotoxic granules positive natural killer cells in patients with pancreatic cancer, gastric cancer, and colorectal cancer. *J. Transl. Med.* **2013**, *11*, 262. [CrossRef]
59. Kaur, K.; Chang, H.-H.; Topchyan, P.; Cook, J.M.; Barkhordarian, A.; Eibl, G.; Jewett, A. Deficiencies in Natural Killer Cell Numbers, Expansion, and Function at the Pre-Neoplastic Stage of Pancreatic Cancer by KRAS Mutation in the Pancreas of Obese Mice. *Front. Immunol.* **2018**, *9*, 1229. [CrossRef]
60. Huber, M.; Brehm, C.U.; Gress, T.M.; Buchholz, M.; Alashkar Alhamwe, B.; von Strandmann, E.P.; Slater, E.P.; Bartsch, J.W.; Bauer, C.; Lauth, M. The Immune Microenvironment in Pancreatic Cancer. *Int. J. Mol. Sci.* **2020**, *21*, 7307. [CrossRef]
61. Lim, S.A.; Kim, J.; Jeon, S.; Shin, M.H.; Kwon, J.; Kim, T.-J.; Im, K.; Han, Y.; Kwon, W.; Kim, S.-W.; et al. Defective Localization With Impaired Tumor Cytotoxicity Contributes to the Immune Escape of NK Cells in Pancreatic Cancer Patients. *Front. Immunol.* **2019**, *10*, 496. [CrossRef]
62. Bähr, I.; Spielmann, J.; Quandt, D.; Kielstein, H. Obesity-Associated Alterations of Natural Killer Cells and Immunosurveillance of Cancer. *Front. Immunol.* **2020**, *11*, 245. [CrossRef]
63. Wu, S.-Y.; Fu, T.; Jiang, Y.-Z.; Shao, Z.-M. Natural killer cells in cancer biology and therapy. *Mol. Cancer* **2020**, *19*, 120. [CrossRef]
64. Hodgins, J.J.; Khan, S.T.; Park, M.M.; Auer, R.C.; Ardolino, M. Killers 2.0: NK cell therapies at the forefront of cancer control. *J. Clin. Investig.* **2019**, *129*, 3499–3510. [CrossRef] [PubMed]
65. Cervantes-Villagrana, R.D.; Albores-García, D.; Cervantes-Villagrana, A.R.; García-Acevez, S.J. Tumor-induced neurogenesis and immune evasion as targets of innovative anti-cancer therapies. *Signal Transduct. Target. Ther.* **2020**, *5*, 99. [CrossRef]
66. Marcon, F.; Zuo, J.; Pearce, H.; Nicol, S.; Margielewska-Davies, S.; Farhat, M.; Mahon, B.; Middleton, G.; Brown, R.; Roberts, K.J.; et al. NK cells in pancreatic cancer demonstrate impaired cytotoxicity and a regulatory IL-10 phenotype. *Oncoimmunology* **2020**, *9*, 1845424. [CrossRef] [PubMed]
67. Husain, Z.; Huang, Y.; Seth, P.; Sukhatme, V.P. Tumor-derived lactate modifies antitumor immune response: Effect on myeloid-derived suppressor cells and NK cells. *J. Immunol.* **2013**, *191*, 1486–1495. [CrossRef] [PubMed]
68. Li, X.; Ni, R.; Chen, J.; Liu, Z.; Xiao, M.; Jiang, F.; Lu, C. The presence of IGHG1 in human pancreatic carcinomas is associated with immune evasion mechanisms. *Pancreas* **2011**, *40*, 753–761. [CrossRef]
69. He, C.; Wang, D.; Shukla, S.K.; Hu, T.; Thakur, R.; Fu, X.; King, R.J.; Kollala, S.S.; Attri, K.S.; Murthy, D.; et al. Vitamin B6 Competition in the Tumor Microenvironment Hampers Antitumor Functions of NK Cells. *Cancer Discov.* **2024**, *14*, 176–193. [CrossRef]
70. Janakiram, N.B.; Mohammed, A.; Bryant, T.; Ritchie, R.; Stratton, N.; Jackson, L.; Lightfoot, S.; Benbrook, D.M.; Asch, A.S.; Lang, M.L.; et al. Loss of natural killer T cells promotes pancreatic cancer in LSL-KrasG12D/+ mice. *Immunology* **2017**, *152*, 36–51. [CrossRef]
71. Kobayashi, H.; Dubois, S.; Sato, N.; Sabzevari, H.; Sakai, Y.; Waldmann, T.A.; Tagaya, Y. Role of trans-cellular IL-15 presentation in the activation of NK cell-mediated killing, which leads to enhanced tumor immunosurveillance. *Blood* **2005**, *105*, 721–727. [CrossRef] [PubMed]

72. Kopp, H.-G.; Placke, T.; Salih, H.R. Platelet-derived transforming growth factor-beta down-regulates NKG2D thereby inhibiting natural killer cell antitumor reactivity. *Cancer Res.* **2009**, *69*, 7775–7783. [CrossRef] [PubMed]
73. Placke, T.; Örgel, M.; Schaller, M.; Jung, G.; Rammensee, H.-G.; Kopp, H.-G.; Salih, H.R. Platelet-derived MHC class I confers a pseudonormal phenotype to cancer cells that subverts the antitumor reactivity of natural killer immune cells. *Cancer Res.* **2012**, *72*, 440–448. [CrossRef]
74. Hoshikawa, M.; Aoki, T.; Matsushita, H.; Karasaki, T.; Hosoi, A.; Odaira, K.; Fujieda, N.; Kobayashi, Y.; Kambara, K.; Ohara, O.; et al. NK cell and IFN signatures are positive prognostic biomarkers for resectable pancreatic cancer. *Biochem. Biophys. Res. Commun.* **2018**, *495*, 2058–2065. [CrossRef]
75. van Audenaerde, J.R.M.; Roeyen, G.; Darcy, P.K.; Kershaw, M.H.; Peeters, M.; Smits, E.L.J. Natural killer cells and their therapeutic role in pancreatic cancer: A systematic review. *Pharmacol. Ther.* **2018**, *189*, 31–44. [CrossRef]
76. Brooks, J.; Fleischmann-Mundt, B.; Woller, N.; Niemann, J.; Ribback, S.; Peters, K.; Demir, I.E.; Armbrecht, N.; Ceyhan, G.O.; Manns, M.P.; et al. Perioperative, Spatiotemporally Coordinated Activation of T and NK Cells Prevents Recurrence of Pancreatic Cancer. *Cancer Res.* **2018**, *78*, 475–488. [CrossRef]
77. Koh, C.Y.; Blazar, B.R.; George, T.; Welniak, L.A.; Capitini, C.M.; Raziuddin, A.; Murphy, W.J.; Bennett, M. Augmentation of antitumor effects by NK cell inhibitory receptor blockade in vitro and in vivo. *Blood* **2001**, *97*, 3132–3137. [CrossRef] [PubMed]
78. McKenna, D.H.; Sumstad, D.; Bostrom, N.; Kadidlo, D.M.; Fautsch, S.; McNearney, S.; Dewaard, R.; McGlave, P.B.; Weisdorf, D.J.; Wagner, J.E.; et al. Good manufacturing practices production of natural killer cells for immunotherapy: A six-year single-institution experience. *Transfusion* **2007**, *47*, 520–528. [CrossRef]
79. van den Eynde, A.; Gehrcken, L.; Verhezen, T.; Lau, H.W.; Hermans, C.; Lambrechts, H.; Flieswasser, T.; Quatannens, D.; Roex, G.; Zwaenepoel, K.; et al. IL-15-secreting CAR natural killer cells directed toward the pan-cancer target CD70 eliminate both cancer cells and cancer-associated fibroblasts. *J. Hematol. Oncol.* **2024**, *17*, 8. [CrossRef]
80. DeNardo, D.G.; Ruffell, B. Macrophages as regulators of tumour immunity and immunotherapy. *Nat. Rev. Immunol.* **2019**, *19*, 369–382. [CrossRef]
81. Lankadasari, M.B.; Mukhopadhyay, P.; Mohammed, S.; Harikumar, K.B. TAMing pancreatic cancer: Combat with a double edged sword. *Mol. Cancer* **2019**, *18*, 48. [CrossRef] [PubMed]
82. Zhu, Y.; Herndon, J.M.; Sojka, D.K.; Kim, K.-W.; Knolhoff, B.L.; Zuo, C.; Cullinan, D.R.; Luo, J.; Bearden, A.R.; Lavine, K.J.; et al. Tissue-Resident Macrophages in Pancreatic Ductal Adenocarcinoma Originate from Embryonic Hematopoiesis and Promote Tumor Progression. *Immunity* **2017**, *47*, 323–338.e6. [CrossRef]
83. Clark, C.E.; Hingorani, S.R.; Mick, R.; Combs, C.; Tuveson, D.A.; Vonderheide, R.H. Dynamics of the Immune Reaction to Pancreatic Cancer from Inception to Invasion. *Cancer Res.* **2007**, *67*, 9518–9527. [CrossRef] [PubMed]
84. Väyrynen, S.A.; Zhang, J.; Yuan, C.; Väyrynen, J.P.; Dias Costa, A.; Williams, H.; Morales-Oyarvide, V.; Lau, M.C.; Rubinson, D.A.; Dunne, R.F.; et al. Composition, Spatial Characteristics, and Prognostic Significance of Myeloid Cell Infiltration in Pancreatic Cancer. Clin. *Cancer Res.* **2021**, *27*, 1069–1081. [CrossRef]
85. Baer, J.M.; Zuo, C.; Kang, L.-I.; de la Lastra, A.A.; Borcherding, N.C.; Knolhoff, B.L.; Bogner, S.J.; Zhu, Y.; Yang, L.; Laurent, J.; et al. Fibrosis induced by resident macrophages has divergent roles in pancreas inflammatory injury and PDAC. *Nat. Immunol.* **2023**, *24*, 1443–1457. [CrossRef]
86. Caronni, N.; La Terza, F.; Vittoria, F.M.; Barbiera, G.; Mezzanzanica, L.; Cuzzola, V.; Barresi, S.; Pellegatta, M.; Canevazzi, P.; Dunsmore, G.; et al. IL-1β+ macrophages fuel pathogenic inflammation in pancreatic cancer. *Nature* **2023**, *623*, 415–422. [CrossRef]
87. Liu, M.; Ren, Y.; Zhou, Z.; Yang, J.; Shi, X.; Cai, Y.; Arreola, A.X.; Luo, W.; Fung, K.-M.; Xu, C.; et al. The crosstalk between macrophages and cancer cells potentiates pancreatic cancer cachexia. *Cancer Cell* **2024**, *42*, 885–903.e4. [CrossRef]
88. Crezee, T.; Rabold, K.; de Jong, L.; Jaeger, M.; Netea-Maier, R.T. Metabolic programming of tumor associated macrophages in the context of cancer treatment. *Ann. Transl. Med.* **2020**, *8*, 1028. [CrossRef]
89. Hörhold, F.; Eisel, D.; Oswald, M.; Kolte, A.; Röll, D.; Osen, W.; Eichmüller, S.B.; König, R. Reprogramming of macrophages employing gene regulatory and metabolic network models. *PLoS Comput. Biol.* **2020**, *16*, e1007657. [CrossRef]
90. Tan, Z.; Xie, N.; Cui, H.; Moellering, D.R.; Abraham, E.; Thannickal, V.J.; Liu, G. Pyruvate dehydrogenase kinase 1 participates in macrophage polarization via regulating glucose metabolism. *J. Immunol.* **2015**, *194*, 6082–6089. [CrossRef]
91. Zhang, M.; Pan, X.; Fujiwara, K.; Jurcak, N.; Muth, S.; Zhou, J.; Xiao, Q.; Li, A.; Che, X.; Li, Z.; et al. Pancreatic cancer cells render tumor-associated macrophages metabolically reprogrammed by a GARP and DNA methylation-mediated mechanism. *Signal Transduct. Target. Ther.* **2021**, *6*, 366. [CrossRef] [PubMed]
92. Halbrook, C.J.; Pontious, C.; Kovalenko, I.; Lapienyte, L.; Dreyer, S.; Lee, H.-J.; Thurston, G.; Zhang, Y.; Lazarus, J.; Sajjakulnukit, P.; et al. Macrophage-Released Pyrimidines Inhibit Gemcitabine Therapy in Pancreatic Cancer. *Cell Metab.* **2019**, *29*, 1390–1399.e6. [CrossRef] [PubMed]
93. Mantovani, A.; Allavena, P.; Marchesi, F.; Garlanda, C. Macrophages as tools and targets in cancer therapy. *Nat. Rev. Drug Discov.* **2022**, *21*, 799–820. [CrossRef]

94. O'Hara, M.H.; O'Reilly, E.M.; Varadhachary, G.; Wolff, R.A.; Wainberg, Z.A.; Ko, A.H.; Fisher, G.; Rahma, O.; Lyman, J.P.; Cabanski, C.R.; et al. CD40 agonistic monoclonal antibody APX005M (sotigalimab) and chemotherapy, with or without nivolumab, for the treatment of metastatic pancreatic adenocarcinoma: An open-label, multicentre, phase 1b study. *Lancet Oncol.* **2021**, *22*, 118–131. [CrossRef]
95. Beatty, G.L.; Torigian, D.A.; Chiorean, E.G.; Saboury, B.; Brothers, A.; Alavi, A.; Troxel, A.B.; Sun, W.; Teitelbaum, U.R.; Vonderheide, R.H.; et al. A phase I study of an agonist CD40 monoclonal antibody (CP-870,893) in combination with gemcitabine in patients with advanced pancreatic ductal adenocarcinoma. Clin. *Cancer Res.* **2013**, *19*, 6286–6295. [CrossRef] [PubMed]
96. Cervera, R. *Autoimmunity: From Bench to Bedside*; Editorial Universidad del Rosario: Bogotá, Colombia, 2013; ISBN 978-958-738-366-9.
97. Jagannathan-Bogdan, M.; Zon, L.I. Hematopoiesis. *Development* **2013**, *140*, 2463–2467. [CrossRef]
98. Shortman, K.; Liu, Y. Mouse and human dendritic cell subtypes. *Nat. Rev. Immunol.* **2002**, *2*, 151–161. [CrossRef]
99. Collin, M.; Milne, P. Langerhans cell origin and regulation. *Curr. Opin. Hematol.* **2016**, *23*, 28–35. [CrossRef]
100. Collin, M.; Bigley, V. Human dendritic cell subsets: An update. *Immunology* **2018**, *154*, 3–20. [CrossRef]
101. Arlt, E.; Kindermann, A.; Fritsche, A.-K.; Navarrete Santos, A.; Kielstein, H.; Bazwinsky-Wutschke, I. A Flow Cytometry-Based Examination of the Mouse White Blood Cell Differential in the Context of Age and Sex. *Cells* **2024**, *13*, 1583. [CrossRef]
102. Balan, S.; Saxena, M.; Bhardwaj, N. Dendritic cell subsets and locations. *Int. Rev. Cell Mol. Biol.* **2019**, *348*, 1–68. [CrossRef] [PubMed]
103. Villani, A.-C.; Satija, R.; Reynolds, G.; Sarkizova, S.; Shekhar, K.; Fletcher, J.; Griesbeck, M.; Butler, A.; Zheng, S.; Lazo, S.; et al. Single-cell RNA-seq reveals new types of human blood dendritic cells, monocytes, and progenitors. *Science* **2017**, *356*, eaah4573. [CrossRef] [PubMed]
104. Yin, G.; Du, J.; Cao, H.; Liu, X.; Xu, Q.; Xiang, M. Reg3g Promotes Pancreatic Carcinogenesis in a Murine Model of Chronic Pancreatitis. *Dig. Dis. Sci.* **2015**, *60*, 3656–3668. [CrossRef] [PubMed]
105. Liu, X.; Zhou, Z.; Cheng, Q.; Wang, H.; Cao, H.; Xu, Q.; Tuo, Y.; Jiang, L.; Zou, Y.; Ren, H.; et al. Acceleration of pancreatic tumorigenesis under immunosuppressive microenvironment induced by Reg3g overexpression. *Cell Death Dis.* **2017**, *8*, e3033. [CrossRef]
106. Ochi, A.; Nguyen, A.H.; Bedrosian, A.S.; Mushlin, H.M.; Zarbakhsh, S.; Barilla, R.; Zambirinis, C.P.; Fallon, N.C.; Rehman, A.; Pylayeva-Gupta, Y.; et al. MyD88 inhibition amplifies dendritic cell capacity to promote pancreatic carcinogenesis via Th2 cells. *J. Exp. Med.* **2012**, *209*, 1671–1687. [CrossRef]
107. Kim, H.-J.; Kim, H.; Lee, J.-H.; Hwangbo, C. Toll-like receptor 4 (TLR4): New insight immune and aging. *Immun. Ageing* **2023**, *20*, 67. [CrossRef]
108. Lin, J.H.; Huffman, A.P.; Wattenberg, M.M.; Walter, D.M.; Carpenter, E.L.; Feldser, D.M.; Beatty, G.L.; Furth, E.E.; Vonderheide, R.H. Type 1 conventional dendritic cells are systemically dysregulated early in pancreatic carcinogenesis. *J. Exp. Med.* **2020**, *217*, e20190673. [CrossRef]
109. Falcomatà, C.; Bärthel, S.; Schneider, G.; Rad, R.; Schmidt-Supprian, M.; Saur, D. Context-Specific Determinants of the Immunosuppressive Tumor Microenvironment in Pancreatic Cancer. *Cancer Discov.* **2023**, *13*, 278–297. [CrossRef]
110. Justus, C.R.; Dong, L.; Yang, L.V. Acidic tumor microenvironment and pH-sensing G protein-coupled receptors. *Front. Physiol.* **2013**, *4*, 354. [CrossRef]
111. Zhang, B.; Ohuchida, K.; Tsutsumi, C.; Shimada, Y.; Mochida, Y.; Oyama, K.; Iwamoto, C.; Sheng, N.; Fei, S.; Shindo, K.; et al. Dynamic glycolytic reprogramming effects on dendritic cells in pancreatic ductal adenocarcinoma. *J. Exp. Clin. Cancer Res.* **2024**, *43*, 271. [CrossRef]
112. Jang, J.-E.; Hajdu, C.H.; Liot, C.; Miller, G.; Dustin, M.L.; Bar-Sagi, D. Crosstalk between Regulatory T Cells and Tumor-Associated Dendritic Cells Negates Anti-tumor Immunity in Pancreatic Cancer. *Cell Rep.* **2017**, *20*, 558–571. [CrossRef]
113. Kenkel, J.A.; Tseng, W.W.; Davidson, M.G.; Tolentino, L.L.; Choi, O.; Bhattacharya, N.; Seeley, E.S.; Winer, D.A.; Reticker-Flynn, N.E.; Engleman, E.G. An Immunosuppressive Dendritic Cell Subset Accumulates at Secondary Sites and Promotes Metastasis in Pancreatic Cancer. *Cancer Res.* **2017**, *77*, 4158–4170. [CrossRef] [PubMed]
114. Basso, D.; Fogar, P.; Falconi, M.; Fadi, E.; Sperti, C.; Frasson, C.; Greco, E.; Tamburrino, D.; Teolato, S.; Moz, S.; et al. Pancreatic tumors and immature immunosuppressive myeloid cells in blood and spleen: Role of inhibitory co-stimulatory molecules PDL1 and CTLA4. An in vivo and in vitro study. *PLoS ONE* **2013**, *8*, e54824. [CrossRef] [PubMed]
115. Tjomsland, V.; Niklasson, L.; Sandström, P.; Borch, K.; Druid, H.; Bratthäll, C.; Messmer, D.; Larsson, M.; Spångeus, A. The desmoplastic stroma plays an essential role in the accumulation and modulation of infiltrated immune cells in pancreatic adenocarcinoma. *Clin. Dev. Immunol.* **2011**, *2011*, 212810. [CrossRef] [PubMed]
116. Xu, M.; Zhou, B.P.; Tao, M.; Liu, J.; Li, W. The Role of Stromal Components in Pancreatic Cancer Progression. *Anti-Cancer Agents Med. Chem.* **2016**, *16*, 1117–1124. [CrossRef]

117. Mahadevan, K.K.; Dyevoich, A.M.; Chen, Y.; Li, B.; Sugimoto, H.; Sockwell, A.M.; McAndrews, K.M.; Sthanam, L.K.; Wang, H.; Shalapour, S.; et al. Type I conventional dendritic cells facilitate immunotherapy in pancreatic cancer. *Science* **2024**, *384*, eadh4567. [CrossRef]
118. Hu, Z.I.; O'Reilly, E.M. Therapeutic developments in pancreatic cancer. *Nat. Rev. Gastroenterol. Hepatol.* **2024**, *21*, 7–24. [CrossRef]
119. Cappello, P.; Tomaino, B.; Chiarle, R.; Ceruti, P.; Novarino, A.; Castagnoli, C.; Migliorini, P.; Perconti, G.; Giallongo, A.; Milella, M.; et al. An integrated humoral and cellular response is elicited in pancreatic cancer by alpha-enolase, a novel pancreatic ductal adenocarcinoma-associated antigen. *Int. J. Cancer* **2009**, *125*, 639–648. [CrossRef]
120. Tjomsland, V.; Sandström, P.; Spångeus, A.; Messmer, D.; Emilsson, J.; Falkmer, U.; Falkmer, S.; Magnusson, K.-E.; Borch, K.; Larsson, M. Pancreatic adenocarcinoma exerts systemic effects on the peripheral blood myeloid and plasmacytoid dendritic cells: An indicator of disease severity? *BMC Cancer* **2010**, *10*, 87. [CrossRef]
121. Lunardi, S.; Muschel, R.J.; Brunner, T.B. The stromal compartments in pancreatic cancer: Are there any therapeutic targets? *Cancer Lett.* **2014**, *343*, 147–155. [CrossRef]
122. Plesca, I.; Benešová, I.; Beer, C.; Sommer, U.; Müller, L.; Wehner, R.; Heiduk, M.; Aust, D.; Baretton, G.; Bachmann, M.P.; et al. Clinical Significance of Tumor-Infiltrating Conventional and Plasmacytoid Dendritic Cells in Pancreatic Ductal Adenocarcinoma. *Cancers* **2022**, *14*, 1216. [CrossRef]
123. Tjomsland, V.; Spångeus, A.; Sandström, P.; Borch, K.; Messmer, D.; Larsson, M. Semi mature blood dendritic cells exist in patients with ductal pancreatic adenocarcinoma owing to inflammatory factors released from the tumor. *PLoS ONE* **2010**, *5*, e13441. [CrossRef]
124. Hiraoka, N.; Yamazaki-Itoh, R.; Ino, Y.; Mizuguchi, Y.; Yamada, T.; Hirohashi, S.; Kanai, Y. CXCL17 and ICAM2 are associated with a potential anti-tumor immune response in early intraepithelial stages of human pancreatic carcinogenesis. *Gastroenterology* **2011**, *140*, 310–321. [CrossRef]
125. Elieh Ali Komi, D.; Wöhrl, S.; Bielory, L. Mast Cell Biology at Molecular Level: A Comprehensive Review. *Clin. Rev. Allergy Immunol.* **2020**, *58*, 342–365. [CrossRef] [PubMed]
126. Reber, L.L.; Sibilano, R.; Mukai, K.; Galli, S.J. Potential effector and immunoregulatory functions of mast cells in mucosal immunity. *Mucosal Immunol.* **2015**, *8*, 444–463. [CrossRef]
127. Frossi, B.; Mion, F.; Sibilano, R.; Danelli, L.; Pucillo, C.E.M. Is it time for a new classification of mast cells? What do we know about mast cell heterogeneity? *Immunol. Rev.* **2018**, *282*, 35–46. [CrossRef] [PubMed]
128. Gri, G.; Frossi, B.; D'Inca, F.; Danelli, L.; Betto, E.; Mion, F.; Sibilano, R.; Pucillo, C. Mast cell: An emerging partner in immune interaction. *Front. Immunol.* **2012**, *3*, 120. [CrossRef]
129. Tsai, M.; Valent, P.; Galli, S.J. KIT as a master regulator of the mast cell lineage. *J. Allergy Clin. Immunol.* **2022**, *149*, 1845–1854. [CrossRef] [PubMed]
130. Vukman, K.V.; Försönits, A.; Oszvald, Á.; Tóth, E.Á.; Buzás, E.I. Mast cell secretome: Soluble and vesicular components. *Semin. Cell Dev. Biol.* **2017**, *67*, 65–73. [CrossRef]
131. Theoharides, T.C.; Conti, P. Mast cells: The Jekyll and Hyde of tumor growth. *Trends Immunol.* **2004**, *25*, 235–241. [CrossRef]
132. Ribatti, D.; Crivellato, E. The controversial role of mast cells in tumor growth. *Int. Rev. Cell Mol. Biol.* **2009**, *275*, 89–131. [CrossRef] [PubMed]
133. Aponte-López, A.; Muñoz-Cruz, S. Mast Cells in the Tumor Microenvironment. *Adv. Exp. Med. Biol.* **2020**, *1273*, 159–173. [CrossRef]
134. Wang, B.; Li, L.; Liao, Y.; Li, J.; Yu, X.; Zhang, Y.; Xu, J.; Rao, H.; Chen, S.; Zhang, L.; et al. Mast cells expressing interleukin 17 in the muscularis propria predict a favorable prognosis in esophageal squamous cell carcinoma. *Cancer Immunol. Immunother.* **2013**, *62*, 1575–1585. [CrossRef]
135. Chan, J.K.; Magistris, A.; Loizzi, V.; Lin, F.; Rutgers, J.; Osann, K.; DiSaia, P.J.; Samoszuk, M. Mast cell density, angiogenesis, blood clotting, and prognosis in women with advanced ovarian cancer. *Gynecol. Oncol.* **2005**, *99*, 20–25. [CrossRef] [PubMed]
136. Hedström, G.; Berglund, M.; Molin, D.; Fischer, M.; Nilsson, G.; Thunberg, U.; Book, M.; Sundström, C.; Rosenquist, R.; Roos, G.; et al. Mast cell infiltration is a favourable prognostic factor in diffuse large B-cell lymphoma. *Br. J. Haematol.* **2007**, *138*, 68–71. [CrossRef] [PubMed]
137. Pittoni, P.; Tripodo, C.; Piconese, S.; Mauri, G.; Parenza, M.; Rigoni, A.; Sangaletti, S.; Colombo, M.P. Mast cell targeting hampers prostate adenocarcinoma development but promotes the occurrence of highly malignant neuroendocrine cancers. *Cancer Res.* **2011**, *71*, 5987–5997. [CrossRef]
138. Ribatti, D.; Ennas, M.G.; Vacca, A.; Ferreli, F.; Nico, B.; Orru, S.; Sirigu, P. Tumor vascularity and tryptase-positive mast cells correlate with a poor prognosis in melanoma. *Eur. J. Clin. Investig.* **2003**, *33*, 420–425. [CrossRef]
139. Somasundaram, R.; Connelly, T.; Choi, R.; Choi, H.; Samarkina, A.; Li, L.; Gregorio, E.; Chen, Y.; Thakur, R.; Abdel-Mohsen, M.; et al. Tumor-infiltrating mast cells are associated with resistance to anti-PD-1 therapy. *Nat. Commun.* **2021**, *12*, 346. [CrossRef]

40. Reddy, S.M.; Reuben, A.; Barua, S.; Jiang, H.; Zhang, S.; Wang, L.; Gopalakrishnan, V.; Hudgens, C.W.; Tetzlaff, M.T.; Reuben, J.M.; et al. Poor Response to Neoadjuvant Chemotherapy Correlates with Mast Cell Infiltration in Inflammatory Breast Cancer. *Cancer Immunol. Res.* **2019**, *7*, 1025–1035. [CrossRef]
41. Rajput, A.B.; Turbin, D.A.; Cheang, M.C.; Voduc, D.K.; Leung, S.; Gelmon, K.A.; Gilks, C.B.; Huntsman, D.G. Stromal mast cells in invasive breast cancer are a marker of favourable prognosis: A study of 4,444 cases. *Breast Cancer Res. Treat.* **2008**, *107*, 249–257. [CrossRef]
42. Sammarco, G.; Varricchi, G.; Ferraro, V.; Ammendola, M.; de Fazio, M.; Altomare, D.F.; Luposella, M.; Maltese, L.; Currò, G.; Marone, G.; et al. Mast Cells, Angiogenesis and Lymphangiogenesis in Human Gastric Cancer. *Int. J. Mol. Sci.* **2019**, *20*, 2106. [CrossRef] [PubMed]
43. Yano, H.; Kinuta, M.; Tateishi, H.; Nakano, Y.; Matsui, S.; Monden, T.; Okamura, J.; Sakai, M.; Okamoto, S. Mast cell infiltration around gastric cancer cells correlates with tumor angiogenesis and metastasis. *Gastric Cancer* **1999**, *2*, 26–32. [CrossRef] [PubMed]
44. Guo, J.; Wang, S.; Gao, Q. An integrated overview of the immunosuppression features in the tumor microenvironment of pancreatic cancer. *Front. Immunol.* **2023**, *14*, 1258538. [CrossRef]
45. Cai, S.-W.; Yang, S.-Z.; Gao, J.; Pan, K.; Chen, J.-Y.; Wang, Y.-L.; Wei, L.-X.; Dong, J.-H. Prognostic significance of mast cell count following curative resection for pancreatic ductal adenocarcinoma. *Surgery* **2011**, *149*, 576–584. [CrossRef]
46. Chang, D.Z.; Ma, Y.; Ji, B.; Wang, H.; Deng, D.; Liu, Y.; Abbruzzese, J.L.; Liu, Y.; Logsdon, C.D.; Hwu, P. Mast cells in tumor microenvironment promotes the in vivo growth of pancreatic ductal adenocarcinoma. *Clin. Cancer Res.* **2011**, *17*, 7015–7023. [CrossRef] [PubMed]
47. Strouch, M.J.; Cheon, E.C.; Salabat, M.R.; Krantz, S.B.; Gounaris, E.; Melstrom, L.G.; Dangi-Garimella, S.; Wang, E.; Munshi, H.G.; Khazaie, K.; et al. Crosstalk between mast cells and pancreatic cancer cells contributes to pancreatic tumor progression. *Clin. Cancer Res.* **2010**, *16*, 2257–2265. [CrossRef]
48. Tóth, T.; Tóth-Jakatics, R.; Jimi, S.; Takebayashi, S. Increased density of interstitial mast cells in amyloid A renal amyloidosis. *Mod. Pathol.* **2000**, *13*, 1020–1028. [CrossRef]
49. Sawatsubashi, M.; Yamada, T.; Fukushima, N.; Mizokami, H.; Tokunaga, O.; Shin, T. Association of vascular endothelial growth factor and mast cells with angiogenesis in laryngeal squamous cell carcinoma. *Virchows Arch.* **2000**, *436*, 243–248. [CrossRef]
50. Coussens, L.M.; Raymond, W.W.; Bergers, G.; Laig-Webster, M.; Behrendtsen, O.; Werb, Z.; Caughey, G.H.; Hanahan, D. Inflammatory mast cells up-regulate angiogenesis during squamous epithelial carcinogenesis. *Genes Dev.* **1999**, *13*, 1382–1397. [CrossRef]
51. Soucek, L.; Lawlor, E.R.; Soto, D.; Shchors, K.; Swigart, L.B.; Evan, G.I. Mast cells are required for angiogenesis and macroscopic expansion of Myc-induced pancreatic islet tumors. *Nat. Med.* **2007**, *13*, 1211–1218. [CrossRef]
52. Norrby, K. Mast cells and angiogenesis. *J. Pathol. Microbiol. Immunol.* **2002**, *110*, 355–371. [CrossRef] [PubMed]
53. Hiromatsu, Y.; Toda, S. Mast cells and angiogenesis. *Microsc. Res. Tech.* **2003**, *60*, 64–69. [CrossRef] [PubMed]
54. McHale, C.; Mohammed, Z.; Gomez, G. Human Skin-Derived Mast Cells Spontaneously Secrete Several Angiogenesis-Related Factors. *Front. Immunol.* **2019**, *10*, 1445. [CrossRef] [PubMed]
55. Longo, V.; Tamma, R.; Brunetti, O.; Pisconti, S.; Argentiero, A.; Silvestris, N.; Ribatti, D. Mast cells and angiogenesis in pancreatic ductal adenocarcinoma. *Clin. Exp. Med.* **2018**, *18*, 319–323. [CrossRef]
56. Guo, X.; Zhai, L.; Xue, R.; Shi, J.; Zeng, Q.; Gao, C. Mast Cell Tryptase Contributes to Pancreatic Cancer Growth through Promoting Angiogenesis via Activation of Angiopoietin-1. *Int. J. Mol. Sci.* **2016**, *17*, 834. [CrossRef]
57. Wroblewski, M.; Bauer, R.; Cubas Córdova, M.; Udonta, F.; Ben-Batalla, I.; Legler, K.; Hauser, C.; Egberts, J.; Janning, M.; Velthaus, J.; et al. Mast cells decrease efficacy of anti-angiogenic therapy by secreting matrix-degrading granzyme B. *Nat. Commun.* **2017**, *8*, 269. [CrossRef]
58. Ma, Y.; Hwang, R.F.; Logsdon, C.D.; Ullrich, S.E. Dynamic mast cell-stromal cell interactions promote growth of pancreatic cancer. *Cancer Res.* **2013**, *73*, 3927–3937. [CrossRef]
59. Wu, Y.; Zhang, C.; Jiang, K.; Werner, J.; Bazhin, A.V.; D'Haese, J.G. The Role of Stellate Cells in Pancreatic Ductal Adenocarcinoma: Targeting Perspectives. *Front. Oncol.* **2020**, *10*, 621937. [CrossRef]
60. Lichterman, J.N.; Reddy, S.M. Mast Cells: A New Frontier for Cancer Immunotherapy. *Cells* **2021**, *10*, 1270. [CrossRef]
61. Dubreuil, P.; Letard, S.; Ciufolini, M.; Gros, L.; Humbert, M.; Castéran, N.; Borge, L.; Hajem, B.; Lermet, A.; Sippl, W.; et al. Masitinib (AB1010), a potent and selective tyrosine kinase inhibitor targeting KIT. *PLoS ONE* **2009**, *4*, e7258. [CrossRef]
62. Deplanque, G.; Demarchi, M.; Hebbar, M.; Flynn, P.; Melichar, B.; Atkins, J.; Nowara, E.; Moyé, L.; Piquemal, D.; Ritter, D.; et al. A randomized, placebo-controlled phase III trial of masitinib plus gemcitabine in the treatment of advanced pancreatic cancer. *Ann. Oncol.* **2015**, *26*, 1194–1200. [CrossRef] [PubMed]
63. Mitry, E.; Hammel, P.; Deplanque, G.; Mornex, F.; Levy, P.; Seitz, J.-F.; Moussy, A.; Kinet, J.-P.; Hermine, O.; Rougier, P.; et al. Safety and activity of masitinib in combination with gemcitabine in patients with advanced pancreatic cancer. *Cancer Chemother. Pharmacol.* **2010**, *66*, 395–403. [CrossRef] [PubMed]
64. Dancey, J.T.; Deubelbeiss, K.A.; Harker, L.A.; Finch, C.A. Neutrophil kinetics in man. *J. Clin. Investig.* **1976**, *58*, 705–715. [CrossRef]

165. Ho-Tin-Noé, B.; Boulaftali, Y.; Camerer, E. Platelets and vascular integrity: How platelets prevent bleeding in inflammation. *Blood* **2018**, *131*, 277–288. [CrossRef]
166. Thanabalasuriar, A.; Scott, B.N.V.; Peiseler, M.; Willson, M.E.; Zeng, Z.; Warrener, P.; Keller, A.E.; Surewaard, B.G.J.; Dozier, E.A.; Korhonen, J.T.; et al. Neutrophil Extracellular Traps Confine Pseudomonas aeruginosa Ocular Biofilms and Restrict Brain Invasion. *Cell Host Microbe* **2019**, *25*, 526–536.e4. [CrossRef] [PubMed]
167. Drummond, R.A.; Lionakis, M.S. Measuring In Vivo Neutrophil Trafficking Responses During Fungal Infection Using Mixed Bone Marrow Chimeras. *Methods Mol. Biol.* **2021**, *2260*, 179–196. [CrossRef]
168. Iversen, M.B.; Reinert, L.S.; Thomsen, M.K.; Bagdonaite, I.; Nandakumar, R.; Cheshenko, N.; Prabakaran, T.; Vakhrushev, S.Y.; Krzyzowska, M.; Kratholm, S.K.; et al. An innate antiviral pathway acting before interferons at epithelial surfaces. *Nat. Immunol.* **2016**, *17*, 150–158. [CrossRef]
169. Castanheira, F.V.S.; Kubes, P. Neutrophils and NETs in modulating acute and chronic inflammation. *Blood* **2019**, *133*, 2178–2185. [CrossRef]
170. Fridlender, Z.G.; Sun, J.; Kim, S.; Kapoor, V.; Cheng, G.; Ling, L.; Worthen, G.S.; Albelda, S.M. Polarization of tumor-associated neutrophil phenotype by TGF-beta: "N1" versus "N2" TAN. *Cancer Cell* **2009**, *16*, 183–194. [CrossRef]
171. Sandoval, D.; Gukovskaya, A.; Reavey, P.; Gukovsky, S.; Sisk, A.; Braquet, P.; Pandol, S.J.; Poucell-Hatton, S. The role of neutrophils and platelet-activating factor in mediating experimental pancreatitis. *Gastroenterology* **1996**, *111*, 1081–1091. [CrossRef]
172. Felix, K.; Gaida, M.M. Neutrophil-Derived Proteases in the Microenvironment of Pancreatic Cancer -Active Players in Tumor Progression. *Int. J. Biol. Sci.* **2016**, *12*, 302–313. [CrossRef]
173. Gaida, M.M.; Steffen, T.G.; Günther, F.; Tschaharganeh, D.F.; Felix, K.; Bergmann, F.; Schirmacher, P.; Hänsch, G.M. Polymorphonuclear neutrophils promote dyshesion of tumor cells and elastase-mediated degradation of E-cadherin in pancreatic tumors. *Eur. J. Immunol.* **2012**, *42*, 3369–3380. [CrossRef]
174. Brinkmann, V.; Reichard, U.; Goosmann, C.; Fauler, B.; Uhlemann, Y.; Weiss, D.S.; Weinrauch, Y.; Zychlinsky, A. Neutrophil extracellular traps kill bacteria. *Science* **2004**, *303*, 1532–1535. [CrossRef] [PubMed]
175. Adrover, J.M.; McDowell, S.A.C.; He, X.-Y.; Quail, D.F.; Egeblad, M. NETworking with cancer: The bidirectional interplay between cancer and neutrophil extracellular traps. *Cancer Cell* **2023**, *41*, 505–526. [CrossRef]
176. Jung, H.S.; Gu, J.; Kim, J.-E.; Nam, Y.; Song, J.W.; Kim, H.K. Cancer cell-induced neutrophil extracellular traps promote both hypercoagulability and cancer progression. *PLoS ONE* **2019**, *14*, e0216055. [CrossRef]
177. Zhang, Y.; Chandra, V.; Riquelme Sanchez, E.; Dutta, P.; Quesada, P.R.; Rakoski, A.; Zoltan, M.; Arora, N.; Baydogan, S.; Horne, W.; et al. Interleukin-17–induced neutrophil extracellular traps mediate resistance to checkpoint blockade in pancreatic cancer. *J. Exp. Med.* **2020**, *217*, e20190354. [CrossRef] [PubMed]
178. Schoeps, B.; Eckfeld, C.; Prokopchuk, O.; Böttcher, J.; Häußler, D.; Steiger, K.; Demir, I.E.; Knolle, P.; Soehnlein, O.; Jenne, D.E. et al. TIMP1 Triggers Neutrophil Extracellular Trap Formation in Pancreatic Cancer. *Cancer Res.* **2021**, *81*, 3568–3579. [CrossRef] [PubMed]
179. Jin, W.; Yin, H.; Li, H.; Yu, X.-J.; Xu, H.-X.; Liu, L. Neutrophil extracellular DNA traps promote pancreatic cancer cells migration and invasion by activating EGFR/ERK pathway. *J. Cell. Mol. Med.* **2021**, *25*, 5443–5456. [CrossRef]
180. Munir, H.; Jones, J.O.; Janowitz, T.; Hoffmann, M.; Euler, M.; Martins, C.P.; Welsh, S.J.; Shields, J.D. Stromal-driven and Amyloid β-dependent induction of neutrophil extracellular traps modulates tumor growth. *Nat. Commun.* **2021**, *12*, 683. [CrossRef]
181. Fuchs, T.A.; Brill, A.; Duerschmied, D.; Schatzberg, D.; Monestier, M.; Myers, D.D.; Wrobleski, S.K.; Wakefield, T.W.; Hartwig, J.H.; Wagner, D.D. Extracellular DNA traps promote thrombosis. *Proc. Natl. Acad. Sci. USA* **2010**, *107*, 15880–15885. [CrossRef]
182. Frere, C.; Bournet, B.; Gourgou, S.; Fraisse, J.; Canivet, C.; Connors, J.M.; Buscail, L.; Farge, D. Incidence of Venous Thromboembolism in Patients With Newly Diagnosed Pancreatic Cancer and Factors Associated With Outcomes. *Gastroenterology* **2020**, *158*, 1346–1358.e4. [CrossRef] [PubMed]
183. Lasser, S.A.; Ozbay Kurt, F.G.; Arkhypov, I.; Utikal, J.; Umansky, V. Myeloid-derived suppressor cells in cancer and cancer therapy. *Nat. Rev. Clin. Oncol.* **2024**, *21*, 147–164. [CrossRef] [PubMed]
184. Gabrilovich, D.I.; Ostrand-Rosenberg, S.; Bronte, V. Coordinated regulation of myeloid cells by tumours. *Nat. Rev. Immunol.* **2012**, *12*, 253–268. [CrossRef]
185. Marigo, I.; Bosio, E.; Solito, S.; Mesa, C.; Fernandez, A.; Dolcetti, L.; Ugel, S.; Sonda, N.; Bicciato, S.; Falisi, E.; et al. Tumor-induced tolerance and immune suppression depend on the C/EBPbeta transcription factor. *Immunity* **2010**, *32*, 790–802. [CrossRef]
186. Bayne, L.J.; Beatty, G.L.; Jhala, N.; Clark, C.E.; Rhim, A.D.; Stanger, B.Z.; Vonderheide, R.H. Tumor-derived granulocyte-macrophage colony-stimulating factor regulates myeloid inflammation and T cell immunity in pancreatic cancer. *Cancer Cell* **2012**, *21*, 822–835. [CrossRef]
187. Pylayeva-Gupta, Y.; Lee, K.E.; Hajdu, C.H.; Miller, G.; Bar-Sagi, D. Oncogenic Kras-induced GM-CSF production promotes the development of pancreatic neoplasia. *Cancer Cell* **2012**, *21*, 836–847. [CrossRef]

188. Mace, T.A.; Ameen, Z.; Collins, A.; Wojcik, S.; Mair, M.; Young, G.S.; Fuchs, J.R.; Eubank, T.D.; Frankel, W.L.; Bekaii-Saab, T.; et al. Pancreatic cancer-associated stellate cells promote differentiation of myeloid-derived suppressor cells in a STAT3-dependent manner. *Cancer Res.* **2013**, *73*, 3007–3018. [CrossRef] [PubMed]
189. Vasquez-Dunddel, D.; Pan, F.; Zeng, Q.; Gorbounov, M.; Albesiano, E.; Fu, J.; Blosser, R.L.; Tam, A.J.; Bruno, T.; Zhang, H.; et al. STAT3 regulates arginase-I in myeloid-derived suppressor cells from cancer patients. *J. Clin. Investig.* **2013**, *123*, 1580–1589. [CrossRef]
190. Menjivar, R.E.; Nwosu, Z.C.; Du, W.; Donahue, K.L.; Hong, H.S.; Espinoza, C.; Brown, K.; Velez-Delgado, A.; Yan, W.; Lima, F.; et al. Arginase 1 is a key driver of immune suppression in pancreatic cancer. *eLife* **2023**, *12*, e80721. [CrossRef]
191. Panni, R.Z.; Sanford, D.E.; Belt, B.A.; Mitchem, J.B.; Worley, L.A.; Goetz, B.D.; Mukherjee, P.; Wang-Gillam, A.; Link, D.C.; DeNardo, D.G.; et al. Tumor-induced STAT3 activation in monocytic myeloid-derived suppressor cells enhances stemness and mesenchymal properties in human pancreatic cancer. *Cancer Immunol. Immunother.* **2014**, *63*, 513–528. [CrossRef]
192. Porembka, M.R.; Mitchem, J.B.; Belt, B.A.; Hsieh, C.-S.; Lee, H.-M.; Herndon, J.; Gillanders, W.E.; Linehan, D.C.; Goedegebuure, P. Pancreatic adenocarcinoma induces bone marrow mobilization of myeloid-derived suppressor cells which promote primary tumor growth. *Cancer Immunol. Immunother.* **2012**, *61*, 1373–1385. [CrossRef] [PubMed]
193. Sanford, D.E.; Porembka, M.R.; Panni, R.Z.; Mitchem, J.B.; Belt, B.A.; Plambeck-Suess, S.M.; Lin, G.; DeNardo, D.G.; Fields, R.C.; Hawkins, W.G.; et al. A Study of Zoledronic Acid as Neo-Adjuvant, Perioperative Therapy in Patients with Resectable Pancreatic Ductal Adenocarcinoma. *J. Cancer Ther.* **2013**, *4*, 797–803. [CrossRef] [PubMed]
194. Huang, B.; Pan, P.-Y.; Li, Q.; Sato, A.I.; Levy, D.E.; Bromberg, J.; Divino, C.M.; Chen, S.-H. Gr-1^{+}CD115^{+} immature myeloid suppressor cells mediate the development of tumor-induced T regulatory cells and T-cell anergy in tumor-bearing host. *Cancer Res.* **2006**, *66*, 1123–1131. [CrossRef]
195. Siret, C.; Collignon, A.; Silvy, F.; Robert, S.; Cheyrol, T.; André, P.; Rigot, V.; Iovanna, J.; van de Pavert, S.; Lombardo, D.; et al. Deciphering the Crosstalk Between Myeloid-Derived Suppressor Cells and Regulatory T Cells in Pancreatic Ductal Adenocarcinoma. *Front. Immunol.* **2019**, *10*, 3070. [CrossRef]
196. Sarhan, D.; Eisinger, S.; He, F.; Bergsland, M.; Pelicano, C.; Driescher, C.; Westberg, K.; Benitez, I.I.; Humoud, R.; Palano, G.; et al. Targeting myeloid suppressive cells revives cytotoxic anti-tumor responses in pancreatic cancer. *iScience* **2022**, *25*, 105317. [CrossRef] [PubMed]
197. Liu, C.; Yu, S.; Kappes, J.; Wang, J.; Grizzle, W.E.; Zinn, K.R.; Zhang, H.-G. Expansion of spleen myeloid suppressor cells represses NK cell cytotoxicity in tumor-bearing host. *Blood* **2007**, *109*, 4336–4342. [CrossRef]
198. Sinha, P.; Clements, V.K.; Bunt, S.K.; Albelda, S.M.; Ostrand-Rosenberg, S. Cross-talk between myeloid-derived suppressor cells and macrophages subverts tumor immunity toward a type 2 response. *J. Immunol.* **2007**, *179*, 977–983. [CrossRef]
199. Suzuki, E.; Kapoor, V.; Jassar, A.S.; Kaiser, L.R.; Albelda, S.M. Gemcitabine selectively eliminates splenic Gr-1+/CD11b+ myeloid suppressor cells in tumor-bearing animals and enhances antitumor immune activity. *Clin. Cancer Res.* **2005**, *11*, 6713–6721. [CrossRef]
200. Sun, R.; Sun, Y.; Wu, C.; Liu, Y.; Zhou, M.; Dong, Y.; Du, G.; Luo, H.; Shi, B.; Jiang, H.; et al. CXCR4-modified CAR-T cells suppresses MDSCs recruitment via STAT3/NF-κB/SDF-1α axis to enhance efficacy against pancreatic cancer. *Mol. Ther.* **2023**, *31*, 3193–3209. [CrossRef]
201. Diaz-Montero, C.M.; Salem, M.L.; Nishimura, M.I.; Garrett-Mayer, E.; Cole, D.J.; Montero, A.J. Increased circulating myeloid-derived suppressor cells correlate with clinical cancer stage, metastatic tumor burden, and doxorubicin-cyclophosphamide chemotherapy. *Cancer Immunol. Immunother.* **2009**, *58*, 49–59. [CrossRef]
202. Takeuchi, S.; Baghdadi, M.; Tsuchikawa, T.; Wada, H.; Nakamura, T.; Abe, H.; Nakanishi, S.; Usui, Y.; Higuchi, K.; Takahashi, M.; et al. Chemotherapy-Derived Inflammatory Responses Accelerate the Formation of Immunosuppressive Myeloid Cells in the Tissue Microenvironment of Human Pancreatic Cancer. *Cancer Res.* **2015**, *75*, 2629–2640. [CrossRef] [PubMed]
203. Ogawa, M. Differentiation and proliferation of hematopoietic stem cells. *Blood* **1993**, *81*, 2844–2853. [CrossRef] [PubMed]
204. Gardner, F.H.; Cohen, P. Platelet Life Span. *Transfusion* **1966**, *6*, 23–31. [CrossRef]
205. Yun, S.-H.; Sim, E.-H.; Goh, R.-Y.; Park, J.-I.; Han, J.-Y. Platelet Activation: The Mechanisms and Potential Biomarkers. *BioMed Res. Int.* **2016**, *2016*, 9060143. [CrossRef] [PubMed]
206. Haemmerle, M.; Stone, R.L.; Menter, D.G.; Afshar-Kharghan, V.; Sood, A.K. The Platelet Lifeline to Cancer: Challenges and Opportunities. *Cancer Cell* **2018**, *33*, 965–983. [CrossRef]
207. Bottsford-Miller, J.; Choi, H.-J.; Dalton, H.J.; Stone, R.L.; Cho, M.S.; Haemmerle, M.; Nick, A.M.; Pradeep, S.; Zand, B.; Previs, R.A.; et al. Differential platelet levels affect response to taxane-based therapy in ovarian cancer. *Clin. Cancer Res.* **2015**, *21*, 602–610. [CrossRef]
208. Haemmerle, M.; Bottsford-Miller, J.; Pradeep, S.; Taylor, M.L.; Choi, H.-J.; Hansen, J.M.; Dalton, H.J.; Stone, R.L.; Cho, M.S.; Nick, A.M.; et al. FAK regulates platelet extravasation and tumor growth after antiangiogenic therapy withdrawal. *J. Clin. Investig.* **2016**, *126*, 1885–1896. [CrossRef]

209. Haemmerle, M.; Taylor, M.L.; Gutschner, T.; Pradeep, S.; Cho, M.S.; Sheng, J.; Lyons, Y.M.; Nagaraja, A.S.; Dood, R.L.; Wen, Y.; et al. Platelets reduce anoikis and promote metastasis by activating YAP1 signaling. *Nat. Commun.* **2017**, *8*, 310. [CrossRef]
210. Ali, R.A.; Wuescher, L.M.; Worth, R.G. Platelets: Essential components of the immune system. *Curr. Trends Immunol.* **2015**, *16*, 65–78.
211. Nicolai, L.; Gaertner, F.; Massberg, S. Platelets in Host Defense: Experimental and Clinical Insights. *Trends Immunol.* **2019**, *40*, 922–938. [CrossRef]
212. Dib, P.R.B.; Quirino-Teixeira, A.C.; Merij, L.B.; Pinheiro, M.B.M.; Rozini, S.V.; Andrade, F.B.; Hottz, E.D. Innate immune receptors in platelets and platelet-leukocyte interactions. *J. Leukoc. Biol.* **2020**, *108*, 1157–1182. [CrossRef]
213. Chapman, L.M.; Aggrey, A.A.; Field, D.J.; Srivastava, K.; Ture, S.; Yui, K.; Topham, D.J.; Baldwin, W.M.; Morrell, C.N. Platelets present antigen in the context of MHC class I. *J. Immunol.* **2012**, *189*, 916–923. [CrossRef] [PubMed]
214. Pitchford, S.C.; Momi, S.; Giannini, S.; Casali, L.; Spina, D.; Page, C.P.; Gresele, P. Platelet P-selectin is required for pulmonary eosinophil and lymphocyte recruitment in a murine model of allergic inflammation. *Blood* **2005**, *105*, 2074–2081. [CrossRef] [PubMed]
215. Pitchford, S.C.; Yano, H.; Lever, R.; Riffo-Vasquez, Y.; Ciferri, S.; Rose, M.J.; Giannini, S.; Momi, S.; Spina, D.; O'connor, B.; et al. Platelets are essential for leukocyte recruitment in allergic inflammation. *J. Allergy Clin. Immunol.* **2003**, *112*, 109–118. [CrossRef]
216. de Stoppelaar, S.F.; van't Veer, C.; Claushuis, T.A.M.; Albersen, B.J.A.; Roelofs, J.J.T.H.; van der Poll, T. Thrombocytopenia impairs host defense in gram-negative pneumonia-derived sepsis in mice. *Blood* **2014**, *124*, 3781–3790. [CrossRef]
217. van den Boogaard, F.E.; Schouten, M.; de Stoppelaar, S.F.; Roelofs, J.J.T.H.; Brands, X.; Schultz, M.J.; van't Veer, C.; van der Poll, T. Thrombocytopenia impairs host defense during murine Streptococcus pneumoniae pneumonia. *Crit. Care Med.* **2015**, *43*, e75–e83. [CrossRef] [PubMed]
218. Nieswandt, B.; Hafner, M.; Echtenacher, B.; Männel, D.N. Lysis of tumor cells by natural killer cells in mice is impeded by platelets. *Cancer Res.* **1999**, *59*, 1295–1300.
219. Maurer, S.; Kropp, K.N.; Klein, G.; Steinle, A.; Haen, S.P.; Walz, J.S.; Hinterleitner, C.; Märklin, M.; Kopp, H.-G.; Salih, H.R. Platelet-mediated shedding of NKG2D ligands impairs NK cell immune-surveillance of tumor cells. *Oncoimmunology* **2018**, *7*, e1364827. [CrossRef]
220. Clar, K.L.; Hinterleitner, C.; Schneider, P.; Salih, H.R.; Maurer, S. Inhibition of NK Reactivity Against Solid Tumors by Platelet-Derived RANKL. *Cancers* **2019**, *11*, 277. [CrossRef]
221. Kissel, K.; Berber, S.; Nockher, A.; Santoso, S.; Bein, G.; Hackstein, H. Human platelets target dendritic cell differentiation and production of proinflammatory cytokines. *Transfusion* **2006**, *46*, 818–827. [CrossRef]
222. Langer, H.F.; Daub, K.; Braun, G.; Schönberger, T.; May, A.E.; Schaller, M.; Stein, G.M.; Stellos, K.; Bueltmann, A.; Siegel-Axel, D.; et al. Platelets recruit human dendritic cells via Mac-1/JAM-C interaction and modulate dendritic cell function in vitro. *Arterioscler. Thromb. Vasc. Biol.* **2007**, *27*, 1463–1470. [CrossRef]
223. Carestia, A.; Mena, H.A.; Olexen, C.M.; Ortiz Wilczyñski, J.M.; Negrotto, S.; Errasti, A.E.; Gómez, R.M.; Jenne, C.N.; Carrera Silva, E.A.; Schattner, M. Platelets Promote Macrophage Polarization toward Pro-inflammatory Phenotype and Increase Survival of Septic Mice. *Cell Rep.* **2019**, *28*, 896–908.e5. [CrossRef] [PubMed]
224. Chen, Y.; Zhou, J.; Liu, Z.; Wu, T.; Li, S.; Zhang, Y.; Yin, X.; Yang, G.; Zhang, G. Tumor cell-induced platelet aggregation accelerates hematogenous metastasis of malignant melanoma by triggering macrophage recruitment. *J. Exp. Clin. Cancer Res.* **2023**, *42*, 277. [CrossRef]
225. Gleissner, C.A.; Shaked, I.; Little, K.M.; Ley, K. CXC chemokine ligand 4 induces a unique transcriptome in monocyte-derived macrophages. *J. Immunol.* **2010**, *184*, 4810–4818. [CrossRef] [PubMed]
226. Lucotti, S.; Ogitani, Y.; Kenific, C.M.; Geri, J.; Kim, Y.H.; Gu, J.; Balaji, U.; Bojmar, L.; Shaashua, L.; Song, Y.; et al. Extracellular vesicles from the lung pro-thrombotic niche drive cancer-associated thrombosis and metastasis via integrin beta 2. *Cell* **2025**, *188*, 1642–1661.e24. [CrossRef]
227. Santoso, S.; Sachs, U.J.H.; Kroll, H.; Linder, M.; Ruf, A.; Preissner, K.T.; Chavakis, T. The junctional adhesion molecule 3 (JAM-3) on human platelets is a counterreceptor for the leukocyte integrin Mac-1. *J. Exp. Med.* **2002**, *196*, 679–691. [CrossRef]
228. Haselmayer, P.; Grosse-Hovest, L.; von Landenberg, P.; Schild, H.; Radsak, M.P. TREM-1 ligand expression on platelets enhances neutrophil activation. *Blood* **2007**, *110*, 1029–1035. [CrossRef] [PubMed]
229. Rahman, M.; Zhang, S.; Chew, M.; Ersson, A.; Jeppsson, B.; Thorlacius, H. Platelet-derived CD40L (CD154) mediates neutrophil upregulation of Mac-1 and recruitment in septic lung injury. *Ann. Surg.* **2009**, *250*, 783–790. [CrossRef]
230. Zuchtriegel, G.; Uhl, B.; Puhr-Westerheide, D.; Pörnbacher, M.; Lauber, K.; Krombach, F.; Reichel, C.A. Platelets Guide Leukocytes to Their Sites of Extravasation. *PLoS Biol.* **2016**, *14*, e1002459. [CrossRef]
231. Massberg, S.; Grahl, L.; von Bruehl, M.-L.; Manukyan, D.; Pfeiler, S.; Goosmann, C.; Brinkmann, V.; Lorenz, M.; Bidzhekov, K.; Khandagale, A.B.; et al. Reciprocal coupling of coagulation and innate immunity via neutrophil serine proteases. *Nat. Med.* **2010**, *16*, 887–896. [CrossRef]

232. von Brühl, M.-L.; Stark, K.; Steinhart, A.; Chandraratne, S.; Konrad, I.; Lorenz, M.; Khandoga, A.; Tirniceriu, A.; Coletti, R.; Köllnberger, M.; et al. Monocytes, neutrophils, and platelets cooperate to initiate and propagate venous thrombosis in mice in vivo. *J. Exp. Med.* **2012**, *209*, 819–835. [CrossRef] [PubMed]
233. Rosell, A.; Martinod, K.; Mackman, N.; Thålin, C. Neutrophil extracellular traps and cancer-associated thrombosis. *Thromb. Res.* **2022**, *213* (Suppl. 1), S35–S41. [CrossRef]
234. Clark, S.R.; Ma, A.C.; Tavener, S.A.; McDonald, B.; Goodarzi, Z.; Kelly, M.M.; Patel, K.D.; Chakrabarti, S.; McAvoy, E.; Sinclair, G.D.; et al. Platelet TLR4 activates neutrophil extracellular traps to ensnare bacteria in septic blood. *Nat. Med.* **2007**, *13*, 463–469. [CrossRef]
235. Etulain, J.; Martinod, K.; Wong, S.L.; Cifuni, S.M.; Schattner, M.; Wagner, D.D. P-selectin promotes neutrophil extracellular trap formation in mice. *Blood* **2015**, *126*, 242–246. [CrossRef]
236. Maugeri, N.; Campana, L.; Gavina, M.; Covino, C.; De Metrio, M.; Panciroli, C.; Maiuri, L.; Maseri, A.; D'Angelo, A.; Bianchi, M.E.; et al. Activated platelets present high mobility group box 1 to neutrophils, inducing autophagy and promoting the extrusion of neutrophil extracellular traps. *J. Thromb. Haemost.* **2014**, *12*, 2074–2088. [CrossRef] [PubMed]
237. Joseph, R.; Soundararajan, R.; Vasaikar, S.; Yang, F.; Allton, K.L.; Tian, L.; den Hollander, P.; Isgandarova, S.; Haemmerle, M.; Mino, B.; et al. $CD8^+$ T cells inhibit metastasis and CXCL4 regulates its function. *Br. J. Cancer* **2021**, *125*, 176–189. [CrossRef]
238. Servais, L.; Wéra, O.; Dibato Epoh, J.; Delierneux, C.; Bouznad, N.; Rahmouni, S.; Mazzucchelli, G.; Baiwir, D.; Delvenne, P.; Lancellotti, P.; et al. Platelets contribute to the initiation of colitis-associated cancer by promoting immunosuppression. *J. Thromb. Haemost.* **2018**, *16*, 762–777. [CrossRef] [PubMed]
239. Karhausen, J.; Choi, H.W.; Maddipati, K.R.; Mathew, J.P.; Ma, Q.; Boulaftali, Y.; Lee, R.H.; Bergmeier, W.; Abraham, S.N. Platelets trigger perivascular mast cell degranulation to cause inflammatory responses and tissue injury. *Sci. Adv.* **2020**, *6*, eaay6314. [CrossRef]
240. de Giovanni, M.; Dang, E.V.; Chen, K.Y.; An, J.; Madhani, H.D.; Cyster, J.G. Platelets and mast cells promote pathogenic eosinophil recruitment during invasive fungal infection via the 5-HIAA-GPR35 ligand-receptor system. *Immunity* **2023**, *56*, 1548–1560.e5. [CrossRef]
241. Xu, H.; He, A.; Liu, A.; Tong, W.; Cao, D. Evaluation of the prognostic role of platelet-lymphocyte ratio in cancer patients treated with immune checkpoint inhibitors: A systematic review and meta-analysis. *Int. Immunopharmacol.* **2019**, *77*, 105957. [CrossRef]
242. Cho, M.S.; Lee, H.; Gonzalez-Delgado, R.; Li, D.; Sasano, T.; Carlos-Alcalde, W.; Ma, Q.; Liu, J.; Sood, A.K.; Afshar-Kharghan, V. Platelets Increase the Expression of PD-L1 in Ovarian Cancer. *Cancers* **2022**, *14*, 2498. [CrossRef] [PubMed]
243. Guo, Q.; Malloy, M.W.; Roweth, H.G.; McAllister, S.S.; Italiano, J.E.; Battinelli, E.M. Platelets upregulate tumor cell programmed death ligand 1 in an epidermal growth factor receptor-dependent manner in vitro. *Blood Adv.* **2022**, *6*, 5668–5675. [CrossRef] [PubMed]
244. Cui, J.-W.; Li, Y.; Yang, Y.; Yang, H.-K.; Dong, J.-M.; Xiao, Z.-H.; He, X.; Guo, J.-H.; Wang, R.-Q.; Dai, B.; et al. Tumor immunotherapy resistance: Revealing the mechanism of PD-1/PD-L1-mediated tumor immune escape. *Biomed. Pharmacother.* **2024**, *171*, 116203. [CrossRef]
245. Zaslavsky, A.B.; Adams, M.P.; Cao, X.; Maj, T.; Choi, J.E.; Stangl-Kremser, J.; Patel, S.; Putelo, A.; Lee, S.K.; Nallandhighal, S.; et al. Platelet PD-L1 suppresses anti-cancer immune cell activity in PD-L1 negative tumors. *Sci. Rep.* **2020**, *10*, 19296. [CrossRef] [PubMed]
246. Hinterleitner, C.; Strähle, J.; Malenke, E.; Hinterleitner, M.; Henning, M.; Seehawer, M.; Bilich, T.; Heitmann, J.; Lutz, M.; Mattern, S.; et al. Platelet PD-L1 reflects collective intratumoral PD-L1 expression and predicts immunotherapy response in non-small cell lung cancer. *Nat. Commun.* **2021**, *12*, 7005. [CrossRef]
247. Lutz, M.S.; Klimovich, B.; Maurer, S.; Heitmann, J.S.; Märklin, M.; Zekri, L.; Jung, G.; Salih, H.R.; Hinterleitner, C. Platelets subvert antitumor efficacy of T cell-recruiting bispecific antibodies. *J. Immunother. Cancer* **2022**, *10*, e003655. [CrossRef]
248. Rachidi, S.; Metelli, A.; Riesenberg, B.; Wu, B.X.; Nelson, M.H.; Wallace, C.; Paulos, C.M.; Rubinstein, M.P.; Garrett-Mayer, E.; Hennig, M.; et al. Platelets subvert T cell immunity against cancer via GARP-TGFβ axis. *Sci. Immunol.* **2017**, *2*, eaai7911. [CrossRef]
249. Motz, G.T.; Santoro, S.P.; Wang, L.-P.; Garrabrant, T.; Lastra, R.R.; Hagemann, I.S.; Lal, P.; Feldman, M.D.; Benencia, F.; Coukos, G. Tumor endothelium FasL establishes a selective immune barrier promoting tolerance in tumors. *Nat. Med.* **2014**, *20*, 607–615. [CrossRef]
250. Yang, J.; Yamashita-Kanemaru, Y.; Morris, B.I.; Contursi, A.; Trajkovski, D.; Xu, J.; Patrascan, I.; Benson, J.; Evans, A.C.; Conti, A.G.; et al. Aspirin prevents metastasis by limiting platelet TXA2 suppression of T cell immunity. *Nature* **2025**, *640*, 1052–1061. [CrossRef]
251. Liu, X.; Song, J.; Zhang, H.; Liu, X.; Zuo, F.; Zhao, Y.; Zhao, Y.; Yin, X.; Guo, X.; Wu, X.; et al. Immune checkpoint HLA-E:CD94-NKG2A mediates evasion of circulating tumor cells from NK cell surveillance. *Cancer Cell* **2023**, *41*, 272–287.e9. [CrossRef]
252. Heinmöller, E.; Schropp, T.; Kisker, O.; Simon, B.; Seitz, R.; Weinel, R.J. Tumor cell-induced platelet aggregation in vitro by human pancreatic cancer cell lines. *Scand. J. Gastroenterol.* **1995**, *30*, 1008–1016. [CrossRef] [PubMed]

253. Wang, J.-G.; Geddings, J.E.; Aleman, M.M.; Cardenas, J.C.; Chantrathammachart, P.; Williams, J.C.; Kirchhofer, D.; Bogdanov, V.Y. Bach, R.R.; Rak, J.; et al. Tumor-derived tissue factor activates coagulation and enhances thrombosis in a mouse xenograft model of human pancreatic cancer. *Blood* **2012**, *119*, 5543–5552. [CrossRef]
254. Hisada, Y.; Ay, C.; Auriemma, A.C.; Cooley, B.C.; Mackman, N. Human pancreatic tumors grown in mice release tissue factor-positive microvesicles that increase venous clot size. *J. Thromb. Haemost.* **2017**, *15*, 2208–2217. [CrossRef]
255. Ansari, D.; Ansari, D.; Andersson, R.; Andrén-Sandberg, Å. Pancreatic cancer and thromboembolic disease, 150 years after Trousseau. *Hepatobiliary Surg. Nutr.* **2015**, *4*, 325–335. [CrossRef]
256. Brown, K.M.; Domin, C.; Aranha, G.V.; Yong, S.; Shoup, M. Increased preoperative platelet count is associated with decreased survival after resection for adenocarcinoma of the pancreas. *Am. J. Surg.* **2005**, *189*, 278–282. [CrossRef] [PubMed]
257. Chadha, A.S.; Kocak-Uzel, E.; Das, P.; Minsky, B.D.; Delclos, M.E.; Mahmood, U.; Guha, S.; Ahmad, M.; Varadhachary, G.R.; Javle M.; et al. Paraneoplastic thrombocytosis independently predicts poor prognosis in patients with locally advanced pancreatic cancer. *Acta Oncol.* **2015**, *54*, 971–978. [CrossRef]
258. Iodice, S.; Gandini, S.; Löhr, M.; Lowenfels, A.B.; Maisonneuve, P. Venous thromboembolic events and organ-specific occult cancers: A review and meta-analysis. *J. Thromb. Haemost.* **2008**, *6*, 781–788. [CrossRef] [PubMed]
259. Song, W.; Tian, C.; Wang, K.; Zhang, R.-J.; Zou, S.-B. Preoperative platelet lymphocyte ratio as independent predictors of prognosis in pancreatic cancer: A systematic review and meta-analysis. *PLoS ONE* **2017**, *12*, e0178762. [CrossRef]
260. Shirai, Y.; Shiba, H.; Haruki, K.; Horiuchi, T.; Saito, N.; Fujiwara, Y.; Sakamoto, T.; Uwagawa, T.; Yanaga, K. Preoperative Platelet-to-Albumin Ratio Predicts Prognosis of Patients with Pancreatic Ductal Adenocarcinoma After Pancreatic Resection *Anticancer. Res.* **2017**, *37*, 787–794. [CrossRef]
261. Best, M.G.; Sol, N.; Kooi, I.; Tannous, J.; Westerman, B.A.; Rustenburg, F.; Schellen, P.; Verschueren, H.; Post, E.; Koster, J.; et al RNA-Seq of Tumor-Educated Platelets Enables Blood-Based Pan-Cancer, Multiclass, and Molecular Pathway Cancer Diagnostics *Cancer Cell* **2015**, *28*, 666–676. [CrossRef]
262. Assoian, R.K.; Komoriya, A.; Meyers, C.A.; Miller, D.M.; Sporn, M.B. Transforming growth factor-beta in human platelets Identification of a major storage site, purification, and characterization. *J. Biol. Chem.* **1983**, *258*, 7155–7160. [CrossRef]
263. Tindall, R.R.; Bailey-Lundberg, J.M.; Cao, Y.; Ko, T.C. The TGF-β superfamily as potential therapeutic targets in pancreatic cancer *Front. Oncol.* **2024**, *14*, 1362247. [CrossRef] [PubMed]
264. Shek, F.W.-T.; Benyon, R.C.; Walker, F.M.; McCrudden, P.R.; Pender, S.L.F.; Williams, E.J.; Johnson, P.A.; Johnson, C.D.; Bateman A.C.; Fine, D.R.; et al. Expression of Transforming Growth Factor-β1 by Pancreatic Stellate Cells and Its Implications for Matrix Secretion and Turnover in Chronic Pancreatitis. *Am. J. Pathol.* **2002**, *160*, 1787–1798. [CrossRef] [PubMed]
265. Chuvin, N.; Vincent, D.F.; Pommier, R.M.; Alcaraz, L.B.; Gout, J.; Caligaris, C.; Yacoub, K.; Cardot, V.; Roger, E.; Kaniewski B.; et al. Acinar-to-Ductal Metaplasia Induced by Transforming Growth Factor Beta Facilitates KRAS G12D -driven Pancreatic Tumorigenesis. *Cell. Mol. Gastroenterol. Hepatol.* **2017**, *4*, 263–282. [CrossRef] [PubMed]
266. Lindemann, S.; Tolley, N.D.; Dixon, D.A.; McIntyre, T.M.; Prescott, S.M.; Zimmerman, G.A.; Weyrich, A.S. Activated platelets mediate inflammatory signaling by regulated interleukin 1beta synthesis. *J. Cell Biol.* **2001**, *154*, 485–490. [CrossRef] [PubMed]
267. Pennings, G.J.; Reddel, C.J.; Traini, M.; Lam, M.; Kockx, M.; Chen, V.M.; Kritharides, L. Rapid Release of Interleukin-1β from Human Platelets Is Independent of NLRP3 and Caspase. *Thromb. Haemost.* **2022**, *122*, 517–528. [CrossRef]
268. Takahashi, R.; Macchini, M.; Sunagawa, M.; Jiang, Z.; Tanaka, T.; Valenti, G.; Renz, B.W.; White, R.A.; Hayakawa, Y.; Westphalen C.B.; et al. Interleukin-1β-induced pancreatitis promotes pancreatic ductal adenocarcinoma via B lymphocyte-mediated immune suppression. *Gut* **2021**, *70*, 330–341. [CrossRef]
269. Marrache, F.; Tu, S.P.; Bhagat, G.; Pendyala, S.; Osterreicher, C.H.; Gordon, S.; Ramanathan, V.; Penz-Osterreicher, M.; Betz, K.S. Song, Z.; et al. Overexpression of interleukin-1beta in the murine pancreas results in chronic pancreatitis. *Gastroenterology* **2008** *135*, 1277–1287. [CrossRef]
270. Li, H.; Jiang, W.; Zhang, S.-R.; Li, P.-C.; Li, T.-J.; Jin, W.; Xu, H.-X.; Yu, X.-J.; Liu, L. The platelet pannexin 1-IL-1β axis orchestrates pancreatic ductal adenocarcinoma invasion and metastasis. *Oncogene* **2023**, *42*, 1453–1465. [CrossRef]
271. Zhao, J.-G.; Li, Y.-J.; Wu, Y.; Zhang, K.; Peng, L.-J.; Chen, H. Revealing platelet-related subtypes and prognostic signature in pancreatic adenocarcinoma. *BMC Med. Genom.* **2023**, *16*, 106. [CrossRef]
272. Malehmir, M.; Pfister, D.; Gallage, S.; Szydlowska, M.; Inverso, D.; Kotsiliti, E.; Leone, V.; Peiseler, M.; Surewaard, B.G.J.; Rath, D. et al. Platelet GPIbα is a mediator and potential interventional target for NASH and subsequent liver cancer. *Nat. Med.* **2019**, *25* 641–655. [CrossRef] [PubMed]
273. Buckland, G.R.; Wilding, S.A.; McDonnell, D.; Hamady, Z.Z.R. The role of aspirin in the prevention of pancreatic cancer: A nested case-control study in the UK Biobank. *Pancreatology* **2024**, *24*, 947–953. [CrossRef] [PubMed]
274. Dong, H.; Gao, M.; Lu, L.; Gui, R.; Fu, Y. Doxorubicin-Loaded Platelet Decoys for Enhanced Chemoimmunotherapy Against Triple-Negative Breast Cancer in Mice Model. *Int. J. Nanomed.* **2023**, *18*, 3577–3593. [CrossRef] [PubMed]

275. Mai, X.; Zhang, Y.; Fan, H.; Song, W.; Chang, Y.; Chen, B.; Shi, J.; Xin, X.; Teng, Z.; Sun, J.; et al. Integration of immunogenic activation and immunosuppressive reversion using mitochondrial-respiration-inhibited platelet-mimicking nanoparticles. *Biomaterials* **2020**, *232*, 119699. [CrossRef]
276. Chen, C.; Chen, N.; Qi, Y.; Lyu, M.; Wu, C.; Xie, C.; Yu, H. Copper-Based Single-Atom Nanozyme System Mimicking Platelet Cells for Enhancing the Outcome of Radioimmunotherapy. *Int. J. Nanomed.* **2024**, *19*, 403–414. [CrossRef]
277. Yang, Y.; Wang, Y.; Yao, Y.; Wang, S.; Zhang, Y.; Dotti, G.; Yu, J.; Gu, Z. T cell-mimicking platelet-drug conjugates. *Matter* **2023**, *6*, 2340–2355. [CrossRef]
278. Kött, J.; Zell, T.; Zimmermann, N.; Rünger, A.; Smit, D.J.; Abeck, F.; Geidel, G.; Hansen-Abeck, I.; Heidrich, I.; Weichenthal, M.; et al. Improved survival of advanced melanoma patients receiving immunotherapy with concomitant antithrombotic therapy—A multicenter study on 2419 patients from the prospective skin cancer registry ADOReg. *Eur. J. Cancer* **2024**, *214*, 115159. [CrossRef]
279. Wculek, S.K.; Cueto, F.J.; Mujal, A.M.; Melero, I.; Krummel, M.F.; Sancho, D. Dendritic cells in cancer immunology and immunotherapy. *Nat. Rev. Immunol.* **2020**, *20*, 7–24. [CrossRef]
280. Gupta, Y.H.; Khanom, A.; Acton, S.E. Control of Dendritic Cell Function Within the Tumour Microenvironment. *Front. Immunol.* **2022**, *13*, 733800. [CrossRef]
281. Crouse, J.; Xu, H.C.; Lang, P.A.; Oxenius, A. NK cells regulating T cell responses: Mechanisms and outcome. *Trends Immunol.* **2015**, *36*, 49–58. [CrossRef]
282. Krieger, T.G.; Le Blanc, S.; Jabs, J.; Ten, F.W.; Ishaque, N.; Jechow, K.; Debnath, O.; Leonhardt, C.-S.; Giri, A.; Eils, R.; et al. Single-cell analysis of patient-derived PDAC organoids reveals cell state heterogeneity and a conserved developmental hierarchy. *Nat. Commun.* **2021**, *12*, 5826. [CrossRef] [PubMed]
283. Lin, W.; Noel, P.; Borazanci, E.H.; Lee, J.; Amini, A.; Han, I.W.; Heo, J.S.; Jameson, G.S.; Fraser, C.; Steinbach, M.; et al. Single-cell transcriptome analysis of tumor and stromal compartments of pancreatic ductal adenocarcinoma primary tumors and metastatic lesions. *Genome Med.* **2020**, *12*, 80. [CrossRef] [PubMed]
284. Peng, J.; Sun, B.-F.; Chen, C.-Y.; Zhou, J.-Y.; Chen, Y.-S.; Chen, H.; Liu, L.; Huang, D.; Jiang, J.; Cui, G.-S.; et al. Single-cell RNA-seq highlights intra-tumoral heterogeneity and malignant progression in pancreatic ductal adenocarcinoma. *Cell Res.* **2019**, *29*, 725–738. [CrossRef] [PubMed]
285. Steele, N.G.; Carpenter, E.S.; Kemp, S.B.; Sirihorachai, V.R.; The, S.; Delrosario, L.; Lazarus, J.; Amir, E.-A.D.; Gunchick, V.; Espinoza, C.; et al. Multimodal Mapping of the Tumor and Peripheral Blood Immune Landscape in Human Pancreatic Cancer. *Nat. Cancer* **2020**, *1*, 1097–1112. [CrossRef]
286. Liudahl, S.M.; Betts, C.B.; Sivagnanam, S.; Morales-Oyarvide, V.; Da Silva, A.; Yuan, C.; Hwang, S.; Grossblatt-Wait, A.; Leis, K.R.; Larson, W.; et al. Leukocyte Heterogeneity in Pancreatic Ductal Adenocarcinoma: Phenotypic and Spatial Features Associated with Clinical Outcome. *Cancer Discov.* **2021**, *11*, 2014–2031. [CrossRef]
287. Elyada, E.; Bolisetty, M.; Laise, P.; Flynn, W.F.; Courtois, E.T.; Burkhart, R.A.; Teinor, J.A.; Belleau, P.; Biffi, G.; Lucito, M.S.; et al. Cross-Species Single-Cell Analysis of Pancreatic Ductal Adenocarcinoma Reveals Antigen-Presenting Cancer-Associated Fibroblasts. *Cancer Discov.* **2019**, *9*, 1102–1123. [CrossRef]
288. Grünwald, B.T.; Devisme, A.; Andrieux, G.; Vyas, F.; Aliar, K.; McCloskey, C.W.; Macklin, A.; Jang, G.H.; Denroche, R.; Romero, J.M.; et al. Spatially confined sub-tumor microenvironments in pancreatic cancer. *Cell* **2021**, *184*, 5577–5592.e18. [CrossRef]
289. Pei, G.; Min, J.; Rajapakshe, K.I.; Branchi, V.; Liu, Y.; Selvanesan, B.C.; Thege, F.; Sadeghian, D.; Zhang, D.; Cho, K.S.; et al. Spatial mapping of transcriptomic plasticity in metastatic pancreatic cancer. *Nature* **2025**. [CrossRef]
290. Zhou, D.C.; Jayasinghe, R.G.; Chen, S.; Herndon, J.M.; Iglesia, M.D.; Navale, P.; Wendl, M.C.; Caravan, W.; Sato, K.; Storrs, E.; et al. Spatially restricted drivers and transitional cell populations cooperate with the microenvironment in untreated and chemo-resistant pancreatic cancer. *Nat. Genet.* **2022**, *54*, 1390–1405. [CrossRef]

cancers

MDPI

Review

From Genes to Environment: Elucidating Pancreatic Carcinogenesis Through Genetically Engineered and Risk Factor-Integrated Mouse Models

Bin Yan [1,†], Anne-Kristin Fritsche [2,3,†], Erik Haußner [4], Tanvi Vikrant Inamdar [5], Helmut Laumen [5], Michael Boettcher [4], Martin Gericke [3], Patrick Michl [1,*] and Jonas Rosendahl [5,*]

1 Department of Internal Medicine IV, Heidelberg University Hospital, 69120 Heidelberg, Germany; bin.yan@med.uni-heidelberg.de
2 Institute of Anatomy and Cell Biology, Martin-Luther-University Halle-Wittenberg, 06120 Halle (Saale), Germany; anne-kristin.fritsche@medizin.uni-leipzig.de
3 Institute of Anatomy, Leipzig University, 04103 Leipzig, Germany; martin.gericke@medizin.uni-leipzig.de
4 Institute of Molecular Medicine, Section for Molecular Medicine of Signal Transduction, Faculty of Medicine, Martin-Luther-University Halle-Wittenberg, 06120 Halle (Saale), Germany; erik.haussner@uk-halle.de (E.H.); michael.boettcher@medizin.uni-halle.de (M.B.)
5 Department of Internal Medicine I, Martin-Luther-University Halle-Wittenberg, 06120 Halle (Saale), Germany; tanvivikrant.inamdar@uk-halle.de (T.V.I.); helmut.laumen@medizin.uni-halle.de (H.L.)
* Correspondence: patrick.michl@med.uni-heidelberg.de (P.M.); jonas.rosendahl@uk-halle.de (J.R.)
† These authors contributed equally to this work.

Simple Summary: Pancreatic cancer remains one of the deadliest malignancies. This review summarizes preclinical mouse models in early pancreatic cancer research, focusing on genetically engineered models ranging from transgenic to inducible gene editing approaches. These models offer diverse platforms for deciphering carcinogenesis mechanisms and testing therapeutic strategies. We emphasize their applications in investigating environmental risk factors, aiming to provide researchers with a better understanding of their utility and limitations in translational pancreatic cancer research.

Abstract: Pancreatic cancer is characterized by late diagnosis, therapy resistance, and poor prognosis, necessitating the exploration of early carcinogenesis and prevention methods. Preclinical mouse models have evolved from cell line-based to human tumor tissue- or organoid-derived xenografts, now to humanized mouse models and genetically engineered mouse models (GEMMs). GEMMs, primarily driven by oncogenic Kras mutations and tumor suppressor gene alterations, offer a realistic platform for investigating pancreatic cancer initiation, progression, and metastasis. The incorporation of inducible somatic mutations and CRISPR-Cas9 screening methods has expanded their utility. To better recapitulate tumor initiation triggered by inflammatory cues, common pancreatic risk factors are being integrated into model designs. This approach aims to decipher the role of environmental factors as secondary or parallel triggers of tumor initiation alongside oncogenic burdens. Emerging models exploring pancreatitis, obesity, diabetes, and other risk factors offer significant translational potential. This review describes current mouse models for studying pancreatic carcinogenesis, their combination with inflammatory factors, and their utility in evaluating pathogenesis, providing guidance for selecting the most suitable models for pancreatic cancer research.

Keywords: genetically engineered mouse models; pancreatic cancer; carcinogenesis; risk factors; pancreatitis; obesity; diabetes

1. Introduction

Pancreatic cancer remains a tremendous challenge in oncology, ranking the third leading cause of cancer deaths [1]. Despite modest improvements in recent years, the 5-year relative survival rate for pancreatic cancer stands at 13%. Pancreatic ductal adenocarcinoma (PDAC), the most prevalent type of pancreatic cancer, is characterized by its aggressive nature, lack of early detection methods, and an immunosuppressive tumor microenvironment [2,3]. These factors contribute to a narrow therapeutic window, underscoring the critical need for research focused on risk factors and early carcinogenesis. Understanding the key genetic and environmental risk factors that drive pancreatic cancer development is essential for improving early detection strategies, prevention approaches, and treatment outcomes.

Epidemiological studies have identified several well-established risk factors for pancreatic cancer, including both modifiable lifestyle/environmental factors and non-modifiable factors such as age and genetic predisposition [4] (Figure 1). Among the modifiable factors, smoking is one of the most significant with the highest risk observed in heavy smokers compared to non-smokers, and the elevated risk persists for at least 10 years after cessation [5]. Alcohol consumption is also associated with increased risk, either through direct genotoxic effects on the pancreas or indirectly via the induction of pancreatitis [6]. Pancreatitis, particularly chronic pancreatitis, significantly elevates pancreatic cancer risk, with acute pancreatitis also contributing to short-term risk within the first three years after diagnosis [7,8]. Furthermore, obesity is another major modifiable risk factor, often associated with poor prognosis and treatment outcomes in pancreatic cancer patients [9,10]. Obesity-induced insulin resistance can lead to type 2 diabetes, which—along with non-obese diabetes—is a recognized risk factor. Infections with pathogens such as Hepatitis B and C viruses and Helicobacter pylori have also been implicated in pancreatic cancer development, suggesting a role for microbiome alterations in disease progression [11,12].

In addition to modifiable factors, non-modifiable contributors also play a significant role. Aging is strongly associated with pancreatic cancer incidence, with most PDAC diagnoses occurring between 60 and 80 years of age [13]. The accumulation of oncogenic mutations over time, along with inherited genetic predispositions, further increases susceptibility.

Understanding how these risk factors influence the molecular progression of pancreatic carcinogenesis is critical. Pancreatic carcinogenesis typically progresses through a series of sequential steps, often beginning with acinar-to-ductal metaplasia (ADM), which is initially reversible [14]. However, with persistent inflammation or injury, as induced by the risk factors described above, ADM can progress to premalignant pancreatic intraepithelial neoplasias (PanINs). These PanINs are graded from low-grade (PanIN-1 and PanIN-2) to high-grade (PanIN-3) lesions, which can ultimately develop into invasive PDAC [15]. This progression is induced or accompanied by the accumulation of genetic alterations, including activating mutations in the *Kras* oncogene (in >90% of PDAC cases) and inactivation of tumor suppressor genes such as *CDKN2A*, *TP53*, and *SMAD4* [16]. Alternative precursor lesions, including intraductal papillary mucinous neoplasms (IPMNs) and mucinous cystic neoplasms (MCNs), represent additional routes to PDAC [17].

While existing preclinical mouse models have significantly advanced our understanding of pancreatic tumor biology and therapy, many fail to accurately replicate the early events of tumorigenesis or to include risk factors [18]. Traditional xenograft models using established cell lines typically represent advanced disease states and lack the immune components [19] (Figure 2A). Patient-derived xenografts (PDXs) and patient-derived organoid xenografts (PDOXs) have further improved the retention of parental tumor features such as heterogeneity, but they also rely on immunodeficient hosts and fail to replicate PDAC development in the context of native inflammatory and immune environment [20] (Figure 2B). To better capture tumor–immune dynamics, humanized mouse models, syngeneic models, and GEMMs have been developed. Humanized mouse models, lacking B, T, and NK cell activities, allow the engraftment of human tumor tissue and immune cells, thereby restoring some human-specific immune–tumor interactions while retaining interpatient tumor heterogeneity (Figure 2C). These models, however, exhibit mismatched stromal environments and do not recapitulate de novo tumor initiation [21,22]. Syngeneic models, involving the implantation of Panc02 [23] or $Kras^{G12D}$; $Trp53^{R172H}$; *Pdx-1-Cre* (KPC)-derived cell lines into immunocompetent mice, allow for the study of tumor-immune interactions in genetically matched hosts [24] (Figure 2D). Nevertheless, these models remain implantation-based and genetically uniform. In contrast, GEMMs support spontaneous tumor initiation and progression, capturing dynamic tumor–stroma–immune interactions. Yet, they are typically based on engineered mutations and may not incorporate the full spectrum of environmental, metabolic, or inflammatory factors that drive human disease. Constructing GEMMs can be labor-intensive and costly, requiring specialized equipment and expertise, and the success rate of generating GEMMs can also vary depending on the specific genetic alterations and the strain of mice used [25]. Despite these challenges, GEMMs remain a cornerstone of PDAC research, offering valuable insights into the molecular mechanisms of PDAC, particularly when used in conjunction with relevant risk factors.

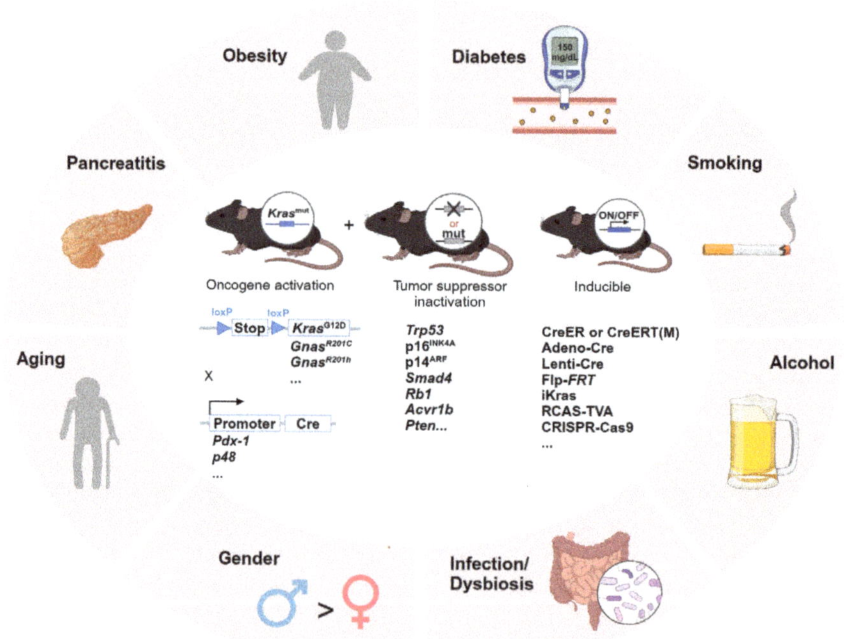

Figure 1. Integrating environmental risk factors into pancreatic carcinogenesis research using GEMMs. Summary of the commonly investigated environmental risk factors in PDAC research and GEMMs of transgenic or inducible oncogene activation and/or tumor suppressor gene inactivation. Adeno-Cre: adenoviral-Cre; Lenti-Cre: lentiviral-Cre; Flp-FRT: flippase-FRT; iKras: doxycycline-inducible Kras; RCAS: replication-competent avian sarcoma-leukosis virus long terminal repeat with splice acceptor; TVA: tumor virus A; CRISPR: clustered regularly interspaced short palindromic repeats; Cas9: CRISPR-associated 9.

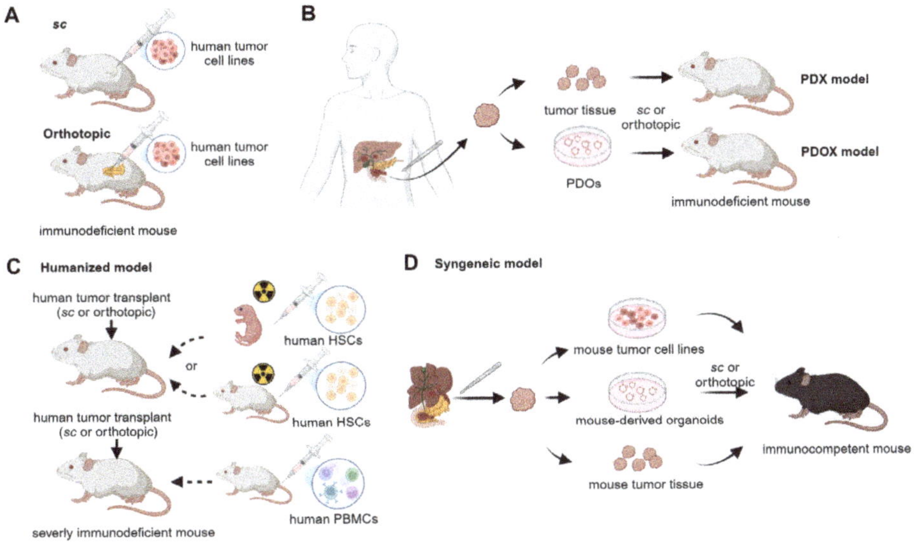

Figure 2. Transplantation-based mouse models studying PDAC. (**A**) Subcutaneous (*sc*) and orthotopic models are generated in immunodeficient mice through the injection of tumor cells under the skin and into the pancreas, respectively. (**B**) Immunocompromised mice are transplanted either subcutaneously or orthotopically with human tumor tissues for PDX (patient-derived xenografts) models or with PDOs (patient-derived organoids) for PDOX (patient-derived organoid xenografts) models. (**C**) Humanized mouse models are developed by first injecting peripheral blood mononuclear cells (PBMCs) into an adult severely immunodeficient mouse or by first engrafting hematopoietic stem cells (HSCs) into irradiated neonatal or adult severely immunodeficient mice. Then, the mice are transplanted with human tumor tissues (cell line, PDX, PDOX, etc.). (**D**) Syngeneic mouse models are generated by injecting mouse tumor materials subcutaneously or orthotopically. These materials include cell lines, PDX (patient-derived xenografts), and PDOX (patient-derived orthotopic xenografts) developed from mouse tumors.

This review aims to provide an overview of the most widely used and promising GEMMs in pancreatic carcinogenesis, with a further emphasis on their applications in studying modifiable risk factors such as pancreatitis, obesity, and diabetes, which represent major modifiable risk factors for human PDAC. Additionally, we will explore the cutting-edge engineering methods including genome-wide and targeted CRISPR screening methods that have expanded the utility of animal models, enabling more precise and comprehensive studies of pancreatic cancer biology.

2. GEMMs

GEMMs have been instrumental in elucidating the mechanisms of PDAC initiation and progression. While comprehensive overviews of existing GEMMs are available elsewhere [26,27], here we briefly highlight the most relevant models that form the basis for studying genetic changes in PDAC, especially those that can later be used to explore how risk factors affect the disease.

Pioneering animal studies first utilized the elastase (EL) promoter controlled SV40 T-antigen [28], c-H-*ras* [29], Myc [30], and TGF-α [31] to study the roles of these genes during early cancer development. Among these, only TGF-α activation can induce ADM followed by fibrosis and eventually advanced PDAC, while the other genes primarily affect acinar cells. Moreover, these mice did not develop PDAC through well-defined PanIN. The discovery that *KRAS* mutations—especially the G12D isoform—occur in over

90% of PanIN-1 lesions [32] and increase with disease stage led to the development of the Lox-Stop-Lox (LSL)-*Kras*$^{G12D/+}$ model (KC mice), controlled by Cre recombinase under pancreas-specific promoter *Pdx-1* or *p48* (*Ptf1a*) [33]. This model faithfully recapitulates human PanIN progression with the PanIN-1 lesions appearing by 8 weeks of age but rarely advances to invasive PDAC without additional genetic events or environmental stimulus.

Concomitant expression of heterozygous *Trp53*^{R172H} and *Kras*^{G12D} in the mouse pancreas, known as the KPC model, induce invasive and widely metastatic PDAC [34], while mice with homozygous *Trp53* mutations (KPPC) develop more aggressive tumors with faster growth and shorter survival [35]. In contrast, mice with *Trp53* depletion and *Kras*$^{G12D/+}$ develop similar PanIN lesions and tumor stages as KPC mice but show significantly less metastasis [36]. Other combinations, such as *Rb1* loss [37] or *Ink4a/Arf* deletion [38] with *Kras*^{G12D}, also result in aggressive tumorigenesis due to the disruption of cell cycle regulation pathways.

Notably, concomitant deletion of *Smad4* with mutant *Kras*^{G12D} promotes tumor progression via IPMN/MCN lesions [39]. This SMAD4-dependent phenotype may be influenced by TGF-β superfamily ligands such as activin, as loss of activin receptor 1B (ACVR1B) accelerates IPMN-to-PDAC progression in the context of oncogenic *Kras* [40]. Interestingly, inactivation of TGFβR2, an upstream receptor of SMAD4, also enhances PanIN and PDAC development in a SMAD4-independent manner [41]. While TGF-β generally acts as a tumor suppressor, it may shift to a tumor-promoting role during later stages through interaction with the stroma, underscoring the complex and context-dependent role of TGF-β signaling in PDAC [42]. Similarly, *Gnas* gain-of-function mutation (R201C [43] or R201H [44]) induces low-grade IPMN that, when combined with oncogenic *Kras*, results in accelerated progression to invasive PDAC.

GEMMs also serve as valuable platforms for evaluating therapeutic strategies targeting the tumor microenvironment in PDAC. For example, stromal depletion through sonic hedgehog (SHH) loss [45] or αSMA+ myofibroblast ablation [46] enhances tumor aggressiveness in the background of oncogenic *Kras*, challenging classical views of the stroma as predominantly tumor-promoting [47]. Moreover, GEMMs enable preclinical testing of immunotherapies, such as checkpoint inhibitors (α-CTLA-4 and α-PD-L1) [48], as well as combination therapies (e.g., gemcitabine plus VEGFR/EGFR inhibitors [26]), which have shown encouraging outcomes. These models are thus critical for translating mechanistic findings into therapeutic advances, as reviewed in depth by Gopinathan et al. [49].

Although GEMMs may not fully capture the high mutation burden and abundant neoantigens seen in human PDAC, they offer unique advantages in modeling specific genetic alterations and their functional consequences. Importantly, these models serve as the foundation for incorporating various environmental and physiological risk factors, which will be discussed in detail in the following sections.

3. Inducible Somatic Gene Editing Models

To more closely mimic the somatic mutations that temporally occur in human pancreatic cancer, different inducible somatic mutation models prompt special tools to control gene expression. One of the most commonly applied tools is the inducible Cre system. The CreER system or the advanced version CreERT(M) utilizes a fusion of Cre recombinase with a modified estrogen receptor that allows tamoxifen-inducible Cre activity. Lee et al. used *Kras*$^{LSL\text{-}G12D}$; *Trp53*$^{flox/flox}$; *Sox9*^{CreERTM} and *Kras*$^{LSL\text{-}G12D}$; *Trp53*$^{flox/flox}$; *Ptf1a*^{CreERTM} to manipulate the gene expressions of adult mice in ductal and acinar cells, respectively, and found that ductal cells are more primed readily to form carcinoma upon oncogenic *Kras* and *Trp53* deletion, while acinar cells require longer period and develop from widespread low-grade PanINs to PDAC [50]. To model PDAC-induced cachexia, *Kras*$^{G12D/+}$; *Ptf1a*$^{ER\text{-}Cre/+}$;

Pten$^{flox/flox}$ (KPP) mice were generated with controlled activation of oncogenic *Kras* and *Pten* depletion post-natally. The mice developed moderate PDAC and also exhibited a progressive wasting phenotype that closely mimics human PDAC-associated cachexia [51]. The Cre recombinase can also be delivered by retrograde pancreatic ductal injection of both adenoviral-Cre (Adeno-Cre) and lentiviral-Cre (Lenti-Cre) vectors to activate the LSL-*Kras*^{G12D} allele in the pancreas [52].

An alternative time- and host-specific recombination system that can be used alongside or instead of Cre-lox is flippase-*FRT* (Flp-*FRT*) [53]. In the *FSF-Kras$^{G12D/++}$; FSF-R26$^{CAG-CreERT2/++}$; Trp53$^{flox/flox}$; Pdx1-Flp* mice, under the control of Pdx1-Flip, oncogenic *Kras* and CreERTM can be induced in the pancreas. After Tamoxifen administration, Cre functions to deplete *Trp53* by the Cre-loxP system. This dual-recombinase system can also be applied to study the tumor microenvironment. For example, in *FSF-Kras$^{G12D/+}$; Trp53$^{frt/frt}$; Pdx1-Flp; αSMA-Cre; Col1a1$^{flox/flox}$* mice, oncogenic *Kras* is controlled by Flp-*FRT* in the pancreas and the Col1a1 is depleted in the myofibroblasts, allowing for more sophisticated spatial genetic manipulations [54].

Additionally, the doxycycline-inducible *Kras* system (iKras) allows for temporary control of the gene expression. Collins et al. generated triple transgenic R26-rtTa-IRES-EGFP; TetO-*Kras^{G12D}*; *p48*-Cre mice [55]. Upon doxycycline administration, the reverse tetracycline transactivator (rtTa)-doxycycline complex, which is specifically expressed in the pancreas controlled by p48-Cre, binds to the tetracycline-responsive element (TRE), allowing downstream *Kras^{G12D}* expression. They found that inactivation of *Kras^{G12D}* in established precursor lesions resulted in regression of these lesions, demonstrating that sustained *Kras^{G12D}* expression is essential for tumor maintenance.

The avian sarcoma-leukosis virus-A-derived vector, namely RCAS (replication-competent avian sarcoma-leukosis virus long terminal repeat with splice acceptor), can deliver cDNA, shRNAs, non-coding RNAs, or CRISPR components to tumor virus A (TVA)-expressing cells under the control of promoters like elastase [56]. The RCAS-TVA system allows for versatile gene delivery in transgenic mice expressing the TVA receptor. In *LSL-Kras^{G12D}; Ptf1a-cre; elastase-tva* mice, injected DF1 chicken fibroblasts producing RCAS-*Wnt1*, -*GFP*, or -*β-catenin^{S37A}* selectively control Wnt signaling in pancreatic tissues already primed for oncogenic *Kras* expression [57]. This approach provides the flexibility to combine multiple genetic alterations for investigating various molecular mechanisms.

CRISPR-based somatic genome engineering has emerged as a powerful method for modeling PDAC with the advantage of increased speed, flexibility, and cost-effectiveness. Two main delivery methods have been developed for in vivo CRISPR editing in PDAC models: viral and non-viral approaches [58]. Viral delivery systems, particularly adeno-associated viruses (AAVs), have been widely adopted. In one common approach, *Kras$^{LSL-G12D}$; Rosa26$^{CAG-LSL-Cas9}$; Ptf1a^{Cre}* mice express oncogenic *Kras*^{G12D} and Cas9 specifically in pancreatic cells. Researchers can then deliver vectors encoding sgRNAs by using self-complementary AAV targeting genes of interest, such as *Trp53*, via retrograde pancreatic ductal injection. Non-viral delivery methods, such as pancreas electroporation, offer an alternative approach with potentially reduced immunogenicity and larger cargo capacity [58]. In this technique, plasmid DNA encoding *Cas9* and sgRNAs is directly introduced into pancreatic cells through electrical pulses. The choice of plasmids often depends on the specific experimental design. In mice that already express Cas9 (e.g., *Rosa26$^{CAG-LSL-Cas9}$* strains), only sgRNAs need to be delivered. Conversely, in wild-type mice, vectors containing both *Cas9* and sgRNAs should be used. These CRISPR-based approaches have significantly accelerated PDAC research, allowing for rapid screening of potential tumor suppressors and oncogenes. The in vivo CRISPR screening method will be further reviewed in the following sections.

4. CRISPR-Cas9 Screening Models

CRISPR-Cas9-based genetic screening is a powerful tool for high-throughput functional genomics. Typically, sgRNA libraries are delivered via lentiviral vectors alongside Cas9 to induce gene knockouts in cell populations, with proliferation-based drop-out assays used to identify fitness or drug-sensitivity genes (Figure 3A) [59–61]. While informative, such systems lack the complexity of in vivo tumor biology. To address this limitation, CRISPR screening has been adapted to in vivo models, where transplantation-based approaches introduce perturbed cell pools derived from xenografts or established lines into host animals, offering a level of robustness comparable to in vitro systems [62–64] (Figure 3B). This enables assessment of gene function under physiological conditions and has revealed both conserved and context-specific metabolic dependencies. For example, in vivo screens, compared with in vitro screens, have identified genes regulating heme metabolism, oxidative phosphorylation, nucleotide synthesis, and antigen presentation as crucial for tumor formation [65]. Additionally, immune profiling using immunocompetent versus immunodeficient mice identified interferon-γ (IFNγ) as a key mediator of immune evasion and tumor suppression in pancreatic cancer [66]. Drug-assisted in vivo CRISPR screens using this platform have also uncovered targets that enhance the efficacy of gemcitabine or MEK inhibition, highlighting its therapeutic relevance [67].

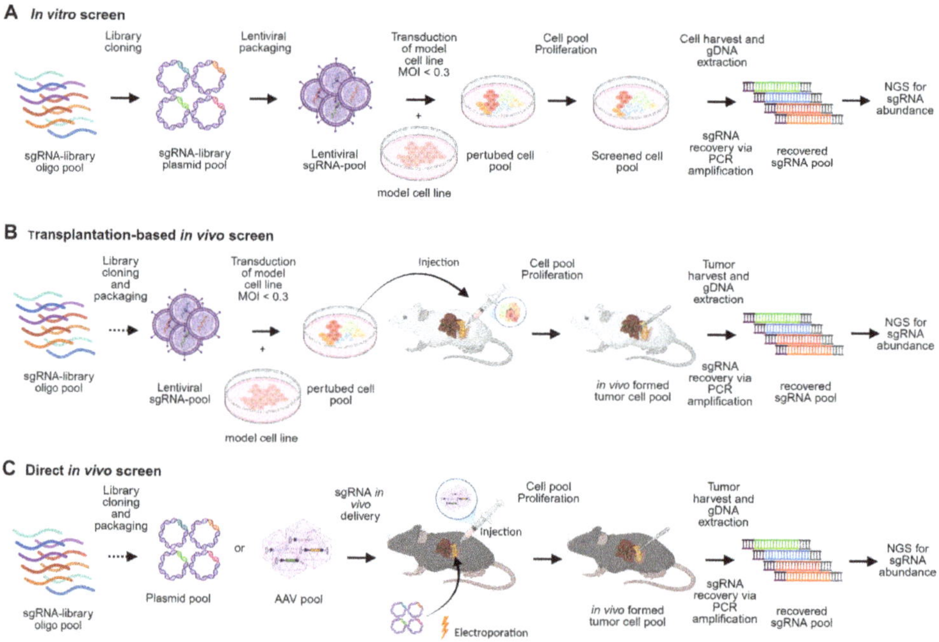

Figure 3. Screening methods in PDAC research. (**A**) CRISPR in vitro screening begins with cloning an sgRNA pool into a library, which is used to produce a lentiviral pool. The model cell line is transduced at a multiplicity of infection (MOI) < 0.3 to ensure only one sgRNA integrates per cell. The perturbed cell pool is then expanded for the required number of doublings, followed by genomic DNA extraction and PCR amplification of sgRNA sequences to determine their abundance. (**B**) For in vivo screens using transplantation-based methods, the perturbed cell pool is injected intravenously, subcutaneously, or orthotopically into the host model. (**C**) Alternatively, somatic in vivo screening methods deliver sgRNA libraries directly into pancreatic tissue through electroporation or AAV injection. In both cases, tumor formation is monitored, and sgRNA abundance is analyzed post-harvest.

More recently, somatic CRISPR screening using GEMMs has enabled direct analysis of gene function during tumor initiation (Figure 3C). In these models, sgRNA libraries are delivered via electroporation or AAV into pancreatic tissue, allowing in situ gene editing within a native microenvironment [68]. For instance, a recent study used an in vivo screening method with an adeno-associated virus-sgRNA library targeting 125 recurrently mutated PDAC genes [69]. Using KC mice with inducible Kras and Cas9-GFP, the study identified accelerated tumor formation upon Cas9-mediated knockout of suppressor genes such as *Cdkn2a*, *Rnf43*, and *Fbxw7*, validating the somatic screen's effectiveness in phenotyping relevant PanIN development hits. Notably, novel tumor progression regulators, SCAF1 and USP15, were discovered, shown to be suppressive in pancreatic tumorigenesis. These findings significantly contribute to understanding early PDAC carcinogenesis mechanisms, providing more insights into key regulators and pathways like TGF-β regulation, MAPK signaling, and NF-κB signaling. Although this method is pivotal for addressing tumor suppressors in early PDAC development, the library size was limited due to constraints such as viral titer and transduction efficiency. To ensure each cell received only one sgRNA and to maintain statistical robustness, infection efficiencies were optimized at low levels, which inherently restricted the number of sgRNAs that could be screened.

Emerging systems like organoids, either directly cultured from patient tissue such as IPMNs [70] or derived from induced pluripotent stem cells (iPSCs) [71], offer advantages over traditional 2D cell culture by better mimicking cancer heterogeneity, making them clinically relevant for transplantation-based screening methods. However, challenges such as sgRNA efficiency, clonal heterogeneity [72], and variability in transduction efficiency and proliferation among clones [73] lead to high false-positive rates. While such approaches hold promise for functional studies, they are not yet established for pancreatic or iPSC-derived organoids. Furthermore, most in vivo screens rely on CRISPR/Cas9 or RNAi, but the rapidly expanding CRISPR toolbox offers even greater potential. Emerging technologies such as CRISPR interference (CRISPRi), CRISPR activation (CRISPRa) [74], and prime editing [75], which allows precise base conversion without double-strand breaks, enable refined modulation of gene function. Additionally, CRISPR base editing has been applied in PDAC models to correct oncogenic *KRAS* mutations in organoids and cell lines, offering a potential tool for early intervention [76]. TALENs (transcription activator-like effector nucleases), though less widely used in PDAC research, remain a valuable alternative for precise gene editing, particularly when off-target minimization is critical [77]. Alternative CRISPR systems such as Cas12 [78] and Cas13 [79] also hold promise for refined gene regulation studies in vivo. Additionally, applying CRISPR screening to in vivo models that incorporate risk factors such as pancreatitis, obesity, or diabetes as discussed in the flowing sections could provide valuable insights into early PDAC carcinogenesis.

5. Risk Factor: Pancreatitis

Pancreatitis is a well-established risk factor for pancreatic cancer [80,81]. While evidence regarding acute pancreatitis (AP) as a risk factor remains inconsistent [8,82], numerous studies have shown that chronic pancreatitis (CP) is particularly significant in increasing the risk of PDAC [83–85]. CP is a complex disease influenced by factors such as smoking [86], alcohol abuse [87], pancreatic duct obstruction [88], autoimmunity [89], and genetic mutations [90–92]. Hereditary CP typically begins with recurrent episodes of AP that progress to CP over 10–15 years, significantly increasing the risk of PDAC in affected individuals by creating a chronic inflammatory microenvironment. This hereditary form, often caused by mutations in genes encoding protease serine 1 (PRSS1), chymotrypsin C (CTRC), serine protease inhibitor Kazal type 1 (SPINK1), and/or carboxypeptidase A1

(CPA1), serves as a genetic background for studying the mechanisms underlying pancreatitis and its progression to PDAC.

The p.R122H mutation in the *PRSS1* gene that encodes the human cationic trypsinogen is the first reported mutation that was identified in hereditary CP [90]. In the subsequent years, several mutations like the p.N21I [93] and p.A16V [94,95] in the *PRSS1* gene were also linked to hereditary CP. All these mutations lead to elevated levels of intrapancreatic trypsin that causes damage to the organ. Trypsin is produced and secreted by the pancreas in an inactive form called trypsinogen. Trypsinogen is converted to the active form by proteolysis of its activation peptide. This proteolysis occurs by enterokinase or trypsin itself. However, mutations in trypsinogen or the effector proteins of the protective mechanisms can disturb the homeostasis and lead to pancreatitis. Several studies also reported that increased autoactivation of trypsinogen is the underlying mechanism of action for other cationic trypsinogen mutations [96,97]. The first transgenic mouse model expressing the PRSS1 mutant p.R122H was generated by Archer et al., mimicking key features of human pancreatitis, including acinar cell damage, fibrosis, and inflammation [98]. However, the penetrance of the p.R122H mutation in this model was only 40%, compared to 80% in hereditary pancreatitis patients. Another model system, developed by Athwal et al. [99], expressed human PRSS1 wild-type protein or mutants (p.R122H and p.N29I), predisposing mice to pancreatitis. Upon stimulation with low-dose cerulein, these mice progressed to PDAC. Additionally, mutations that increase trypsinogen autoactivation, such as p.D23A [100] and p.D22N/K24R [101], have been used to generate mouse models that replicate hallmarks of pancreatitis, including inflammatory cell infiltration and acinar cell necrosis. These preclinical models provide valuable tools for studying pancreatitis and early steps of PDAC.

In humans, mutations in the *CTRC* gene are strongly associated with chronic pancreatitis [102,103]. Under normal physiological conditions, CTRC protects against pancreatitis by degrading intrapancreatic trypsinogen. Loss-of-function mutations in CTRC impair this protective mechanism, increasing susceptibility to pancreatitis. Interestingly, C57BL/6N mice naturally lack CTRC expression, with chymotrypsin B1 (CTRB1) serving as the major chymotrypsin isoform in these mice. Using CRISPR-Cas9 technology, Jancsó et al. [104] generated a *Ctrb1*-deficient mouse model, which exhibited more severe cerulein-induced pancreatitis compared to controls due to elevated intrapancreatic trypsin activation. These findings highlight the critical role of chymotrypsin in maintaining protease homeostasis in the pancreas.

Another defense strategy of the pancreas against trypsinogen autoactivation is the enzyme SPINK1, which inactivates prematurely activated trypsin and protects against pancreatitis [105]. Over 20 SPINK1 variants have been reported, with the p.N34S mutation being the most frequent [91]. Given SPINK1's critical role in the human pancreas, several mouse models have been developed to elucidate its mechanisms and explore its potential as a therapeutic target. It is important to note that the mouse ortholog of human SPINK1 shares 63% amino acid sequence identity with the human protein, while rats possess homologous proteins known as pancreatic secretory trypsin inhibitors I and II (PSTI-I and -II) [106]. While *Spink1*-null mice (previously referred to as Spink3-null) did not survive beyond two weeks [107], heterozygous *Spink1*-deficient mice exhibited reduced SPINK1 expression without altered susceptibility to transient cerulein-induced pancreatitis. However, recent studies demonstrated that prolonged cerulein hyperstimulation in *Spink1-KO^{het}* mice led to hallmarks of acute pancreatitis, underscoring SPINK1's protective role in trypsin-dependent pancreatitis [108]. Furthermore, when crossed with trypsinogen mutant strains (T7D23A or T7D22N/K24R), which spontaneously develop CP, *Spink1-KO^{het}* mice exhibited accelerated CP progression, suggesting that even slightly reduced SPINK1 levels can exacerbate CP development [108]. These findings underscore SPINK1's significance as a disease modifier in pancreatitis and its potential relevance to therapeutic strategies.

Recent studies have shown that CP can also occur through mechanisms independent of trypsin-dependent pathways. The second most abundant enzyme in pancreatic juice, procarboxypeptidase A1 (proCPA1) [109], is activated to its functional form, CPA1, by trypsin and CTRC [110]. DNA sequencing of 944 individuals with CP showed that loss-of-function CPA1 variants play a role in the development of CP. Forty-one percent of individuals with functionally impaired CPA1 variants carried the c.768C > G (p.Asn256Lys) mutation [92]. In 2019, a mouse model that recapitulated CPA1-associated CP was developed [111]. Experiments using this model demonstrated that misfolding of the mutant CPA1 protein induces endoplasmic reticulum (ER) stress, leading to CP. Importantly, this model differs from trypsin-dependent models by highlighting ER stress as a distinct mechanism in CP pathogenesis, underscoring the complexity of the disease and the need to investigate multiple molecular pathways.

Cerulein, a cholecystokinin analogue, is the most commonly used agent to induce acute or chronic pancreatitis in rodents. The severity of pancreatic damage in cerulein-induced models is directly proportional to the dose and duration of administration, making it a reproducible and widely used experimental system. Studies by Guerra et al. indicate that activation of oncogenic $Kras^{G12V}$ in adult acinar cells alone does not lead to PDAC; however, pretreatment with cerulein to induce CP results in PDAC development, suggesting that cerulein sensitizes the pancreas for tumorigenesis [112]. Nonetheless, a major drawback of cerulein-induced mouse models is that they do not represent the clinical situation, where various factors such as alcohol abuse, gallstones, or genetic predisposition contribute to pancreatitis.

Several important factors must be considered when selecting a mouse model to study the role of CP in PDAC. The model should faithfully replicate the stages of human disease and allow disease induction with minimal artificial intervention. For instance, mouse models that develop pancreatitis while harboring genetic predispositions to PDAC provide a more patient-relevant platform. It is also important to note that early steps of PDAC and CP share similar histopathological features such as ADM and inflammatory cell infiltration, and hence these mouse models offer the opportunity to understand the different stages of the diseases in a context-dependent manner. Furthermore, CP and PDAC develop over years in humans, involving mutation accumulation, DNA damage, and neoplastic lesion formation. Mouse models offer the advantage of recapitulating these processes under controlled conditions, enabling comprehensive studies of genetic and environmental influences on disease progression. Combining the described genetic or chemically induced pancreatitis models with well-established cancer models, such as inducible $Kras^{\mathrm{G12D}}$ mice, can enhance our understanding of CP as a risk factor for PDAC and provide insights into the molecular mechanisms driving this progression.

6. Risk Factor: Obesity

Obesity is a chronic disease characterized by abnormal and excessive fat accumulation, posing significant health risks worldwide. Since 1990, adult obesity rates have more than doubled, while adolescent obesity has quadrupled globally, contributing to a growing public health crisis [113]. A hallmark of obesity is hypertrophic and dysfunctional adipose tissue, which acts not only as an energy storage depot but also as an endocrine and immunologically active organ [114]. By releasing adipokines, it influences both local microenvironments and distant organs systemically [115]. Consequently, obesity is associated with systemic and chronic low-grade inflammation [116].

Over recent decades, obesity has been identified as a significant risk factor for numerous chronic diseases, including cardiovascular conditions, type 2 diabetes, and various cancers such as PDAC [9,117,118]. Additionally, obesity elevates the risk of developing pancreatic precancerous lesions [119]. Preclinical studies suggest several mechanisms by which obesity promotes pancreatic tumorigenesis, including hyperinsulinaemia and insulin resistance, hyperglycaemia, inflammation, altered cellular metabolism, hormone dysregulation, cellular stress, microbial dysbiosis, as well as activation of oncogenic drivers [120–122] (Figure 4A).

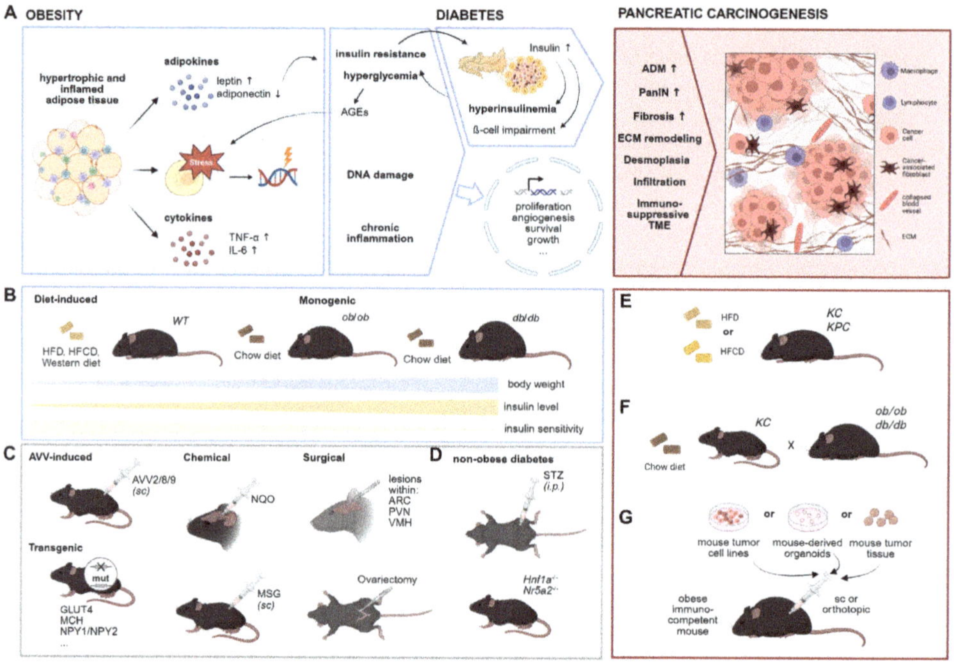

Figure 4. Animal models to investigate the impact of obesity on PDAC. (**A**) Selected hypothesized links between obesity and early pancreatic carcinogenesis. Dysfunctional adipose tissue results in cellular stress and altered hormone and cytokine secretion causing DNA damage and a status of chronic inflammation, respectively (**left**). Obesity can further result in diabetes (**middle**) in which insulin resistance causes increased insulin production within pancreatic islets, which in turn leads to hyperinsulinaemia and β-cell impairment. The resulting hyperglycaemia promotes the generation of advanced glycation end products (AGEs) which further fuel cellular stress. The mentioned links may promote altered gene expression of processes associated with carcinogenesis, promoting features of early pancreatic carcinogenesis (**right**). ADM: acinar to ductal metaplasia, PanIN: pancreatic intraepithelial neoplasia, ECM: extracellular matrix, TME: tumor microenvironment. (**B**) Common obesity mouse models. HFD: high-fat diet, HFCD: high-fat, high-calorie diet. (**C**) Additional models to induce obesity in rodents. AVV: adeno-associated virus vector, *sc*: subcutaneous, NQO: 4-nitroquinoline 1-oxide, MSG: monosodium glutamate, ARC: arcuate nucleus, PVN: paraventricular nucleus, VMH: ventromedial hypothalamus. (**D**) Mouse models to induce non-obese diabetes. STZ: streptozotocin, *i.p.*: intraperitoneal (**E**) Combination of genetic obesity and PDAC models. (**F**) Diet-induced obesity in PDAC mouse models. (**G**) Syngeneic models to investigate tumor progression in the context of obesity.

Numerous murine obesity models have been studied in this context [123] and reviewed in detail by Kfoury et al., among others [123–126]. The most commonly used models are genetically engineered or diet-induced obesity (DIO) models (Figure 4B). For example, the *ob/ob* and *db/db* mice are monogenic models that represent mutations in the leptin gene or its receptor, respectively. These mutations lead to hyperphagia, resulting in severe early-onset obesity and, in the case of *db/db* mice, diabetes [127]. The *ob/ob* mice exhibit impaired glucose tolerance and insulin sensitivity reflecting a more pre-diabetic stage, whereas *db/db* mice are insulin resistant and display hyperinsulinemia as well as hyperleptinaemia. Obesity can also be modeled using other approaches, including nutritional, surgical, chemical, and AAV methods (Figure 4C), which differ from non-obese diabetes models (Figure 4D) that will be discussed in the following section.

To investigate the effect of obesity on pancreatic carcinogenesis, recent studies have combined obesity models with PDAC models. For instance, crossing *ob/ob* mice with KC mice generates KCO mice (Figure 4E) [128], which develop early-onset obesity and show increased pancreatic tumor burden. Chung et al. have detailed the impact of obesity on early pancreatic carcinogenesis and demonstrated that weight loss—induced either by caloric restriction or exogenous AAV-leptin administration—can reverse these effects [128]. They also identified an endocrine–exocrine signaling pathway involving cholecystokinin derived from stressed β-cells in pancreatic islets, highlighting local obesity-associated changes as pivotal in early pancreatic carcinogenesis. However, several studies have highlighted leptin as an adipokine with both systemic and obesity-independent effects, acting as a potent anti-apoptotic, proliferative, and inflammatory agent [129,130], which significantly influences the immune response [131,132] and thus may directly impact tumorigenesis. In vitro studies further showed that leptin increases the migratory capacity of pancreatic cancer cells [133–135]. Given these findings, models based on modifications in leptin signaling, such as *ob/ob* mice, may not accurately reflect the microenvironment of pre-neoplastic lesions or pancreatic cancer. Additionally, *db/db* mice are less suitable for studying obesity-related pancreatic carcinogenesis due to confounding effects from diabetes. Non-diabetic obesity models are therefore recommended to ensure more accurate results.

Another commonly used model to investigate obesity-related effects on pancreatic carcinogenesis is the DIO model (Figure 4F). These models involve feeding wild-type or transgenic mice high-caloric diets, resulting in a slower onset of obesity compared to *ob/ob* and *db/db* mice, which more closely mimics the human pathogenesis of obesity. Chronic high-fat diet (HFD) consumption in mice leads to glucose intolerance, impaired insulin sensitivity, and enhanced β-cell mass and proliferation [136–139], reflecting a pre-diabetic stage that progressively worsens over time. Several studies have demonstrated that HFD-induced obesity promotes pancreatic cancer development in KC and KPC mice [122,128,140–144]. HFD has been shown to increase inflammation, fibrosis, and PanIN lesions while accelerating progression into more aggressive PDAC [122,140,144,145]. Notably, it has been suggested that HFD contributes to pancreatic cancer not only through obesity and pre-diabetes but also by directly affecting carcinogenic processes [146]. However, the HFD of these studies varied in composition, fatty acid (FA) ratio, and duration and onset of intervention. Ead et al. reported that feeding KC mice an HFD with 60% of calories from fat (based on lard; 9:1 n-6:n-3 FA ratio) resulted in only mild effects on early pancreatic ADM without cancer development [142]. In contrast, a high-fat, high-calorie diet with 40% of calories from corn oil (50:1 n-6:n-3 FA ratio) in KC mice led to more advanced PanIN lesions [144] and tumor development already at an age of 3 months [141]. Furthermore, KPC mice fed a HFD (60% calories from fat; source: beef tallow and safflower oil) developed larger primary tumors and exhibited higher metastatic rates [143]. Compared to HFD, a high-carbohydrate diet displayed lower tumorigenic potential, while a high-protein diet was comparable to a normal diet [147]. These findings emphasize the significance of factors such as calorie percentage from fat, fat source, and n-6:n-3 FA ratio in influencing the obese phenotype and metabolic signaling linked to pancreatic carcinogenesis [121].

Additionally, when interpreting results from DIO models, researchers must consider confounding variables such as housing conditions, microbiome composition, age, gender, and feeding duration.

An alternative experimental design involves combining KC mice with gene therapy, where AAV vectors (AVV2/9/8) [140,148–150] are injected into the adipose tissue to induce obesity. Using this strategy, the precise timing of obesity induction based on the experimental design can be controlled, thereby avoiding undesired effects on embryonic development and hormone-related processes [126].

Since in humans, obesity develops gradually over time and pancreatic cancer-driving mutations typically occur in adulthood, GEMMs for PDAC that present mutations from birth may not accurately replicate human disease pathogenesis, especially when combining two GEMMs (e.g., KCO mice). Therefore, inducing pancreatic carcinogenesis in pre-existing obesity models by inducible oncogene mutations [151] or orthotopic implantation models—using PDAC cells, organoids [152] or tumor xeno-/allografts—offer promising tools to study the impact of obesity onset on pancreatic cancer progression (Figure 4G).

7. Risk Factor: Diabetes

Diabetes and pancreatic cancer share some concurrent hereditary predispositions, particularly in subgroups of patients with family history and younger age at diagnosis, and these concomitant genetic susceptibilities have been comprehensively reviewed recently by Popovic et al. [153]. Mutations in *HNF1A, PDX1, and HNF1B*, which affect pancreatic development, have been associated with increased risk of monogenic forms of maturity onset diabetes of the young (MODY types 3, 4, and 5) and pancreatic cancer [154,155]. For instance, by crossing KC mice with $Hnf1a^{flox/flox}$ mice, Kalisz et al. found that *Hnf1a* loss cooperates with the $Kras^{G12D}$ mutation to promote pancreatic carcinogenesis [156]. The nuclear receptor NR5A2 plays a dual role in pancreatic health and disease. Agonistic activation of NR5A2 promotes beta cell regeneration, potentially reversing type 1 diabetes [157]. Conversely, *Nr5a2* heterozygosity sensitizes the pancreas to pancreatitis-induced inflammation, delays the ADM regeneration, and accelerates oncogenic *Kras*-driven carcinogenesis in mice [158,159]. Additionally, *UCP2* gene polymorphisms are associated with both diabetes and PDAC, with UCP2 loss significantly reducing oncogenic *Kras*-induced PDAC growth [160]. These findings collectively indicate that certain genetic factors contribute to both diabetes and pancreatic cancer susceptibility, and designing mouse models for understanding these shared genetic pathways may provide new insights into prevention strategies and targeted therapies for both conditions.

Type 2 diabetes has been associated with an approximately two-fold overall increased risk of pancreatic cancer, with the highest risk observed in the first year following diabetes diagnosis gradually diminishing over time [161,162]. Interestingly, recent studies have revealed that type 1 diabetes patients also exhibit modestly elevated hazard ratios for pancreatic cancer, with men showing a slightly higher risk than women [163]. This similarity in risk profile between type 1 and type 2 diabetes suggests that the underlying mechanism may be related to shared metabolic pathology, likely chronic hyperglycaemia, rather than factors specific to type 2 diabetes. The strong association between hyperglycaemia and pancreatic cancer risk is further supported by the finding that each 0.56 mmol/L (10 mg/dL) increment in fasting glucose is associated with a 14% increase in the incidence rate of pancreatic cancer [164]. Experimental evidence from mouse models has provided mechanistic insights into this relationship. Non-obese-associated diabetes induced by streptozotocin accelerates the PDAC development in KC mice (Figure 4D), an effect that can be prevented by scavenger of reactive carbonyl species (RCS) and advanced glycation end-product (AGE) inhibitor, indicating that hyperglycaemia-derived carbonyl stress plays a crucial role in pancreatic carcinogenesis, particularly in high-risk diabetic individuals [165]. These findings also highlight the importance of glycaemic control and cancer surveillance in all diabetic patients, regardless of diabetes classification.

Diabetes and pancreatic cancer share some common risk factors, such as obesity—as earlier mentioned—highlighting the complexity and overlap of underlying mechanisms [166]. Obesity-induced insulin resistance is a critical link in this relationship, contributing to both diabetes and carcinogenesis [167]. Experimental evidence supports this connection, as obese-associated diabetic *db/db* mice demonstrate accelerated PDAC progression and metastasis [168]. To elucidate the specific role of insulin in PDAC initiation, Zhang et al. generated LSL-$Kras^{G12D}$; $Ins1^{+/-}$; $Ins2^{-/-}$; $Ptf1a^{CreER}$ mice with genetic manipulations of *Ins1* and *Ins2* resulting in a sustained reduction in fasting insulin while maintaining unimpaired glucose homeostasis in female mice. Their findings revealed that HFD-mediated increases in insulin, in the absence of changes in fasting glucose, promoted PanIN development [169]. In a case-control study involving 973 patients with PDAC, Li et al. found that insulin or insulin secretagogues increased the risk of PDAC, while metformin administration in diabetic patients lowered the risk [170]. Preclinical studies have further demonstrated that metformin suppresses PDAC initiation and progression in KC and KPC mice [171]. These findings underscore the importance of further investigating the causal relationship between pharmacological therapies for type 2 diabetes and PDAC development.

New-onset diabetes is significantly associated with an increased incidence of pancreatic cancer compared to long-term diabetes (more than 2 years) prior to pancreatic cancer diagnosis, suggesting a potential reverse causation, where diabetes occurs as a consequence of PDAC development and may present as a subclinical manifestation [172]. Supporting this hypothesis, Parajuli et al. demonstrated in a KC mouse model that TGF-β signaling-activated apoptosis during PDAC progression caused depletion of β-cell mass, resulting in diabetic susceptibility [173]. This evidence that pancreatic cancer can trigger diabetes by damaging islet β-cells further contributes to the complexity.

In summary, it is crucial to recognize that chronic inflammation, hyperglycaemia, and insulin resistance can contribute to pancreatic carcinogenesis, consistent with the observation that long-term type 2 diabetes patients have an increased pancreatic cancer incidence compared to those with short-term type 2 diabetes (2–5 years) [172]. Besides, diabetes is often associated with comorbidities such as obesity and pancreatitis, which are themselves risk factors for pancreatic cancer. This complexity underscores the importance of precisely defining mouse models to avoid confounding factors and clearly delineate specific causal relationships. Conversely, pancreatic cancer development can also cause the onset of diabetes. These bidirectional relationships highlight the importance of carefully designing relevant mouse models to decipher the underlying mechanisms.

8. Other Risk Factors

Other than the previously mentioned risk factors that have been extensively investigated, additional cancer risk factors such as smoking, alcohol consumption, and infections [174] are also explored in GEMMs concerning the epidemiology of pancreatic cancer.

Patients with a history of pancreatitis, especially heavy smokers, exhibit a significantly elevated risk of developing pancreatic cancer [162]. Data regarding the impact of smoking on PDAC carcinogenesis is inconsistent. For instance, KC mice exposed to cigarette smoke for two weeks experienced significant weight loss but showed decreased cell proliferation in pancreatic ductal and acinar cells [175]. However, a six-week exposure to tobacco smoke promoted the formation of PanINs in KC mice, which was further exacerbated by the induction of chronic pancreatitis [176]. This discrepancy may arise from variations in the source, duration, and concentration of cigarette smoke used in different studies. Another investigation exposed KC mice to cigarette smoke for up to 20 weeks and observed overexpression of stem cell features such as *Paf1* and *Sox9*; this stemness may contribute to the expansion of PanINs [177]. Nicotine, the primary addictive substance in cigarette smoke, has been shown to accelerate ADM and tumor formation by activating AKT/ERK/MYC signaling in both KC and KPC mice [178]. When interpreting these results, it is essential to consider confounding factors such as smoking-induced genotoxicity [179] and its interplay with other risk factors like diabetes, obesity, and chronic pancreatitis. These interactions have been extensively reviewed elsewhere [180].

Excessive alcohol consumption is associated with an increased risk of pancreatic cancer [6]. Moderate alcohol intake has been shown to lead to the development of advanced PanIN and subsequent PDAC in KC mice [181]. However, it is important to note that alcohol is also a leading cause of pancreatitis, which can act as a confounding factor in this context.

Infection with pathogens such as Hepatitis B virus and *Helicobacter pylori* has been identified as potential risk factors for PDAC, highlighting the role of microbiome alterations and dysfunction in the disease's development. Studies have investigated the gut microbiome in KC mice [182] and the fecal and tumoral microbiome in KPC mice [183] to better understand the relationship between microbiome composition and PDAC development. Additionally, the oral microbiome, particularly *Porphyromonas gingivalis*, has been linked to an increased risk of pancreatic cancer [184], prompting further investigation using GEMMs. Administration of *Porphyromonas gingivalis* induced pancreatic ADM in wild-type mice and accelerated PDAC progression from PanIN lesions in $Kras^{G12D/+}$; $Ptf1a^{ER\text{-}Cre/+}$ mice, while also altering the intrapancreatic microbiome composition [185]. Furthermore, ablation of the gut microbiome in $Kras^{G12D/+}$; $PTEN^{flox/+}$; *Pdx1-Cre* mice resulted in decreased tumor growth and a reduction in the suppressive immune microenvironment [186]. Beyond these examples, recent studies have manipulated the gut microbiome through methods such as fecal microbial transplants and systemic antibiotics or antifungals in mouse models to explore specific microbiome relationships with pancreatic carcinogenesis. This area of research has been extensively reviewed, emphasizing the potential for microbial modification as a therapeutic strategy against pancreatic cancer [187,188].

9. Conclusions and Perspectives

Preclinical mouse models offer diverse approaches for investigating PDAC tumor development and identifying potential therapeutic targets. While xenograft models derived from PDAC cell lines, tumor tissues, or PDOs allow for genetic manipulation and drug testing in a relatively high-throughput manner, they have limitations in monitoring early carcinogenesis and testing early triggers. Humanized models add another dimension by better mimicking the human immune system but still fall short in replicating the complete process of early tumor development. GEMMs, particularly those manipulating somatic gene expression, are invaluable for exploring genetic alterations in early pancreatic carcinogenesis within the context of a competent immune system. Although often time consuming, these models provide crucial insights into tumor initiation and progression. The new introduction of large-scale CRISPR screening has further extended the utility of GEMMs, enabling unbiased identification of key genetic players in PDAC development.

Recent research has increasingly focused on the role of inflammatory triggers in PDAC initiation. Applying environmental risk factors or targeting underlying mechanisms in GEMMs can broaden our understanding of carcinogenesis, potentially leading to early prevention strategies and the development of druggable targets to halt cancer progression at its earliest stages.

However, caution is necessary when designing and interpreting results from mouse models. While GEMMs like the KPC model display good tumor heterogeneity, they may not consistently correlate with all clinical features seen in PDAC patients, such as cachexia. Off-target effects should also be considered, particularly when using Cre-lox systems. For instance, drivers like PDX-1 and Ptf1a can be expressed in organs other than the pancreas during embryonic development. Notably, the development of thymic tumors in KC mice has been reported and should be accounted for to avoid misinterpretation of results [189]. Furthermore, inflammatory factors are often interconnected and can act as confounders for each other, necessitating the careful interpretation of results. Finally, it is crucial to verify the translational relevance of findings from mouse models in human systems before drawing conclusions.

Author Contributions: Conceptualization, B.Y., A.-K.F., E.H., T.V.I., H.L., M.B., M.G., P.M. and J.R.; writing—original draft preparation, B.Y., A.-K.F., T.V.I. and E.H.; visualization, B.Y., A.-K.F. and E.H.; writing—review and editing, B.Y., A.-K.F., T.V.I., E.H., H.L., M.B., M.G., P.M. and J.R.; funding acquisition, H.L., M.B., M.G., P.M. and J.R. All authors have read and agreed to the published version of the manuscript.

Funding: The work was conducted within the Research Training Group InCuPanc (GRK 2751/1-2022 Project number: 449501615) funded by the DFG.

Acknowledgments: The figures were created with BioRender.com.

Conflicts of Interest: The authors declare no conflicts of interest.

References

1. Siegel, R.L.; Giaquinto, A.N.; Jemal, A. Cancer statistics, 2024. *CA Cancer J. Clin.* **2024**, *74*, 12–49. [CrossRef] [PubMed]
2. Wang, S.; Zheng, Y.; Yang, F.; Zhu, L.; Zhu, X.-Q.; Wang, Z.-F.; Wu, X.-L.; Zhou, C.-H.; Yan, J.-Y.; Hu, B.-Y.; et al. The molecular biology of pancreatic adenocarcinoma: Translational challenges and clinical perspectives. *Signal Transduct. Target. Ther.* **2021**, *6*, 249. [CrossRef] [PubMed]
3. Mizrahi, J.D.; Surana, R.; Valle, J.W.; Shroff, R.T. Pancreatic cancer. *Lancet* **2020**, *395*, 2008–2020. [CrossRef] [PubMed]
4. Capasso, M.; Franceschi, M.; Rodriguez-Castro, K.I.; Crafa, P.; Cambiè, G.; Miraglia, C.; Barchi, A.; Nouvenne, A.; Leandro, G.; Meschi, T.; et al. Epidemiology and risk factors of pancreatic cancer. *Acta Biomed.* **2018**, *89*, 141–146. [CrossRef]
5. Iodice, S.; Gandini, S.; Maisonneuve, P.; Lowenfels, A.B. Tobacco and the risk of pancreatic cancer: A review and meta-analysis. *Langenbeck's Arch. Surg.* **2008**, *393*, 535–545. [CrossRef]
6. Wang, Y.-T.; Gou, Y.-W.; Jin, W.-W.; Xiao, M.; Fang, H.-Y. Association between alcohol intake and the risk of pancreatic cancer: A dose–response meta-analysis of cohort studies. *BMC Cancer* **2016**, *16*, 212. [CrossRef]
7. Gandhi, S.; de la Fuente, J.; Murad, M.H.; Majumder, S. Chronic Pancreatitis Is a Risk Factor for Pancreatic Cancer, and Incidence Increases with Duration of Disease: A Systematic Review and Meta-analysis. *Clin. Transl. Gastroenterol.* **2022**, *13*, e00463. [CrossRef]
8. Ma, D.-M.; Dong, X.-W.; Han, X.; Ling, Z.; Lu, G.-T.; Sun, Y.-Y.; Yin, X.-D. Pancreatitis and Pancreatic Cancer Risk. *Technol. Cancer Res. Treat.* **2023**, *22*, 15330338231164875. [CrossRef]
9. Calle, E.E.; Rodriguez, C.; Walker-Thurmond, K.; Thun, M.J. Overweight, obesity, and mortality from cancer in a prospectively studied cohort of U.S. adults. *N. Engl. J. Med.* **2003**, *348*, 1625–1638. [CrossRef]
10. Berrington de Gonzalez, A.; Sweetland, S.; Spencer, E. A meta-analysis of obesity and the risk of pancreatic cancer. *Br. J. Cancer* **2003**, *89*, 519–523. [CrossRef]
11. Zanini, S.; Renzi, S.; Limongi, A.R.; Bellavite, P.; Giovinazzo, F.; Bermano, G. A review of lifestyle and environment risk factors for pancreatic cancer. *Eur. J. Cancer* **2021**, *145*, 53–70. [CrossRef] [PubMed]
12. Xu, J.H.; Fu, J.J.; Wang, X.L.; Zhu, J.Y.; Ye, X.H.; Chen, S.D. Hepatitis B or C viral infection and risk of pancreatic cancer: A meta-analysis of observational studies. *World J. Gastroenterol.* **2013**, *19*, 4234–4241. [CrossRef]
13. Grigorescu, R.R.; Husar-Sburlan, I.A.; Gheorghe, C. Pancreatic Cancer: A Review of Risk Factors. *Life* **2024**, *14*, 980. [CrossRef] [PubMed]
14. Marstrand-Daucé, L.; Lorenzo, D.; Chassac, A.; Nicole, P.; Couvelard, A.; Haumaitre, C. Acinar-to-Ductal Metaplasia (ADM): On the Road to Pancreatic Intraepithelial Neoplasia (PanIN) and Pancreatic Cancer. *Int. J. Mol. Sci.* **2023**, *24*, 9946. [CrossRef] [PubMed]

15. Guo, J.; Xie, K.; Zheng, S. Molecular Biomarkers of Pancreatic Intraepithelial Neoplasia and Their Implications in Early Diagnosis and Therapeutic Intervention of Pancreatic Cancer. *Int. J. Biol. Sci.* **2016**, *12*, 292–301. [CrossRef]
16. Hu, H.-F.; Ye, Z.; Qin, Y.; Xu, X.-W.; Yu, X.-J.; Zhuo, Q.-F.; Ji, S.-R. Mutations in key driver genes of pancreatic cancer: Molecularly targeted therapies and other clinical implications. *Acta Pharmacol. Sin.* **2021**, *42*, 1725–1741. [CrossRef]
17. de Wilde, R.F.; Hruban, R.H.; Maitra, A.; Offerhaus, G.J.A. Reporting precursors to invasive pancreatic cancer: Pancreatic intraepithelial neoplasia, intraductal neoplasms and mucinous cystic neoplasm. *Diagn. Histopathol.* **2012**, *18*, 17–30. [CrossRef]
18. Mallya, K.; Gautam, S.K.; Aithal, A.; Batra, S.K.; Jain, M. Modeling pancreatic cancer in mice for experimental therapeutics. *Biochim. Biophys. Acta Rev. Cancer* **2021**, *1876*, 188554. [CrossRef]
19. Fernandez, J.L.; Årbogen, S.; Sadeghinia, M.J.; Haram, M.; Snipstad, S.; Torp, S.H.; Einen, C.; Mühlenpfordt, M.; Maardalen, M.; Vikedal, K.; et al. A Comparative Analysis of Orthotopic and Subcutaneous Pancreatic Tumour Models: Tumour Microenvironment and Drug Delivery. *Cancers* **2023**, *15*, 5415. [CrossRef]
20. Wang, E.; Xiang, K.; Zhang, Y.; Wang, X.-F. Patient-derived organoids (PDOs) and PDO-derived xenografts (PDOXs): New opportunities in establishing faithful pre-clinical cancer models. *J. Natl. Cancer Cent.* **2022**, *2*, 263–276. [CrossRef]
21. He, M.; Henderson, M.; Muth, S.; Murphy, A.; Zheng, L. Preclinical mouse models for immunotherapeutic and non-immunotherapeutic drug development for pancreatic ductal adenocarcinoma. *Ann. Pancreat. Cancer* **2020**, *3*, 7. [CrossRef] [PubMed]
22. Guil-Luna, S.; Sedlik, C.; Piaggio, E. Humanized Mouse Models to Evaluate Cancer Immunotherapeutics. *Annu. Rev. Cancer Biol.* **2021**, *5*, 119–136. [CrossRef]
23. Corbett, T.H.; Roberts, B.J.; Leopold, W.R.; Peckham, J.C.; Wilkoff, L.J.; Griswold, D.P., Jr.; Schabel, F.M., Jr. Induction and chemotherapeutic response of two transplantable ductal adenocarcinomas of the pancreas in C57BL/6 mice. *Cancer Res.* **1984**, *44*, 717–726.
24. Torres, M.P.; Rachagani, S.; Souchek, J.J.; Mallya, K.; Johansson, S.L.; Batra, S.K. Novel Pancreatic Cancer Cell Lines Derived from Genetically Engineered Mouse Models of Spontaneous Pancreatic Adenocarcinoma: Applications in Diagnosis and Therapy. *PLoS ONE* **2013**, *8*, e80580. [CrossRef] [PubMed]
25. Kersten, K.; de Visser, K.E.; van Miltenburg, M.H.; Jonkers, J. Genetically engineered mouse models in oncology research and cancer medicine. *EMBO Mol. Med.* **2017**, *9*, 137–153. [CrossRef]
26. Westphalen, C.B.; Olive, K.P. Genetically engineered mouse models of pancreatic cancer. *Cancer J.* **2012**, *18*, 502–510. [CrossRef]
27. Vudatha, V.; Herremans, K.M.; Freudenberger, D.C.; Liu, C.; Trevino, J.G. Chapter Three—In vivo models of pancreatic ductal adenocarcinoma. In *Advances in Cancer Research*; Emdad, L., Atfi, A., Gogna, R., Trevino, J.G., Fisher, P.B., Eds.; Academic Press: New York, NY, USA, 2023; Volume 159, pp. 75–112.
28. Ornitz, D.M.; Hammer, R.E.; Messing, A.; Palmiter, R.D.; Brinster, R.L. Pancreatic Neoplasia Induced by SV40 T-Antigen Expression in Acinar Cells of Transgenic Mice. *Science* **1987**, *238*, 188–193. [CrossRef]
29. Quaife, C.J.; Pinkert, C.A.; Ornitz, D.M.; Palmiter, R.D.; Brinster, R.L. Pancreatic neoplasia induced by ras expression in acinar cells of transgenic mice. *Cell* **1987**, *48*, 1023–1034. [CrossRef]
30. Sandgren, E.P.; Quaife, C.J.; Paulovich, A.G.; Palmiter, R.D.; Brinster, R.L. Pancreatic tumor pathogenesis reflects the causative genetic lesion. *Proc. Natl. Acad. Sci. USA* **1991**, *88*, 93–97. [CrossRef]
31. Sandgren, E.P.; Luetteke, N.C.; Palmiter, R.D.; Brinster, R.L.; Lee, D.C. Overexpression of TGFα in transgenic mice: Induction of epithelial hyperplasia, pancreatic metaplasia, and carcinoma of the breast. *Cell* **1990**, *61*, 1121–1135. [CrossRef]
32. Kanda, M.; Matthaei, H.; Wu, J.; Hong, S.M.; Yu, J.; Borges, M.; Hruban, R.H.; Maitra, A.; Kinzler, K.; Vogelstein, B.; et al. Presence of somatic mutations in most early-stage pancreatic intraepithelial neoplasia. *Gastroenterology* **2012**, *142*, 730–733.e739. [CrossRef] [PubMed]
33. Hingorani, S.R.; Petricoin, E.F.; Maitra, A.; Rajapakse, V.; King, C.; Jacobetz, M.A.; Ross, S.; Conrads, T.P.; Veenstra, T.D.; Hitt, B.A.; et al. Preinvasive and invasive ductal pancreatic cancer and its early detection in the mouse. *Cancer Cell* **2003**, *4*, 437–450. [CrossRef]
34. Hingorani, S.R.; Wang, L.; Multani, A.S.; Combs, C.; Deramaudt, T.B.; Hruban, R.H.; Rustgi, A.K.; Chang, S.; Tuveson, D.A. Trp53R172H and KrasG12D cooperate to promote chromosomal instability and widely metastatic pancreatic ductal adenocarcinoma in mice. *Cancer Cell* **2005**, *7*, 469–483. [CrossRef] [PubMed]
35. Hirth, M.; Xie, Y.; Höper, C.; Prats, A.; Hackert, T.; Ebert, M.P.; Kuner, R. Genetic Mouse Models to Study Pancreatic Cancer-Induced Pain and Reduction in Well-Being. *Cells* **2022**, *11*, 2634. [CrossRef]
36. Morton, J.P.; Timpson, P.; Karim, S.A.; Ridgway, R.A.; Athineos, D.; Doyle, B.; Jamieson, N.B.; Oien, K.A.; Lowy, A.M.; Brunton, V.G.; et al. Mutant p53 drives metastasis and overcomes growth arrest/senescence in pancreatic cancer. *Proc. Natl. Acad. Sci. USA* **2010**, *107*, 246–251. [CrossRef]
37. Carrière, C.; Gore, A.J.; Norris, A.M.; Gunn, J.R.; Young, A.L.; Longnecker, D.S.; Korc, M. Deletion of Rb Accelerates Pancreatic Carcinogenesis by Oncogenic Kras and Impairs Senescence in Premalignant Lesions. *Gastroenterology* **2011**, *141*, 1091–1101. [CrossRef] [PubMed]

38. Aguirre, A.J.; Bardeesy, N.; Sinha, M.; Lopez, L.; Tuveson, D.A.; Horner, J.; Redston, M.S.; DePinho, R.A. Activated Kras and Ink4a/Arf deficiency cooperate to produce metastatic pancreatic ductal adenocarcinoma. *Genes Dev.* **2003**, *17*, 3112–3126. [CrossRef]
39. Izeradjene, K.; Combs, C.; Best, M.; Gopinathan, A.; Wagner, A.; Grady, W.M.; Deng, C.-X.; Hruban, R.H.; Adsay, N.V.; Tuveson, D.A.; et al. KrasG12D and Smad4/Dpc4 Haploinsufficiency Cooperate to Induce Mucinous Cystic Neoplasms and Invasive Adenocarcinoma of the Pancreas. *Cancer Cell* **2007**, *11*, 229–243. [CrossRef]
40. Qiu, W.; Tang, S.M.; Lee, S.; Turk, A.T.; Sireci, A.N.; Qiu, A.; Rose, C.; Xie, C.; Kitajewski, J.; Wen, H.-J.; et al. Loss of Activin Receptor Type 1B Accelerates Development of Intraductal Papillary Mucinous Neoplasms in Mice with Activated KRAS. *Gastroenterology* **2016**, *150*, 218–228.e212. [CrossRef]
41. Ijichi, H.; Chytil, A.; Gorska, A.E.; Aakre, M.E.; Fujitani, Y.; Fujitani, S.; Wright, C.V.; Moses, H.L. Aggressive pancreatic ductal adenocarcinoma in mice caused by pancreas-specific blockade of transforming growth factor-beta signaling in cooperation with active Kras expression. *Genes Dev.* **2006**, *20*, 3147–3160. [CrossRef] [PubMed]
42. Costanza, B.; Umelo, I.A.; Bellier, J.; Castronovo, V.; Turtoi, A. Stromal Modulators of TGF-β in Cancer. *J. Clin. Med.* **2017**, *6*, 7. [CrossRef] [PubMed]
43. Ideno, N.; Yamaguchi, H.; Ghosh, B.; Gupta, S.; Okumura, T.; Steffen, D.J.; Fisher, C.G.; Wood, L.D.; Singhi, A.D.; Nakamura, M.; et al. GNAS(R201C) Induces Pancreatic Cystic Neoplasms in Mice That Express Activated KRAS by Inhibiting YAP1 Signaling. *Gastroenterology* **2018**, *155*, 1593–1607.e1512. [CrossRef] [PubMed]
44. Taki, K.; Ohmuraya, M.; Tanji, E.; Komatsu, H.; Hashimoto, D.; Semba, K.; Araki, K.; Kawaguchi, Y.; Baba, H.; Furukawa, T. GNAS(R201H) and Kras(G12D) cooperate to promote murine pancreatic tumorigenesis recapitulating human intraductal papillary mucinous neoplasm. *Oncogene* **2016**, *35*, 2407–2412. [CrossRef]
45. Rhim, A.D.; Oberstein, P.E.; Thomas, D.H.; Mirek, E.T.; Palermo, C.F.; Sastra, S.A.; Dekleva, E.N.; Saunders, T.; Becerra, C.P.; Tattersall, I.W.; et al. Stromal Elements Act to Restrain, Rather Than Support, Pancreatic Ductal Adenocarcinoma. *Cancer Cell* **2014**, *25*, 735–747. [CrossRef]
46. Özdemir, B.C.; Pentcheva-Hoang, T.; Carstens, J.L.; Zheng, X.; Wu, C.-C.; Simpson, T.R.; Laklai, H.; Sugimoto, H.; Kahlert, C.; Novitskiy, S.V.; et al. Depletion of Carcinoma-Associated Fibroblasts and Fibrosis Induces Immunosuppression and Accelerates Pancreas Cancer with Reduced Survival. *Cancer Cell* **2014**, *25*, 719–734. [CrossRef] [PubMed]
47. Polani, F.; Grierson, P.M.; Lim, K.H. Stroma-targeting strategies in pancreatic cancer: Past lessons, challenges and prospects. *World J. Gastroenterol.* **2021**, *27*, 2105–2121. [CrossRef] [PubMed]
48. Feig, C.; Jones, J.O.; Kraman, M.; Wells, R.J.B.; Deonarine, A.; Chan, D.S.; Connell, C.M.; Roberts, E.W.; Zhao, Q.; Caballero, O.L.; et al. Targeting CXCL12 from FAP-expressing carcinoma-associated fibroblasts synergizes with anti–PD-L1 immunotherapy in pancreatic cancer. *Proc. Natl. Acad. Sci. USA* **2013**, *110*, 20212–20217. [CrossRef]
49. Gopinathan, A.; Morton, J.P.; Jodrell, D.I.; Sansom, O.J. GEMMs as preclinical models for testing pancreatic cancer therapies. *Dis. Model. Mech.* **2015**, *8*, 1185–1200. [CrossRef]
50. Lee, A.Y.L.; Dubois, C.L.; Sarai, K.; Zarei, S.; Schaeffer, D.F.; Sander, M.; Kopp, J.L. Cell of origin affects tumour development and phenotype in pancreatic ductal adenocarcinoma. *Gut* **2019**, *68*, 487–498. [CrossRef]
51. Talbert, E.E.; Cuitiño, M.C.; Ladner, K.J.; Rajasekerea, P.V.; Siebert, M.; Shakya, R.; Leone, G.W.; Ostrowski, M.C.; Paleo, B.; Weisleder, N.; et al. Modeling Human Cancer-induced Cachexia. *Cell Rep.* **2019**, *28*, 1612–1622.e1614. [CrossRef]
52. Chiou, S.H.; Winters, I.P.; Wang, J.; Naranjo, S.; Dudgeon, C.; Tamburini, F.B.; Brady, J.J.; Yang, D.; Grüner, B.M.; Chuang, C.H.; et al. Pancreatic cancer modeling using retrograde viral vector delivery and in vivo CRISPR/Cas9-mediated somatic genome editing. *Genes Dev.* **2015**, *29*, 1576–1585. [CrossRef] [PubMed]
53. Schönhuber, N.; Seidler, B.; Schuck, K.; Veltkamp, C.; Schachtler, C.; Zukowska, M.; Eser, S.; Feyerabend, T.B.; Paul, M.C.; Eser, P.; et al. A next-generation dual-recombinase system for time- and host-specific targeting of pancreatic cancer. *Nat. Med.* **2014**, *20*, 1340–1347. [CrossRef] [PubMed]
54. Chen, Y.; Kim, J.; Yang, S.; Wang, H.; Wu, C.-J.; Sugimoto, H.; LeBleu, V.S.; Kalluri, R. Type I collagen deletion in αSMA+ myofibroblasts augments immune suppression and accelerates progression of pancreatic cancer. *Cancer Cell* **2021**, *39*, 548–565.e546. [CrossRef]
55. Collins, M.A.; Bednar, F.; Zhang, Y.; Brisset, J.-C.; Galbán, S.; Galbán, C.J.; Rakshit, S.; Flannagan, K.S.; Adsay, N.V.; Pasca di Magliano, M. Oncogenic Kras is required for both the initiation and maintenance of pancreatic cancer in mice. *J. Clin. Investig.* **2012**, *122*, 639–653. [CrossRef]
56. Wang, W.; Dong, B.; Ittmann, M.M.; Yang, F. A Versatile Gene Delivery System for Efficient and Tumor Specific Gene Manipulation in vivo. *Discoveries* **2016**, *4*, e58. [CrossRef]
57. Sano, M.; Driscoll, D.R.; De Jesus-Monge, W.E.; Klimstra, D.S.; Lewis, B.C. Activated Wnt Signaling in Stroma Contributes to Development of Pancreatic Mucinous Cystic Neoplasms. *Gastroenterology* **2014**, *146*, 257–267. [CrossRef]

58. Kaltenbacher, T.; Löprich, J.; Maresch, R.; Weber, J.; Müller, S.; Oellinger, R.; Groß, N.; Griger, J.; de Andrade Krätzig, N.; Avramopoulos, P.; et al. CRISPR somatic genome engineering and cancer modeling in the mouse pancreas and liver. *Nat. Protoc.* **2022**, *17*, 1142–1188. [CrossRef] [PubMed]
59. Hanna, R.E.; Doench, J.G. Design and analysis of CRISPR–Cas experiments. *Nat. Biotechnol.* **2020**, *38*, 813–823. [CrossRef]
60. Doench, J.G.; Fusi, N.; Sullender, M.; Hegde, M.; Vaimberg, E.W.; Donovan, K.F.; Smith, I.; Tothova, Z.; Wilen, C.; Orchard, R.; et al. Optimized sgRNA design to maximize activity and minimize off-target effects of CRISPR-Cas9. *Nat. Biotechnol.* **2016**, *34*, 184–191. [CrossRef]
61. Oktriani, R.; Pirona, A.C.; Kalmár, L.; Rahadian, A.S.; Miao, B.; Bauer, A.S.; Hoheisel, J.D.; Boettcher, M.; Du, H. Genome-Wide CRISPR Screen Identifies Genes Involved in Metastasis of Pancreatic Ductal Adenocarcinoma. *Cancers* **2024**, *16*, 3684. [CrossRef]
62. Chen, S.; Sanjana, N.E.; Zheng, K.; Shalem, O.; Lee, K.; Shi, X.; Scott, D.A.; Song, J.; Pan, J.Q.; Weissleder, R.; et al. Genome-wide CRISPR Screen in a Mouse Model of Tumor Growth and Metastasis. *Cell* **2015**, *160*, 1246–1260. [CrossRef]
63. Braun, C.J.; Adames, A.C.; Saur, D.; Rad, R. Tutorial: Design and execution of CRISPR in vivo screens. *Nat. Protoc.* **2022**, *17*, 1903–1925. [CrossRef] [PubMed]
64. Hulton, C.H.; Costa, E.A.; Shah, N.S.; Quintanal-Villalonga, A.; Heller, G.; de Stanchina, E.; Rudin, C.M.; Poirier, J.T. Direct genome editing of patient-derived xenografts using CRISPR-Cas9 enables rapid in vivo functional genomics. *Nat. Cancer* **2020**, *1*, 359–369. [CrossRef]
65. Zhu, X.G.; Chudnovskiy, A.; Baudrier, L.; Prizer, B.; Liu, Y.; Ostendorf, B.N.; Yamaguchi, N.; Arab, A.; Tavora, B.; Timson, R.; et al. Functional Genomics In Vivo Reveal Metabolic Dependencies of Pancreatic Cancer Cells. *Cell Metab.* **2021**, *33*, 211–221.e216. [CrossRef] [PubMed]
66. Dubrot, J.; Du, P.P.; Lane-Reticker, S.K.; Kessler, E.A.; Muscato, A.J.; Mehta, A.; Freeman, S.S.; Allen, P.M.; Olander, K.E.; Ockerman, K.M.; et al. In vivo CRISPR screens reveal the landscape of immune evasion pathways across cancer. *Nat. Immunol.* **2022**, *23*, 1495–1506. [CrossRef] [PubMed]
67. Szlachta, K.; Kuscu, C.; Tufan, T.; Adair, S.J.; Shang, S.; Michaels, A.D.; Mullen, M.G.; Fischer, N.L.; Yang, J.; Liu, L.; et al. CRISPR knockout screening identifies combinatorial drug targets in pancreatic cancer and models cellular drug response. *Nat. Commun.* **2018**, *9*, 4275. [CrossRef]
68. Maresch, R.; Mueller, S.; Veltkamp, C.; Öllinger, R.; Friedrich, M.; Heid, I.; Steiger, K.; Weber, J.; Engleitner, T.; Barenboim, M.; et al. Multiplexed pancreatic genome engineering and cancer induction by transfection-based CRISPR/Cas9 delivery in mice. *Nat. Commun.* **2016**, *7*, 10770. [CrossRef]
69. Martinez, S.; Wu, S.; Geuenich, M.; Malik, A.; Weber, R.; Woo, T.; Zhang, A.; Jang, G.H.; Dervovic, D.; Al-Zahrani, K.N.; et al. In vivo CRISPR screens reveal SCAF1 and USP15 as drivers of pancreatic cancer. *Nat. Commun.* **2024**, *15*, 5266. [CrossRef] [PubMed]
70. Beato, F.; Reverón, D.; Dezsi, K.B.; Ortiz, A.; Johnson, J.O.; Chen, D.-T.; Ali, K.; Yoder, S.J.; Jeong, D.; Malafa, M.; et al. Establishing a living biobank of patient-derived organoids of intraductal papillary mucinous neoplasms of the pancreas. *Lab. Investig.* **2021**, *101*, 204–217. [CrossRef]
71. Ungricht, R.; Guibbal, L.; Lasbennes, M.-C.; Orsini, V.; Beibel, M.; Waldt, A.; Cuttat, R.; Carbone, W.; Basler, A.; Roma, G.; et al. Genome-wide screening in human kidney organoids identifies developmental and disease-related aspects of nephrogenesis. *Cell Stem Cell* **2022**, *29*, 160–175.e167. [CrossRef]
72. Michels, B.E.; Mosa, M.H.; Streibl, B.I.; Zhan, T.; Menche, C.; Abou-El-Ardat, K.; Darvishi, T.; Członka, E.; Wagner, S.; Winter, J.; et al. Pooled In Vitro and In Vivo CRISPR-Cas9 Screening Identifies Tumor Suppressors in Human Colon Organoids. *Cell Stem Cell* **2020**, *26*, 782–792.e787. [CrossRef] [PubMed]
73. Ringel, T.; Frey, N.; Ringnalda, F.; Janjuha, S.; Cherkaoui, S.; Butz, S.; Srivatsa, S.; Pirkl, M.; Russo, G.; Villiger, L.; et al. Genome-Scale CRISPR Screening in Human Intestinal Organoids Identifies Drivers of TGF-β Resistance. *Cell Stem Cell* **2020**, *26*, 431–440.e438. [CrossRef]
74. Gilbert, L.A.; Horlbeck, M.A.; Adamson, B.; Villalta, J.E.; Chen, Y.; Whitehead, E.H.; Guimaraes, C.; Panning, B.; Ploegh, H.L.; Bassik, M.C.; et al. Genome-Scale CRISPR-Mediated Control of Gene Repression and Activation. *Cell* **2014**, *159*, 647–661. [CrossRef] [PubMed]
75. Anzalone, A.V.; Randolph, P.B.; Davis, J.R.; Sousa, A.A.; Koblan, L.W.; Levy, J.M.; Chen, P.J.; Wilson, C.; Newby, G.A.; Raguram, A.; et al. Search-and-replace genome editing without double-strand breaks or donor DNA. *Nature* **2019**, *576*, 149–157. [CrossRef] [PubMed]
76. Sayed, S.; Sidorova, O.A.; Hennig, A.; Augsburg, M.; Cortés Vesga, C.P.; Abohawya, M.; Schmitt, L.T.; Sürün, D.; Stange, D.E.; Mircetic, J.; et al. Efficient Correction of Oncogenic KRAS and TP53 Mutations through CRISPR Base Editing. *Cancer Res.* **2022**, *82*, 3002–3015. [CrossRef]
77. Joung, J.K.; Sander, J.D. TALENs: A widely applicable technology for targeted genome editing. *Nat. Rev. Mol. Cell Biol.* **2013**, *14*, 49–55. [CrossRef]

78. DeWeirdt, P.C.; Sanson, K.R.; Sangree, A.K.; Hegde, M.; Hanna, R.E.; Feeley, M.N.; Griffith, A.L.; Teng, T.; Borys, S.M.; Strand, C.; et al. Optimization of AsCas12a for combinatorial genetic screens in human cells. *Nat. Biotechnol.* **2021**, *39*, 94–104. [CrossRef]
79. Konermann, S.; Lotfy, P.; Brideau, N.J.; Oki, J.; Shokhirev, M.N.; Hsu, P.D. Transcriptome Engineering with RNA-Targeting Type VI-D CRISPR Effectors. *Cell* **2018**, *173*, 665–676.e614. [CrossRef]
80. Lowenfels, A.B.; Maisonneuve, P.; Cavallini, G.; Ammann, R.W.; Lankisch, P.G.; Andersen, J.R.; Dimagno, E.P.; Andrén-Sandberg, A.; Domellöf, L. Pancreatitis and the risk of pancreatic cancer. International Pancreatitis Study Group. *N. Engl. J. Med.* **1993**, *328*, 1433–1437. [CrossRef]
81. Kim, H.S.; Gweon, T.-G.; Park, S.H.; Kim, T.H.; Kim, C.W.; Chang, J.H. Incidence and risk of pancreatic cancer in patients with chronic pancreatitis: Defining the optimal subgroup for surveillance. *Sci. Rep.* **2023**, *13*, 106. [CrossRef]
82. Kirkegård, J.; Cronin-Fenton, D.; Heide-Jørgensen, U.; Mortensen, F.V. Acute Pancreatitis and Pancreatic Cancer Risk: A Nationwide Matched-Cohort Study in Denmark. *Gastroenterology* **2018**, *154*, 1729–1736. [CrossRef]
83. Park, S.M.; Kim, K.B.; Han, J.-H.; Kim, N.; Kang, T.U.; Swan, H.; Kim, H.J. Incidence and risk of pancreatic cancer in patients with acute or chronic pancreatitis: A population-based cohort study. *Sci. Rep.* **2023**, *13*, 18930. [CrossRef] [PubMed]
84. Malka, D.; Hammel, P.; Maire, F.; Rufat, P.; Madeira, I.; Pessione, F.; Lévy, P.; Ruszniewski, P. Risk of pancreatic adenocarcinoma in chronic pancreatitis. *Gut* **2002**, *51*, 849–852. [CrossRef] [PubMed]
85. Ueda, J.; Tanaka, M.; Ohtsuka, T.; Tokunaga, S.; Shimosegawa, T.; Research Committee of Intractable Diseases of the Pancreas. Surgery for chronic pancreatitis decreases the risk for pancreatic cancer: A multicenter retrospective analysis. *Surgery* **2013**, *153*, 357–364. [CrossRef]
86. Yadav, D.; Hawes, R.H.; Brand, R.E.; Anderson, M.A.; Money, M.E.; Banks, P.A.; Bishop, M.D.; Baillie, J.; Sherman, S.; DiSario, J.; et al. Alcohol consumption, cigarette smoking, and the risk of recurrent acute and chronic pancreatitis. *Arch. Intern. Med.* **2009**, *169*, 1035–1045. [CrossRef]
87. Pandol, S.J.; Gorelick, F.S.; Gerloff, A.; Lugea, A. Alcohol abuse, endoplasmic reticulum stress and pancreatitis. *Dig. Dis.* **2010**, *28*, 776–782. [CrossRef]
88. Tanaka, T.; Miura, Y.; Matsugu, Y.; Ichiba, Y.; Ito, H.; Dohi, K. Pancreatic duct obstruction is an aggravating factor in the canine model of chronic alcoholic pancreatitis. *Gastroenterology* **1998**, *115*, 1248–1253. [CrossRef]
89. Okazaki, K.; Chiba, T. Autoimmune related pancreatitis. *Gut* **2002**, *51*, 1–4. [CrossRef] [PubMed]
90. Whitcomb, D.C.; Gorry, M.C.; Preston, R.A.; Furey, W.; Sossenheimer, M.J.; Ulrich, C.D.; Martin, S.P.; Gates, L.K.; Amann, S.T.; Toskes, P.P.; et al. Hereditary pancreatitis is caused by a mutation in the cationic trypsinogen gene. *Nat. Genet.* **1996**, *14*, 141–145. [CrossRef] [PubMed]
91. Witt, H.; Luck, W.; Hennies, H.C.; Classen, M.; Kage, A.; Lass, U.; Landt, O.; Becker, M. Mutations in the gene encoding the serine protease inhibitor, Kazal type 1 are associated with chronic pancreatitis. *Nat. Genet.* **2000**, *25*, 213–216. [CrossRef]
92. Witt, H.; Beer, S.; Rosendahl, J.; Chen, J.-M.; Chandak, G.R.; Masamune, A.; Bence, M.; Szmola, R.; Oracz, G.; Macek, M.; et al. Variants in CPA1 are strongly associated with early onset chronic pancreatitis. *Nat. Genet.* **2013**, *45*, 1216–1220. [CrossRef]
93. Gorry, M.C.; Gabbaizedeh, D.; Furey, W.; Gates, L.K.; Preston, R.A.; Aston, C.E.; Zhang, Y.; Ulrich, C.; Ehrlich, G.D.; Whitcomb, D.C. Mutations in the cationic trypsinogen gene are associated with recurrent acute and chronic pancreatitis. *Gastroenterology* **1997**, *113*, 1063–1068. [CrossRef] [PubMed]
94. Grocock, C.J.; Rebours, V.; Delhaye, M.N.; Andrén-Sandberg, A.; Weiss, F.U.; Mountford, R.; Harcus, M.J.; Niemczyck, E.; Vitone, L.J.; Dodd, S.; et al. The variable phenotype of the p.A16V mutation of cationic trypsinogen (PRSS1) in pancreatitis families. *Gut* **2010**, *59*, 357–363. [CrossRef] [PubMed]
95. Witt, H.; Luck, W.; Becker, M. A signal peptide cleavage site mutation in the cationic trypsinogen gene is strongly associated with chronic pancreatitis. *Gastroenterology* **1999**, *117*, 7–10. [CrossRef] [PubMed]
96. Teich, N.; Nemoda, Z.; Köhler, H.; Heinritz, W.; Mössner, J.; Keim, V.; Sahin-Tóth, M. Gene conversion between functional trypsinogen genes PRSS1 and PRSS2 associated with chronic pancreatitis in a six-year-old girl. *Hum. Mutat.* **2005**, *25*, 343–347. [CrossRef]
97. Sahin-Tóth, M.; Tóth, M. Gain-of-function mutations associated with hereditary pancreatitis enhance autoactivation of human cationic trypsinogen. *Biochem. Biophys. Res. Commun.* **2000**, *278*, 286–289. [CrossRef]
98. Archer, H.; Jura, N.; Keller, J.; Jacobson, M.; Bar-Sagi, D. A mouse model of hereditary pancreatitis generated by transgenic expression of R122H trypsinogen. *Gastroenterology* **2006**, *131*, 1844–1855. [CrossRef]
99. Athwal, T.; Huang, W.; Mukherjee, R.; Latawiec, D.; Chvanov, M.; Clarke, R.; Smith, K.; Campbell, F.; Merriman, C.; Criddle, D.; et al. Expression of human cationic trypsinogen (PRSS1) in murine acinar cells promotes pancreatitis and apoptotic cell death. *Cell Death Dis.* **2014**, *5*, e1165. [CrossRef]
100. Geisz, A.; Sahin-Tóth, M. A preclinical model of chronic pancreatitis driven by trypsinogen autoactivation. *Nat. Commun.* **2018**, *9*, 5033. [CrossRef]
101. Demcsák, A.; Sahin-Tóth, M. Rate of Autoactivation Determines Pancreatitis Phenotype in Trypsinogen Mutant Mice. *Gastroenterology* **2022**, *163*, 761–763. [CrossRef]

102. Rosendahl, J.; Witt, H.; Szmola, R.; Bhatia, E.; Ozsvári, B.; Landt, O.; Schulz, H.-U.; Gress, T.M.; Pfützer, R.; Löhr, M.; et al. Chymotrypsin C (CTRC) variants that diminish activity or secretion are associated with chronic pancreatitis. *Nat. Genet.* **2008**, *40*, 78–82. [CrossRef] [PubMed]
103. Masson, E.; Chen, J.-M.; Scotet, V.; Le Maréchal, C.; Férec, C. Association of rare chymotrypsinogen C (CTRC) gene variations in patients with idiopathic chronic pancreatitis. *Hum. Genet.* **2008**, *123*, 83–91. [CrossRef] [PubMed]
104. Jancsó, Z.; Hegyi, E.; Sahin-Tóth, M. Chymotrypsin Reduces the Severity of Secretagogue-Induced Pancreatitis in Mice. *Gastroenterology* **2018**, *155*, 1017–1021. [CrossRef]
105. Laskowski, M.; Kato, I. Protein inhibitors of proteinases. *Annu. Rev. Biochem.* **1980**, *49*, 593–626. [CrossRef]
106. Romac, J.M.J.; Ohmuraya, M.; Bittner, C.; Majeed, M.F.; Vigna, S.R.; Que, J.; Fee, B.E.; Wartmann, T.; Yamamura, K.-I.; Liddle, R.A. Transgenic expression of pancreatic secretory trypsin inhibitor-1 rescues SPINK3-deficient mice and restores a normal pancreatic phenotype. *Am. J. Physiol. Gastrointest. Liver Physiol.* **2010**, *298*, G518–G524. [CrossRef]
107. Ohmuraya, M.; Hirota, M.; Araki, M.; Mizushima, N.; Matsui, M.; Mizumoto, T.; Haruna, K.; Kume, S.; Takeya, M.; Ogawa, M.; et al. Autophagic cell death of pancreatic acinar cells in serine protease inhibitor Kazal type 3-deficient mice. *Gastroenterology* **2005**, *129*, 696–705. [CrossRef]
108. Demcsák, A.; Sahin-Tóth, M. Heterozygous Spink1 Deficiency Promotes Trypsin-dependent Chronic Pancreatitis in Mice. *Cell. Mol. Gastroenterol. Hepatol.* **2024**, *18*, 101361. [CrossRef] [PubMed]
109. Scheele, G.; Bartelt, D.; Bieger, W. Characterization of human exocrine pancreatic proteins by two-dimensional isoelectric focusing/sodium dodecyl sulfate gel electrophoresis. *Gastroenterology* **1981**, *80*, 461–473. [CrossRef]
110. Szmola, R.; Bence, M.; Carpentieri, A.; Szabó, A.; Costello, C.E.; Samuelson, J.; Sahin-Tóth, M. Chymotrypsin C is a co-activator of human pancreatic procarboxypeptidases A1 and A2. *J. Biol. Chem.* **2011**, *286*, 1819–1827. [CrossRef]
111. Hegyi, E.; Sahin-Tóth, M. Human CPA1 mutation causes digestive enzyme misfolding and chronic pancreatitis in mice. *Gut* **2019**, *68*, 301–312. [CrossRef]
112. Guerra, C.; Schuhmacher, A.J.; Cañamero, M.; Grippo, P.J.; Verdaguer, L.; Pérez-Gallego, L.; Dubus, P.; Sandgren, E.P.; Barbacid, M. Chronic pancreatitis is essential for induction of pancreatic ductal adenocarcinoma by K-Ras oncogenes in adult mice. *Cancer Cell* **2007**, *11*, 291–302. [CrossRef] [PubMed]
113. Murray, C.J.L.; Aravkin, A.Y.; Zheng, P.; Abbafati, C.; Abbas, K.M.; Abbasi-Kangevari, M.; Abd-Allah, F.; Abdelalim, A.; Abdollahi, M.; Abdollahpour, I.; et al. Global burden of 87 risk factors in 204 countries and territories, 1990–2019: A systematic analysis for the Global Burden of Disease Study 2019. *Lancet* **2020**, *396*, 1223–1249. [CrossRef] [PubMed]
114. Rosen, E.D.; Spiegelman, B.M. What We Talk About When We Talk About Fat. *Cell* **2014**, *156*, 20–44. [CrossRef]
115. Hotamisligil, G.S. Inflammation and metabolic disorders. *Nature* **2006**, *444*, 860–867. [CrossRef] [PubMed]
116. Zatterale, F.; Longo, M.; Naderi, J.; Raciti, G.A.; Desiderio, A.; Miele, C.; Beguinot, F. Chronic Adipose Tissue Inflammation Linking Obesity to Insulin Resistance and Type 2 Diabetes. *Front. Physiol.* **2020**, *10*, 1607. [CrossRef]
117. Quail, D.F.; Dannenberg, A.J. The obese adipose tissue microenvironment in cancer development and progression. *Nat. Rev. Endocrinol.* **2019**, *15*, 139–154. [CrossRef]
118. Bhaskaran, K.; Douglas, I.; Forbes, H.; dos-Santos-Silva, I.; Leon, D.A.; Smeeth, L. Body-mass index and risk of 22 specific cancers: A population-based cohort study of 5·24 million UK adults. *Lancet* **2014**, *384*, 755–765. [CrossRef]
119. Rebours, V.; Gaujoux, S.; d'Assignies, G.; Sauvanet, A.; Ruszniewski, P.; Lévy, P.; Paradis, V.; Bedossa, P.; Couvelard, A. Obesity and Fatty Pancreatic Infiltration Are Risk Factors for Pancreatic Precancerous Lesions (PanIN). *Clin. Cancer Res.* **2015**, *21*, 3522–3528. [CrossRef]
120. El-Tanani, M.; Rabbani, S.A.; Aljabali, A.A.; Matalka, I.I.; El-Tanani, Y.; Rizzo, M.; Tambuwala, M.M. The Complex Connection between Obesity and Cancer: Signaling Pathways and Therapeutic Implications. *Nutr. Cancer* **2024**, *76*, 683–706. [CrossRef]
121. Ruiz, C.F.; Garcia, C.; Jacox, J.B.; Lawres, L.; Muzumdar, M.D. Decoding the obesity–cancer connection: Lessons from preclinical models of pancreatic adenocarcinoma. *Life Sci. Alliance* **2023**, *6*, e202302228. [CrossRef]
122. Philip, B.; Roland, C.L.; Daniluk, J.; Liu, Y.; Chatterjee, D.; Gomez, S.B.; Ji, B.; Huang, H.; Wang, H.; Fleming, J.B.; et al. A high-fat diet activates oncogenic Kras and COX2 to induce development of pancreatic ductal adenocarcinoma in mice. *Gastroenterology* **2013**, *145*, 1449–1458. [CrossRef] [PubMed]
123. Suleiman, J.B.; Mohamed, M.; Bakar, A.B.A. A systematic review on different models of inducing obesity in animals: Advantages and limitations. *J. Adv. Vet. Anim. Res.* **2020**, *7*, 103–114. [CrossRef] [PubMed]
124. Kfoury, S.; Michl, P.; Roth, L. Modeling Obesity-Driven Pancreatic Carcinogenesis-A Review of Current In Vivo and In Vitro Models of Obesity and Pancreatic Carcinogenesis. *Cells* **2022**, *11*, 3170. [CrossRef]
125. Lutz, T.A.; Woods, S.C. Overview of animal models of obesity. *Curr. Protoc. Pharmacol.* **2012**, *58*, 5–61. [CrossRef]
126. Wu, S.-C.; Lin, C.-H. Direct Adeno-associated Viruses Injection of Murine Adipose Tissue. *Bio-Protocol* **2023**, *13*, e4674. [CrossRef] [PubMed]
127. Singh, R.; Gholipourmalekabadi, M.; Shafikhani, S.H. Animal models for type 1 and type 2 diabetes: Advantages and limitations. *Front. Endocrinol.* **2024**, *15*, 1359685. [CrossRef]

28. Chung, K.M.; Singh, J.; Lawres, L.; Dorans, K.J.; Garcia, C.; Burkhardt, D.B.; Robbins, R.; Bhutkar, A.; Cardone, R.; Zhao, X.; et al. Endocrine-Exocrine Signaling Drives Obesity-Associated Pancreatic Ductal Adenocarcinoma. *Cell* **2020**, *181*, 832–847.e818. [CrossRef]
29. Renehan, A.G.; Zwahlen, M.; Egger, M. Adiposity and cancer risk: New mechanistic insights from epidemiology. *Nat. Rev. Cancer* **2015**, *15*, 484–498. [CrossRef]
30. Iyengar, N.M.; Gucalp, A.; Dannenberg, A.J.; Hudis, C.A. Obesity and Cancer Mechanisms: Tumor Microenvironment and Inflammation. *J. Clin. Oncol.* **2016**, *34*, 4270–4276. [CrossRef]
31. Vansaun, M.N. Molecular pathways: Adiponectin and leptin signaling in cancer. *Clin. Cancer Res.* **2013**, *19*, 1926–1932. [CrossRef]
32. Myers, M.G.; Cowley, M.A.; Münzberg, H. Mechanisms of leptin action and leptin resistance. *Annu. Rev. Physiol.* **2008**, *70*, 537–556. [CrossRef] [PubMed]
33. Xu, Y.; Tan, M.; Tian, X.; Zhang, J.; Zhang, J.; Chen, J.; Xu, W.; Sheng, H. Leptin receptor mediates the proliferation and glucose metabolism of pancreatic cancer cells via AKT pathway activation. *Mol. Med. Rep.* **2020**, *21*, 945–952. [CrossRef]
34. Mendonsa, A.M.; Chalfant, M.C.; Gorden, L.D.; Vansaun, M.N. Modulation of the leptin receptor mediates tumor growth and migration of pancreatic cancer cells. *PLoS ONE* **2015**, *10*, e0126686. [CrossRef]
35. Fan, Y.; Gan, Y.; Shen, Y.; Cai, X.; Song, Y.; Zhao, F.; Yao, M.; Gu, J.; Tu, H. Leptin signaling enhances cell invasion and promotes the metastasis of human pancreatic cancer via increasing MMP-13 production. *Oncotarget* **2015**, *6*, 16120–16134. [CrossRef] [PubMed]
36. Mosser, R.E.; Maulis, M.F.; Moullé, V.S.; Dunn, J.C.; Carboneau, B.A.; Arasi, K.; Pappan, K.; Poitout, V.; Gannon, M. High-fat diet-induced β-cell proliferation occurs prior to insulin resistance in C57Bl/6J male mice. *Am. J. Physiol. Endocrinol. Metab.* **2015**, *308*, E573–E582. [CrossRef]
37. Ahren, B.; Pacini, G. Insufficient islet compensation to insulin resistance vs. reduced glucose effectiveness in glucose-intolerant mice. *Am. J. Physiol. Endocrinol. Metab.* **2002**, *283*, E738–E744. [CrossRef] [PubMed]
38. Berglund, E.D.; Li, C.Y.; Poffenberger, G.; Ayala, J.E.; Fueger, P.T.; Willis, S.E.; Jewell, M.M.; Powers, A.C.; Wasserman, D.H. Glucose metabolism in vivo in four commonly used inbred mouse strains. *Diabetes* **2008**, *57*, 1790–1799. [CrossRef]
39. Turner, N.; Kowalski, G.M.; Leslie, S.J.; Risis, S.; Yang, C.; Lee-Young, R.S.; Babb, J.R.; Meikle, P.J.; Lancaster, G.I.; Henstridge, D.C.; et al. Distinct patterns of tissue-specific lipid accumulation during the induction of insulin resistance in mice by high-fat feeding. *Diabetologia* **2013**, *56*, 1638–1648. [CrossRef]
40. Wang, D.; Tai, P.W.L.; Gao, G. Adeno-associated virus vector as a platform for gene therapy delivery. *Nat. Rev. Drug Discov.* **2019**, *18*, 358–378. [CrossRef]
41. Chang, H.-H.; Moro, A.; Takakura, K.; Su, H.-Y.; Mo, A.; Nakanishi, M.; Waldron, R.T.; French, S.W.; Dawson, D.W.; Hines, O.J.; et al. Incidence of pancreatic cancer is dramatically increased by a high fat, high calorie diet in KrasG12D mice. *PLoS ONE* **2017**, *12*, e0184455. [CrossRef]
42. Ead, A.S.; Wirkus, J.; Matsukuma, K.; Mackenzie, G.G. A high-fat diet induces changes in mesenteric adipose tissue accelerating early-stage pancreatic carcinogenesis in mice. *J. Nutr. Biochem.* **2024**, *131*, 109690. [CrossRef]
43. Okumura, T.; Ohuchida, K.; Sada, M.; Abe, T.; Endo, S.; Koikawa, K.; Iwamoto, C.; Miura, D.; Mizuuchi, Y.; Moriyama, T.; et al. Extra-pancreatic invasion induces lipolytic and fibrotic changes in the adipose microenvironment, with released fatty acids enhancing the invasiveness of pancreatic cancer cells. *Oncotarget* **2017**, *8*, 18280–18295. [CrossRef]
44. Dawson, D.W.; Hertzer, K.; Moro, A.; Donald, G.; Chang, H.-H.; Go, V.L.; Pandol, S.J.; Lugea, A.; Gukovskaya, A.S.; Li, G.; et al. High-fat, high-calorie diet promotes early pancreatic neoplasia in the conditional KrasG12D mouse model. *Cancer Prev. Res.* **2013**, *6*, 1064–1073. [CrossRef] [PubMed]
145. Luo, Y.; Yang, Y.; Liu, M.; Wang, D.; Wang, F.; Bi, Y.; Ji, J.; Li, S.; Liu, Y.; Chen, R.; et al. Oncogenic KRAS Reduces Expression of FGF21 in Acinar Cells to Promote Pancreatic Tumorigenesis in Mice on a High-Fat Diet. *Gastroenterology* **2019**, *157*, 1413–1428.e1411. [CrossRef] [PubMed]
146. Ruze, R.; Song, J.; Yin, X.; Chen, Y.; Xu, R.; Wang, C.; Zhao, Y. Mechanisms of obesity- and diabetes mellitus-related pancreatic carcinogenesis: A comprehensive and systematic review. *Signal Transduct. Target. Ther.* **2023**, *8*, 139. [CrossRef]
147. Zhu, L.; Ji, J.; Ma, J.; Wang, D.; Liu, M.; Du, J.X.; Chen, R.; Hou, W.; Abbruzzese, J.L.; Logsdon, C.D.; et al. Differential Effects of Dietary Macronutrients on the Development of Oncogenic KRAS-Mediated Pancreatic Ductal Adenocarcinoma. *Cancers* **2022**, *14*, 2723. [CrossRef]
148. O'Neill, S.M.; Hinkle, C.; Chen, S.-J.; Sandhu, A.; Hovhannisyan, R.; Stephan, S.; Lagor, W.R.; Ahima, R.S.; Johnston, J.C.; Reilly, M.P. Targeting adipose tissue via systemic gene therapy. *Gene Ther.* **2014**, *21*, 653–661. [CrossRef]
149. Uhrig-Schmidt, S.; Geiger, M.; Luippold, G.; Birk, G.; Mennerich, D.; Neubauer, H.; Grimm, D.; Wolfrum, C.; Kreuz, S. Gene delivery to adipose tissue using transcriptionally targeted rAAV8 vectors. *PLoS ONE* **2014**, *9*, e116288. [CrossRef]
150. Bates, R.; Huang, W.; Cao, L. Adipose Tissue: An Emerging Target for Adeno-associated Viral Vectors. *Mol. Ther. Methods Clin. Dev.* **2020**, *19*, 236–249. [CrossRef]

151. Mallya, K.; Haridas, D.; Seshacharyulu, P.; Pothuraju, R.; Junker, W.M.; Krishn, S.R.; Muniyan, S.; Vengoji, R.; Batra, S.K. Rachagani, S. Acinar transformed ductal cells exhibit differential mucin expression in a tamoxifen-induced pancreatic ducta adenocarcinoma mouse model. *Biol. Open* **2020**, *9*, bio052878. [CrossRef] [PubMed]
152. Lupo, F.; Piro, G.; Torroni, L.; Delfino, P.; Trovato, R.; Rusev, B.; Fiore, A.; Filippini, D.; Sanctis, F.d.; Manfredi, M.; et al. Organoid Transplant Model Systems to Study the Effects of Obesity on the Pancreatic Carcinogenesis in vivo. *Front. Cell Dev. Biology* **2020**, *8*, 308. [CrossRef] [PubMed]
153. Popovic, K.; Smolović, B.; Martinović, M.; Vučković, L. The Relationship between Diabetes Mellitus and Pancreatic Cancer—Diabetes Mellitus as a Red Flag for Pancreatic Cancer. *Cancer Epidemiol. Biomark. Prev.* **2023**, *32*, 298–305. [CrossRef]
154. Duvillié, B.; Kourdoughli, R.; Druillennec, S.; Eychène, A.; Pouponnot, C. Interplay Between Diabetes and Pancreatic Ducta Adenocarcinoma and Insulinoma: The Role of Aging, Genetic Factors, and Obesity. *Front. Endocrinol.* **2020**, *11*, 563267. [CrossRef] [PubMed]
155. Amundadottir, L.T. Pancreatic Cancer Genetics. *Int. J. Biol. Sci.* **2016**, *12*, 314–325. [CrossRef]
156. Kalisz, M.; Bernardo, E.; Beucher, A.; Maestro, M.A.; del Pozo, N.; Millán, I.; Haeberle, L.; Schlensog, M.; Safi, S.A.; Knoefel, W.T. et al. HNF1A recruits KDM6A to activate differentiated acinar cell programs that suppress pancreatic cancer. *EMBO J.* **2020**, *39* e102808. [CrossRef]
157. Cobo-Vuilleumier, N.; Lorenzo, P.I.; Rodríguez, N.G.; Herrera Gómez, I.G.; Fuente-Martin, E.; López-Noriega, L.; Mellado-Gil J.M.; Romero-Zerbo, S.Y.; Baquié, M.; Lachaud, C.C.; et al. LRH-1 agonism favours an immune-islet dialogue which protects against diabetes mellitus. *Nat. Commun.* **2018**, *9*, 1488. [CrossRef]
158. Flandez, M.; Cendrowski, J.; Cañamero, M.; Salas, A.; del Pozo, N.; Schoonjans, K.; Real, F.X. Nr5a2 heterozygosity sensitises to and cooperates with, inflammation in KRas(G12V)-driven pancreatic tumourigenesis. *Gut* **2014**, *63*, 647–655. [CrossRef] [PubMed]
159. Cobo, I.; Martinelli, P.; Flández, M.; Bakiri, L.; Zhang, M.; Carrillo-de-Santa-Pau, E.; Jia, J.; Sánchez-Arévalo Lobo, V.J.; Megías, D. Felipe, I.; et al. Transcriptional regulation by NR5A2 links differentiation and inflammation in the pancreas. *Nature* **2018**, *554* 533–537. [CrossRef]
160. Raho, S.; Capobianco, L.; Malivindi, R.; Vozza, A.; Piazzolla, C.; De Leonardis, F.; Gorgoglione, R.; Scarcia, P.; Pezzuto, F.; Agrimi G.; et al. KRAS-regulated glutamine metabolism requires UCP2-mediated aspartate transport to support pancreatic cancer growth. *Nat. Metab.* **2020**, *2*, 1373–1381. [CrossRef]
161. Li, D.; Tang, H.; Hassan, M.M.; Holly, E.A.; Bracci, P.M.; Silverman, D.T. Diabetes and risk of pancreatic cancer: A pooled analysis of three large case–control studies. *Cancer Causes Control* **2011**, *22*, 189–197. [CrossRef]
162. Maisonneuve, P.; Lowenfels, A.B.; Bueno-de-Mesquita, H.B.; Ghadirian, P.; Baghurst, P.A.; Zatonski, W.A.; Miller, A.B.; Duell E.J.; Boffetta, P.; Boyle, P. Past Medical History and Pancreatic Cancer Risk: Results from a Multicenter Case-Control Study. *Ann Epidemiol.* **2010**, *20*, 92–98. [CrossRef]
163. Carstensen, B.; Read, S.H.; Friis, S.; Sund, R.; Keskimäki, I.; Svensson, A.M.; Ljung, R.; Wild, S.H.; Kerssens, J.J.; Harding, J.L.; et al Cancer incidence in persons with type 1 diabetes: A five-country study of 9,000 cancers in type 1 diabetic individuals. *Diabetologia* **2016**, *59*, 980–988. [CrossRef] [PubMed]
164. Liao, W.-C.; Tu, Y.-K.; Wu, M.-S.; Lin, J.-T.; Wang, H.-P.; Chien, K.-L. Blood glucose concentration and risk of pancreatic cancer Systematic review and dose-response meta-analysis. *BMJ* **2015**, *349*, g7371. [CrossRef] [PubMed]
165. Menini, S.; Iacobini, C.; de Latouliere, L.; Manni, I.; Vitale, M.; Pilozzi, E.; Pesce, C.; Cappello, P.; Novelli, F.; Piaggio, G.; et al Diabetes promotes invasive pancreatic cancer by increasing systemic and tumour carbonyl stress in Kras(G12D/+) mice. *J. Exp Clin. Cancer Res.* **2020**, *39*, 152. [CrossRef]
166. van Kruijsdijk, R.C.M.; van der Wall, E.; Visseren, F.L.J. Obesity and Cancer: The Role of Dysfunctional Adipose Tissue. *Cancer Epidemiol. Biomark. Prev.* **2009**, *18*, 2569–2578. [CrossRef]
167. Kahn, S.E.; Hull, R.L.; Utzschneider, K.M. Mechanisms linking obesity to insulin resistance and type 2 diabetes. *Nature* **2006**, *444*, 840–846. [CrossRef] [PubMed]
168. Xu, T.; Xu, X.; Liu, P.-C.; Mao, H.; Ju, S. Transcriptomic Analyses and Potential Therapeutic Targets of Pancreatic Cancer With Concomitant Diabetes. *Front. Oncol.* **2020**, *10*, 563527. [CrossRef]
169. Zhang, A.M.Y.; Magrill, J.; de Winter, T.J.J.; Hu, X.; Skovsø, S.; Schaeffer, D.F.; Kopp, J.L.; Johnson, J.D. Endogenous Hyperinsulinemia Contributes to Pancreatic Cancer Development. *Cell Metab.* **2019**, *30*, 403–404. [CrossRef]
170. Li, D.; Yeung, S.C.J.; Hassan, M.M.; Konopleva, M.; Abbruzzese, J.L. Antidiabetic Therapies Affect Risk of Pancreatic Cancer *Gastroenterology* **2009**, *137*, 482–488. [CrossRef]
171. Chen, K.; Qian, W.; Jiang, Z.; Cheng, L.; Li, J.; Sun, L.; Zhou, C.; Gao, L.; Lei, M.; Yan, B.; et al. Metformin suppresses cancer initiation and progression in genetic mouse models of pancreatic cancer. *Mol. Cancer* **2017**, *16*, 131. [CrossRef]
172. Tan, J.; You, Y.; Guo, F.; Xu, J.; Dai, H.; Bie, P. Association of elevated risk of pancreatic cancer in diabetic patients: A systematic review and meta-analysis. *Oncol. Lett.* **2017**, *13*, 1247–1255. [CrossRef] [PubMed]
173. Parajuli, P.; Nguyen, T.L.; Prunier, C.; Razzaque, M.S.; Xu, K.; Atfi, A. Pancreatic cancer triggers diabetes through TGF-β–mediated selective depletion of islet β-cells. *Life Sci. Alliance* **2020**, *3*, e201900573. [CrossRef] [PubMed]

174. McGuigan, A.; Kelly, P.; Turkington, R.C.; Jones, C.; Coleman, H.G.; McCain, R.S. Pancreatic cancer: A review of clinical diagnosis, epidemiology, treatment and outcomes. *World J. Gastroenterol.* **2018**, *24*, 4846–4861. [CrossRef] [PubMed]
175. Glauert, H.P.; Elliott, R.S.; Han, S.G.; Athey, M.; Lee, E.Y.; Gairola, C.G. Effect of cigarette smoke exposure and mutant Kras overexpression on pancreatic cell proliferation. *Oncol. Lett.* **2017**, *13*, 1939–1943. [CrossRef]
176. Edderkaoui, M.; Grippo, P.J.; Ouhaddi, Y.; Benhaddou, H.; Xu, S.; Pinkerton, K.; Tsukamoto, H.; Knudsen, B.; Gukovskaya, A.S.; Pandol, S. Mouse models of pancreatic cancer induced by chronic pancreatitis and smoking. *J. Clin. Oncol.* **2014**, *32*, 229. [CrossRef]
177. Nimmakayala, R.K.; Seshacharyulu, P.; Lakshmanan, I.; Rachagani, S.; Chugh, S.; Karmakar, S.; Rauth, S.; Vengoji, R.; Atri, P.; Talmon, G.A.; et al. Cigarette Smoke Induces Stem Cell Features of Pancreatic Cancer Cells via PAF1. *Gastroenterology* **2018**, *155*, 892–908.e896. [CrossRef]
178. Hermann, P.C.; Sancho, P.; Cañamero, M.; Martinelli, P.; Madriles, F.; Michl, P.; Gress, T.; de Pascual, R.; Gandia, L.; Guerra, C.; et al. Nicotine promotes initiation and progression of KRAS-induced pancreatic cancer via Gata6-dependent dedifferentiation of acinar cells in mice. *Gastroenterology* **2014**, *147*, 1119–1133.e1114. [CrossRef]
179. Momi, N.; Kaur, S.; Ponnusamy, M.P.; Kumar, S.; Wittel, U.A.; Batra, S.K. Interplay between Smoking-induced Genotoxicity and Altered Signaling in Pancreatic Carcinogenesis. *Carcinogenesis* **2012**, *33*, 1617–1628. [CrossRef]
180. Weissman, S.; Takakura, K.; Eibl, G.; Pandol, S.J.; Saruta, M. The Diverse Involvement of Cigarette Smoking in Pancreatic Cancer Development and Prognosis. *Pancreas* **2020**, *49*, 612–620. [CrossRef]
181. Asahina, K.; Balog, S.; Hwang, E.; Moon, E.; Wan, E.; Skrypek, K.; Chen, Y.; Fernandez, J.; Romo, J.; Yang, Q.; et al. Moderate alcohol intake promotes pancreatic ductal adenocarcinoma development in mice expressing oncogenic Kras. *Am. J. Physiol. Gastrointest. Liver Physiol.* **2020**, *318*, G265–G276. [CrossRef]
182. Kaune, T.; Griesmann, H.; Theuerkorn, K.; Hämmerle, M.; Laumen, H.; Krug, S.; Plumeier, I.; Kahl, S.; Junca, H.; Gustavo Dos Anjos Borges, L.; et al. Gender-specific changes of the gut microbiome correlate with tumor development in murine models of pancreatic cancer. *iScience* **2023**, *26*, 106841. [CrossRef] [PubMed]
183. Pfisterer, N.; Ammer-Herrmenau, C.; Antweiler, K.; Küffer, S.; Ellenrieder, V.; Neesse, A. Dynamics of intestinal and intratumoral microbiome signatures in genetically engineered mice and human pancreatic ductal adenocarcinoma. *Pancreatology* **2023**, *23*, 663–673. [CrossRef] [PubMed]
184. Michaud, D.S.; Izard, J.; Wilhelm-Benartzi, C.S.; You, D.H.; Grote, V.A.; Tjønneland, A.; Dahm, C.C.; Overvad, K.; Jenab, M.; Fedirko, V.; et al. Plasma antibodies to oral bacteria and risk of pancreatic cancer in a large European prospective cohort study. *Gut* **2013**, *62*, 1764–1770. [CrossRef]
185. Saba, E.; Farhat, M.; Daoud, A.; Khashan, A.; Forkush, E.; Menahem, N.H.; Makkawi, H.; Pandi, K.; Angabo, S.; Kawasaki, H.; et al. Oral bacteria accelerate pancreatic cancer development in mice. *Gut* **2024**, *73*, 770–786. [CrossRef] [PubMed]
186. Thomas, R.M.; Gharaibeh, R.Z.; Gauthier, J.; Beveridge, M.; Pope, J.L.; Guijarro, M.V.; Yu, Q.; He, Z.; Ohland, C.; Newsome, R.; et al. Intestinal microbiota enhances pancreatic carcinogenesis in preclinical models. *Carcinogenesis* **2018**, *39*, 1068–1078. [CrossRef]
187. Sexton, R.E.; Uddin, M.H.; Bannoura, S.; Khan, H.Y.; Mzannar, Y.; Li, Y.; Aboukameel, A.; Al-Hallak, M.N.; Al-Share, B.; Mohamed, A.; et al. Connecting the Human Microbiome and Pancreatic Cancer. *Cancer Metastasis Rev.* **2022**, *41*, 317–331. [CrossRef]
188. Attebury, H.; Daley, D. The Gut Microbiome and Pancreatic Cancer Development and Treatment. *Cancer J.* **2023**, *29*, 49–56. [CrossRef]
189. Liot, S.; El Kholti, N.; Balas, J.; Genestier, L.; Verrier, B.; Valcourt, U.; Lambert, E. Development of thymic tumor in [LSL:KrasG12D.; Pdx1-CRE] mice, an adverse effect associated with accelerated pancreatic carcinogenesis. *Sci. Rep.* **2021**, *11*, 15075. [CrossRef]

cancers

MDPI

Review

Long Non-Coding RNAs and RNA-Binding Proteins in Pancreatic Cancer Development and Progression

Pit Preckwinkel [1], Khursheed Ul Islam Mir [2], Florian W. Otto [3,4], Hend Elrewany [2], Andrea Sinz [3,4], Stefan Hüttelmaier [2], Nadine Bley [2,*] and Tony Gutschner [1,*]

1 Section for RNA Biology and Pathogenesis, Institute of Molecular Medicine, Faculty of Medicine, Martin Luther University Halle-Wittenberg, 06120 Halle (Saale), Germany; pit.preckwinkel@uk-halle.de
2 Section for Molecular Cell Biology, Institute of Molecular Medicine, Faculty of Medicine, Martin Luther University Halle-Wittenberg, 06120 Halle (Saale), Germany; khursheed.mir@medizin.uni-halle.de (K.U.I.M.); hend.elrewany@medizin.uni-halle.de (H.E.); stefan.huettelmaier@medizin.uni-halle.de (S.H.)
3 Department of Pharmaceutical Chemistry and Bioanalytics, Institute of Pharmacy, Faculty of Natural Sciences I, Martin Luther University Halle-Wittenberg, 06120 Halle (Saale), Germany; florian.otto@pharmazie.uni-halle.de (F.W.O.); andrea.sinz@pharmazie.uni-halle.de (A.S.)
4 Center for Structural Mass Spectrometry, Martin Luther University Halle-Wittenberg, 06120 Halle (Saale), Germany
* Correspondence: nadine.stoehr@medizin.uni-halle.de (N.B.); tony.gutschner@uk-halle.de (T.G.)

Simple Summary: Pancreatic cancer is a deadly disease which is often detected at advanced stages. Novel and innovative approaches are urgently needed to improve diagnosis and personalized treatment strategies to achieve significant clinical benefits. Here, we introduce two interesting yet largely understudied classes of disease-associated molecules, i.e., long non-coding RNAs and RNA-binding proteins. We highlight their potential as biomarkers as well as therapeutic targets, and we provide examples of their functional diversity contributing to pancreatic cancer development and progression.

Abstract: Pancreatic ductal adenocarcinoma (PDAC) is the most common type of pancreatic cancer and is responsible for about 467,000 cancer deaths annually. An oftentimes asymptomatic early phase of this disease results in a delayed diagnosis, and patients often present with advanced disease. Current treatment options have limited survival benefits, and only a minor patient population carries actionable genomic alterations. Hence, innovative personalized treatment strategies that consider molecular, cellular and functional analyses are urgently needed for pancreatic cancer patients. However, the majority of the genetic alterations found in PDAC are currently undruggable, or patients' response is not as expected. Therefore, non-genomic biomarkers and alternative molecular targets should be considered in order to advance the clinical management of PDAC patients. In line with this, recent gene expression and single-cell transcriptome analyses have identified molecular subtypes and transcriptional cell states that affect disease progression and drug efficiency. In this review, we will introduce long non-coding RNAs (lncRNAs) as well as RNA-binding proteins (RBPs) that are able to modulate the transcriptome of a cell through diverse mechanisms, thereby contributing to disease progression. We will provide a brief overview about the general functions of lncRNAs and RBPs, respectively. Subsequently, we will highlight selected lncRNAs and RBPs that have been shown to play a role in PDAC development, progression and drug response. Finally, we will present strategies aiming to interfere with the expression and function of lncRNAs and RBPs.

Keywords: HuR; IGF2BP1; KRAS; LINC00261; LncRNA; MAPK; PDAC; RBP; TGF-β

1. Introduction

The most recent global cancer statistics for the year 2022 estimate a total of almost 20 million new cancer cases and about 9.7 million cancer deaths [1]. With nearly 510,716 new cases and 467,000 deaths, pancreatic cancer ranks at position 12 and 6 in terms of incidence and mortality, respectively. Pancreatic ductal adenocarcinoma (PDAC), the most common type of pancreatic cancer, is a devastating disease with an overall 5-year survival rate of approximately 13% [2]. An oftentimes asymptomatic early phase leading to a delayed diagnosis of PDAC in patients presenting with advanced and metastatic disease, in conjunction with a high resistance to currently available therapies, is a critical factor responsible for this high mortality rate. Of note, surgery as well as chemotherapy and radiotherapy is the major treatment option, and despite advances in surgical and perioperative approaches, high recurrence rates (up to 79% after three years) after curative intended surgery are observed [3]. Importantly, somatic mutations in key cancer genes such as *KRAS*, *TP53*, *CDKN2A*, and *SMAD4* as well as a large number of genomic and epigenetic passenger alterations generate a remarkable inter- and intratumoural heterogeneity, which induces a considerable variation in responses to anticancer therapies [4]. Moreover, the performance status and comorbidities of the patient often dictate the choice of regimen and limit the application of non-specific and toxic chemotherapy, thereby affecting therapy resistance and tumour progression. Hence, for pancreatic cancer patients, personalized treatment strategies that consider molecular, cellular and functional analyses are urgently needed to overcome these limitations. However, only 12–25% of pancreatic cancer cases harbour actionable genomic alterations [5]. For example, about 7% of patients carry *BRCA1/2* germline mutations that sensitize their tumours to the PARP inhibitor olaparib, which was shown to extend progression-free survival in metastatic pancreatic adenocarcinoma [6]. Additional targeted therapies for rare molecular pancreatic cancer subgroups like *NTRK*-fusion-positive, the $KRAS^{G12C}$ mutant, DNA mismatch repair-deficient, or microsatellite-instable (MSI^{high}) tumours might be viable options as well [7–10]. However, the majority of the genetic alterations found in PDAC are currently undruggable, or patients' response is not as expected despite targeting actionable mutations with tailored drugs. Therefore, non-genomic biomarkers and alternative molecular targets should be considered in order to advance the clinical management of PDAC patients. In line with this, recent gene expression and single-cell transcriptome analyses have identified molecular subtypes and transcriptional cell states that affect disease progression and drug efficiency [11–14].

In this review, we will introduce long non-coding RNAs (lncRNAs) as well as RNA-binding proteins (RBPs), which have been shown to be associated with certain PDAC subtypes and are able to modulate the transcriptome of a cell through diverse mechanisms [15–18]. We will provide a brief overview about the general functions of lncRNAs and RBPs, respectively. Subsequently, we will highlight selected lncRNAs and RBPs that have been shown to play a role in PDAC development, progression, and drug response. Last but not least, we will present strategies aiming to interfere with the expression and function of lncRNAs and RBPs.

2. Role of lncRNAs in PDAC Development and Progression

Even though less than 2% of the human genome consists of protein-coding genes, transcription is pervasive, and modern RNA sequencing technologies have shown that transcripts are generated from 75 to 85% of the genome [19,20]. Some of these non-protein-coding RNAs (ncRNAs), such as ribosomal RNAs, transfer RNAs and microRNAs (miRNAs), can be categorized into classes based on their specific functions. What remains is a vast number of mostly RNA polymerase II (Pol II)-derived transcripts that vary in size, function and distribution. LncRNAs are somewhat arbitrarily, as they are defined as transcripts that are longer than 500 nucleotides (nts) [21]. More than 100,000 human lncRNAs have been recorded, exceeding the ~20,000 protein-coding genes in number. Their lengths range from one to tens of thousands of nucleotides, and they can occupy various genomic locations [22–24]. Intergenic lncRNAs are derived from regions devoid of coding potential, while intronic and sense/antisense lncRNAs are co-localized with protein-coding genes. Bidirectional lncRNAs share promoters with protein-coding genes and are transcribed in the antisense direction. Many lncRNAs share features with messenger RNAs (mRNAs) in that they are often polyadenylated and 5′capped, tend to comprise multiple exons and undergo alternative splicing [25,26]. Major differences lie in their overall lower degree of sequence conservation between species and their more restricted expression patterns, often being limited to specific cell types or developmental stages [27,28].

On a molecular level, lncRNAs can form complex secondary and tertiary structures that can interface with DNA, proteins and other RNAs and may be found in both nucleus and cytoplasm, enabling them to regulate gene expression on every level [29]. Through RNA-DNA interactions, they can alter the chromatin architecture and control transcription [30,31]. Via RNA-RNA actions, they affect the processing, splicing, editing, stability and localization of RNAs, in general, as well as influence the translation rates of mRNAs [32–35]. Finally, they can regulate protein localization, turnover and modification through RNA–protein interactions and serve as scaffolds for large protein complexes and biomolecular condensates [36–40]. When it comes to classifying lncRNAs based on their functions, the broadest approach is to differentiate between cis-acting and trans-acting lncRNAs. Cis-acting lncRNAs accumulate at and interact with the locus from which they are transcribed [41]. Many lncRNAs are found associated with the chromatin, tethered to their transcriptional origins by Pol II, and these proximity-based mechanisms may offset their often low expression levels [42,43]. Other lncRNAs vacate their sites of transcription to operate in trans and exert their functions in other nuclear regions or the cytoplasm. Table 1 lists a selection of common modes of action that have been found for lncRNAs acting in both cis and trans. Notably, a given lncRNA can have multiple interaction partners and functional modes depending on the biological context.

Table 1. Overview of common modes of action of long non-coding RNAs (lncRNAs).

Function	Mode of Action	Description	Examples
Enhancer action	cis/trans	A total of 30–60% of lncRNAs are transcribed from enhancer regions, and enhancer activity is modulated by the active transcription and splicing of enhancer lncRNAs [44–46]. These transcripts may potentiate enhancer activity by recruiting proteins that participate in the formation of chromatin loops between distal enhancers and their promoters or direct the recruitment of transcriptional activators to gene-proximal enhancers [47–49]. Similar mechanisms can also result in the repression of enhancer activity when lncRNA loci compete for enhancers with protein-coding genes [50].	*Hand2os1* [47,48] *CCAT1-L* [49] *PVT1* [50]
Chromatin architecture modulation	cis/trans	The process of X chromosome inactivation is dependent on the *cis*-acting lncRNA *XIST*, which spreads along and coats the inactive chromosome, ensuring dosage compensation [31,51]. Additionally, association with chromatin remodelling complexes is a common feature among lncRNAs [52]. The polycomp repressive complex 2 (PRC2) in particular is functionally dependent on RNAs and has been shown to interact with ~20% of human lncRNAs [52,53].	*HOTAIR* [30,54] *XIST* [31,51]
Biomolecular condensate formation	trans	Intracellular condensates are formed from RNA and protein interactions through liquid–liquid phase separation. Many of these compartments depend on architectural lncRNAs for their structures, compositions and functions [55].	*NORAD* [36] *NEAT1* [40] *MALAT1* [56]
miRNA sponge	trans	The target sites of miRNAs are found in mRNAs but are also present in many types of ncRNAs including lncRNAs. This has led to the hypothesis that all transcripts sharing binding sites for a particular miRNA may regulate each other by competing against each other [57]. An extensive number of publications have focused on the action of lncRNAs as competing endogenous RNAs (ceRNAs), but the hypothesis has also received criticism relating to the stoichiometries needed to support ceRNA regulatory networks [58].	*LINCMD1* [59], *PTENP1* [60,61]

Importantly, lncRNAs have been associated with a broad spectrum of human diseases, and it was discovered that the vast majority (~99%) of somatic single-nucleotide variations (SNVs) occur in non-coding regions including lncRNA loci [62]. Importantly, gene expression analyses uncovered a frequent dysregulation of lncRNAs in cancer, and functional studies identified individual non-coding transcripts controlling cancer hallmarks [63–65]. Accordingly, lncRNAs have gained relevance as biomarkers for the early detection of cancer, prognostic markers and therapeutic targets [66]. Their expression patterns also have the tendency to be more cancer-type specific compared to pseudogenes and protein-coding genes, further underscoring their diagnostic value [67]. Given the dire trajectory of pancreatic cancer incidence and mortality, the potential for new biomarkers and therapeutic avenues offered by lncRNAs holds great potential. Of note, a large selection of lncRNAs has been found to be dysregulated in pancreatic tumours and PDAC cell lines and was shown to be associated with clinical disease parameters [68–72]. Many of these transcripts are upregulated in PDAC acting as oncogenes, promoting proliferation, survival and invasiveness. Several lncRNAs that were previously known to promote tumours in other cancer types have also been found to be increased in PDAC, e.g., H19, *MALAT1* and *HOTAIR* [73–75]. Tumour-suppressive lncRNAs have also been identified, with examples including *DGCR5*, *MEG3* and *lnc-PCTST* [76–78]. In the following paragraphs, we will highlight individual lncRNAs that have been linked with PDAC development and oncogenic signalling pathways underlying pancreatic cancer progression.

2.1. LncRNAs Associated with PDAC Initiation and Early Development

Frequently, dysregulated lncRNAs in PDAC are identified by comparing the gene expression signatures of late-stage tumour samples and normal pancreatic tissues. In order to gain insights into the early stages of carcinogenesis, precursor lesions or preceding benign pancreatic diseases should be included in such analyses, and liquid biopsy samples might be considered for early biomarker discovery. In fact, the lncRNAs *ABHD11-AS1* and *HULC* were both detected in the serum of pancreatic cancer patients with increasing levels following the disease's progression from healthy patients to those with benign diseases like chronic pancreatitis, as well as to those with fully developed pancreatic cancer [79,80]. Another study focused on intraductal papillary mucinous neoplasms (IPMNs), a common type of cystic PDAC precursor lesion. LncRNA signatures in the plasma from a cohort of IPMN cases could differentiate both IPMNs from non-disease controls as well as aggressive IPMNs from benign precursors [81]. However, patient biopsies from early-stage PDAC cases are often difficult to obtain due to the late diagnosis of the disease. Here, genetically engineered mouse models (GEMMs) present a powerful tool to follow the entire progression, from precursor to metastatic cancer, and study the role of lncRNAs in this cascade. For example, Mello et al. used a mouse model with pancreas-specific expression of oncogenic $Kras^{G12D}$ to study the role of the lncRNA *Neat1* in tumour initiation. In this model, *Neat1* proved critical in suppressing the development of premalignant pancreatic intraepithelial neoplasia (PanIN) and cystic lesions [82]. Of note, this conserved lncRNA has been implicated in a variety of cellular functions and is best known for its architectural role in nuclear paraspeckles, a type of nuclear body which is itself multifunctional [83]. It is therefore perhaps not surprising that its role in cancer is also multifaceted, promoting or suppressing tumour development depending on the cancer type and context. Indeed, in developed pancreatic cancer and fully transformed PDAC cell lines, human *NEAT1* has mostly been assigned oncogenic roles [84–86]. The example of *NEAT1* highlights the importance of resolving the functions of lncRNAs in early cancer stages to gain a complete mechanistic understanding of the disease and the stage-specific contributions of lncRNAs.

2.2. LncRNAs Associated with Oncogenic KRAS Signalling

In the majority of PDAC cases, mutations cause a molecular switch in KRAS to assume a constitutive 'ON' state, resulting in a constant stream of proliferation and survival signals. The G12D and G12V mutations in the *KRAS* gene are sufficient to initiate the development of precursor lesions, and the gene dosage of mutant *KRAS* remains relevant throughout the full progression of the disease up to the growth and maintenance of metastases [87–89]. Interestingly, some lncRNAs have been found to regulate the expression and activity of *KRAS*. For example, *MALAT1* and *NUTF2P3-01* were both found to be overexpressed in pancreatic cancer, and their knockdown led to a reduction in KRAS protein level. Both lncRNAs share miRNA binding sites with the *KRAS* mRNA, suggesting a ceRNA network that is involved in tuning intracellular *KRAS* expression [90,91]. Additionally, several studies have reported the upregulation of the lncRNA *UCA1* in PDAC tissues and cell lines [92]. One of these studies observed that *UCA1* promoted the interaction between the KRAS and hnRNPAB1 proteins [93]. This interaction had previously been shown to positively regulate the activation of PI3K/AKT/mTOR signalling through oncogenic KRAS [94]. The authors also observed that *UCA1* knockdown decreased KRAS expression, and KRAS depletion reduced *UCA1* levels, indicating a positive feedback loop [93]. Furthermore, *UCA1* was found to modulate the downstream signalling pathways of KRAS. In particular, MAPK/ERK signalling was shown to be positively regulated by *UCA1*, which increased mitochondrial dynamics and thereby affected the migratory ability of pancreatic cancer cells [95]. Another study corroborated the enhancement of ERK signalling by *UCA1* and revealed that *CUDR*, an alternative transcript variant of *UCA1*, could promote the migration and invasion of pancreatic cancer cells by activating AKT/FAK and ERK signalling to induce an epithelial-to-mesenchymal transition (EMT) [96,97].

In addition to *UCA1*, several other lncRNAs have been shown to modulate KRAS downstream signalling in pancreatic cancer. For example, *ABHD11-AS1* and *SNHG1* are both overexpressed in PDAC and promote the proliferation and survival of cancer cells by up-regulating PI3K/AKT signalling [98,99]. In addition, the lncRNA *LUCAT1* was found to increase both AKT- and p38-mediated MAPK signalling, thereby supporting proliferation and invasion [100,101]. One lncRNA that has been studied in more detail on the mechanistic level is *LINC01232*. Like *UCA1*, it has also been shown to interact with hnRNPAB1 [102]. In addition to the *KRAS* mRNA, hnRNPAB1 also binds to the pre-mRNA of the downstream effector *ARAF* and regulates its splicing. This interaction favours the generation of the full-length, kinase-proficient ARAF protein [103]. *LINC01232* stabilizes hnRNPAB1 by reducing its ubiquitination and proteasomal degradation, thereby promoting the splicing of the active ARAF isoform and subsequent downstream MAPK signalling [102].

In addition to PDAC-associated lncRNAs that regulate KRAS and its downstream pathways, several studies have also identified non-coding transcripts whose expression is regulated by these signalling cues. For instance, a recent study systematically deactivated MAPK/ERK signalling in a panel of PDAC cell lines and performed comparative transcriptome analyses to identify MAPK-associated lncRNAs [104]. Out of a list of 45 candidates, *LINC00941* showed the most consistent downregulation upon MAPK abrogation, and the authors identified a binding site for the MAPK-activated transcription factor ETS-1 in its promoter region [104]. *LINC00941* has been linked to PDAC progression in several studies and has been implicated in enhancing aerobic glycolysis by modulating the Hippo pathway and inducing AKT/FAK signalling by binding and stabilizing the ANXA2 protein [105,106]. Overall, these findings highlight the intimate link between lncRNAs and KRAS/MAPK/ERK and their associated downstream signalling in PDAC.

2.3. LncRNAs Associated with Oncogenic and Tumour-Suppressive TGF-β Signalling

TGF-β signalling has an ambivalent role throughout PDAC carcinogenesis. In the early stages of the disease, it presents a serious impediment to cancer progression by blocking the cell cycle and inducing apoptosis. In contrast, advanced tumours benefit from TGF-β-mediated immune evasion and the increased cell motility and metastatic potential stemming from a TGF-β-mediated epigenetic and transcriptional reprogramming that leads to EMT [107]. The loss of the TGF-β downstream signalling protein and tumour suppressor SMAD4, which occurs in up to 60% of PDAC, is often instrumental in this switch [108–111]. Many of the tumour suppressive effects of TGF-β are mediated by SMAD4, while the oncogenic pathways are mostly SMAD4-independent [112]. Intriguingly, recent studies identified regulatory lncRNAs that modulate the expression of SMAD4 in pancreatic cancer cells. One prominent lncRNA that has been extensively studied in cancer, in part due to the close proximity of its genomic locus to the well-known *MYC* oncogene, is *PVT1* [113,114]. Increased levels of *PVT1* were detected in PDAC tissues and cell lines, and its depletion inhibited TGF-β/SMAD signalling, including the phosphorylation of SMAD2 and SMAD3, as well as the expression of TGF-β1, but at the same time, it increased SMAD4 levels. Conversely, transient overexpression of *PVT1* decreased SMAD4 levels, enhanced cellular proliferation and activated an EMT programme, thereby promoting cell migration and invasion [115]. In addition, *LINC00909* was recently identified as an upregulated lncRNA in PDAC tissues compared to a normal pancreas, and its expression was associated with poor clinicopathological features and patient outcomes. Importantly, experimental studies revealed a cytoplasmic localization of this lncRNA in PDAC cell lines, and the modulation of its expression inversely affected the stability of the *SMAD4* mRNA. Hence, this study established *LINC00909* as an important regulator of pluripotency factors, cancer stemness and metastasis by inhibiting *SMAD4* expression [116].

While the downregulation or inactivation of *SMAD4* is important for PDAC progression, the TGF-β pathway has several other members whose expression or activity could be modulated by lncRNAs. In fact, several studies have identified lncRNAs that apply diverse modes of action in order to promote or inhibit TGF-β signalling in PDAC. Two lncRNAs, namely *BC037916* and *LINC00462*, were found to be upregulated in PDAC, and they positively regulate the core TGF-β pathway, as evaluated by the increased phosphorylation of SMAD2/3 [117,118]. *BC037916* was shown to activate JAK/STAT in addition to SMAD signalling, thereby promoting an EMT programme that increased cellular invasion and metastasis in xenograft models [117]. In contrast, *LINC00462* was found to sequester miR-665, thereby upregulating TGFBR1 and TGFBR2 protein levels and activating migration and invasion through EMT induction [118].

In addition to these oncogenic lncRNAs, previous studies also highlighted the role of lncRNAs acting as tumour suppressors by modulating TGF-β signalling. For example, *LINC-PINT* was found to be downregulated in PDAC, and low plasma *LINC-PINT* expression might serve as a biomarker for early pancreatic cancer detection, whereas low levels of *LINC-PINT* in tumour tissues correlated with a poor prognosis after pancreatectomy [119,120]. Of note, the plasma levels of *LINC-PINT* and TGF-β1 were positively correlated in early-stage PDAC patients but not in healthy controls. Furthermore, the overexpression of *LINC-PINT* upregulated TGF-β1 expression in a pancreatic cancer cell line but not in telomerase-immortalized pancreatic ductal cells [120]. Importantly, *LINC-PINT* overexpression as well as exogenous TGF-β1 stimulation specifically reduced the proliferation of the pancreatic cancer cell line without affecting the growth of the non-malignant immortalized cells. The inhibitory effects of both *LINC-PINT* and TGF-β1 could be blocked by the simultaneous application of SD-208, a TGFBR1 inhibitor [120]. In conclusion, *LINC-PINT* may inhibit early-stage PDAC growth through TGF-β pathway activation. Last but not least, our own studies have identified *LINC00261* as a TGF-β-regulated tumour-suppressive lncRNA that is involved in maintaining a pro-epithelial cell state, which is associated with a favourable disease outcome. We showed that the depletion of *LINC00261* induced the expression of EMT-related genes, decreased E-cadherin levels and increased cell migration and invasion [121].

These examples underscore the diagnostic potential and functional relevance of lncRNAs in modulating the oncogenic as well as tumour-suppressive properties of the TGF-β signalling pathway in pancreatic cancer cells. Table 2 lists and Figure 1 schematically summarizes the findings on lncRNAs associated with KRAS and TGF-β signalling that have been described in this section. These principal cellular pathways controlling early PDAC progression evidently undergo regulation by lncRNAs on many levels.

Table 2. LncRNAs associated with KRAS/MAPK and TGF-β signalling in pancreatic cancer.

LncRNA	Expression in PDAC	Clinical Association	Function and Mechanism	References
NUTF2P3-01	upregulated	high expression correlates with tumour size; poor tumour differentiation; the tumour, node and metastasis (TNM) stage; lymphatic invasion; distant metastasis; and shorter overall survival (OS)	promotes proliferation, invasion, xenograft tumour growth and hepatic metastasis and acts as a ceRNA to sequester miR-3923 and increase KRAS expression	[90]
MALAT1	upregulated	high expression is associated with shorter OS	promotes proliferation, migration, invasion, and xenograft growth; reduces apoptosis; and acts as a ceRNA to sequester miR-217 and increase KRAS expression	[91]
UCA1/CUDR	upregulated	high expression correlates with an advanced T and N stage and is associated with poor OS	promotes proliferation, migration, drug resistance and xenograft tumour growth; reduces apoptosis; positively regulates MAPK/ERK and AKT/FAK signalling; enhances the interaction between KRAS and hnRNPA2/B1; and acts as a ceRNA to sequester miR-590-3p and increase KRAS expression	[93,95,96]
ABHD11-AS1	upregulated	expression correlates with poor OS and disease-free survival (DFS), an advanced TNM stage, increased distant metastasis and poor tumour differentiation	promotes proliferation and migration, reduces apoptosis and positively regulates PI3K/AKT signalling and EMT	[98]
SNHG1	upregulated	expression correlates with an advanced TNM stage and a larger tumour size	promotes proliferation, invasion and xenograft tumour growth; reduces apoptosis; and positively regulates PI3K/AKT signalling	[99]
LUCAT1	upregulated	increased expression linked to a larger tumour size and lymphatic invasion	promotes proliferation, invasion and xenograft tumour growth; reduces apoptosis; and positively regulates AKT and p38-MAPK signalling and the sponge of miR-539	[100,101]
LINC01232	upregulated	expression is positively correlated with nerve invasion, and high *LINC01232* levels are associated with worse outcomes	promotes migration and invasion and regulates the alternative splicing of ARAF by stabilizing hnRNPA2/B1, thereby activating MAPK/ERK signalling	[102]
LINC00941	upregulated	high expression is associated with a poor prognosis	promotes proliferation, is a downstream target of MAPK/ETS-1 signalling and increases E2F7	[104]
PVT1	upregulated	high expression is associated with an advanced clinical stage and lymph node metastasis (LNM)	promotes cell adhesion, viability, migration and invasion; enhances EMT via TGF-β/SMAD signalling; and downregulates SMAD4 and p21	[115,122]

Table 2. *Cont.*

LncRNA	Expression in PDAC	Clinical Association	Function and Mechanism	References
LINC00909	upregulated	high expression is associated with poor OS and DFS and correlates with an advanced TNM stage, a larger tumour size, poor differentiation and LNM	promotes cell viability, colony formation, migration and xenograft tumour growth and metastasis; inhibits apoptosis; upregulates the expression of pluripotency factors; promotes the pancreatic cancer stem cell phenotype; activates the MAPK/JNK pathway; and destabilizes the *SMAD4* mRNA	[116]
BC037916	upregulated	increased expression correlates with a clinical stage and advanced T and N stages and is associated with poor OS	promotes proliferation, invasion and xenograft tumour growth; reduces apoptosis; positively regulates EMT via SMAD2/3 signalling; and upregulates JAK/STAT signalling	[117]
LINC00462	upregulated	expression is associated with a larger tumour size, poor tumour differentiation, a TNM stage and distant metastasis	promotes proliferation, migration, invasion, xenograft growth and invasion; reduces apoptosis and cellular adhesion; induces EMT through the activation of the TGF-β pathway via the upregulation of TGFBR1/2; and acts as a ceRNA to sequester miR-665	[118]
LINC-PINT	downregulated	Low plasma levels correlate with tumour recurrence and are associated with tumour size; a low *LINC-PINT* level in tumour tissues correlates with a poor prognosis after pancreatectomy	reduces cell proliferation and increases TGF-β1 expression in a pancreatic cancer cell line	[119,120]
LINC00261	downregulated	expression is subtype-dependent and shows an inverse correlation with tumour grade and stage, and high expression is associated with better OS	inhibits cell migration and invasion; TGF-β stimulation decreases *LINC00261* levels, and its genetic ablation leads to the downregulation of the E-cadherin mRNA and protein and the induction of an EMT programme	[121]

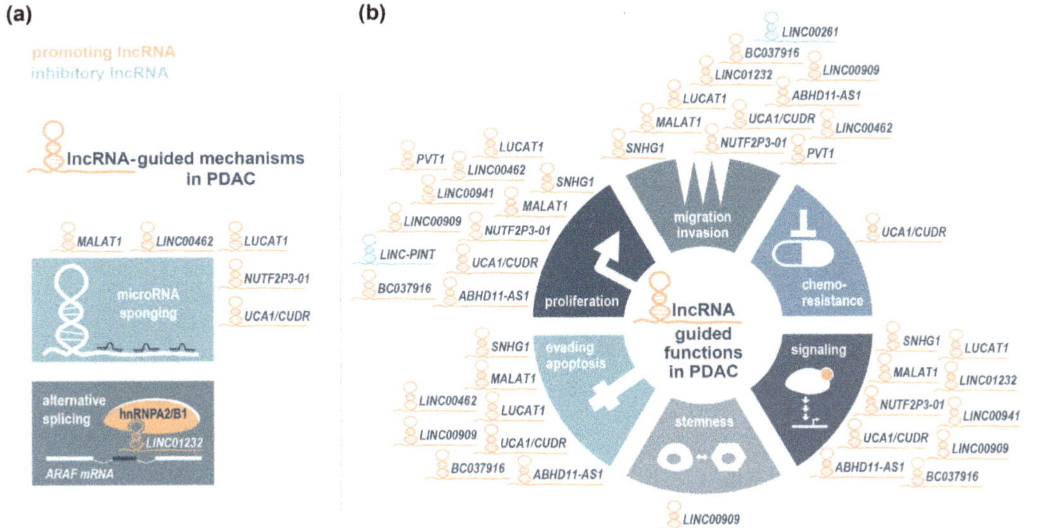

Figure 1. Long non-coding RNA (lncRNA)-guided functions and regulatory mechanisms involved in PDAC development and progression. Identified mechanisms (**a**) and cellular functions (**b**) of selected lncRNAs in pancreatic cancer, specifically in the context of KRAS/MAPK and TGF-/SMAD signalling, have been described in the main text and are summarized here schematically, with implicated promoting (orange) or inhibitory (turquois) lncRNAs assigned to their respective function. For more details about the clinical relevance and the mode of action of these lncRNAs, see Table 2.

The large number and functional versatility of lncRNAs, in general, suggest that this list is by no means completed yet. Systematic approaches towards mapping lncRNA dependencies could reveal many more potential biomarkers and therapeutic targets. Future work should incorporate samples from patients with benign precursor lesions and early-stage cancer models whenever possible. As illustrated by the examples of *NEAT1* and the TGF-β pathway, the roles of lncRNAs and the processes involving them may change dynamically as pancreatic cancer progresses.

3. Role of RNA-Binding Proteins in PDAC

RNA-binding proteins are essential regulators of RNA biology, overseeing key stages of RNA life, including RNA splicing, processing, transport, stability, turnover and translation [123–125]. These multifunctional proteins are integral for maintaining cellular homeostasis and, consequently, human health. However, RBPs can become dysregulated, contributing to various diseases including cancer [126]. In PDAC, several RBPs are considered as disease drivers with prognostic relevance [127]. Some RBPs like LIN28A/B, ELAVL1, IGF2BP or MUSASHI proteins also exhibit long-standing and well-characterized roles in carcinogenesis or tumour suppression in other cancer types. In these cases, small-molecule inhibitors have been developed and employed to target malignant phenotypes. Despite these advancements, novel cancer-related functions for RBPs have recently been identified, continuously increasing the portfolio of RBP-based therapeutic strategies. This is particularly relevant in the context of PDAC where emerging evidence links specific RBPs to disease progression. In this section, we explore recent pancreatic cancer-related findings of selected RBPs, delving into the molecular mechanisms that underpin their influence on tumour growth, survival and metastasis (Figure 2). We will provide an overview of the regulatory pathways affected by the selected RBPs and summarize the potential of targeting these proteins.

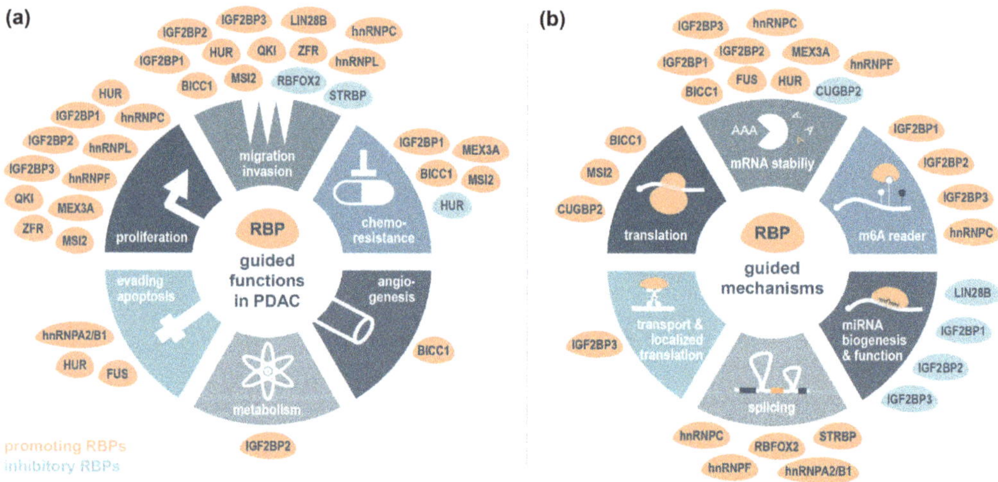

Figure 2. RNA-binding protein-guided functions and regulatory mechanisms involved in PDAC development and progression. Indicated cellular (**a**) and molecular functions (**b**) are depicted schematically with implicated promoting (orange) or inhibitory (turquois) RBPs assigned to their respective functions. Importantly, several RBPs have been shown to modulate cancer hallmarks by applying one or more modes of action to regulate their target transcripts.

3.1. ELAV-Like RNA Binding Protein 1 (ELAVL1)

ELAVL1, also known as human antigen R (HuR), plays a crucial role in the post-transcriptional regulation of numerous mRNAs involved in proliferation, cell survival, the stress response and chemoresistance. The protein is primarily located in the nucleus but shuttles to the cytoplasm to control the expression of its target transcripts. HuR binds to AU- or U-rich elements in the 3′ untranslated regions (3′UTRs) of target mRNAs to stabilize and/or enhance the translation of the respective transcripts [128]. HuR was initially discovered to be overexpressed in various cancer entities associated with a poor prognosis [129,130]. In PDAC, the HuR protein was detected in the nucleus and cytoplasm, and its cytoplasmic localization was associated with the tumour (T) stage. Interestingly, high cytoplasmic expression of HuR was associated with a favourable outcome in patients who received adjuvant therapy with gemcitabine [131]. Mechanistically, it was shown that HuR promotes the expression of DCK, an enzyme that activates gemcitabine, by stabilizing the *DCK* mRNA and enhancing its translation [132]. However, a retrospective study conducted in a cohort of 175 patients with resected periampullary adenocarcinomas, including pancreatic cancer, could not confirm the association between HuR and DCK expression and found that high HuR levels or a high HuR cytoplasmic-to-nuclear ratio is associated with poor survival in patients that received gemcitabine [133]. This finding is well in line with other reports that have assigned tumour-promoting functions to HuR. For instance, HuR was shown to stabilize the *GPRC5A* mRNA, encoding an orphan G-protein-coupled receptor, which is upregulated by gemcitabine and contributes to resistance mechanisms in pancreatic cancer cells [134].

Furthermore, HuR was identified as a regulator of proliferation, the cell cycle and apoptotic pathways in PDAC-derived cells under normal and stress conditions. In detail, the treatment of pancreatic cancer cells with DNA-damaging agents led to an accumulation of HuR in the cytoplasm and silenced expression-sensitized cells to these agents. Mechanistically, HuR was identified as a post-transcriptional regulator of the mitotic inhibitor kinase WEE1 by stabilizing the corresponding mRNA of this kinase, especially after DNA damage. Importantly, the upregulation of WEE1 induces a G2/M cell cycle arrest that enables cancer cells to repair their DNA [135]. Another study confirmed this DNA repair-promoting function of HuR by regulating the expression of *BARD1* mRNA, thereby ensuring effective DNA repair via the homologous recombination repair pathway [136].

In addition to these DNA damage response-related functions, HuR was also shown to enhance the resilience of PDAC cells to cope with metabolic stress. For example, the depletion of HuR-sensitized pancreatic cancer cells to glucose deprivation led to increased apoptosis and reduced anchorage-independent colony formation. Interestingly, glucose deprivation induced the cytoplasmic translocation of HuR and allowed for the binding of this RBP to mRNAs encoding for several metabolic enzymes, including GPI, PRPS2 and IDH1. Of note, the depletion of HuR reduced the transcript and protein abundance of these metabolic enzymes in three pancreatic cancer cell lines, suggesting a critical role of HuR in modulating pancreatic cancer cell metabolism and survival under acute glucose deprivation [137]. This pro-survival effect of HuR in pancreatic cancer cells was observed in several other studies, and additional HuR target genes like *YAP1* and *DR5/TNFRSF10B* as well as their associated pathways have been shown to be activated or inhibited by HuR [138,139].

Besides proliferation and apoptosis, HuR has been shown to promote cancer cell migration, invasion and metastasis as well as stem cell properties through its regulation of key genes, such as *SNAI1*, that play a role in EMT [140]. Intriguingly, the interruption of the HuR-RNA interaction by a novel compound called KH-3 reduced PDAC cell viability, EMT and metastatic potential both in vitro and in vivo [140].

In addition to the aforementioned tumour cell intrinsic functions, HuR was also shown to contribute to the remodelling of the tumour microenvironment (TME) by regulating the secretion of PDGFA, which led to increased collagen deposition and stromal activation in PDAC [141].

In summary, given its multifaceted role in promoting PDAC cell growth and survival, drug resistance and DNA repair, metabolic adaptation, EMT as well as metastasis, HuR represents an interesting as well as challenging therapeutic target. Inhibiting HuR alone or in combination with, e.g., DNA-damaging agents or WEE1 inhibitors, may alter therapy responses and patient outcomes in pancreatic cancer.

3.2. *Insulin-Like Growth Factor II mRNA-Binding Proteins (IGF2BPs)*

The family of oncofetal IGF2BPs, commonly upregulated or de novo expressed in various solid cancers, is notably active in several types of cancer, including PDAC, where these RBPs regulate a range of cellular processes such as proliferation, migration, invasion, metabolic pathways, chemoresistance and interactions within the TME [142,143]. As highly conserved regulators of mRNA turnover and translation, IGF2BPs can act as N6-methyladenosine (m6A) readers, binding predominantly to the 3′UTR of target mRNAs [144,145]. Through this binding, IGF2BPs protect mRNAs from miRNA-mediated decay, thereby influencing the stability and translation efficiency of various oncogenic transcripts [146]. In detail, IGF2BP1 has been identified as a key player in pancreatic cancer and was found to be significantly upregulated in this malignancy [147,148]. The overexpression of IGF2BP1 was correlated with tumour size and shorter overall survival (OS) in pancreatic cancer patients, highlighting its clinical relevance as a prognostic marker [147,148]. Mechanistically, IGF2BP1 was shown to promote cell cycle progression and proliferation via CDC25A and E2F1 and by activating AKT signalling [147–150]. Moreover, IGF2BP1 was shown to contribute to gemcitabine resistance of pancreatic cancer cells via multiple mechanisms. One study unravelled a complex RNA regulatory network that is controlled by the interaction of IGF2BP1 with m6A-modified SH3BP5-AS1, which increased the expression and stability of this lncRNA. In turn, SH3BP5-AS1 activated the WNT signalling pathway by sponging miR-139-5p, upregulated CTBP1 expression and thereby contributed to increased pancreatic cancer cell invasion, migration and stemness, as well as enhanced resistance to gemcitabine [151]. Another study could show that gemcitabine treatment inhibited pancreatic cancer cell proliferation and migration and decreased the overall m6A level potentially via the treatment-induced downregulation of the m6A writer WTAP [152]. The reduction in WTAP led to a downregulation of the m6A-modified *MYC* mRNA as well as the MYC protein. Since the *MYC* mRNA is known to be bound and stabilized by IGF2BP1 in a m6A-dependent manner, the authors speculated that gemcitabine might interfere with the WTAP/MYC/IGF2BP1 axis to inhibit pancreatic cancer progression [152,153].

The second member of the IGF2BP family, namely IGF2BP2, was found to be overexpressed in pancreatic cancer tissues as well, where it has been associated with significantly shorter OS [154,155]. The overexpression of IGF2BP2 might be driven by multiple mechanisms, including the loss of tumour-suppressive miRNAs, gene amplification and upregulation mediated by the lncRNA *LINC00901* [154,156]. Interestingly, high IGF2BP2 expression is often found in high-risk tumours that exhibit lower immune response activity [157]. Moreover, a negative correlation with immune signature markers and a direct association with the expression of PD-L1, a key immune checkpoint protein, have been described for IGF2BP2. In fact, by regulating PD-L1 expression, IGF2BP2 may contribute to immune evasion, further promoting tumour survival in the immune-suppressive microenvironment of pancreatic cancer [158]. In addition, IGF2BP2 was shown to promote cell proliferation and metabolic reprogramming to support rapid tumour growth through the activation of the PI3K/AKT signalling pathway as well as through the stimulation of the glycolytic activity in PDAC cells by stabilizing the mRNA of *GLUT1/SLC2A1*, thus enhancing its expression level and facilitating increased glucose uptake [154,159].

Last but not least, the third family member, IGF2BP3, is most frequently used as a biomarker for solid tumours [160]. In 1997, IGF2BP3 was discovered in a large-scale screen for differentially expressed genes in pancreatic cancer, and it was cloned and initially named as a KH domain-containing protein overexpressed in cancer (KOC) [161]. Later studies confirmed its overexpression and revealed the prognostic relevance of IGF2BP3 in PDAC [161–165]. Importantly, based on biopsies or microdissections, IGF2BP3 is considered as a biomarker that detects early pancreatic lesions with high sensitivity and specificity [162–168]. Similar to IGF2BP2, IGF2BP3 is part of a prognostic five-gene signature that allows for the stratification of patients into low-risk and high-risk groups. The latter shows a high tumour mutational burden with lower response rates to immune checkpoint therapies [157]. Furthermore, elevated IGF2BP3 levels are associated with increased cell proliferation, migration and invasion, although its exact mechanisms remain incompletely understood. A recent study suggested that IGF2BP3 might act by blocking or mediating the interaction of specific transcripts with the RNA-induced silencing complex (RISC), thereby modulating their susceptibility to miRNA-mediated post-transcriptional gene silencing [169]. Further data suggest that IGF2BP3 might facilitate pancreatic cancer cell invasion and metastasis through additional mechanisms, including the regulation of localized translation at cell protrusions, altered adhesion by controlling CD44 expression or by stabilizing the *SMS* mRNA [170–173]. Furthermore, IGF2BP3 was shown to upregulate UBE2K, which reinforces the proliferation and stem cell-like phenotype in PDAC [174].

Collectively, these studies highlight the functional relevance of the individual IGF2BP family members in pancreatic cancer by employing overlapping as well as specific regulatory mechanisms to activate oncogenic pathways while at the same time inhibiting tumour suppressive genes and immune cell functions. Hence, these proteins are prime candidates for drug development efforts, and their oncofetal expression patterns should allow for cancer-specific targeting with minimal side effects.

3.3. BicC Family RNA-Binding Protein 1 (BICC1)

BICC1 plays a crucial role in regulating cell fate through post-transcriptional mechanisms [175]. Originally identified in *Drosophila melanogaster*, *BICC1* was recognized as a gene associated with maternal-effect mutations that cause a double-abdomen phenotype [176,177]. Later it was shown that the RBP BICC1 regulates anterior–posterior patterning in early development by controlling the localized translation of *oskar*, a key mRNA in Drosophila axis formation [178]. Recent studies highlight the upregulation of BICC1 in PDAC, particularly in lymph node metastases. Elevated BICC1 expression might affect immune cell infiltration and was shown to correlate with oncogenic pathways like EMT, TNFα/NF-kB and TGF-β signalling, which might underlie the poor prognosis of pancreatic cancer patients that express high levels of BICC1 in their tumours [179]. Mechanistically, BICC1 is able to influences tumour growth and progression through its post-transcriptional control of several molecular targets and pathways. In pancreatic cancer, BICC1 was shown to facilitate angiogenesis in a VEGF-independent manner [180]. In detail, an AU-rich sequence within the 3′UTR of the *LCN2* mRNA was recognized by BICC1, and this stabilizing interaction increased the expression of the LCN2 protein. Elevated levels of LCN2 subsequently activated the JAK2/STAT3 signalling pathway and resulted in the enhanced expression and secretion of the pro-angiogenic factor CXCL1. Intriguingly, the anti-tumour effect of gemcitabine could be improved by treating patient-derived xenograft models with elevated BICC1 expression with an anti-LCN2 antibody but not with the anti-VEGF antibody Bevacizumab [180]. Another possibility to improve gemcitabine efficacy in PDAC by targeting BICC1 and its downstream signalling was recently described. In particular, BICC1 has been identified as an activator of tryptophan catabolism by increasing the expression of IDO1 [181]. The resulting increase in tryptophan metabolites contributes to the synthesis of nicotinamide adenine dinucleotide (NAD+) and promotes oxidative phosphorylation, creating a metabolic environment conducive to a stem cell-like phenotype in cancer cells. Notably, the inhibition of the BICC1/IDO1/tryptophan metabolic axis has shown potential in improving the efficacy of gemcitabine by reducing drug resistance and limiting the stem cell-like qualities of tumour cells [181]. Hence, BICC1 emerges as a multifaceted regulator in pancreatic cancer, influencing processes such as EMT, immune infiltration, angiogenesis, chemoresistance and stemness. Its regulatory impact on *LCN2* and *IDO1* expression highlights its potential as a therapeutic target to overcome VEGF inhibitor resistance and improve responses to chemotherapy in PDAC.

Taken together, the RBPs introduced in this section highlight the important contribution of post-transcriptional regulators in modulating gene expression programmes in pancreatic cancers. Table 3 provides a comprehensive overview about additional pancreatic cancer-associated RBPs. While these RBPs represent interesting targets to treat PDAC, only a limited number of inhibitors targeting a specific RBP have been developed so far. In the final section, we will provide a general overview about the diverse opportunities that enable interference with RBPs as well as lncRNAs.

Table 3. RNA-binding proteins and their roles in pancreatic cancer.

RBP	Roles in PDAC	References
ELAVL1 (HuR)	upregulated in PDAC; associated with a poor prognosis; promotes proliferation, the cell cycle, migration and invasion; inhibits apoptosis; and might mediate gemcitabine sensitivity induced by promoting DCK expression; stabilized mRNAs in PDAC: *BARD1, DCK, DR5/TNFRSF10B, GPRC5A, IDH1, PRPS2, PDGFA, SNAI1, WEE1* and *YAP1*	[128,131–141,182]
IGF2BP1	upregulated in PDAC; associated with a poor prognosis; promotes proliferation, cell cycle progression, EMT, metastasis and gemcitabine resistance; is an m6A reader; and stabilized RNAs in PDAC: *SH3BP5-AS, E2F1* and *CDC25A*	[142–144,146–150,183]
IGF2BP2	upregulated in PDAC; associated with a poor prognosis; promotes proliferation and glucose metabolism; associated with an immune-suppressive microenvironment; is an m6A reader; and stabilized mRNAs in PDAC: *SLC2A1* and *CD274*	[142,143,154–159,183]
IGF2BP3	upregulated in PDAC; associated with a poor prognosis; frequently used as a biomarker (needle biopsy); promotes proliferation, adhesion, migration and invasion; associated with an immune suppressive microenvironment; is an m6A reader; and stabilized mRNAs in PDAC: *ARF6, ARHGEF4, CD44, SMS* and *UBE2K*	[142,143,157,161,162,164–174,183]
BICC1	upregulated in PDAC; expression associated with EMT and immune infiltration; and supports angiogenesis and chemoresistance by promoting LCN2 and CXCL1 expression	[176–181]
CELF2 (CUGBP2)	enhances stability but represses the translation of *VEGF* and *COX2* mRNAs and induced by curcumin	[184]
CSDE1 (UNR)	biomarker associated with a favourable prognosis and the immunogenic subtype	[185]
FUS	upregulated in PDAC, stabilizes the *NRF2* mRNA and suppresses oxidative stress and ferroptosis	[186]
hnRNPA2/B1	upregulated in early PDAC stages; inhibits apoptosis by suppressing *BCL-X(S)* splicing; regulates splicing of ARAF; and interacts with KRAS	[93,102,187,188]
hnRNPC	controls the mRNA stability of *IQGAP3* to promote cell proliferation, migration, invasion and metastasis	[189]
hnRNPF	part of a druggable super-enhancer network that promotes PDAC cell and tumour growth and stabilizes the *PRMT1* mRNA to promote *MYC* expression	[190]

Table 3. *Cont.*

RBP	Roles in PDAC	References
hnRNPL	upregulated in PDAC, associated with a poor prognosis and promotes migration and EMT	[191]
LIN28B	upregulated in PDAC, associated with metastasis and a poor prognosis; promotes proliferation, stemness, migration and EMT; targets in PDAC (via de-regulating let-7): *MYC, HMGA2, KRAS, TET3, WNT5A* and *PCSK9*	[192–194]
MEX3A	upregulated in PDAC, expression correlates with disease progression in human and mice; promotes cell cycle and gemcitabine resistance and stabilized mRNAs in PDAC: *CDK6*	[195]
MSI2	upregulated in PDAC; associated with metastasis and a poor prognosis; promotes proliferation, metastasis and chemoresistance; transcriptionally suppressed by KLF4; and controls HIPPO signalling by suppressing SAV1 and MOB1 translation; mRNA targets in PDAC: *NUMB, MOB1, SAV1*	[196–199]
QKI	upregulated in PDAC tumour cells and fibroblasts and promotes proliferation, EMT and metastasis	[200]
RBFOX2	prevents PDAC progression and metastasis and controls the splicing of *ABI1* mRNA to inhibit migration	[201]
RBM10	downregulated in PDAC; the RBM10 mutation in advanced-stage tumours is associated with favourable survival; regulates the splicing of *hTERT*	[202,203]
STRBP	Binds to the *HSATII* RNA to prevent EMT and invasion and controls isoform switching of *CLSTN1*	[204]
ZFR	upregulated in PDAC and promotes proliferation, cell cycle progression and invasion	[205]

4. Strategies to Target lncRNAs and RBPs

In general, targeting lncRNAs or RBPs in human PDAC patients is not a trivial task, and commonly applied strategies try to modulate the expression or interfere with molecular interactions. More recently, small molecules that mediate the selective degradation of RNAs and proteins have been developed and represent an innovative and promising opportunity (Figure 3). In this section, we will briefly introduce these strategies in more detail, and we discuss their advantages as well as their limitations.

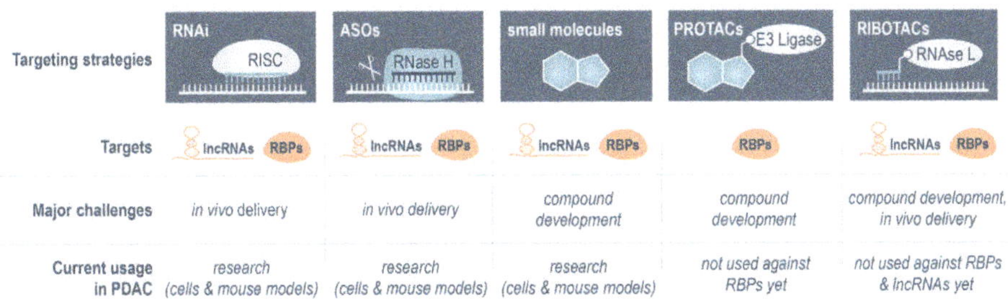

Figure 3. Summary of RBP- and lncRNA-directed therapeutic strategies and their current application in pancreatic cancer. Most strategies are currently at the early stages and have been tested in cell lines and pre-clinical mouse models. The targeting strategies can be divided into two groups. RNA interference (RNAi) and antisense oligonucleotides (ASOs). Ribonuclease-targeting chimeras (RIBOTACs) are generally RNA-directed approaches and can be used to degrade RBP-encoding mRNAs as well as lncRNAs. In contrast, small molecules and proteolysis-targeting chimeras (PROTACs) aim to target the RNA-binding protein directly and can be used to either interfere with its molecular interactions, i.e., binding to RNA, or to recruit an E3 ubiquitin ligase to induce the destruction of the RBP via the ubiquitin–proteasome system. Small molecules can also be directed against structural elements in lncRNAs to interfere with molecular interactions. The identification of specific and high-affinity binding compounds and the tumour-specific delivery of these substances pose major challenges for their clinical application in PDAC patients.

4.1. RNA Interference-Based Targeting Approaches

RNA interference (RNAi) is a conserved cellular mechanism that utilizes small, double-stranded RNA molecules, such as small interfering RNA (siRNA), short hairpin RNA (shRNA) or miRNAs, to silence gene expression by targeting complementary RNA sequences [206]. This mechanism provides a versatile and fairly specific method for reducing lncRNA and RBP expression by effectively eliminating the respective transcripts that are mainly found in the cytoplasm. The specificity of the method minimizes the risk of off-target effects, which can be a concern with other therapeutic approaches. Furthermore, RNAi-based therapies offer the flexibility to inhibit multiple targets simultaneously, enabling a more comprehensive treatment design tailored to the complexities of the disease. Hence, this multifaceted approach can potentially address various pathways that contribute to tumour growth and resistance, enhancing overall treatment efficacy. However, despite its promising capabilities, RNA-based therapy faces significant challenges, particularly concerning delivery mechanisms. RNAi agents, such as siRNA and shRNA, are highly susceptible to rapid degradation in the bloodstream, which can significantly diminish their therapeutic potential. To achieve the effective silencing of target genes within PDAC cells, RNAi agents often require the use of specialized delivery vectors, such as lipid nanoparticles or viral vectors. These vectors play a crucial role in enhancing the stability of RNAi agents and facilitating their successful delivery to target cells. Consequently, ongoing research aims at improving the delivery and stability of RNAi agents, which is essential for advancing the clinical applicability of RNAi in cancer therapy [207]. For example, novel exosome-based delivery systems have been engineered to carry siRNAs or shRNAs that targeted mutant $KRAS^{G12D}$ in multiple mouse models of pancreatic cancer [208].

In summary, RNAi offers a precise and flexible approach for gene silencing, providing a strategy for overcoming treatment resistance and enhancing chemotherapy efficacy by targeting lncRNAs and RBPs highlighted herein. While challenges related to delivery and stability persist, advancements in RNAi technologies hold promise for translating this innovative approach into effective clinical therapies for PDAC patients.

4.2. Antisense Oligonucleotides to Target lncRNAs and RBPs

Antisense oligonucleotides (ASOs) represent a powerful therapeutic strategy for targeting lncRNAs and RBPs. These short, single-stranded nucleic acids are designed to bind to complementary RNA sequences, providing a means to modulate gene expression at the transcript level. Importantly, their precise mechanisms of action depend on the specific design and chemical modification of ASOs. A major mechanism by which ASOs exert their effects is through their interaction with ribonuclease H (RNase H). This endogenous enzyme cleaves the RNA strand in RNA-DNA hybrids, and ASOs designed to leverage this interaction therefore contain a central DNA region flanked by chemically modified nucleotides [207,209]. Because RNase H cleavage occurs in the nucleus and cytoplasm, ASOs might be the preferred agents to manipulate the expression of lncRNAs that reside in the nucleus [209,210]. Another clinically relevant mechanism of action involves the regulation of alternative splicing by ASOs [211]. By binding to splice sites or regulatory sequences, ASOs can modulate the splicing patterns of target genes. Similarly, ASOs can function as steric blockers to prevent intra- and intermolecular RNA-RNA as well as RNA-DNA and RNA–protein interactions. This mode of action could be harnessed to inhibit mRNA translation, regulate polyadenylation or interfere with miRNA-mediated RNAi. Hence, ASOs similar to RNAi agents offer high specificity and versatility, and their design can be tailored for particular applications, enhancing their therapeutic potential. Furthermore, ASOs generally have manageable toxicity profiles, as they can be engineered to avoid interactions with non-targeted RNAs and proteins. Nevertheless, ASO-based therapies also face similar limitations like other RNA-based agents, particularly regarding their specific delivery. ASOs are often susceptible to rapid degradation in the bloodstream, which can hinder their effectiveness. To reach target cells, ASOs may require specialized delivery systems, such as nanoparticle-based carriers or conjugation to cell-penetrating peptides [207,212]. Thus, advancements in delivery strategies are crucial for improving the therapeutic efficacy of ASOs and ensuring that they effectively reach their intended targets within cancer cells.

In conclusion, ASOs are powerful agents that enable the targeting of nuclear and cytoplasmic protein-coding and non-coding transcripts. By inhibiting the expression of critical PDAC-associated lncRNAs and RBPs, ASOs can potentially disrupt the pathways that support tumour growth and survival. However, innovative ASO delivery systems need to be developed to enhance the effectiveness of these therapies in the fight against pancreatic cancer.

4.3. Small-Molecule Inhibitors

In addition to the aforementioned oligonucleotide-based targeting strategies, small molecules comprise another interesting approach to target lncRNAs and RBPs. These molecules are either rationally designed to bind to specific regions within their targets or they can be discovered using unbiased screening approaches. The major mechanism of action of such small-molecule inhibitors is to interfere with intra- and/or intermolecular interactions, thereby, for example, causing RNA misfolding or blocking the interaction between RBPs and their target transcripts. Indeed, several small-molecule inhibitors have been developed in recent years, and interested readers are referred to excellent reviews on this exciting topic [17,213–218]. Importantly, small-molecule inhibitors offer several advantages in targeting lncRNAs and RBPs. For example, by designing small molecules that bind to specific domains or structural elements only present in the target lncRNA or RBP, these molecules can be engineered for specificity, allowing for targeted inhibition with potentially minimal impact on non-target RNAs or proteins. Furthermore, many small-molecule inhibitors are designed for oral bioavailability and are optimized for pharmacokinetics and pharmacodynamics, which can simplify their administration and improve patient compliance. Compared to oligonucleotides and viral delivery systems, small molecules are typically easier and cheaper to synthesize and modify. Nevertheless, the identification of specific and effective small-molecule inhibitors to target RNAs and RBPs is not a trivial task given the lack of enzymatic activities that would provide an easy read-out for measuring on-target activity. Moreover, the lack of suitable binding pockets within most RBPs as well as the conserved structure of commonly found RNA-binding domains and therefore the lack of RBP-specific structural motifs as a suitable target region to disrupt intermolecular interactions complicates the rational design of small molecules. Moreover, combinatorial recognition of target RNA sequences or structures may be a common phenomenon, which makes it difficult to design small molecules that are able to block multiple binding sites. In the case of lncRNAs, structural information is often not available, and functionally relevant regions within the transcript are often unknown. Last but not least, a small molecule binding to its lncRNA or RBP target might not be sufficient to interfere with the activity of the respective target. However, once identified, specific small molecule binders can be converted to degraders as will be discussed in the next paragraph.

4.4. Targeting of lncRNAs and RBPs via Proximity-Inducing Bifunctional Molecules

The targeted degradation of disease-relevant proteins is a therapeutic concept that has gained lots of attention in recent years and has been transferred recently to the RNA world as well. The general idea is to induce proximity between a target molecule, e.g., RBP or lncRNA, and a machinery that is able to degrade the target. In order to achieve targeted protein degradation (TPD), so-called proteolysis-targeting chimeras (PROTACs) have been developed. These are heterobifunctional small molecules consisting of two ligands: one that binds a specific target protein and another one that binds an E3 ubiquitin ligase. Both ligands are joined by a linker, and the simultaneous binding of both ligands to their intended proteins induces the ubiquitination and subsequent degradation of the target protein [219]. This concept was recently applied to degrade the splicing factor SF3B1 as well as the eukaryotic translation initiation factor EIF4E [220,221]. An interesting variation of this concept, called RNA-PROTAC, has been developed and applied to degrade two RBPs, namely LIN28A and RBFOX1 [222]. The RNA-PROTAC approach requires a chimeric molecule which consists of a short oligo-ribonucleotide corresponding to the consensus binding sequence of the RBP that is conjugated to a peptide derived from HIF1A, thereby enabling the recruitment of VHL, an E3 ubiquitin ligase. The adaptation of the concept of proximity-induced degradation to eliminate specific RNAs led to the development of ribonuclease-targeting chimeras (RIBOTACs). Here, small molecules that bind to the RNA of interest are modified to carry a short 2′-5′oligoadenylate or another small molecule that binds to and locally activates RNase L [223–225]. This approach was recently leveraged to convert strong yet inactive binding interactions into potent and specific modulators of RNA function [226]. Of note, additional ASO and aptamer-based strategies have been invented to engage RNase L in targeted RNA degradation [227–230]. Thus, the field is rapidly evolving, and the development and application of PROTACs and RIBOTACs to target RBPs and lncRNAs in pancreatic cancer might change the trajectories of this devastating disease.

In summary, several strategies enable the targeting of lncRNAs and RBPs, thereby opening new avenues for biomedical research and development. However, targeting these new classes of molecules comes with additional clinical challenges and limitations. For example, targeting RBPs with housekeeping functions, e.g., regulators of splicing or translation, might cause systemic on-target toxicities that need to be carefully assessed using appropriate preclinical models. In addition, off-target toxicities of the therapeutic molecules could also occur and should be taken into account. Furthermore, genes with redundant functions, e.g., members of a specific RBP family, might require concurrent targeting in order to achieve therapeutic effects and avoid treatment resistance. Hence, potential resistance mechanisms, which are hard to predict, should be investigated early on using in vitro and in vivo approaches including unbiased functional genetic screens and molecular studies in order to understand the mode of action and drug resistance. This could also enable the development of companion diagnostics to enhance safety and efficacy. Last but not least, it is unlikely that single-target/single-agent strategies will achieve an enduring and deep clinical response in cancer therapy. Therefore, targeting a specific RBP or lncRNA in combination with already approved treatment regimen, e.g., gemcitabine/nab-paclitaxel in the case of PDAC, might be a promising strategy that should be explored systematically.

5. Conclusions and Future Perspectives

LncRNAs and RBPs are critical regulators of chemoresistance, cancer stem cell properties and oncogenic signalling in PDAC, making them compelling candidates for therapeutic interventions and disease biomarkers. In particular, the oncofetal expression pattern of individual RBPs and the tissue- and cell-type specific expression of certain lncRNAs represent unique opportunities for making future therapies more specific and early detection more sensitive. Therefore, future research should focus, on the one hand, on elucidating the molecular functions of individual, disease-associated lncRNAs and RBPs as well as their interconnections to better understand the complex regulatory networks that drive PDAC progression. Importantly, interfering with these interactions could be a valid therapeutic strategy. For example, targeting *LINC01232* or *UCA1* might affect hnRNPA2/B1 expression and its oncogenic functions [93,102]. Alternatively, preventing the m6A-dependent interaction between *LINC00941* and IGF2BP2 could be a valid strategy to impair pancreatic cancer cell migration and invasion [231]. Additionally, *LINC00261* was shown to compete with the *MYC* mRNA for binding to IGF2BP1, suggesting that the overexpression of *LINC00261*, or maybe just parts of it, could be used to decrease oncogenic MYC protein expression in PDAC [232].

On the other hand, there is an urgent need for novel sensitive and specific biomarkers, since the only Food and Drug Administration (FDA)-approved blood biomarker CA 19-9 is limited in its applicability for surveillance due to its variability among different ethnic populations and its insufficient sensitivity and specificity [233,234]. Thus, prospective studies should explore several sources, e.g., blood, saliva, urine and exosomes, and analyze different molecular classes, as well as potentially combine multiple approaches, especially transcriptomics and proteomics, in order to evaluate lncRNAs and RBPs as early disease biomarkers for patient identification and stratification. In addition, high-risk populations, like patients diagnosed with chronic pancreatitis, should also be considered and thoroughly investigated in order to identify RBPs and lncRNAs that are associated with predisposing conditions [235,236].

With ongoing research and improvements in targeting and drug delivery, the inhibition of lncRNAs and RBPs holds great potential, and novel combinatorial approaches involving lncRNA- or RBP-targeting drugs as well as conventional (chemo)therapies or other targeted agents may enhance their therapeutic efficacy and pave the way for more effective treatments against one of the most challenging cancers.

Author Contributions: Conceptualization, A.S., N.B., S.H. and T.G.; investigation, P.P., F.W.O., H.E. and K.U.I.M.; writing—original draft preparation, P.P., F.W.O., H.E., K.U.I.M., N.B., S.H. and T.G.; writing—review and editing, N.B. and T.G.; visualization, N.B.; supervision, T.G.; funding acquisition, A.S., N.B., S.H. and T.G. All authors have read and agreed to the published version of the manuscript.

Funding: This work was conducted within the Research Training Group InCuPanc (RTG2751) funded by Deutsche Forschungsgemeinschaft (DFG), grant number 449501615.

Acknowledgments: The authors want to thank Sina Krehahn and Nico Hesselbarth for their administrative support within the RTG 2751.

Conflicts of Interest: The authors declare no conflicts of interest. The funders had no role in the design of the study; in the collection, analyses, or interpretation of data; in the writing of the manuscript; or in the decision to publish the results.

References

1. Bray, F.; Laversanne, M.; Sung, H.; Ferlay, J.; Siegel, R.L.; Soerjomataram, I.; Jemal, A. Global cancer statistics 2022: GLOBOCAN estimates of incidence and mortality worldwide for 36 cancers in 185 countries. *CA Cancer J. Clin.* **2024**, *74*, 229–263. [CrossRef] [PubMed]
2. Siegel, R.L.; Giaquinto, A.N.; Jemal, A. Cancer statistics, 2024. *CA Cancer J. Clin.* **2024**, *74*, 12–49. [CrossRef]
3. Conroy, T.; Hammel, P.; Hebbar, M.; Ben Abdelghani, M.; Wei, A.C.; Raoul, J.L.; Chone, L.; Francois, E.; Artru, P.; Biagi, J.J.; et al. FOLFIRINOX or Gemcitabine as Adjuvant Therapy for Pancreatic Cancer. *N. Engl. J. Med.* **2018**, *379*, 2395–2406. [CrossRef]
4. Beutel, A.K.; Ekizce, M.; Ettrich, T.J.; Seufferlein, T.; Lindenmayer, J.; Gout, J.; Kleger, A. Organoid-based precision medicine in pancreatic cancer. *United Eur. Gastroenterol. J.* **2024**, *13*, 21–33. [CrossRef] [PubMed]

5. Pishvaian, M.J.; Blais, E.M.; Brody, J.R.; Lyons, E.; DeArbeloa, P.; Hendifar, A.; Mikhail, S.; Chung, V.; Sahai, V.; Sohal, D.P.S.; et a Overall survival in patients with pancreatic cancer receiving matched therapies following molecular profiling: A retrospectiv analysis of the Know Your Tumor registry trial. *Lancet Oncol.* **2020**, *21*, 508–518. [CrossRef] [PubMed]
6. Golan, T.; Hammel, P.; Reni, M.; Van Cutsem, E.; Macarulla, T.; Hall, M.J.; Park, J.O.; Hochhauser, D.; Arnold, D.; Oh, D.Y.; et a Maintenance Olaparib for Germline BRCA-Mutated Metastatic Pancreatic Cancer. *N. Engl. J. Med.* **2019**, *381*, 317–327. [CrossRef
7. Anisetti, B.; Coston, T.W.; Ahmed, A.K.; Mahadevia, H.J.; Edgar, M.A.; Starr, J.S.; Babiker, H.M. An Excellent Response o Microsatellite Instability-High Pancreatic Adenocarcinoma to Pembrolizumab Treatment: The Role of Circulating Tumor DN Testing. *Cureus* **2023**, *15*, e37239. [CrossRef]
8. Drilon, A.; Laetsch, T.W.; Kummar, S.; DuBois, S.G.; Lassen, U.N.; Demetri, G.D.; Nathenson, M.; Doebele, R.C.; Farago, A.F Pappo, A.S.; et al. Efficacy of Larotrectinib in TRK Fusion-Positive Cancers in Adults and Children. *N. Engl. J. Med.* **2018**, *378* 731–739. [CrossRef]
9. Hu, Z.I.; Shia, J.; Stadler, Z.K.; Varghese, A.M.; Capanu, M.; Salo-Mullen, E.; Lowery, M.A.; Diaz, L.A., Jr.; Mandelker, D.; Yu, K.H et al. Evaluating Mismatch Repair Deficiency in Pancreatic Adenocarcinoma: Challenges and Recommendations. *Clin. Cance Res.* **2018**, *24*, 1326–1336. [CrossRef]
10. Strickler, J.H.; Satake, H.; George, T.J.; Yaeger, R.; Hollebecque, A.; Garrido-Laguna, I.; Schuler, M.; Burns, T.F.; Coveler, A.L Falchook, G.S.; et al. Sotorasib in KRAS p.G12C-Mutated Advanced Pancreatic Cancer. *N. Engl. J. Med.* **2023**, *388*, 33–4 [CrossRef]
11. Bailey, P.; Chang, D.K.; Nones, K.; Johns, A.L.; Patch, A.M.; Gingras, M.C.; Miller, D.K.; Christ, A.N.; Bruxner, T.J.; Quinn, M.C et al. Genomic analyses identify molecular subtypes of pancreatic cancer. *Nature* **2016**, *531*, 47–52. [CrossRef]
12. Collisson, E.A.; Sadanandam, A.; Olson, P.; Gibb, W.J.; Truitt, M.; Gu, S.; Cooc, J.; Weinkle, J.; Kim, G.E.; Jakkula, L.; et al. Subtype of pancreatic ductal adenocarcinoma and their differing responses to therapy. *Nat. Med.* **2011**, *17*, 500–503. [CrossRef] [PubMed
13. Moffitt, R.A.; Marayati, R.; Flate, E.L.; Volmar, K.E.; Loeza, S.G.; Hoadley, K.A.; Rashid, N.U.; Williams, L.A.; Eaton, S.C.; Chung A.H.; et al. Virtual microdissection identifies distinct tumor- and stroma-specific subtypes of pancreatic ductal adenocarcinom *Nat. Genet.* **2015**, *47*, 1168–1178. [CrossRef]
14. Raghavan, S.; Winter, P.S.; Navia, A.W.; Williams, H.L.; DenAdel, A.; Lowder, K.E.; Galvez-Reyes, J.; Kalekar, R.L.; Mulugeta N.; Kapner, K.S.; et al. Microenvironment drives cell state, plasticity, and drug response in pancreatic cancer. *Cell* **2021**, *184* 6119–6137.e6126. [CrossRef] [PubMed]
15. Glass, M.; Dorn, A.; Huttelmaier, S.; Haemmerle, M.; Gutschner, T. Comprehensive Analysis of LincRNAs in Classical and Basal-Like Subtypes of Pancreatic Cancer. *Cancers* **2020**, *12*, 2077. [CrossRef]
16. Henninger, J.E.; Young, R.A. An RNA-centric view of transcription and genome organization. *Mol. Cell* **2024**, *84*, 3627–3643 [CrossRef] [PubMed]
17. Singh, V.; Singh, A.; Liu, A.J.; Fuchs, S.Y.; Sharma, A.K.; Spiegelman, V.S. RNA Binding Proteins as Potential Therapeutic Targets in Colorectal Cancer. *Cancers* **2024**, *16*, 3502. [CrossRef]
18. Weisse, J.; Rosemann, J.; Krauspe, V.; Kappler, M.; Eckert, A.W.; Haemmerle, M.; Gutschner, T. RNA-Binding Proteins as Regulators of Migration, Invasion and Metastasis in Oral Squamous Cell Carcinoma. *Int. J. Mol. Sci.* **2020**, *21*, 6835. [CrossRef]
19. Djebali, S.; Davis, C.A.; Merkel, A.; Dobin, A.; Lassmann, T.; Mortazavi, A.; Tanzer, A.; Lagarde, J.; Lin, W.; Schlesinger, F.; et al Landscape of transcription in human cells. *Nature* **2012**, *489*, 101–108. [CrossRef]
20. International Human Genome Sequencing Consortium. Finishing the euchromatic sequence of the human genome. *Nature* **2004** *431*, 931–945. [CrossRef]
21. Mattick, J.S.; Amaral, P.P.; Carninci, P.; Carpenter, S.; Chang, H.Y.; Chen, L.L.; Chen, R.; Dean, C.; Dinger, M.E.; Fitzgerald, K.A. et al. Long non-coding RNAs: Definitions, functions, challenges and recommendations. *Nat. Rev. Mol. Cell Biol.* **2023**, *24*, 430–447 [CrossRef]
22. Mattick, J.S. Challenging the dogma: The hidden layer of non-protein-coding RNAs in complex organisms. *Bioessays* **2003**, *25* 930–939. [CrossRef] [PubMed]
23. Melo, C.A.; Drost, J.; Wijchers, P.J.; van de Werken, H.; de Wit, E.; Oude Vrielink, J.A.; Elkon, R.; Melo, S.A.; Leveille, N.; Kalluri R.; et al. eRNAs are required for p53-dependent enhancer activity and gene transcription. *Mol. Cell* **2013**, *49*, 524–535. [CrossRef]
24. Zhao, L.; Wang, J.; Li, Y.; Song, T.; Wu, Y.; Fang, S.; Bu, D.; Li, H.; Sun, L.; Pei, D.; et al. NONCODEV6: An updated database dedicated to long non-coding RNA annotation in both animals and plants. *Nucleic Acids Res.* **2021**, *49*, D165–D171. [CrossRef] [PubMed]
25. Deveson, I.W.; Brunck, M.E.; Blackburn, J.; Tseng, E.; Hon, T.; Clark, T.A.; Clark, M.B.; Crawford, J.; Dinger, M.E.; Nielsen, L.K. et al. Universal Alternative Splicing of Noncoding Exons. *Cell Syst.* **2018**, *6*, 245–255.e245. [CrossRef]
26. Iyer, M.K.; Niknafs, Y.S.; Malik, R.; Singhal, U.; Sahu, A.; Hosono, Y.; Barrette, T.R.; Prensner, J.R.; Evans, J.R.; Zhao, S.; et al. The landscape of long noncoding RNAs in the human transcriptome. *Nat. Genet.* **2015**, *47*, 199–208. [CrossRef] [PubMed]
27. Gloss, B.S.; Dinger, M.E. The specificity of long noncoding RNA expression. *Biochim. Biophys. Acta* **2016**, *1859*, 16–22. [CrossRef]

28. Quinn, J.J.; Zhang, Q.C.; Georgiev, P.; Ilik, I.A.; Akhtar, A.; Chang, H.Y. Rapid evolutionary turnover underlies conserved lncRNA-genome interactions. *Genes. Dev.* **2016**, *30*, 191–207. [CrossRef]
29. Guttman, M.; Rinn, J.L. Modular regulatory principles of large non-coding RNAs. *Nature* **2012**, *482*, 339–346. [CrossRef]
30. Bhan, A.; Mandal, S.S. LncRNA HOTAIR: A master regulator of chromatin dynamics and cancer. *Biochim. Biophys. Acta* **2015**, *1856*, 151–164. [CrossRef]
31. Sahakyan, A.; Yang, Y.; Plath, K. The Role of Xist in X-Chromosome Dosage Compensation. *Trends Cell Biol.* **2018**, *28*, 999–1013. [CrossRef]
32. Faghihi, M.A.; Modarresi, F.; Khalil, A.M.; Wood, D.E.; Sahagan, B.G.; Morgan, T.E.; Finch, C.E.; St Laurent, G., 3rd; Kenny, P.J.; Wahlestedt, C. Expression of a noncoding RNA is elevated in Alzheimer's disease and drives rapid feed-forward regulation of beta-secretase. *Nat. Med.* **2008**, *14*, 723–730. [CrossRef] [PubMed]
33. Gong, C.; Maquat, L.E. lncRNAs transactivate STAU1-mediated mRNA decay by duplexing with 3′ UTRs via Alu elements. *Nature* **2011**, *470*, 284–288. [CrossRef] [PubMed]
34. Romero-Barrios, N.; Legascue, M.F.; Benhamed, M.; Ariel, F.; Crespi, M. Splicing regulation by long noncoding RNAs. *Nucleic Acids Res.* **2018**, *46*, 2169–2184. [CrossRef]
35. Toki, N.; Takahashi, H.; Sharma, H.; Valentine, M.N.Z.; Rahman, F.M.; Zucchelli, S.; Gustincich, S.; Carninci, P. SINEUP long non-coding RNA acts via PTBP1 and HNRNPK to promote translational initiation assemblies. *Nucleic Acids Res.* **2020**, *48*, 11626–11644. [CrossRef] [PubMed]
36. Elguindy, M.M.; Mendell, J.T. NORAD-induced Pumilio phase separation is required for genome stability. *Nature* **2021**, *595*, 303–308. [CrossRef]
37. Guo, C.J.; Ma, X.K.; Xing, Y.H.; Zheng, C.C.; Xu, Y.F.; Shan, L.; Zhang, J.; Wang, S.; Wang, Y.; Carmichael, G.G.; et al. Distinct Processing of lncRNAs Contributes to Non-conserved Functions in Stem Cells. *Cell* **2020**, *181*, 621–636.e622. [CrossRef]
38. Liu, B.; Sun, L.; Liu, Q.; Gong, C.; Yao, Y.; Lv, X.; Lin, L.; Yao, H.; Su, F.; Li, D.; et al. A cytoplasmic NF-kappaB interacting long noncoding RNA blocks IkappaB phosphorylation and suppresses breast cancer metastasis. *Cancer Cell* **2015**, *27*, 370–381. [CrossRef]
39. Lyu, Q.; Xu, S.; Lyu, Y.; Choi, M.; Christie, C.K.; Slivano, O.J.; Rahman, A.; Jin, Z.G.; Long, X.; Xu, Y.; et al. SENCR stabilizes vascular endothelial cell adherens junctions through interaction with CKAP4. *Proc. Natl. Acad. Sci. USA* **2019**, *116*, 546–555. [CrossRef]
40. Yamazaki, T.; Souquere, S.; Chujo, T.; Kobelke, S.; Chong, Y.S.; Fox, A.H.; Bond, C.S.; Nakagawa, S.; Pierron, G.; Hirose, T. Functional Domains of NEAT1 Architectural lncRNA Induce Paraspeckle Assembly through Phase Separation. *Mol. Cell* **2018**, *70*, 1038–1053.e1037. [CrossRef]
41. Gil, N.; Ulitsky, I. Regulation of gene expression by cis-acting long non-coding RNAs. *Nat. Rev. Genet.* **2020**, *21*, 102–117. [CrossRef] [PubMed]
42. Derrien, T.; Johnson, R.; Bussotti, G.; Tanzer, A.; Djebali, S.; Tilgner, H.; Guernec, G.; Martin, D.; Merkel, A.; Knowles, D.G.; et al. The GENCODE v7 catalog of human long noncoding RNAs: Analysis of their gene structure, evolution, and expression. *Genome Res.* **2012**, *22*, 1775–1789. [CrossRef]
43. Werner, M.S.; Ruthenburg, A.J. Nuclear Fractionation Reveals Thousands of Chromatin-Tethered Noncoding RNAs Adjacent to Active Genes. *Cell Rep.* **2015**, *12*, 1089–1098. [CrossRef]
44. Arner, E.; Daub, C.O.; Vitting-Seerup, K.; Andersson, R.; Lilje, B.; Drablos, F.; Lennartsson, A.; Ronnerblad, M.; Hrydziuszko, O.; Vitezic, M.; et al. Transcribed enhancers lead waves of coordinated transcription in transitioning mammalian cells. *Science* **2015**, *347*, 1010–1014. [CrossRef] [PubMed]
45. Tan, J.Y.; Marques, A.C. The activity of human enhancers is modulated by the splicing of their associated lncRNAs. *PLoS Comput. Biol.* **2022**, *18*, e1009722. [CrossRef]
46. Vucicevic, D.; Corradin, O.; Ntini, E.; Scacheri, P.C.; Orom, U.A. Long ncRNA expression associates with tissue-specific enhancers. *Cell Cycle* **2015**, *14*, 253–260. [CrossRef]
47. Anderson, K.M.; Anderson, D.M.; McAnally, J.R.; Shelton, J.M.; Bassel-Duby, R.; Olson, E.N. Transcription of the non-coding RNA upperhand controls Hand2 expression and heart development. *Nature* **2016**, *539*, 433–436. [CrossRef] [PubMed]
48. Han, X.; Zhang, J.; Liu, Y.; Fan, X.; Ai, S.; Luo, Y.; Li, X.; Jin, H.; Luo, S.; Zheng, H.; et al. The lncRNA Hand2os1/Uph locus orchestrates heart development through regulation of precise expression of Hand2. *Development* **2019**, *146*, dev176198. [CrossRef]
49. Xiang, J.F.; Yin, Q.F.; Chen, T.; Zhang, Y.; Zhang, X.O.; Wu, Z.; Zhang, S.; Wang, H.B.; Ge, J.; Lu, X.; et al. Human colorectal cancer-specific CCAT1-L lncRNA regulates long-range chromatin interactions at the MYC locus. *Cell Res.* **2014**, *24*, 513–531. [CrossRef]
50. Cho, S.W.; Xu, J.; Sun, R.; Mumbach, M.R.; Carter, A.C.; Chen, Y.G.; Yost, K.E.; Kim, J.; He, J.; Nevins, S.A.; et al. Promoter of lncRNA Gene PVT1 Is a Tumor-Suppressor DNA Boundary Element. *Cell* **2018**, *173*, 1398–1412.e1322. [CrossRef]
51. Penny, G.D.; Kay, G.F.; Sheardown, S.A.; Rastan, S.; Brockdorff, N. Requirement for Xist in X chromosome inactivation. *Nature* **1996**, *379*, 131–137. [CrossRef]

52. Khalil, A.M.; Guttman, M.; Huarte, M.; Garber, M.; Raj, A.; Rivea Morales, D.; Thomas, K.; Presser, A.; Bernstein, B.E.; van Oudenaarden, A.; et al. Many human large intergenic noncoding RNAs associate with chromatin-modifying complexes and affect gene expression. *Proc. Natl. Acad. Sci. USA* **2009**, *106*, 11667–11672. [CrossRef] [PubMed]
53. Long, Y.; Hwang, T.; Gooding, A.R.; Goodrich, K.J.; Rinn, J.L.; Cech, T.R. RNA is essential for PRC2 chromatin occupancy and function in human pluripotent stem cells. *Nat. Genet.* **2020**, *52*, 931–938. [CrossRef] [PubMed]
54. Rinn, J.L.; Kertesz, M.; Wang, J.K.; Squazzo, S.L.; Xu, X.; Brugmann, S.A.; Goodnough, L.H.; Helms, J.A.; Farnham, P.J.; Segal, E.; et al. Functional demarcation of active and silent chromatin domains in human HOX loci by noncoding RNAs. *Cell* **2007**, *129*, 1311–1323. [CrossRef]
55. Roden, C.; Gladfelter, A.S. RNA contributions to the form and function of biomolecular condensates. *Nat. Rev. Mol. Cell Biol.* **2021**, *22*, 183–195. [CrossRef] [PubMed]
56. Miyagawa, R.; Tano, K.; Mizuno, R.; Nakamura, Y.; Ijiri, K.; Rakwal, R.; Shibato, J.; Masuo, Y.; Mayeda, A.; Hirose, T.; et al. Identification of cis- and trans-acting factors involved in the localization of MALAT-1 noncoding RNA to nuclear speckles. *RNA* **2012**, *18*, 738–751. [CrossRef]
57. Salmena, L.; Poliseno, L.; Tay, Y.; Kats, L.; Pandolfi, P.P. A ceRNA hypothesis: The Rosetta Stone of a hidden RNA language? *Cell* **2011**, *146*, 353–358. [CrossRef]
58. Denzler, R.; Agarwal, V.; Stefano, J.; Bartel, D.P.; Stoffel, M. Assessing the ceRNA hypothesis with quantitative measurements of miRNA and target abundance. *Mol. Cell* **2014**, *54*, 766–776. [CrossRef]
59. Cesana, M.; Cacchiarelli, D.; Legnini, I.; Santini, T.; Sthandier, O.; Chinappi, M.; Tramontano, A.; Bozzoni, I. A long noncoding RNA controls muscle differentiation by functioning as a competing endogenous RNA. *Cell* **2011**, *147*, 358–369. [CrossRef]
60. Poliseno, L.; Salmena, L.; Zhang, J.; Carver, B.; Haveman, W.J.; Pandolfi, P.P. A coding-independent function of gene and pseudogene mRNAs regulates tumour biology. *Nature* **2010**, *465*, 1033–1038. [CrossRef]
61. Vitiello, M.; Evangelista, M.; Zhang, Y.; Salmena, L.; Pandolfi, P.P.; Poliseno, L. PTENP1 is a ceRNA for PTEN: It's CRISPR clear. *J. Hematol. Oncol.* **2020**, *13*, 73. [CrossRef]
62. Khurana, E.; Fu, Y.; Colonna, V.; Mu, X.J.; Kang, H.M.; Lappalainen, T.; Sboner, A.; Lochovsky, L.; Chen, J.; Harmanci, A.; et al. Integrative annotation of variants from 1092 humans: Application to cancer genomics. *Science* **2013**, *342*, 1235587. [CrossRef] [PubMed]
63. Gutschner, T.; Diederichs, S. The hallmarks of cancer: A long non-coding RNA point of view. *RNA Biol.* **2012**, *9*, 703–719. [CrossRef]
64. Vancura, A.; Gutierrez, A.H.; Hennig, T.; Pulido-Quetglas, C.; Slack, F.J.; Johnson, R.; Haefliger, S. Is Evolutionary Conservation a Useful Predictor for Cancer Long Noncoding RNAs? Insights from the Cancer LncRNA Census 3. *Noncoding RNA* **2022**, *8*, 82. [CrossRef]
65. Yang, M.; Lu, H.; Liu, J.; Wu, S.; Kim, P.; Zhou, X. lncRNAfunc: A knowledgebase of lncRNA function in human cancer. *Nucleic Acids Res.* **2022**, *50*, D1295–D1306. [CrossRef]
66. Gutschner, T.; Richtig, G.; Haemmerle, M.; Pichler, M. From biomarkers to therapeutic targets-the promises and perils of long non-coding RNAs in cancer. *Cancer Metastasis Rev.* **2018**, *37*, 83–105. [CrossRef] [PubMed]
67. Yan, X.; Hu, Z.; Feng, Y.; Hu, X.; Yuan, J.; Zhao, S.D.; Zhang, Y.; Yang, L.; Shan, W.; He, Q.; et al. Comprehensive Genomic Characterization of Long Non-coding RNAs across Human Cancers. *Cancer Cell* **2015**, *28*, 529–540. [CrossRef]
68. Ashrafizadeh, M.; Rabiee, N.; Kumar, A.P.; Sethi, G.; Zarrabi, A.; Wang, Y. Long noncoding RNAs (lncRNAs) in pancreatic cancer progression. *Drug Discov. Today* **2022**, *27*, 2181–2198. [CrossRef] [PubMed]
69. Duguang, L.; Jin, H.; Xiaowei, Q.; Peng, X.; Xiaodong, W.; Zhennan, L.; Jianjun, Q.; Jie, Y. The involvement of lncRNAs in the development and progression of pancreatic cancer. *Cancer Biol. Ther.* **2017**, *18*, 927–936. [CrossRef]
70. Ghafouri-Fard, S.; Fathi, M.; Zhai, T.; Taheri, M.; Dong, P. LncRNAs: Novel Biomarkers for Pancreatic Cancer. *Biomolecules* **2021**, *11*, 1665. [CrossRef]
71. Huang, X.; Zhi, X.; Gao, Y.; Ta, N.; Jiang, H.; Zheng, J. LncRNAs in pancreatic cancer. *Oncotarget* **2016**, *7*, 57379–57390. [CrossRef]
72. Xu, J.; Xu, J.; Liu, X.; Jiang, J. The role of lncRNA-mediated ceRNA regulatory networks in pancreatic cancer. *Cell Death Discov.* **2022**, *8*, 287. [CrossRef] [PubMed]
73. Kim, K.; Jutooru, I.; Chadalapaka, G.; Johnson, G.; Frank, J.; Burghardt, R.; Kim, S.; Safe, S. HOTAIR is a negative prognostic factor and exhibits pro-oncogenic activity in pancreatic cancer. *Oncogene* **2013**, *32*, 1616–1625. [CrossRef] [PubMed]
74. Ma, C.; Nong, K.; Zhu, H.; Wang, W.; Huang, X.; Yuan, Z.; Ai, K. H19 promotes pancreatic cancer metastasis by derepressing let-7′s suppression on its target HMGA2-mediated EMT. *Tumour Biol.* **2014**, *35*, 9163–9169. [CrossRef] [PubMed]
75. Pang, E.J.; Yang, R.; Fu, X.B.; Liu, Y.F. Overexpression of long non-coding RNA MALAT1 is correlated with clinical progression and unfavorable prognosis in pancreatic cancer. *Tumour Biol.* **2015**, *36*, 2403–2407. [CrossRef]
76. Li, X.; Zhou, S.; Fan, T.; Feng, X. lncRNA DGCR 5/miR-27a-3p/BNIP3 promotes cell apoptosis in pancreatic cancer by regulating the p38 MAPK pathway. *Int. J. Mol. Med.* **2020**, *46*, 729–739. [CrossRef]

77. Ma, L.; Wang, F.; Du, C.; Zhang, Z.; Guo, H.; Xie, X.; Gao, H.; Zhuang, Y.; Kornmann, M.; Gao, H.; et al. Long non-coding RNA MEG3 functions as a tumour suppressor and has prognostic predictive value in human pancreatic cancer. *Oncol. Rep.* **2018**, *39*, 1132–1140. [CrossRef]
78. Wang, Y.; Ding, X.; Hu, H.; He, Y.; Lu, Z.; Wu, P.; Tian, L.; Xia, T.; Yin, J.; Yuan, H.; et al. Long non-coding RNA lnc-PCTST predicts prognosis through inhibiting progression of pancreatic cancer by downregulation of TACC-3. *Int. J. Cancer* **2018**, *143*, 3143–3154. [CrossRef]
79. Liu, Y.; Feng, W.; Liu, W.; Kong, X.; Li, L.; He, J.; Wang, D.; Zhang, M.; Zhou, G.; Xu, W.; et al. Circulating lncRNA ABHD11-AS1 serves as a biomarker for early pancreatic cancer diagnosis. *J. Cancer* **2019**, *10*, 3746–3756. [CrossRef]
80. Ou, Z.L.; Luo, Z.; Lu, Y.B. Long non-coding RNA HULC as a diagnostic and prognostic marker of pancreatic cancer. *World J. Gastroenterol.* **2019**, *25*, 6728–6742. [CrossRef]
81. Permuth, J.B.; Chen, D.T.; Yoder, S.J.; Li, J.; Smith, A.T.; Choi, J.W.; Kim, J.; Balagurunathan, Y.; Jiang, K.; Coppola, D.; et al. Linc-ing Circulating Long Non-coding RNAs to the Diagnosis and Malignant Prediction of Intraductal Papillary Mucinous Neoplasms of the Pancreas. *Sci. Rep.* **2017**, *7*, 10484. [CrossRef] [PubMed]
82. Mello, S.S.; Sinow, C.; Raj, N.; Mazur, P.K.; Bieging-Rolett, K.; Broz, D.K.; Imam, J.F.C.; Vogel, H.; Wood, L.D.; Sage, J.; et al. Neat1 is a p53-inducible lincRNA essential for transformation suppression. *Genes. Dev.* **2017**, *31*, 1095–1108. [CrossRef] [PubMed]
83. Ingram, H.B.; Fox, A.H. Unveiling the intricacies of paraspeckle formation and function. *Curr. Opin. Cell Biol.* **2024**, *90*, 102399. [CrossRef] [PubMed]
84. Cao, J.; Zhang, Y.; Yang, J.; He, S.; Li, M.; Yan, S.; Chen, Y.; Qu, C.; Xu, L. NEAT1 regulates pancreatic cancer cell growth, invasion and migration though mircroRNA-335-5p/c-met axis. *Am. J. Cancer Res.* **2016**, *6*, 2361–2374.
85. Feng, Y.; Gao, L.; Cui, G.; Cao, Y. LncRNA NEAT1 facilitates pancreatic cancer growth and metastasis through stabilizing ELF3 mRNA. *Am. J. Cancer Res.* **2020**, *10*, 237–248.
86. Huang, B.; Liu, C.; Wu, Q.; Zhang, J.; Min, Q.; Sheng, T.; Wang, X.; Zou, Y. Long non-coding RNA NEAT1 facilitates pancreatic cancer progression through negative modulation of miR-506-3p. *Biochem. Biophys. Res. Commun.* **2017**, *482*, 828–834. [CrossRef]
87. Hingorani, S.R.; Petricoin, E.F.; Maitra, A.; Rajapakse, V.; King, C.; Jacobetz, M.A.; Ross, S.; Conrads, T.P.; Veenstra, T.D.; Hitt, B.A.; et al. Preinvasive and invasive ductal pancreatic cancer and its early detection in the mouse. *Cancer Cell* **2003**, *4*, 437–450. [CrossRef]
88. Mueller, S.; Engleitner, T.; Maresch, R.; Zukowska, M.; Lange, S.; Kaltenbacher, T.; Konukiewitz, B.; Ollinger, R.; Zwiebel, M.; Strong, A.; et al. Evolutionary routes and KRAS dosage define pancreatic cancer phenotypes. *Nature* **2018**, *554*, 62–68. [CrossRef]
89. Guerra, C.; Schuhmacher, A.J.; Canamero, M.; Grippo, P.J.; Verdaguer, L.; Perez-Gallego, L.; Dubus, P.; Sandgren, E.P.; Barbacid, M. Chronic pancreatitis is essential for induction of pancreatic ductal adenocarcinoma by K-Ras oncogenes in adult mice. *Cancer Cell* **2007**, *11*, 291–302. [CrossRef]
90. Li, X.; Deng, S.J.; Zhu, S.; Jin, Y.; Cui, S.P.; Chen, J.Y.; Xiang, C.; Li, Q.Y.; He, C.; Zhao, S.F.; et al. Hypoxia-induced lncRNA-NUTF2P3-001 contributes to tumorigenesis of pancreatic cancer by derepressing the miR-3923/KRAS pathway. *Oncotarget* **2016**, *7*, 6000–6014. [CrossRef]
91. Liu, P.; Yang, H.; Zhang, J.; Peng, X.; Lu, Z.; Tong, W.; Chen, J. The lncRNA MALAT1 acts as a competing endogenous RNA to regulate KRAS expression by sponging miR-217 in pancreatic ductal adenocarcinoma. *Sci. Rep.* **2017**, *7*, 5186. [CrossRef] [PubMed]
92. Sun, C.C.; Li, L.; Jiang, Z.C.; Liu, Z.C.; Wang, L.; Wang, H.J. The Functional Role of LncRNA UCA1 in Pancreatic Cancer: A mini-review. *J. Cancer* **2023**, *14*, 275–280. [CrossRef] [PubMed]
93. Liu, Y.; Feng, W.; Gu, S.; Wang, H.; Zhang, Y.; Chen, W.; Xu, W.; Lin, C.; Gong, A.; Xu, M. The UCA1/KRAS axis promotes human pancreatic ductal adenocarcinoma stem cell properties and tumor growth. *Am. J. Cancer Res.* **2019**, *9*, 496–510.
94. Barcelo, C.; Etchin, J.; Mansour, M.R.; Sanda, T.; Ginesta, M.M.; Sanchez-Arevalo Lobo, V.J.; Real, F.X.; Capella, G.; Estanyol, J.M.; Jaumot, M.; et al. Ribonucleoprotein HNRNPA2B1 interacts with and regulates oncogenic KRAS in pancreatic ductal adenocarcinoma cells. *Gastroenterology* **2014**, *147*, 882–892.e888. [CrossRef] [PubMed]
95. Wang, H.; Ding, Y.; He, Y.; Yu, Z.; Zhou, Y.; Gong, A.; Xu, M. LncRNA UCA1 promotes pancreatic cancer cell migration by regulating mitochondrial dynamics via the MAPK pathway. *Arch. Biochem. Biophys.* **2023**, *748*, 109783. [CrossRef]
96. Liang, X.; Qi, M.; Wu, R.; Liu, A.; Chen, D.; Tang, L.; Chen, J.; Hu, X.; Li, W.; Zhan, L.; et al. Long non-coding RNA CUDR promotes malignant phenotypes in pancreatic ductal adenocarcinoma via activating AKT and ERK signaling pathways. *Int. J. Oncol.* **2018**, *53*, 2671–2682. [CrossRef]
97. Wang, Y.; Chen, W.; Yang, C.; Wu, W.; Wu, S.; Qin, X.; Li, X. Long non-coding RNA UCA1a(CUDR) promotes proliferation and tumorigenesis of bladder cancer. *Int. J. Oncol.* **2012**, *41*, 276–284. [CrossRef]
98. Qiao, X.; Lv, S.X.; Qiao, Y.; Li, Q.P.; Ye, B.; Wang, C.C.; Miao, L. Long noncoding RNA ABHD11-AS1 predicts the prognosis of pancreatic cancer patients and serves as a promoter by activating the PI3K-AKT pathway. *Eur. Rev. Med. Pharmacol. Sci.* **2018**, *22*, 8630–8639. [CrossRef]

99. Zhang, Y.; Zhang, R.; Luo, G.; Ai, K. Long noncoding RNA SNHG1 promotes cell proliferation through PI3K/AKT signaling pathway in pancreatic ductal adenocarcinoma. *J. Cancer* **2018**, *9*, 2713–2722. [CrossRef]
100. Cao, W.; Zhang, H.F.; Ding, X.L.; Zhu, S.Z.; Zhou, G.X. The progression of pancreatic cancer cells is promoted by a long non-coding RNA LUCAT1 by activating AKT phosphorylation. *Eur. Rev. Med. Pharmacol. Sci.* **2021**, *25*, 738–748. [CrossRef]
101. Nai, Y.; Pan, C.; Hu, X.; Ma, Y. LncRNA LUCAT1 contributes to cell proliferation and migration in human pancreatic ductal adenocarcinoma via sponging miR-539. *Cancer Med.* **2020**, *9*, 757–767. [CrossRef]
102. Meng, L.D.; Shi, G.D.; Ge, W.L.; Huang, X.M.; Chen, Q.; Yuan, H.; Wu, P.F.; Lu, Y.C.; Shen, P.; Zhang, Y.H.; et al. Linc01232 promotes the metastasis of pancreatic cancer by suppressing the ubiquitin-mediated degradation of HNRNPA2B1 and activating the A-Raf-induced MAPK/ERK signaling pathway. *Cancer Lett.* **2020**, *494*, 107–120. [CrossRef] [PubMed]
103. Shilo, A.; Ben Hur, V.; Denichenko, P.; Stein, I.; Pikarsky, E.; Rauch, J.; Kolch, W.; Zender, L.; Karni, R. Splicing factor hnRNP A2 activates the Ras-MAPK-ERK pathway by controlling A-Raf splicing in hepatocellular carcinoma development. *RNA* **2014**, *20*, 505–515. [CrossRef]
104. Ishikawa, T.; Fukushige, S.; Saiki, Y.; Hirose, K.; Hiyoshi, T.; Ogawa, T.; Katori, Y.; Furukawa, T. Long Non-Coding RNAs Associated with Mitogen-Activated Protein Kinase in Human Pancreatic Cancer. *Cancers* **2023**, *15*, 303. [CrossRef] [PubMed]
105. Wang, J.; He, Z.; Liu, X.; Xu, J.; Jiang, X.; Quan, G.; Jiang, J. LINC00941 promotes pancreatic cancer malignancy by interacting with ANXA2 and suppressing NEDD4L-mediated degradation of ANXA2. *Cell Death Dis.* **2022**, *13*, 718. [CrossRef] [PubMed]
106. Xu, M.; Cui, R.; Ye, L.; Wang, Y.; Wang, X.; Zhang, Q.; Wang, K.; Dong, C.; Le, W.; Chen, B. LINC00941 promotes glycolysis in pancreatic cancer by modulating the Hippo pathway. *Mol. Ther. Nucleic Acids* **2021**, *26*, 280–294. [CrossRef]
107. Shen, W.; Tao, G.Q.; Zhang, Y.; Cai, B.; Sun, J.; Tian, Z.Q. TGF-beta in pancreatic cancer initiation and progression: Two sides of the same coin. *Cell Biosci.* **2017**, *7*, 39. [CrossRef]
108. Hahn, S.A.; Schutte, M.; Hoque, A.T.; Moskaluk, C.A.; da Costa, L.T.; Rozenblum, E.; Weinstein, C.L.; Fischer, A.; Yeo, C.J.; Hruban, R.H.; et al. DPC4, a candidate tumor suppressor gene at human chromosome 18q21.1. *Science* **1996**, *271*, 350–353. [CrossRef]
109. McCarthy, A.J.; Chetty, R. Smad4/DPC4. *J. Clin. Pathol.* **2018**, *71*, 661–664. [CrossRef]
110. Tascilar, M.; Skinner, H.G.; Rosty, C.; Sohn, T.; Wilentz, R.E.; Offerhaus, G.J.; Adsay, V.; Abrams, R.A.; Cameron, J.L.; Kern, S.E.; et al. The SMAD4 protein and prognosis of pancreatic ductal adenocarcinoma. *Clin. Cancer Res.* **2001**, *7*, 4115–4121.
111. Yamada, S.; Fujii, T.; Shimoyama, Y.; Kanda, M.; Nakayama, G.; Sugimoto, H.; Koike, M.; Nomoto, S.; Fujiwara, M.; Nakao, A.; et al. SMAD4 expression predicts local spread and treatment failure in resected pancreatic cancer. *Pancreas* **2015**, *44*, 660–664. [CrossRef] [PubMed]
112. Xia, X.; Wu, W.; Huang, C.; Cen, G.; Jiang, T.; Cao, J.; Huang, K.; Qiu, Z. SMAD4 and its role in pancreatic cancer. *Tumour Biol.* **2015**, *36*, 111–119. [CrossRef] [PubMed]
113. Derderian, C.; Orunmuyi, A.T.; Olapade-Olaopa, E.O.; Ogunwobi, O.O. PVT1 Signaling Is a Mediator of Cancer Progression. *Front. Oncol.* **2019**, *9*, 502. [CrossRef]
114. Li, R.; Wang, X.; Zhu, C.; Wang, K. lncRNA PVT1: A novel oncogene in multiple cancers. *Cell Mol. Biol. Lett.* **2022**, *27*, 84. [CrossRef]
115. Zhang, X.; Feng, W.; Zhang, J.; Ge, L.; Zhang, Y.; Jiang, X.; Peng, W.; Wang, D.; Gong, A.; Xu, M. Long non-coding RNA PVT1 promotes epithelial-mesenchymal transition via the TGF-beta/Smad pathway in pancreatic cancer cells. *Oncol. Rep.* **2018**, *40*, 1093–1102. [CrossRef]
116. Li, Z.; Ma, Z.; Wang, S.; Yan, Q.; Zhuang, H.; Zhou, Z.; Liu, C.; Chen, Y.; Han, M.; Wu, Z.; et al. LINC00909 up-regulates pluripotency factors and promotes cancer stemness and metastasis in pancreatic ductal adenocarcinoma by targeting SMAD4. *Biol. Direct* **2024**, *19*, 24. [CrossRef]
117. Chen, G.; Xu, L.; Ye, G.; Lin, J.; Meng, Z.; Shen, Y. Overexpression of a Long Non-Coding RNA BC037916 is Associated with Pancreatic Tumorigenesis and Poor Prognosis. *Onco Targets Ther.* **2020**, *13*, 13451–13463. [CrossRef]
118. Zhou, B.; Guo, W.; Sun, C.; Zhang, B.; Zheng, F. Linc00462 promotes pancreatic cancer invasiveness through the miR-665/TGFBR1-TGFBR2/SMAD2/3 pathway. *Cell Death Dis.* **2018**, *9*, 706. [CrossRef] [PubMed]
119. Li, L.; Zhang, G.Q.; Chen, H.; Zhao, Z.J.; Chen, H.Z.; Liu, H.; Wang, G.; Jia, Y.H.; Pan, S.H.; Kong, R.; et al. Plasma and tumor levels of Linc-pint are diagnostic and prognostic biomarkers for pancreatic cancer. *Oncotarget* **2016**, *7*, 71773–71781. [CrossRef]
120. Lu, H.; Yang, D.; Zhang, L.; Lu, S.; Ye, J.; Li, M.; Hu, W. Linc-pint inhibits early stage pancreatic ductal adenocarcinoma growth through TGF-beta pathway activation. *Oncol. Lett.* **2019**, *17*, 4633–4639. [CrossRef]
121. Dorn, A.; Glass, M.; Neu, C.T.; Heydel, B.; Huttelmaier, S.; Gutschner, T.; Haemmerle, M. LINC00261 Is Differentially Expressed in Pancreatic Cancer Subtypes and Regulates a Pro-Epithelial Cell Identity. *Cancers* **2020**, *12*, 1227. [CrossRef]
122. Wu, B.Q.; Jiang, Y.; Zhu, F.; Sun, D.L.; He, X.Z. Long Noncoding RNA PVT1 Promotes EMT and Cell Proliferation and Migration Through Downregulating p21 in Pancreatic Cancer Cells. *Technol. Cancer Res. Treat.* **2017**, *16*, 819–827. [CrossRef] [PubMed]
123. Gebauer, F.; Schwarzl, T.; Valcarcel, J.; Hentze, M.W. RNA-binding proteins in human genetic disease. *Nat. Rev. Genet.* **2021**, *22*, 185–198. [CrossRef] [PubMed]

124. Gerstberger, S.; Hafner, M.; Tuschl, T. A census of human RNA-binding proteins. *Nat. Rev. Genet.* **2014**, *15*, 829–845. [CrossRef]
125. Hentze, M.W.; Castello, A.; Schwarzl, T.; Preiss, T. A brave new world of RNA-binding proteins. *Nat. Rev. Mol. Cell Biol.* **2018**, *19*, 327–341. [CrossRef]
126. Pereira, B.; Billaud, M.; Almeida, R. RNA-Binding Proteins in Cancer: Old Players and New Actors. *Trends Cancer* **2017**, *3*, 506–528. [CrossRef]
127. Glass, M.; Michl, P.; Huttelmaier, A.S. RNA Binding Proteins as Drivers and Therapeutic Target Candidates in Pancreatic Ductal Adenocarcinoma. *Int. J. Mol. Sci.* **2020**, *21*, 4190. [CrossRef] [PubMed]
128. Grammatikakis, I.; Abdelmohsen, K.; Gorospe, M. Posttranslational control of HuR function. *Wiley Interdiscip. Rev. RNA* **2017**, *8*, e1372. [CrossRef]
129. Finan, J.M.; Sutton, T.L.; Dixon, D.A.; Brody, J.R. Targeting the RNA-Binding Protein HuR in Cancer. *Cancer Res.* **2023**, *83*, 3507–3516. [CrossRef]
130. Srikantan, S.; Gorospe, M. HuR function in disease. *Front. Biosci.* **2012**, *17*, 189–205. [CrossRef]
131. Richards, N.G.; Rittenhouse, D.W.; Freydin, B.; Cozzitorto, J.A.; Grenda, D.; Rui, H.; Gonye, G.; Kennedy, E.P.; Yeo, C.J.; Brody, J.R.; et al. HuR status is a powerful marker for prognosis and response to gemcitabine-based chemotherapy for resected pancreatic ductal adenocarcinoma patients. *Ann. Surg.* **2010**, *252*, 499–505; discussion 505–506. [CrossRef]
132. Costantino, C.L.; Witkiewicz, A.K.; Kuwano, Y.; Cozzitorto, J.A.; Kennedy, E.P.; Dasgupta, A.; Keen, J.C.; Yeo, C.J.; Gorospe, M.; Brody, J.R. The role of HuR in gemcitabine efficacy in pancreatic cancer: HuR Up-regulates the expression of the gemcitabine metabolizing enzyme deoxycytidine kinase. *Cancer Res.* **2009**, *69*, 4567–4572. [CrossRef] [PubMed]
133. Elebro, J.; Ben Dror, L.; Heby, M.; Nodin, B.; Jirstrom, K.; Eberhard, J. Prognostic effect of hENT1, dCK and HuR expression by morphological type in periampullary adenocarcinoma, including pancreatic cancer. *Acta Oncol.* **2016**, *55*, 286–296. [CrossRef] [PubMed]
134. Zhou, H.; Telonis, A.G.; Jing, Y.; Xia, N.L.; Biederman, L.; Jimbo, M.; Blanco, F.; Londin, E.; Brody, J.R.; Rigoutsos, I. GPRC5A is a potential oncogene in pancreatic ductal adenocarcinoma cells that is upregulated by gemcitabine with help from HuR. *Cell Death Dis.* **2016**, *7*, e2294. [CrossRef]
135. Lal, S.; Burkhart, R.A.; Beeharry, N.; Bhattacharjee, V.; Londin, E.R.; Cozzitorto, J.A.; Romeo, C.; Jimbo, M.; Norris, Z.A.; Yeo, C.J.; et al. HuR posttranscriptionally regulates WEE1: Implications for the DNA damage response in pancreatic cancer cells. *Cancer Res.* **2014**, *74*, 1128–1140. [CrossRef]
136. Jain, A.; McCoy, M.; Coats, C.; Brown, S.Z.; Addya, S.; Pelz, C.; Sears, R.C.; Yeo, C.J.; Brody, J.R. HuR Plays a Role in Double-Strand Break Repair in Pancreatic Cancer Cells and Regulates Functional BRCA1-Associated-Ring-Domain-1(BARD1) Isoforms. *Cancers* **2022**, *14*, 1848. [CrossRef]
137. Burkhart, R.A.; Pineda, D.M.; Chand, S.N.; Romeo, C.; Londin, E.R.; Karoly, E.D.; Cozzitorto, J.A.; Rigoutsos, I.; Yeo, C.J.; Brody, J.R.; et al. HuR is a post-transcriptional regulator of core metabolic enzymes in pancreatic cancer. *RNA Biol.* **2013**, *10*, 1312–1323. [CrossRef] [PubMed]
138. Brown, S.Z.; McCarthy, G.A.; Carroll, J.R.; Di Niro, R.; Pelz, C.; Jain, A.; Sutton, T.L.; Holly, H.D.; Nevler, A.; Schultz, C.W.; et al. The RNA-Binding Protein HuR Posttranscriptionally Regulates the Protumorigenic Activator YAP1 in Pancreatic Ductal Adenocarcinoma. *Mol. Cell Biol.* **2022**, *42*, e0001822. [CrossRef]
139. Pineda, D.M.; Rittenhouse, D.W.; Valley, C.C.; Cozzitorto, J.A.; Burkhart, R.A.; Leiby, B.; Winter, J.M.; Weber, M.C.; Londin, E.R.; Rigoutsos, I.; et al. HuR's post-transcriptional regulation of Death Receptor 5 in pancreatic cancer cells. *Cancer Biol. Ther.* **2012**, *13*, 946–955. [CrossRef]
140. Dong, R.; Chen, P.; Polireddy, K.; Wu, X.; Wang, T.; Ramesh, R.; Dixon, D.A.; Xu, L.; Aube, J.; Chen, Q. An RNA-Binding Protein, Hu-antigen R, in Pancreatic Cancer Epithelial to Mesenchymal Transition, Metastasis, and Cancer Stem Cells. *Mol. Cancer Ther.* **2020**, *19*, 2267–2277. [CrossRef]
141. McCarthy, G.A.; Di Niro, R.; Finan, J.M.; Jain, A.; Guo, Y.; Wyatt, C.R.; Guimaraes, A.R.; Waugh, T.A.; Keith, D.; Morgan, T.K.; et al. Deletion of the mRNA stability factor ELAVL1 (HuR) in pancreatic cancer cells disrupts the tumor microenvironment integrity. *NAR Cancer* **2023**, *5*, zcad016. [CrossRef]
142. Bell, J.L.; Wachter, K.; Muhleck, B.; Pazaitis, N.; Kohn, M.; Lederer, M.; Huttelmaier, S. Insulin-like growth factor 2 mRNA-binding proteins (IGF2BPs): Post-transcriptional drivers of cancer progression? *Cell Mol. Life Sci.* **2013**, *70*, 2657–2675. [CrossRef] [PubMed]
143. Duan, M.; Liu, H.; Xu, S.; Yang, Z.; Zhang, F.; Wang, G.; Wang, Y.; Zhao, S.; Jiang, X. IGF2BPs as novel m(6)A readers: Diverse roles in regulating cancer cell biological functions, hypoxia adaptation, metabolism, and immunosuppressive tumor microenvironment. *Genes. Dis.* **2024**, *11*, 890–920. [CrossRef] [PubMed]
144. Glass, M.; Misiak, D.; Bley, N.; Muller, S.; Hagemann, S.; Busch, B.; Rausch, A.; Huttelmaier, S. IGF2BP1, a Conserved Regulator of RNA Turnover in Cancer. *Front. Mol. Biosci.* **2021**, *8*, 632219. [CrossRef] [PubMed]
145. Huang, H.; Weng, H.; Sun, W.; Qin, X.; Shi, H.; Wu, H.; Zhao, B.S.; Mesquita, A.; Liu, C.; Yuan, C.L.; et al. Recognition of RNA N(6)-methyladenosine by IGF2BP proteins enhances mRNA stability and translation. *Nat. Cell Biol.* **2018**, *20*, 285–295. [CrossRef]

146. Muller, S.; Bley, N.; Glass, M.; Busch, B.; Rousseau, V.; Misiak, D.; Fuchs, T.; Lederer, M.; Huttelmaier, S. IGF2BP1 enhances an aggressive tumor cell phenotype by impairing miRNA-directed downregulation of oncogenic factors. *Nucleic Acids Res.* **2018**, *46*, 6285–6303. [CrossRef]
147. Wan, B.S.; Cheng, M.; Zhang, L. Insulin-like growth factor 2 mRNA-binding protein 1 promotes cell proliferation via activation of AKT and is directly targeted by microRNA-494 in pancreatic cancer. *World J. Gastroenterol.* **2019**, *25*, 6063–6076. [CrossRef]
148. Di Fusco, D.; Segreto, M.T.; Di Maggio, G.; Iannucci, A.; Maresca, C.; Di Grazia, A.; Colella, M.; Stolfi, C.; Monteleone, G.; Monteleone, I. Insulin-like Growth Factor II mRNA-Binding Protein 1 Regulates Pancreatic Cancer Cell Growth through the Surveillance of CDC25A mRNA. *Cancers* **2023**, *15*, 4983. [CrossRef]
149. Zhang, Z.; Yu, H.; Yao, W.; Zhu, N.; Miao, R.; Liu, Z.; Song, X.; Xue, C.; Cai, C.; Cheng, M.; et al. RRP9 promotes gemcitabine resistance in pancreatic cancer via activating AKT signaling pathway. *Cell Commun. Signal* **2022**, *20*, 188. [CrossRef]
150. Muller, S.; Bley, N.; Busch, B.; Glass, M.; Lederer, M.; Misiak, C.; Fuchs, T.; Wedler, A.; Haase, J.; Bertoldo, J.B.; et al. The oncofetal RNA-binding protein IGF2BP1 is a druggable, post-transcriptional super-enhancer of E2F-driven gene expression in cancer. *Nucleic Acids Res.* **2020**, *48*, 8576–8590. [CrossRef]
151. Lin, C.; Wang, Y.; Dong, Y.; Lai, S.; Wang, L.; Weng, S.; Zhang, X. N6-methyladenosine-mediated SH3BP5-AS1 upregulation promotes GEM chemoresistance in pancreatic cancer by activating the Wnt signaling pathway. *Biol. Direct* **2022**, *17*, 33. [CrossRef]
152. Cao, P.; Zhang, W.; Qiu, J.; Tang, Z.; Xue, X.; Feng, T. Gemcitabine Inhibits the Progression of Pancreatic Cancer by Restraining the WTAP/MYC Chain in an m6A-Dependent Manner. *Cancer Res. Treat.* **2024**, *56*, 259–271. [CrossRef] [PubMed]
153. Zhu, S.; Wang, J.Z.; Chen, D.; He, Y.T.; Meng, N.; Chen, M.; Lu, R.X.; Chen, X.H.; Zhang, X.L.; Yan, G.R. An oncopeptide regulates m(6)A recognition by the m(6)A reader IGF2BP1 and tumorigenesis. *Nat. Commun.* **2020**, *11*, 1685. [CrossRef]
154. Xu, X.; Yu, Y.; Zong, K.; Lv, P.; Gu, Y. Up-regulation of IGF2BP2 by multiple mechanisms in pancreatic cancer promotes cancer proliferation by activating the PI3K/Akt signaling pathway. *J. Exp. Clin. Cancer Res.* **2019**, *38*, 497. [CrossRef] [PubMed]
155. Dahlem, C.; Barghash, A.; Puchas, P.; Haybaeck, J.; Kessler, S.M. The Insulin-Like Growth Factor 2 mRNA Binding Protein IMP2/IGF2BP2 is Overexpressed and Correlates with Poor Survival in Pancreatic Cancer. *Int. J. Mol. Sci.* **2019**, *20*, 3204. [CrossRef] [PubMed]
156. Peng, W.X.; Liu, F.; Jiang, J.H.; Yuan, H.; Zhang, Z.; Yang, L.; Mo, Y.Y. N6-methyladenosine modified LINC00901 promotes pancreatic cancer progression through IGF2BP2/MYC axis. *Genes. Dis.* **2023**, *10*, 554–567. [CrossRef]
157. Yao, Y.; Luo, L.; Xiang, G.; Xiong, J.; Ke, N.; Tan, C.; Chen, Y.; Liu, X. The expression of m(6)A regulators correlated with the immune microenvironment plays an important role in the prognosis of pancreatic ductal adenocarcinoma. *Gland. Surg.* **2022**, *11*, 147–165. [CrossRef]
158. Deng, H.; Yao, H.; Zhou, S.; He, C.; Huang, Y.; Li, Y.; Chen, H.; Shu, J. Pancancer analysis uncovers an immunological role and prognostic value of the m6A reader IGF2BP2 in pancreatic cancer. *Mol. Cell Probes* **2024**, *73*, 101948. [CrossRef]
159. Huang, S.; Wu, Z.; Cheng, Y.; Wei, W.; Hao, L. Insulin-like growth factor 2 mRNA binding protein 2 promotes aerobic glycolysis and cell proliferation in pancreatic ductal adenocarcinoma via stabilizing GLUT1 mRNA. *Acta Biochim. Biophys. Sin.* **2019**, *51*, 743–752. [CrossRef]
160. Liu, X.; Chen, J.; Chen, W.; Xu, Y.; Shen, Y.; Xu, X. Targeting IGF2BP3 in Cancer. *Int. J. Mol. Sci.* **2023**, *24*, 9423. [CrossRef]
161. Mueller-Pillasch, F.; Lacher, U.; Wallrapp, C.; Micha, A.; Zimmerhackl, F.; Hameister, H.; Varga, G.; Friess, H.; Buchler, M.; Beger, H.G.; et al. Cloning of a gene highly overexpressed in cancer coding for a novel KH-domain containing protein. *Oncogene* **1997**, *14*, 2729–2733. [CrossRef]
162. Wang, B.J.; Wang, L.; Yang, S.Y.; Liu, Z.J. Expression and clinical significance of IMP3 in microdissected premalignant and malignant pancreatic lesions. *Clin. Transl. Oncol.* **2015**, *17*, 215–222. [CrossRef]
163. Senoo, J.; Mikata, R.; Kishimoto, T.; Hayashi, M.; Kusakabe, Y.; Yasui, S.; Yamato, M.; Ohyama, H.; Sugiyama, H.; Tsuyuguchi, T.; et al. Immunohistochemical analysis of IMP3 and p53 expression in endoscopic ultrasound-guided fine needle aspiration and resected specimens of pancreatic diseases. *Pancreatology* **2018**, *18*, 176–183. [CrossRef]
164. Johnson, B.; Khalil, M.; Blansfield, J.; Lin, F.; Zhu, S.; Kirchner, H.L.; Weir, A.B., 3rd. Investigating the prognostic value of KOC (K homology domain containing protein overexpressed in cancer) overexpression after curative intent resection of pancreatic ductal adenocarcinoma. *J. Gastrointest. Oncol.* **2016**, *7*, E113–E117. [CrossRef] [PubMed]
165. Li, H.; Wang, X.; Fang, Y.; Huo, Z.; Lu, X.; Zhan, X.; Deng, X.; Peng, C.; Shen, B. Integrated expression profiles analysis reveals novel predictive biomarker in pancreatic ductal adenocarcinoma. *Oncotarget* **2017**, *8*, 52571–52583. [CrossRef] [PubMed]
166. Yantiss, R.K.; Cosar, E.; Fischer, A.H. Use of IMP3 in identification of carcinoma in fine needle aspiration biopsies of pancreas. *Acta Cytol.* **2008**, *52*, 133–138. [CrossRef]
167. Wachter, D.L.; Schlabrakowski, A.; Hoegel, J.; Kristiansen, G.; Hartmann, A.; Riener, M.O. Diagnostic value of immunohistochemical IMP3 expression in core needle biopsies of pancreatic ductal adenocarcinoma. *Am. J. Surg. Pathol.* **2011**, *35*, 873–877. [CrossRef] [PubMed]

168. Mikata, R.; Yasui, S.; Kishimoto, T.; Kouchi, Y.; Shingyoji, A.; Senoo, J.; Takahashi, K.; Nagashima, H.; Kusakabe, Y.; Ohyama, H.; et al. Diagnostic value of IMP3 and p53 immunohistochemical staining in EUS-guided fine-needle aspiration for solid pancreatic tumors. *Sci. Rep.* **2021**, *11*, 17257. [CrossRef]
169. Ennajdaoui, H.; Howard, J.M.; Sterne-Weiler, T.; Jahanbani, F.; Coyne, D.J.; Uren, P.J.; Dargyte, M.; Katzman, S.; Draper, J.M.; Wallace, A.; et al. IGF2BP3 Modulates the Interaction of Invasion-Associated Transcripts with RISC. *Cell Rep.* **2016**, *15*, 1876–1883. [CrossRef]
170. Guo, Z.; Zhang, X.; Lin, C.; Huang, Y.; Zhong, Y.; Guo, H.; Zheng, Z.; Weng, S. METTL3-IGF2BP3-axis mediates the proliferation and migration of pancreatic cancer by regulating spermine synthase m6A modification. *Front. Oncol.* **2022**, *12*, 962204. [CrossRef]
171. Pasiliao, C.C.; Chang, C.W.; Sutherland, B.W.; Valdez, S.M.; Schaeffer, D.; Yapp, D.T.; Ng, S.S. The involvement of insulin-like growth factor 2 binding protein 3 (IMP3) in pancreatic cancer cell migration, invasion, and adhesion. *BMC Cancer* **2015**, *15*, 266. [CrossRef] [PubMed]
172. Taniuchi, K.; Furihata, M.; Hanazaki, K.; Saito, M.; Saibara, T. IGF2BP3-mediated translation in cell protrusions promotes cell invasiveness and metastasis of pancreatic cancer. *Oncotarget* **2014**, *5*, 6832–6845. [CrossRef] [PubMed]
173. Taniuchi, K.; Furihata, M.; Saibara, T. KIF20A-mediated RNA granule transport system promotes the invasiveness of pancreatic cancer cells. *Neoplasia* **2014**, *16*, 1082–1093. [CrossRef]
174. Fu, W.; Lei, X.; Lu, Q.; Zhang, J.; Guo, J.; Zhao, J.; Tong, X.; Hu, X. UBE2K regulated by IGF2BP3 promotes cell proliferation and stemness in pancreatic ductal adenocarcinoma. *Int. J. Oncol.* **2023**, *62*, 52. [CrossRef] [PubMed]
175. Dowdle, M.E.; Kanzler, C.R.; Harder, C.R.K.; Moffet, S.; Walker, M.N.; Sheets, M.D. Bicaudal-C Post-transcriptional regulator of cell fates and functions. *Front. Cell Dev. Biol.* **2022**, *10*, 981696. [CrossRef]
176. Mahone, M.; Saffman, E.E.; Lasko, P.F. Localized Bicaudal-C RNA encodes a protein containing a KH domain, the RNA binding motif of FMR1. *EMBO J.* **1995**, *14*, 2043–2055. [CrossRef]
177. Mohler, J.; Wieschaus, E.F. Dominant maternal-effect mutations of Drosophila melanogaster causing the production of double-abdomen embryos. *Genetics* **1986**, *112*, 803–822. [CrossRef]
178. Saffman, E.E.; Styhler, S.; Rother, K.; Li, W.; Richard, S.; Lasko, P. Premature translation of oskar in oocytes lacking the RNA-binding protein bicaudal-C. *Mol. Cell Biol.* **1998**, *18*, 4855–4862. [CrossRef]
179. Meng, F.; Hua, S.; Chen, X.; Meng, N.; Lan, T. Lymph node metastasis related gene BICC1 promotes tumor progression by promoting EMT and immune infiltration in pancreatic cancer. *BMC Med. Genom.* **2023**, *16*, 263. [CrossRef]
180. Huang, C.; Li, H.; Xu, Y.; Xu, C.; Sun, H.; Li, Z.; Ge, Y.; Wang, H.; Zhao, T.; Gao, S.; et al. BICC1 drives pancreatic cancer progression by inducing VEGF-independent angiogenesis. *Signal Transduct. Target. Ther.* **2023**, *8*, 271. [CrossRef]
181. Sun, H.; Li, H.; Guan, Y.; Yuan, Y.; Xu, C.; Fu, D.; Xie, P.; Li, J.; Zhao, T.; Wang, X.; et al. BICC1 drives pancreatic cancer stemness and chemoresistance by facilitating tryptophan metabolism. *Sci. Adv.* **2024**, *10*, eadj8650. [CrossRef] [PubMed]
182. Pu, J.; Zhang, X.; Luo, H.; Xu, L.; Lu, X.; Lu, J. Adrenaline promotes epithelial-to-mesenchymal transition via HuR-TGFbeta regulatory axis in pancreatic cancer cells and the implication in cancer prognosis. *Biochem. Biophys. Res. Commun.* **2017**, *493*, 1273–1279. [CrossRef] [PubMed]
183. Hu, X.; Lei, X.; Guo, J.; Fu, W.; Sun, W.; Lu, Q.; Su, W.; Xu, Q.; Tu, K. The Emerging Role of RNA N6-Methyladenosine Modification in Pancreatic Cancer. *Front. Oncol.* **2022**, *12*, 927640. [CrossRef]
184. Subramaniam, D.; Ramalingam, S.; Linehan, D.C.; Dieckgraefe, B.K.; Postier, R.G.; Houchen, C.W.; Jensen, R.A.; Anant, S. RNA binding protein CUGBP2/CELF2 mediates curcumin-induced mitotic catastrophe of pancreatic cancer cells. *PLoS ONE* **2011**, *6*, e16958. [CrossRef] [PubMed]
185. Martinez-Useros, J.; Georgiev-Hristov, T.; Fernandez-Acenero, M.J.; Borrero-Palacios, A.; Indacochea, A.; Guerrero, S.; Li, W.; Cebrian, A.; Gomez Del Pulgar, T.; Puime-Otin, A.; et al. UNR/CDSE1 expression as prognosis biomarker in resectable pancreatic ductal adenocarcinoma patients: A proof-of-concept. *PLoS ONE* **2017**, *12*, e0182044. [CrossRef]
186. Zhang, L.; Yang, L.; Du, K. Exosomal HSPB1, interacting with FUS protein, suppresses hypoxia-induced ferroptosis in pancreatic cancer by stabilizing Nrf2 mRNA and repressing P450. *J. Cell Mol. Med.* **2024**, *28*, e18209. [CrossRef]
187. Yan-Sanders, Y.; Hammons, G.J.; Lyn-Cook, B.D. Increased expression of heterogeneous nuclear ribonucleoprotein A2/B1 (hnRNP) in pancreatic tissue from smokers and pancreatic tumor cells. *Cancer Lett.* **2002**, *183*, 215–220. [CrossRef]
188. Chen, Z.Y.; Cai, L.; Zhu, J.; Chen, M.; Chen, J.; Li, Z.H.; Liu, X.D.; Wang, S.G.; Bie, P.; Jiang, P.; et al. Fyn requires HnRNPA2B1 and Sam68 to synergistically regulate apoptosis in pancreatic cancer. *Carcinogenesis* **2011**, *32*, 1419–1426. [CrossRef]
189. Yang, N.; Liu, L.; Liu, X.; Chen, Y.; Lu, J.; Wang, Z. hnRNPC Promotes Malignancy in Pancreatic Cancer through Stabilization of IQGAP3. *Biomed. Res. Int.* **2022**, *2022*, 6319685. [CrossRef]
190. Antal, C.E.; Oh, T.G.; Aigner, S.; Luo, E.C.; Yee, B.A.; Campos, T.; Tiriac, H.; Rothamel, K.L.; Cheng, Z.; Jiao, H.; et al. A super-enhancer-regulated RNA-binding protein cascade drives pancreatic cancer. *Nat. Commun.* **2023**, *14*, 5195. [CrossRef]
191. Qiao, L.; Xie, N.; Bai, Y.; Li, Y.; Shi, Y.; Wang, J.; Liu, N. Identification of Upregulated HNRNPs Associated with Poor Prognosis in Pancreatic Cancer. *Biomed. Res. Int.* **2019**, *2019*, 5134050. [CrossRef] [PubMed]

192. Wang, Y.; Li, J.; Guo, S.; Ouyang, Y.; Yin, L.; Liu, S.; Zhao, Z.; Yang, J.; Huang, W.; Qin, H.; et al. Lin28B facilitates the progression and metastasis of pancreatic ductal adenocarcinoma. *Oncotarget* **2017**, *8*, 60414–60428. [CrossRef] [PubMed]
193. Liu, Y.; Wang, D.; Zhou, M.; Chen, H.; Wang, H.; Min, J.; Chen, J.; Wu, S.; Ni, X.; Zhang, Y.; et al. The KRAS/Lin28B axis maintains stemness of pancreatic cancer cells via the let-7i/TET3 pathway. *Mol. Oncol.* **2021**, *15*, 262–278. [CrossRef]
194. Shu, Z.; Fan, M.; Tu, B.; Tang, Z.; Wang, H.; Li, H.; Li, H.; Yuan, M.; Bai, J.; Huo, S.; et al. The Lin28b/Wnt5a axis drives pancreas cancer through crosstalk between cancer associated fibroblasts and tumor epithelium. *Nat. Commun.* **2023**, *14*, 6885. [CrossRef]
195. Panzeri, V.; Manni, I.; Capone, A.; Naro, C.; Sacconi, A.; Di Agostino, S.; de Latouliere, L.; Montori, A.; Pilozzi, E.; Piaggio, G., et al. The RNA-binding protein MEX3A is a prognostic factor and regulator of resistance to gemcitabine in pancreatic ductal adenocarcinoma. *Mol. Oncol.* **2021**, *15*, 579–595. [CrossRef]
196. Sheng, W.; Dong, M.; Chen, C.; Wang, Z.; Li, Y.; Wang, K.; Li, Y.; Zhou, J. Cooperation of Musashi-2, Numb, MDM2, and P53 in drug resistance and malignant biology of pancreatic cancer. *FASEB J.* **2017**, *31*, 2429–2438. [CrossRef] [PubMed]
197. Guo, K.; Cui, J.; Quan, M.; Xie, D.; Jia, Z.; Wei, D.; Wang, L.; Gao, Y.; Ma, Q.; Xie, K. The Novel KLF4/MSI2 Signaling Pathway Regulates Growth and Metastasis of Pancreatic Cancer. *Clin. Cancer Res.* **2017**, *23*, 687–696. [CrossRef]
198. Yang, H.; Hu, J.; Chen, J.; Chen, Z.; Jiao, F.; Cui, J.; Quan, M.; Wang, L. RNA-binding protein Musashi2 regulates Hippo signaling via SAV1 and MOB1 in pancreatic cancer. *Med. Oncol.* **2020**, *37*, 84. [CrossRef]
199. Sheng, W.; Dong, M.; Chen, C.; Li, Y.; Liu, Q.; Dong, Q. Musashi2 promotes the development and progression of pancreatic cancer by down-regulating Numb protein. *Oncotarget* **2017**, *8*, 14359–14373. [CrossRef]
200. Chu, L.; Hu, Y.; Jiang, Y.H.; Xu, C.; Liu, W.C.; Lu, Z.F. Effects of RNA binding protein QKI on pancreatic cancer ductal epithelial cells and surrounding activation fibroblasts. *J. Cell Biochem.* **2019**, *120*, 11551–11561. [CrossRef]
201. Maurin, M.; Ranjouri, M.; Megino-Luque, C.; Newberg, J.Y.; Du, D.; Martin, K.; Miner, R.E., 3rd; Prater, M.S.; Wee, D.K.B., Centeno, B.; et al. RBFOX2 deregulation promotes pancreatic cancer progression and metastasis through alternative splicing. *Nat Commun.* **2023**, *14*, 8444. [CrossRef] [PubMed]
202. Witkiewicz, A.K.; McMillan, E.A.; Balaji, U.; Baek, G.; Lin, W.C.; Mansour, J.; Mollaee, M.; Wagner, K.U.; Koduru, P.; Yopp, A., et al. Whole-exome sequencing of pancreatic cancer defines genetic diversity and therapeutic targets. *Nat. Commun.* **2015**, *6*, 6744 [CrossRef]
203. Xiao, W.; Chen, X.; Li, X.; Deng, K.; Liu, H.; Ma, J.; Wang, Z.; Hu, Y.; Hou, J. RBM10 regulates human TERT gene splicing and inhibits pancreatic cancer progression. *Am. J. Cancer Res.* **2021**, *11*, 157–170. [PubMed]
204. Iwata, T.; Kishikawa, T.; Seimiya, T.; Notoya, G.; Suzuki, T.; Shibata, C.; Miyakawa, Y.; Odawara, N.; Funato, K.; Tanaka, E.; et al Satellite double-stranded RNA induces mesenchymal transition in pancreatic cancer by regulating alternative splicing. *J. Biol. Chem.* **2024**, *300*, 105742. [CrossRef] [PubMed]
205. Zhao, X.; Chen, M.; Tan, J. Knockdown of ZFR suppresses cell proliferation and invasion of human pancreatic cancer. *Biol. Res.* **2016**, *49*, 26. [CrossRef]
206. Fire, A.; Xu, S.; Montgomery, M.K.; Kostas, S.A.; Driver, S.E.; Mello, C.C. Potent and specific genetic interference by double-stranded RNA in Caenorhabditis elegans. *Nature* **1998**, *391*, 806–811. [CrossRef]
207. Tani, H. Recent Advances and Prospects in RNA Drug Development. *Int. J. Mol. Sci.* **2024**, *25*, 12284. [CrossRef]
208. Kamerkar, S.; LeBleu, V.S.; Sugimoto, H.; Yang, S.; Ruivo, C.F.; Melo, S.A.; Lee, J.J.; Kalluri, R. Exosomes facilitate therapeutic targeting of oncogenic KRAS in pancreatic cancer. *Nature* **2017**, *546*, 498–503. [CrossRef]
209. Liang, X.H.; Sun, H.; Nichols, J.G.; Crooke, S.T. RNase H1-Dependent Antisense Oligonucleotides Are Robustly Active in Directing RNA Cleavage in Both the Cytoplasm and the Nucleus. *Mol. Ther.* **2017**, *25*, 2075–2092. [CrossRef]
210. Gutschner, T.; Hammerle, M.; Eissmann, M.; Hsu, J.; Kim, Y.; Hung, G.; Revenko, A.; Arun, G.; Stentrup, M.; Gross, M.; et al. The noncoding RNA MALAT1 is a critical regulator of the metastasis phenotype of lung cancer cells. *Cancer Res.* **2013**, *73*, 1180–1189 [CrossRef]
211. Neil, E.E.; Bisaccia, E.K. Nusinersen: A Novel Antisense Oligonucleotide for the Treatment of Spinal Muscular Atrophy. *J. Pediatr. Pharmacol. Ther.* **2019**, *24*, 194–203. [CrossRef] [PubMed]
212. Ammala, C.; Drury, W.J., 3rd; Knerr, L.; Ahlstedt, I.; Stillemark-Billton, P.; Wennberg-Huldt, C.; Andersson, E.M.; Valeur, E.; Jansson-Lofmark, R.; Janzen, D.; et al. Targeted delivery of antisense oligonucleotides to pancreatic beta-cells. *Sci. Adv.* **2018**, *4*, eaat3386. [CrossRef]
213. Childs-Disney, J.L.; Yang, X.; Gibaut, Q.M.R.; Tong, Y.; Batey, R.T.; Disney, M.D. Targeting RNA structures with small molecules *Nat. Rev. Drug Discov.* **2022**, *21*, 736–762. [CrossRef] [PubMed]
214. Jaiswal, A.K.; Thaxton, M.L.; Scherer, G.M.; Sorrentino, J.P.; Garg, N.K.; Rao, D.S. Small molecule inhibition of RNA binding proteins in haematologic cancer. *RNA Biol.* **2024**, *21*, 276–289. [CrossRef]
215. Li, Q.; Kang, C. Targeting RNA-binding proteins with small molecules: Perspectives, pitfalls and bifunctional molecules. *FEBS Lett.* **2023**, *597*, 2031–2047. [CrossRef]
216. Nguyen, L.D.; Chau, R.K.; Krichevsky, A.M. Small Molecule Drugs Targeting Non-Coding RNAs as Treatments for Alzheimer's Disease and Related Dementias. *Genes* **2021**, *12*, 2005. [CrossRef]

217. Zhao, R.; Fu, J.; Zhu, L.; Chen, Y.; Liu, B. Designing strategies of small-molecule compounds for modulating non-coding RNAs in cancer therapy. *J. Hematol. Oncol.* **2022**, *15*, 14. [CrossRef] [PubMed]
218. Bertoldo, J.B.; Muller, S.; Huttelmaier, S. RNA-binding proteins in cancer drug discovery. *Drug Discov. Today* **2023**, *28*, 103580. [CrossRef]
219. Bekes, M.; Langley, D.R.; Crews, C.M. PROTAC targeted protein degraders: The past is prologue. *Nat. Rev. Drug Discov.* **2022**, *21*, 181–200. [CrossRef]
220. Gama-Brambila, R.A.; Chen, J.; Zhou, J.; Tascher, G.; Munch, C.; Cheng, X. A PROTAC targets splicing factor 3B1. *Cell Chem. Biol.* **2021**, *28*, 1616–1627.e1618. [CrossRef]
221. Kaur, T.; Menon, A.; Garner, A.L. Synthesis of 7-benzylguanosine cap-analogue conjugates for eIF4E targeted degradation. *Eur. J. Med. Chem.* **2019**, *166*, 339–350. [CrossRef] [PubMed]
222. Ghidini, A.; Clery, A.; Halloy, F.; Allain, F.H.T.; Hall, J. RNA-PROTACs: Degraders of RNA-Binding Proteins. *Angew. Chem. Int. Ed. Engl.* **2021**, *60*, 3163–3169. [CrossRef]
223. Costales, M.G.; Matsumoto, Y.; Velagapudi, S.P.; Disney, M.D. Small Molecule Targeted Recruitment of a Nuclease to RNA. *J. Am. Chem. Soc.* **2018**, *140*, 6741–6744. [CrossRef] [PubMed]
224. Costales, M.G.; Aikawa, H.; Li, Y.; Childs-Disney, J.L.; Abegg, D.; Hoch, D.G.; Pradeep Velagapudi, S.; Nakai, Y.; Khan, T.; Wang, K.W.; et al. Small-molecule targeted recruitment of a nuclease to cleave an oncogenic RNA in a mouse model of metastatic cancer. *Proc. Natl. Acad. Sci. USA* **2020**, *117*, 2406–2411. [CrossRef]
225. Meyer, S.M.; Tanaka, T.; Zanon, P.R.A.; Baisden, J.T.; Abegg, D.; Yang, X.; Akahori, Y.; Alshakarchi, Z.; Cameron, M.D.; Adibekian, A.; et al. DNA-Encoded Library Screening to Inform Design of a Ribonuclease Targeting Chimera (RiboTAC). *J. Am. Chem. Soc.* **2022**, *144*, 21096–21102. [CrossRef]
226. Tong, Y.; Lee, Y.; Liu, X.; Childs-Disney, J.L.; Suresh, B.M.; Benhamou, R.I.; Yang, C.; Li, W.; Costales, M.G.; Haniff, H.S.; et al. Programming inactive RNA-binding small molecules into bioactive degraders. *Nature* **2023**, *618*, 169–179. [CrossRef] [PubMed]
227. Cirino, N.M.; Li, G.; Xiao, W.; Torrence, P.F.; Silverman, R.H. Targeting RNA decay with 2′,5′ oligoadenylate-antisense in respiratory syncytial virus-infected cells. *Proc. Natl. Acad. Sci. USA* **1997**, *94*, 1937–1942. [CrossRef]
228. Fang, Y.; Wu, Q.; Wang, F.; Liu, Y.; Zhang, H.; Yang, C.; Zhu, Z. Aptamer-RIBOTAC Strategy Enabling Tumor-Specific Targeted Degradation of MicroRNA for Precise Cancer Therapy. In *Small Methods*; Wiley: New York, NY, USA, 2024; p. e2400349. [CrossRef]
229. Su, X.; Ma, W.; Feng, D.; Cheng, B.; Wang, Q.; Guo, Z.; Zhou, D.; Tang, X. Efficient Inhibition of SARS-CoV-2 Using Chimeric Antisense Oligonucleotides through RNase L Activation. *Angew. Chem. Int. Ed. Engl.* **2021**, *60*, 21662–21667. [CrossRef]
230. Torrence, P.F.; Maitra, R.K.; Lesiak, K.; Khamnei, S.; Zhou, A.; Silverman, R.H. Targeting RNA for degradation with a (2′-5′)oligoadenylate-antisense chimera. *Proc. Natl. Acad. Sci. USA* **1993**, *90*, 1300–1304. [CrossRef]
231. Lu, J.; Yu, L.; Xie, N.; Wu, Y.; Li, B. METTL14 Facilitates the Metastasis of Pancreatic Carcinoma by Stabilizing LINC00941 in an m6A-IGF2BP2-Dependent Manner. *J. Cancer* **2023**, *14*, 1117–1131. [CrossRef]
232. Zhai, S.; Xu, Z.; Xie, J.; Zhang, J.; Wang, X.; Peng, C.; Li, H.; Chen, H.; Shen, B.; Deng, X. Epigenetic silencing of LncRNA LINC00261 promotes c-myc-mediated aerobic glycolysis by regulating miR-222-3p/HIPK2/ERK axis and sequestering IGF2BP1. *Oncogene* **2021**, *40*, 277–291. [CrossRef] [PubMed]
233. Athanasiou, A.; Kureshi, N.; Wittig, A.; Sterner, M.; Huber, R.; Palma, N.A.; King, T.; Schiess, R. Biomarker Discovery for Early Detection of Pancreatic Ductal Adenocarcinoma (PDAC) Using Multiplex Proteomics Technology. *J. Proteome Res.* **2025**, *24*, 315–322. [CrossRef] [PubMed]
234. Khomiak, A.; Brunner, M.; Kordes, M.; Lindblad, S.; Miksch, R.C.; Ohlund, D.; Regel, I. Recent Discoveries of Diagnostic, Prognostic and Predictive Biomarkers for Pancreatic Cancer. *Cancers* **2020**, *12*, 3234. [CrossRef] [PubMed]
235. Bin, W.; Yuan, C.; Qie, Y.; Dang, S. Long non-coding RNAs and pancreatic cancer: A multifaceted view. *Biomed. Pharmacother.* **2023**, *167*, 115601. [CrossRef]
236. von Widdern, J.C.; Rosendahl, J.; Ammer-Herrmenau, C. Chronic and Idiopathic Pancreatitis-A Personalized Treatment Approach. *United Eur. Gastroenterol. J.* **2025**, *13*, 116–124. [CrossRef]

cancers

MDPI

Review

Stromal Cells in Early Inflammation-Related Pancreatic Carcinogenesis—Biology and Its Potential Role in Therapeutic Targeting

Tina Seidel [1,†], Nupur Ohri [2,†], Markus Glaß [3], Yoshiaki Sunami [2], Lutz P. Müller [1,‡] and Jörg Kleeff [2,*,‡]

[1] Department of Internal Medicine, University Hospital Halle, 06120 Halle (Saale), Germany; tina.seidel@uk-halle.de (T.S.); lutz.mueller@uk-halle.de (L.P.M.)
[2] Department of Visceral, Vascular and Endocrine Surgery, University Hospital Halle, 06120 Halle (Saale), Germany; nupur.ohri@uk-halle.de (N.O.); yoshiaki.sunami@uk-halle.de (Y.S.)
[3] Institute of Molecular Medicine, Martin Luther University Halle-Wittenberg, 06108 Halle (Saale), Germany; markuss.glass@medizin.uni.halle.de
* Correspondence: joerg.kleeff@uk-halle.de; Tel.: +49-345-557-2924
† These authors contributed equally to this work.
‡ These authors contributed equally as senior authors.

Simple Summary: The development of pancreatic cancer is strongly influenced by chronic inflammation, which induces changes in the pancreatic stroma—the connective tissue that includes cell types such as fibroblasts, pancreatic stellate cells, and multipotent stromal cells. While it is well established that the stroma plays a significant role in advanced stages of the disease, its contribution during the early, inflammation-driven phases of tumorigenesis remains poorly understood. This review aims to provide deeper insight into the function and transformation of stromal cells during the initial stages of disease development. Gaining this knowledge could support the development of novel therapeutic strategies to prevent cancer at an early stage and drive forward research on the tumor microenvironment.

Abstract: The stroma of healthy pancreases contains various non-hematopoietic, non-endothelial mesenchymal cells. It is altered by chronic inflammation which in turn is a major contributor to the development of pancreatic adenocarcinoma (PDAC). In PDAC, the stroma plays a decisive and well-investigated role for tumor progression and therapy response. This review addresses the central role of stromal cells in the early inflammation-driven development of PDAC. It focuses on major subpopulations of pancreatic mesenchymal cells, i.e., fibroblasts, pancreatic stellate cells, and multipotent stroma cells, particularly their activation and functional alterations upon chronic inflammation including the development of different types of carcinoma-associated fibroblasts. In the second part, the current knowledge on the impact of activated stroma cells on acinar-to-ductal metaplasia and the transition to pancreatic intraepithelial neoplasia is summarized. Finally, putative strategies to target stroma cells and their signaling in early pancreatic carcinogenesis are reflected. In summary, the current data show that the activation of pancreatic stroma cells and the resulting fibrotic changes has pro- and anti-carcinogenetic effects but, overall, creates a carcinogenesis-promoting microenvironment. However, this is a dynamic process and the therapeutic targeting of specific pathways and cells requires in-depth knowledge of the molecular interplay of various cell types.

Keywords: pancreatic adenocarcinoma; cancer-associated fibroblasts; pancreatic stellate cells; mesenchymal stem cells

 https://doi.org/10.3390/cancers17091541

1. Introduction

In healthy pancreases, the stroma serves as a protective environment that provides essential signals to ensure tissue maintenance and function and suppress malignant transformation [1]. However, persistent inflammation induces changes in the phenotype and function of stromal cells, eventually resulting in fibrosis and contributing to carcinogenesis. This is proven not just by murine models [2] but also by the increased risk for developing pancreatic ductal adenocarcinoma (PDAC) in patients with chronic pancreatitis [3]. The chronic inflammatory process does not only involve epithelial cells of the exocrine system and hematopoietic immune cells but also the non-hematopoietic compartment of mesenchymal cells [4]. In the present review, we summarize the current knowledge regarding the differential types of non-hematopoietic mesenchymal cells present in the pancreas and their inflammation-driven alterations contributing to PDAC carcinogenesis. Based on that, we reflect on targeting the altered pancreatic stroma as an approach to prevent inflammation-driven PDAC as well as to provide options for its early treatment.

2. Types of Non-Hematopoietic Mesenchymal Cells in Healthy Pancreas

Fibroblasts, pancreatic stellate cells (PSCs), and multipotent stroma cells (MSCs) have been reported as the major non-hematopoietic, non-endothelial constituents of the stroma in healthy pancreases (Figure 1). However, the distinctions between these cell types are not clearly defined. Thus, it remains questionable whether these cell types uniquely exist in vivo or rather represent different stages of a continuous differentiation process of mesenchymal cells. Still, the existing data and literature justify a distinction between these cell types as they harbor distinct functional characteristics. Based on current data, they appear to coexist in healthy pancreases in a resident, non-activated state (Figure 2).

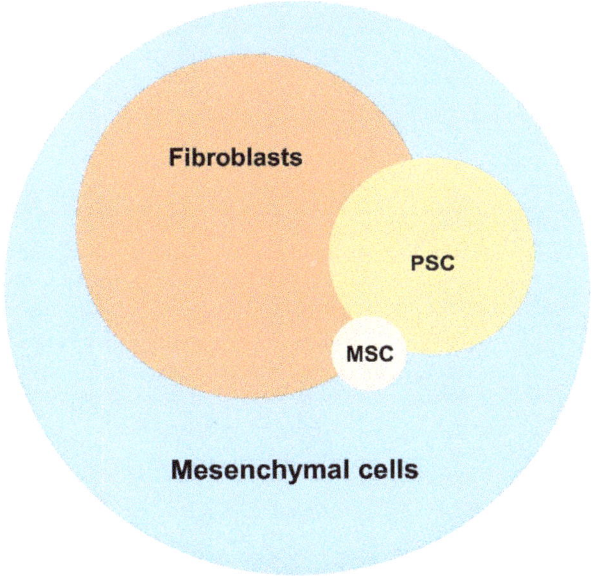

Figure 1. Composition of a healthy pancreatic stroma. The different types of non-hematopoietic stroma cell (fibroblasts, PSCs, and MSCs) as parts of the mesenchymal cell entity is depicted including the reflection of the size of the respective subpopulation. PSC: pancreatic stellate cells; MSC: multipotent stromal cells. Created in https://BioRender.com.

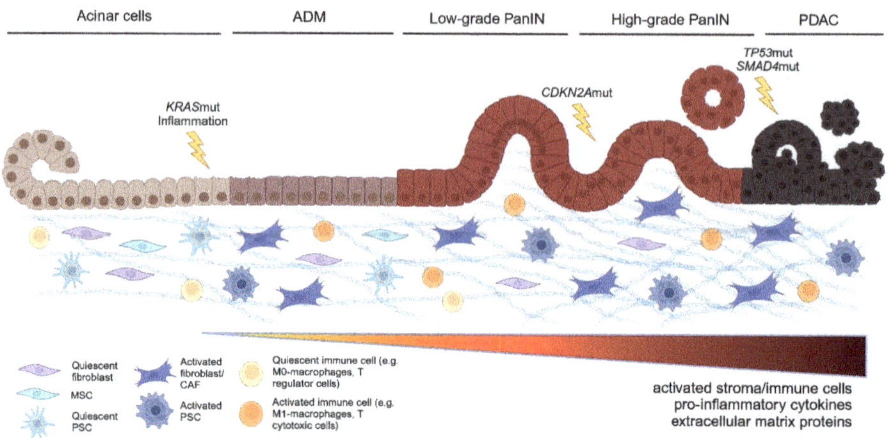

Figure 2. Development of the non-hematopoietic pancreatic stroma during early PDAC carcinogenesis. Depicted is the development of pancreatic adenocarcinoma (PDAC), starting from healthy acinar cells through various precancerous stages to malignant disease including typical mutations and molecular and cellular changes in the microenvironment of the tumor cells. *Acinar cells (healthy pancreas)*: the microenvironment consists of resting fibroblasts, multipotent stromal cells (MSCs), resting pancreatic stellate cells (PSCs), and resting immune cells. *Acinar-to-ductal metaplasia (ADM)*: initiated by activation of KRAS mutations and inflammation. Acinar cells begin to adopt a ductal phenotype. Fibroblasts, MSCs, PSCs, and immune cells are activated, accompanied by immune cell migration and increased extracellular matrix (ECM) production. *Pancreatic intraepithelial neoplasia (PanIN)*: early to advanced precancerous stages with loss of epithelial arrangement and function. The microenvironment shows increased activation of fibroblasts, MSCs, PSCs, and immune cells, as well as increased production of pro-inflammatory cytokines and increasing fibrosis. PDAC: malignant stage with mutations in TP53 and SMAD4. Highly activated tumor microenvironment: pro-inflammatory milieu and pronounced fibrosis. Created in https://BioRender.com.

2.1. Tissue-Resident Fibroblasts in Pancreas—Origin and Markers

Fibroblasts are mesenchymal cells [5], and pancreatic tissue-resident fibroblasts originate from Insulin Gene Enhancer Protein ISL-1-expressing splanchnic mesenchyme during fetal development [6]. Lineage tracing studies in mice have shown that the splanchnic mesenchyme, the fetal cell layer surrounding the endoderm from which the pancreatic epithelium develops, gives rise to the majority of resident pancreatic fibroblasts in the healthy pancreas [6]. These fibroblasts are localized to perivascular regions and the tissue parenchyma, allowing direct interactions with epithelial cells [7]. In general, fibroblasts are spindle-shaped, non-epithelial, non-immune, and non-hematopoietic cells that typically exist in a quiescent or inactive state, with minimal metabolic and transcriptomic activity [8]. Upon activation by factors such as transforming growth factor-β (TGF-β), platelet-derived growth factor (PDGF), or interleukin-6 (IL-6 quiescent fibroblasts transdifferentiate into an activated, myofibroblast-like phenotype [9,10]). This activated state is associated with increased proliferation, migration, enhanced production of growth factors, and extracellular matrix (ECM) components. Activated fibroblasts are characterized by the expression of α-smooth muscle actin (α-SMA, encoded by the *ACTA2* gene) [11,12]. The myofibroblastic differentiation plays a role in wound healing [13], acute and chronic inflammation, and fibrosis [12,13]. Fibroblast-specific protein 1 (FSP1) is often used to identify quiescent, non-proliferating (Ki67-negative) fibroblasts [14]. Markers commonly associated with activated fibroblasts include vimentin, αSMA, fibroblast activation protein (FAP), PDGF receptor-α (PDGFRα), PDGFRβ, and discoidin domain-containing receptor 2 (DDR2) [15]. However, the unambiguous characterization of fibroblasts is often complicated due to the lack of specificity of the aforementioned marker proteins. For instance, FSP1 is also expressed by macrophages and certain cancer cells [16] while FAP is found in subsets of $CD45^+$ immune cells [17].

Recent lineage tracing experiments have identified two distinct fibroblast populations in the healthy pancreas, distinguished by the expression of transcription factors Gli1 and Hoxb6. Gli1, a key target of the Hedgehog signaling pathway [18], is active during embryonic gastrointestinal development but is suppressed during pancreas formation, with low-level signaling persisting for homeostasis and injury recovery [19]. A subset of healthy pancreatic fibroblasts express Gli1, though they do not resemble pancreatic stellate cells [20]. Hoxb6 is broadly expressed in the mesenchyme of the developing pancreas [21] and remains present in a subset of fibroblasts in the adult pancreas. Currently, no unique markers distinguish pancreatic fibroblasts from fibroblasts in other organs [20]. However, lineage-tracing studies highlight their unique embryonic origins, emphasizing the need for further research to identify distinct pancreatic fibroblast markers and better characterize their role in pancreatic homeostasis and disease.

2.2. Pancreatic Stellate Cells—Overlapping and Distinct Characteristics Compared to Pancreatic Fibroblasts

Pancreatic stellate cells (PSCs) are mesenchymal cells with a star-shaped morphology that constitute approximately 7% of the cellular population in the pancreas [22]. They are primarily located around small pancreatic ducts and blood vessels, and in the basolateral regions of pancreatic acinar cells [23]. The developmental origin of PSCs remains a topic of debate, with evidence suggesting contributions from mesenchymal [22,24], endodermal [25], and neuroectodermal lineages [26]. Initially described by Watari in 1982, PSCs were noted for their periacinar localization and their resemblance to hepatic stellate cells. The isolation and culture from rat and human pancreas were optimized in 1998 [23,27] enabling extensive in vitro studies of PSC biology.

In a healthy pancreas, PSCs exist in a quiescent state, characterized by the presence of vitamin A-rich lipid droplets in cytoplasm. The physiological role of vitamin A storage in PSCs remains unclear, but it is hypothesized to contribute to maintaining quiescence [28]. Upon activation in response to injury or inflammation, PSCs lose their lipid droplets presumably due to use of the stored lipids for energy supply and membrane structures [29–31]. This activation is associated with increased proliferation, migration, ECM production, and expression of markers such as α-SMA, FAP, PDGFRα/β, collagens (I and III), fibronectin, ICAM-1, cadherin-11, DDR2, vimentin, GFAP, NGF, NCAM, desmin, nestin, etc. [8,23,28,32–34].

PSCs and pancreatic fibroblasts share similarities, but they also exhibit key differences in their phenotype and biology. Both are of mesenchymal origin and can activate into a myofibroblast-like phenotype, expressing common markers such as α-SMA, PDGFRα/β, and vimentin [15,28]. Additionally, they share roles in tissue homeostasis, wound healing, and ECM remodeling [35]. Besides their ability to store lipid droplets PSC differ from pancreatic fibroblasts on their expression of GFAP, higher ECM production, and unique expression of scavenger receptors, like CD36, CCK1/2 receptors, and the ACh receptor (Acetylcholine receptor) [36,37]. Traditionally, CCK was thought to stimulate pancreatic enzyme secretion via vagus nerve activation. However, an alternative mechanism involves PSCs. These are positioned basolaterally to acinar cells. Upon CCK stimulation, PSCs release ACh, which then acts on muscarinic receptors on acinar cells to promote digestive enzyme secretions [36]. This suggests that quiescent PSCs may play an unappreciated role in pancreatic exocrine regulation. PSCs express desmin, a marker for stellate cells, with over 90% also positive for α-SMA. In contrast, pancreatic fibroblasts show minimal desmin expression, distinguishing them from PSC markers [38,39]. Moreover, the high α-SMA expression in PSCs enhances their contractile properties, allowing them to regulate vascular and ductal tone in the pancreas. Given their localization around blood vessels and ductal structures, PSC-mediated contraction may influence pancreatic blood flow and secretion [28].

In the healthy pancreas, PSCs and fibroblasts contribute to ECM production and remodeling. This dynamic process is essential for tissue development, homeostasis, and repair following injury [35]. ECM homeostasis relies on the balance between ECM synthesis and degradation, mediated by MMPs [40]. PSCs and pancreatic fibroblasts produce key ECM components, including collagen type I, III, IV, and V, laminins, and fibronectin [41]. Additionally, PSCs regulate ECM turnover by also producing MMPs [42], ensuring matrix remodeling.

Beyond ECM regulation, PSCs also participate in immune regulation. They express cell adhesion molecules, such as ICAM-1, which facilitate immune cell recruitment [43]. Furthermore, PSCs express Toll-like receptors (TLRs), including TLR2, TLR4, TLR3, and TLR5, allowing them to recognize bacterial and viral components and activate innate immune responses [44]. Through the phagocytosis of necrotic debris and aged polymorphonuclear cells [45], PSCs contribute to inflammation resolution, tissue repair, and immune homeostasis in the pancreas.

2.3. Multipotent Stroma Cells

Multipotent stroma cells (MSCs)—originally named mesenchymal stem cells—represent a cell type of mesodermal origin and multipotent differentiation potential. According to consensus criteria, the defining minimal characteristics of human MSCs comprise the following: (1) the ability to establish colony-forming unitary fibroblasts (CFU-F) in vitro of spindle-shaped morphologic appearance (similar to fibroblasts); (2) a surface marker profile of $CD105^+$, $CD73^+$, $CD90^+$, $CD45^-$, $CD34^-$, $CD14^-$, $CD11b^-$, $CD79\alpha^-$, $CD19^-$, HLA-DR^-; (3) the ability to differentiate into osteoblasts, adipocytes, and chondroblasts [46,47]. Obviously, these criteria leave space for much heterogeneity and are not suited to define MSCs in vivo. MSCs have originally been described in the bone marrow but can also be isolated from various other tissues of the adult organism, such as cartilage, skeletal muscle, or adipose tissue [48]. It remains open whether the MSCs from different tissues are distinct or represent a uniform cell population. In general, human tissue-resident MSCs are impacted by age and disease [48–50] and serve as progenitor cells for specialized fibroblast subtypes and are involved in fibrosis and immunomodulation [51–54].

Stroma cells fulfilling MSC criteria have been isolated from the human [55] as well as murine [56,57] pancreas. They are mainly found in the perivascular area as well as in the intra- and interlobular stroma tissue, where they surround the glandular structures of the pancreas [55,58,59].

MSCs isolated from human islet fractions (LPI) as a by-product of islet cell transplantation showed typical defining characteristics as MSCs from other sources but exhibited higher expression of nestin and angiogenic markers but a lower expression level of CD146 and a lower adipogenic differentiation potential [55]. MSCs harbor an immunomodulating capacity and in healthy tissue, they support an immunosuppressive environment [60]. This involves the release of soluble factors with anti-inflammatory, anti-oxidative, and anti-apoptotic properties (e. g. IL-6, IL-10, TGF-β, PGE2, CCL2, or VEGF) but also secretion of extracellular vesicles comprising miRNAs, cytokines, growth factors, and cell–cell contact including receptor–ligand interactions (e.g., PD-L1 and PD-L2). To date, there is no clear evidence of the specific relation between MSCs and PSCs.

There are controversial reports on the trans-differentiation of both non-pancreatic and pancreatic MSCs into pancreatic epithelial cells. Cao et al. also report the in vitro differentiation of immortalized MSCs from fetal porcine pancreas into insulin-producing beta cells [61]. In contrast, Seeberger et al. showed that the occurrence of EMT in pancreatic cells is an artifact of in vitro cell culture and does not represent a natural process in pancreatic tissue or tumor development [62]. In our view, despite similarities in surface marker expression [48], pancreatic MSCs and PSCs represent differential cell populations with a differential impact on pancreatic pathobiology.

3. Alterations and Differentiation of Stroma in Pancreatic Inflammation

Based on their clinical course and pathobiology acute and chronic pancreatitis are distinguished. Acute pancreatitis represents a short-term inflammation of the exocrine pancreas and is characterized primarily by an infiltration of granulocytes accompanied by fluid retention [4]. In mild cases, involving only the pancreas, no long-term sequelae are prominent. Severe cases involving a systemic inflammatory response syndrome can lead to necrosis including changes in the pancreatic stroma [63]. In contrast, chronic pancreatitis reflects a recurrent and persistent inflammatory process either preceded by acute pancreatitis [64]. It eventually results in fibrosis, increased stroma presence, loss of functional epithelia, and metaplasia [65]. During this process, the stroma modifies inflammation and is modified itself by inflammation (Figure 3).

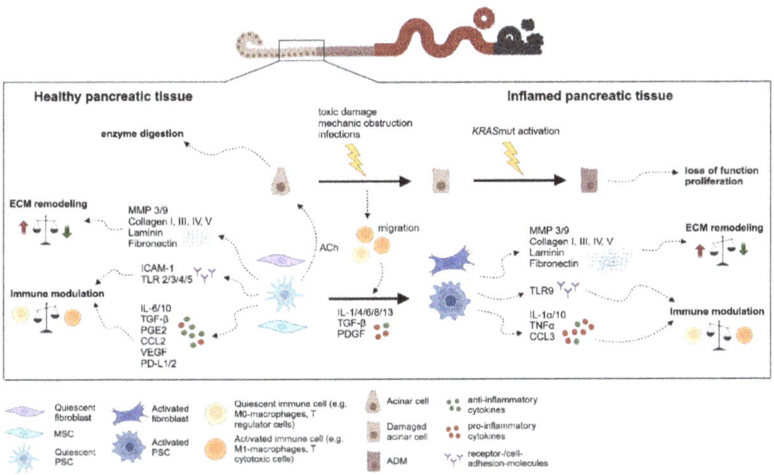

Figure 3. Relevant molecular processes in the pancreatic stroma in chronic pancreatitis as a precursor for PDAC carcinogenesis. The figure illustrates cellular and molecular mechanisms that lead to inflammation in the pancreas. *Healthy pancreatic tissue*: intact acinar cells are responsible for enzyme digestion. Resting fibroblasts, pancreatic stellate cells (PSCs), and multipotent stromal cells (MSCs) ensure functional and immunological homeostasis: the balance between formation and degradation of the extracellular matrix (ECM), including all its components such as collagen, laminin, and fibronectin is maintained. Matrix metalloproteinases (MMPs) regulate the synthesis and degradation of ECM. Anti-inflammatory cytokines, such as IL-6, IL-10, TGF-β, and PGE2, as well as chemotactic factors such as CCL2 and VEGF, promote an immunosuppressive microenvironment. PSCs in particular regulate acinar cell function through acetylcholine (ACh). *Inflamed pancreatic tissue*: toxic damage, mechanical obstruction, and infection lead to cell damage in acinar cells. Activated immune cells migrate into the tissue and promote the differentiation of quiescent mesenchymal cells into activated fibroblasts and PSCs. As a result, collagen and fibronectin are increasingly deposited and MMPs are dysregulated, leading to greater ECM formation than degradation. Pro-inflammatory cytokines such as IL-1α, IL-10, TNFα and CCL3 dominate. TLR9 receptors are activated, which further strengthens the immune response. The consequence is the activation of oncogenic KRAS and increased proliferation of non-functional acinar cells. Created in https://BioRender.com.

The current literature suggests that the pancreatic stroma has a significant impact on the course of inflammatory responses in the pancreas facilitating carcinogenesis of pancreatic ductal adenocarcinoma (PDAC) [66,67].

3.1. Stroma in Acute Pancreatitis

Acute pancreatitis—caused by toxic damage, ductal obstruction, or, in rare cases, infections—represents an acute inflammatory process mostly characterized by the infiltration of hematopoietic cells, particularly granulocytes and fluid retention with subsequent release of pancreatic enzymes into the tissue [68]. Although an activation of PSCs in acute pancreatitis has long be known [69], generally no significant expansion or fibrotic changes in the stroma ensue. In cases of mild injury, the tissue can be rapidly restored by the reactivation of resident progenitor cells that differentiate into new acinar cells, without permanent structural damage and no association with malignant transformation [70].

However, the fact that repeated episodes of acute pancreatitis predispose the development of chronic pancreatitis suggests that pancreatitis represents a dynamic inflammatory process where stroma alterations are present from early on [64,68]. Data on the specific contribution of stroma cells to either the inflammatory process or its containment in acute pancreatitis are sparse. Recent data support the notion that the pancreatic stroma contributes to the inflammatory process in acute pancreatitis. Specifically, resident fibroblasts and PSCs are activated by various inflammatory signals during acute pancreatitis [38]. Based on their known immunosuppressive potential a multitude of studies have explored the therapeutic effects of MSCs or MSC-related products like exosomes in acute pancreatitis [71]. However, it remains speculative whether pancreatic MSCs are decisive for controlling inflammation in acute pancreatitis.

3.2. Stroma in Chronic Pancreatitis

Chronic pancreatitis is often associated with alcohol consumption, smoking, and nutritional factors but also hereditary disposition or efferent duct aberrations [72]. In contrast to acute pancreatitis, it is characterized by an increase in stroma ensuing fibrosis [4] and is a predisposing factor for pancreatic cancer [73].

In general, the chronic inflammatory stimulus with persistent immune cell infiltration leads to dedifferentiation, subsequent re-maturation, and also atrophy of acinar cells [68]. Pancreatic stroma cells may directly impact the inflammation, but data are sparse. For instance, PSCs are a source of cytokines like IL-4Ra ligand which promotes macrophage M2 polarization [74]. The chronic inflammatory response is accompanied by alterations in the proportion and characteristics of pancreatic stroma cells, i.e., pancreatic fibroblasts, PSCs, and probably MSCs as exemplified in Figure 3. Specifically, upon chronic pancreatitis, PSCs and probably other pancreatic stroma cells undergo an activation process mainly induced by pro-inflammatory cytokines like IL-1, IL-4, IL-6, IL-8, IL-13, and many others. In the context of chronic pancreatitis this activation is poorly defined but for PSCs mainly involves a myofibroblastic differentiation with induction of marker genes like a-SMA [75]. For instance, in a feed-forward process, PSC-induced M2 macrophages in turn activate PSCs through IL-4-signaling [74]. Accordingly, the inhibition of IL-4 and IL-13 led to a significant reduction in fibrosis in a model of PSC activation [74]. These activated PSCs and presumably pancreatic stroma cells, in general, are also the main source of ECM which is characteristic of the increased stroma proportion and fibrosis in chronic pancreatitis [4]. The activation of PSCs and probably other pancreatic stroma cells upon chronic pancreatic inflammation may result in a phenotype resembling so-called cancer-associated fibroblasts (CAFs). By definition, CAFs represent differentiated stroma cells in the context of malignant lesions. However, a prominent feature of the dominant CAF subtype is their myofibroblastic differentiation and pro-tumorigenic potential. And a CAF-like state may be induced by chronic inflammation. For instance, activation of TLR9—a major regulator of inflammation—in PSCs results in a pro-tumorigenic phenotype of PSCs with expression of various cytokines like IL1α, IL10, TNFα, CCL3, and CCL11 but also ECM regulators like MMP3 and MMP9 [76]. Thus, the increased risk of pancreatic adenocarcinoma (PDAC) development upon chronic pancreatitis may be, at least partly, due to an early differentiation of PSCs and likely also other pancreatic stroma cells to a pro-tumorigenic, CAF-like phenotype (Figure 3).

Only indirect evidence for the role of MSCs in chronic pancreatitis can be drawn from intervention studies. In animal models of chronic pancreatitis, the transplantation of MSCs had immunosuppressive and antifibrotic effects, qualifying them as a target for therapeutic interventions.

3.3. Activation of Pancreatic Mesenchymal Cells

As mentioned above, inflammatory stimuli and, in particular, their chronic persistence have an impact on pancreatic stroma cells. Current data suggest that this comprises a myofibrogenic differentiation as in other types of chronic inflammation [77]. Regarding PDAC, it appears intriguing to postulate resident pancreatic fibroblasts, PSCs, and pancreatic MSCs on one and CAFs on the opposite pole of a dynamic and continuous process of inflammation-driven stroma, participating in pancreatic carcinogenesis. However, data on this hypothesis is scarce and requires a better understanding of intracellular signaling and intercellular interaction of pancreatic stroma cells. However, recent data on CAFs, in general, and particularly in PDAC have contributed to this hypothesis.

CAFs form a heterogeneous group of mesenchymal cells which can occur in almost all tissues in the context of carcinoma growth [78]. Recent data describe various subtypes of CAFs; however, the current data are not consistent regarding the distinction of their phenotype and function as well as of their presence in different malignancies. Based on studies in PDAC [79], three main subtypes have been classified so far: myofibroblastic CAFs (myCAFs), inflammatory CAFs (iCAFs), and antigen-presenting CAFs (apCAFs) [80]. These subtypes have also been detected in PDAC [78,81].

According to the current knowledge, in pancreatic tissue, CAFs arise via the activation of resident pancreatic stroma cells or infiltrating mesenchymal cells but the precise cellular origin as a determinator of CAF subtypes needs further confirmation [81]. However, myCAFs specifically are derived from PSCs after injury of the pancreas via stimulation by TGF-β, PDGF, or IL-6 and are localized in close proximity to the cancer cells [82]. Activation of PSCs into myCAFs induces a morphological change from star-shaped to spindle-shaped, accompanied by a loss of the intracellular vitamin A droplet and expression of myofibroblast markers like α-SMA [82]. Functionally, myCAFs increasingly produce ECM, promoting the desmoplastic reaction in PDAC. This fibrotic remodeling not only illustrates the connection to the fibrotic reaction seen in chronic pancreatitis and PDAC but also the likely continuum from activated PSCs in chronic pancreatitis to myCAFs in PDAC.

In contrast, iCAFs are located further away from the cancer cells and are characterized by increased secretion of platelet-derived growth factor-α (PDGF-α) as well as chemokines (CXCL1, CXCL2, CCL2, and CXCL12) and interleukins (IL-1, IL-6, and IL-8). Thus, they appear to be involved in the modulation of immune cells [82]. Further, iCAFs specifically express the hyaluronan synthases HAS1 and HAS2.

The third population, apCAF, was defined primarily based on the expression of MHC-II and CD74 and the ability to present antigens to $CD4^+$ T cells in vitro. ApCAFs have been associated with immunomodulation, although it is not fully understood whether they have an immunopromoting or suppressive effect [83].

In a recent work, a CAF classification of four subtypes of proinflammatory CAF (pCAF subtypes A–D) has been suggested [84]. Here, pCAF-A corresponds to myCAF, pCAF-B to iCAF and pCAF-D to apCAF. The additional subgroup of pCAF-C represents a hybrid population between myCAF and iCAF, which both contributes to ECM production and emits inflammatory signals. Moreover, subtypes of CAFs have been assigned based on specific surface markers like $^{Zeb1+}$CAFs, $^{LRRC15+}$CAFs, $^{CD10+/GPR77+}$CAFs, $^{CD105+}$CAFs $^{FAP+/CXCL12+}$CAFs, and $^{Saa3+}$CAFs, but also based on physiological conditions $^{Hypoxia+}$CAFs, ^{Metabolic}CAFs. While all these seem to support PDAC growth, subtypes of $^{CD271+/NGFR+}$CAFs, $^{Gli+}$CAFs, or $^{Meflin+}$CAFs seem to excert a tumor-restraining effect [85,86]. In line with this apparent phenotypic heterogeneity the tumor-promoting or—restraining function of CAF in PDAC is disputed [87–89]. Compared to the vast data on CAFs in fully developed PDAC, little is known about their role in early, only inflammation-driven carcinogenesis.

4. Role of Inflammation-Driven Stroma at Different Stages and Processes of PDAC Carcinogenesis

The relation of pancreatic stroma and fully established PDAC has been explored and reviewed by many studies [90]. In contrast, the role of pancreatic stroma in the carcinogenesis of PDAC and, in particular, at early inflammation-driven stages has been less explored. However, recent data on the interaction of stroma cells with dysplastic pancreatic epithelium as well as pancreatic neuronal and immunoregulatory cells has given some insights into the role of stroma in early stages of PDAC and demonstrates a multitude of changes in pancreatic stroma cells (Figure 4).

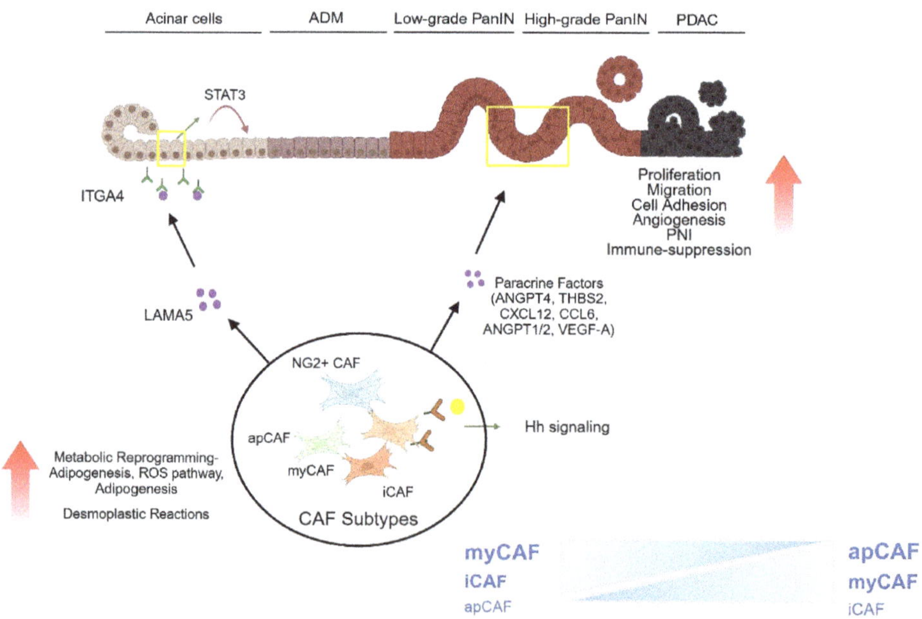

Figure 4. Relevant molecular processes in the pancreatic stroma in early lesions (ADM, PanIN) of PDAC carcinogenesis. Depicted is the development of pancreatic adenocarcinoma (PDAC) and the role of cancer-associated fibroblasts (CAFs) in the tumor microenvironment. The functional heterogeneity of CAFs and their influence on the progression from healthy pancreatic tissue to malignant PDAC via various precursors (ADM, PanIN) are demonstrated. Tumor progression is influenced by signaling pathways, such as STAT3, which contribute to tumor cell activation. The four

CAF subtypes (MyCAFs, iCAFs, apCAFs, and NG2$^+$ CAFs) are dynamically interconverted by the Hedgehog (Hh) signaling pathway. CAFs secrete laminin-α5 (LAMA5), an integrin-α5 (ITGA4) that is bound by acinar cells. This activates signaling pathways, such as STAT3, which contribute to the progression and persistence of ADM. Furthermore, CAFs influence tumor development in higher precancerous stages through paracrine factors (e.g., ANGPT4, THBS2, and VEGF-A) and promote proliferation, migration, cell adhesion, angiogenesis, and immunosuppression in the tumor environment. Additionally, CAFs contribute to the desmoplastic reaction, which means the fibrotic remodeling of the pancreatic tissue characteristic of PDAC. This leads to metabolic reprogramming, adipogenesis, and oxidative stress. Created in https://BioRender.com.

4.1. Impact of Stroma on ADM Development and ADM—PanIN Transition

Acinar-to-ductal metaplasia (ADM), a key initiating-event in pancreatic carcinogenesis, occurs in response to factors such as cell injury, inflammation, or oncogenic *KRAS* mutations [91,92]. It is well established that *KRAS*-mutant cells interact with the desmoplastic stroma, transforming resident fibroblasts into CAFs [93]. While several mechanisms regulating PDAC progression and neoplastic lesions have been extensively studied [94,95], the microenvironment of precursor lesions remains less understood. Oncogenic *KRAS* mutations induce RAS signaling activity, driving sustained ADM, particularly in the presence of inflammatory or growth signals [96]. This persistent activation is amplified by the induction of inflammatory mediators via NF-κB, Cox2, and STAT3 which recruit immune cells [97,98], and activate key receptors, including GPCRs (for cholecystokinin, PGE2), TLRs (TLR4 for LPS), and EGF/HER receptors (for TGF-β, AREG-amphiregulin) [99]. These signaling feedback loops create a self-sustaining environment that promotes ADM persistence and progression to PanIN.

Recent findings using the *iKras* model, which enables inducible and reversible $Kras^{G12D}$ expression in pancreatic epithelial cells, demonstrate that fibroblast reprogramming precedes ADM formation. One-week post-induction, focal ADM lesions emerged despite an otherwise histologically normal pancreas. Notably, just within three days of $Kras^{G12D}$ activation, untransformed acinar cells were already surrounded by infiltrating macrophages and α-SMA$^+$ fibroblasts, highlighting the potential role of activated fibroblasts in ADM initiation [100]. To further investigate the role of reprogrammed fibroblasts in the preinvasive microenvironment, a separate study utilized acinar cells and myCAFs derived from LSL-$Kras^{G12D/+}$; Pdx1Cre (KC) mice compared with wild-type controls. Direct co-culture of pancreatic acinar organoids with myCAFs, as well as indirect co-culture with myCAF-conditioned media, revealed that myCAFs promote ADM. Mechanistically, CAF-secreted laminin α5 (LAMA5) interacts with integrin α4 (ITGA4) on acinar cells, leading to STAT3 activation and acino–ductal transition [101].

4.2. Impact of Stroma on Transition from Low Grade to High Grade PanIN

The presence of CAFs and subtypes in PanIN lesions has been described, suggesting a role in early-stage pancreatic carcinogenesis. Single-cell RNA-seq data demonstrate that myCAFs and iCAFs can be observed in premalignant lesions in both murine models and human samples, suggesting that CAF differentiation occurs early during tumorigenesis [102,103].

Recent studies employing a combinatorial approach—including whole transcriptome analysis from FFPE spatial transcriptomics and single-cell sequencing—have enabled the investigation of rare matched low-grade and high-grade PanIN lesions. This has provided key insights into PDAC evolution and cellular phenotypes. For the first time, the presence of all major CAF subtypes (myCAF, iCAF, and apCAF) has been identified in premalignant human PanIN lesions [102]. Furthermore, these studies suggest a gradual decline in CAF-associated inflammatory and epithelial–mesenchymal transition (EMT)-related pathways during the progression from low-grade to high-grade PanINs. Notably, cancer stem cell

(CSC) markers have been detected in PanIN lesions [102]. Using a combination of bulk sequencing, proteomics/phosphoproteomics, single-cell sequencing, spatial transcriptomics, and high-resolution cellular imaging on 83 PDAC samples, transitional cell populations, including ADM and PanIN cells, alongside non-transformed acinar, ductal, and PDAC cells were identified. Interestingly, a small population of $CD133^+$ iCAFs expressing CSC markers was found within PanIN lesions but not in PDAC. CSCs are known to drive aggressive tumor behavior and are associated with therapy resistance, local recurrence, and metastasis. The presence of CSCs and iCAFs in PanINs suggests that key characteristics linked to therapy resistance in PDAC may develop as early as the PanIN stage [104].

4.3. *Impact on Metabolism of Precursor Lesions*

CAFs play a critical role in PDAC metabolism by supplying essential nutrients to support tumor growth. For instance, CAFs undergo autophagy in response to signals from cancer cells, leading to the secretion of alanine, which can serve as an alternative fuel for tumor cells by feeding into the TCA cycle and supporting the synthesis of nonessential amino acids and lipids [105]. Furthermore, single-cell RNA sequencing has identified a CAF population with activated adipogenesis as marked by ABCA8a expression putatively allowing for lipid transfer to tumor cells to fuel oxidative phosphorylation [106]. However, while the role of CAFs in PDAC metabolism has been extensively studied, their involvement in the metabolic reprogramming of early pancreatic lesions remains underexplored. A recent study examined the transcriptional profiles of fibroblasts isolated from KPC mice at different time points and showed that fibroblasts in KPC mice during early-stage pancreatic carcinogenesis displayed significant upregulation of hallmark metabolic pathways, including ROS signaling, fatty acid metabolism, and adipogenesis [107].

4.4. *Angiogenesis in the Stroma During Early-Stage Pancreatic Carcinogenesis*

Several studies indicate that angiogenic factors are upregulated in the early stages of PanIN. Immunohistochemical analysis of 32 chronic pancreatitis and 38 PDAC patients with PanIN lesions revealed a progressive increase in CEACAM1 and CEACAM5 expression from PanIN-1 to PanIN-3 compared to normal ducts. CEACAMs, members of the GPI-anchored immunoglobulin (Ig) superfamily, are associated with angiogenesis and metastasis [108]. Additionally, other angiogenic factors such as HIF-2α (modulating Wnt signaling) [109], urocortin [110], and neuropeptide Y receptor 2 (Y2R) [111] are upregulated in PanINs, suggesting that angiogenesis is an early event in pancreatic tumorigenesis. However, the specific role of CAFs and stroma cells in mediating angiogenesis or regulating angiogenic factors within the precursor lesion remains less known.

Recent studies identified THBS2 (Thrombospondin-2), a key regulator of cell motility and angiogenesis, as highly expressed in the stroma of PanIN lesions in both KC and KPC mouse models, as well as PDAC patient tumors. THBS2 expression was CAF-specific, first emerging in early PanIN-I and progressively increasing during PDAC progression. Mechanistically, TGF-β1 from pancreatic cancer cells activated CAFs, leading to THBS2 induction via the Smad2/3 pathway. THBS2 in turn promoted cancer cell growth, proliferation, and adhesion by activating MAPK signaling through integrin $\alpha v\beta 3$/CD36 binding. However, its direct role in angiogenesis was not examined in this study [112]. In pancreatic cancer, Hedgehog (HH) signaling functions in a paracrine manner, where tumor epithelial cells secrete HH ligands that signal to stromal cells [113]. The HH coreceptors, GAS1, BOC, and CDON, are expressed in fibroblasts from both normal and KC pancreata. In KC mice three weeks after caerulein-induced acute pancreatitis, these coreceptors were enriched in the stroma surrounding PanIN lesions, with further expansion in later stages. To investigate their role, $Gas1^{-/-}$; $Boc^{-/-}$ double-knockout mouse embryonic fibroblasts (MEFs) were generated and treated with SHH-conditioned medium, confirming attenuated HH-signaling in fibroblasts. In an MEF-transplant tumor model, tumor cells were implanted either alone or co-injected with wild-type MEFs, double-knockout Gas1$^{-/-}$; Boc$^{-/-}$ MEFs, or triple-knockout Gas1$^{-/-}$; Boc$^{-/-}$; Cdon$^{-/-}$ MEFs to assess their impact on tumor development. Stromal deletion of Gas1 and Boc reduced HH pathway activation but paradoxically enhanced tumor growth and angiogenesis, leading to increased expression of VEGFα, ANGPT1, and ANGPT2. While the deletion of all three co-receptors (Gas1, Boc, and Cdon) leads to a near-complete loss of HH-signaling, which in turn severely impairs tumorigenesis and angiogenesis. These findings suggest that CAFs regulate early tumor angiogenesis through HH-signaling, and their dysregulation may drive an angiogenic switch that facilitate PanIN progression [114].

4.5. Impact on Intrapancreatic Nerves and Precursor–Neural Interactions

Sensory neurons transmitting from the pancreas to the CNS and autonomic neurons including sympathetic, parasympathetic, and enteric nerves form a complex network in the pancreas [115]. In rodent models of acute and chronic pancreatitis, blocking sensory neuron fibers from both the nodose and spinal ganglia has been shown to reduce inflammation [116]. In pancreatic carcinogenesis, sensory neurons establish a reciprocal signaling loop between the pancreas and the CNS, driving spinal and pancreatic inflammation, perineural invasion (PNI), and PanIN formation. Markers of spinal cord inflammation were found to be elevated in mice models at both PanIN and PDAC stages. Additionally, in these mice, acinar-derived cells migrated to the dorsal root ganglion during the PanIN stages, indicating that preneoplastic cells interact with sensory neurons. Sensory neuron ablation in these models prevented PNI, reduced glial activation, and neuronal damage, and significantly delayed PanIN formation [117].

Traditionally, neurogenic invasion (NI) has been viewed as a process in which cancer cells invade nerves to facilitate tumor spread. However, recent findings suggest that Schwann cells within the tumor stroma and not malignant cells themselves, may migrate first during the premalignant phase in human and murine PDAC samples [118]. Schwann cell migration occurs in early PanIN lesions and is correlated with a higher frequency of PanIN in the malignant phase [118]. Tumor-associated chemokines, such as CXCL12, recruit Schwann cells to PanIN lesions via CXCR4 and CXCR7 [119]. The pancreatic neuroectodermal–mesenchymal network includes perilesional pericytes—specialized mural cells originating from Nkx3.3-expressing pancreatic mesenchyme—as well as glial cells, i.e., astrocytes. These components contribute to various functions, such as fibrosis scar after tissue injury, local blood flow regulation by adjusting capillary diameter in response to sympathetic adrenergic input, and support of islet basement membranes through ECM production, including laminin [120]. Recent studies using KrasG12D-mutant mice and optically cleared pancreatic tissue allowed for a 3D visualization of PanIN lesion development following repetitive cerulein injections. These studies revealed the clustering of PanINs in spatially organized aggregates, and upregulation of pericyte (NG2^{+}) and glial (GFAP+) markers near PanIN lesions, indicating their activation, and formation of PanIN-islet complexes. Zooming into the PanIN-associated stroma further revealed the presence of NG2^{+} myofibroblast-like cells (α-SMA^{+}/NG2^{+}) around PanIN lesions. This suggest either a pericyte-to-myofibroblast transition or molecular phenotypic changes in stromal cells in response to preneoplastic lesions [121,122]. Hence, dynamic interactions between epithelial transformation, stromal reprogramming, and neurovascular changes contribute to PanIN progression [122].

4.6. Impact on Immune Cell Distribution and Precursor–Immune Cell Interactions

As mentioned above, various CAF subtypes—specifically iCAFs and myCAFs—exhibit distinct functional roles in shaping the tumor microenvironment. Based on current knowledge iCAFs are the key producers of inflammatory cytokines such as IL-6/8/11 and CXCL1/2/12 as well as leukemia inhibitory factor (LIF) [82,83]. In contrast, myCAFs are characterized by their abundant production of ECM components, particularly collagens I, which can act as a physical barrier to immune cells and therapeutic interventions but also potentially restrains preneoplastic lesions from progressing to invasive cancer [87].

Selective depletion of α-SMA$^+$ myCAFs during both the PanIN and PDAC stages weakened immune surveillance, thereby facilitating tumor progression. The impact of depletion was more pronounced at the PanIN stage, where a significant reduction in CD45$^+$ immune cells including CD3$^+$ T cells, CD19$^+$ B cells, and CD4$^+$Foxp3$^-$ effector T cells (Teffs) was observed, along with an increase in immunosuppressive CD4$^+$Foxp3$^+$ Tregs surrounding PanIN lesions [123]. Hence, the formation of PanIN is associated with the infiltration of immunosuppressive cells while cytotoxic cells remain scarce. In accordance with the known role of CD8$^+$-T cells in anti-tumor immunity, their activation at preinvasive stages has been shown to effectively block PanIN progression [124]. Moreover, CD4$^+$CD25$^+$Foxp3$^+$ regulatory T cells (Tregs) progressively accumulate in both mouse and human PanIN and PDAC [124,125]. Given their well-established role in immunosuppression, it was expected that Tregs would actively contribute to immune evasion during early pancreatic carcinogenesis. However, studies using Treg depletion in KC mouse models revealed that Treg depletion failed to relieve immunosuppression and led to accelerated tumor progression. Analysis of single-cell RNA-seq data of mouse PanIN lesions revealed that Tregs serve as key sources of TGFβ1, while both epithelial cells and pancreatic fibroblasts express TGFβ receptors in and around PanINs. The loss of Treg triggers fibroblast reprogramming, probably shifting tumor-restricting α-SMA-high myCAFs into a tumor-promoting inflammatory phenotype, characterized by increased chemokine secretion (*Ccl3*, *Ccl6*, and *Ccl8*) that attracts suppressive myeloid cells and elevated expression of immune-suppressive genes like Arg1 and CD274 (PD-L1). These findings underscore the importance of fibroblast–Treg interactions in the early stages of carcinogenesis. Notably, myCAFs are rare in low-grade dysplastic-IPMNs, but become highly represented in high-grade dysplastic-IPMNs, suggesting a progressive activation of fibroblasts into the myCAF phenotype during preinvasive lesion development. iCAFs are exclusively found in PDAC clusters but are absent in non-invasive IPMNs [126]. Several studies have linked iCAF-derived factors to immune suppression [82,127], indicating that while myCAFs may contribute to fibrosis and immune evasion due in early tumorigenesis, iCAFs later drive immunosuppression through cytokine and chemokine signaling. However, further validation is needed to confirm this transition and its functional implications in PDAC progression. In conclusion, stromal heterogeneity dynamically evolves throughout multistep carcinogenesis, progressively shaping the microenvironment to facilitate the transition from preinvasive IPMN to invasive PDAC. Another CAF subtype, apCAF, has been found adjacent to PanIN lesions, co-localizing with CD4$^+$ T cells, suggesting early-stage precursor–immune cell interactions. As their key feature apCAFs express MHC class II molecules, allowing them to present antigens to CD4$^+$ T cells. However, unlike conventional antigen-presenting cells, apCAFs lack key costimulatory signals required for full T cell activation and proliferation. Moreover, a negative correlation has been observed between apCAF abundance and the effector CD8$^+$ T-cell/Treg ratio in human PDAC. Instead of promoting anti-tumor immunity, MHC-II on apCAFs may function as a decoy receptor, leading to CD4$^+$ T cell dysfunction or inducing their conversion into Treg, thereby reinforcing immune suppression in the tumor microenvironment [83]. While the presence of apCAFs in PanIN lesions suggests a potential immunosuppressive role in early carcinogenesis, further validation is required to fully elucidate their function and therapeutic potential.

5. Current Translation into the Clinical Setting and Outlook

Recent scientific evidence highlights that identifying and selectively targeting tumor-promoting CAFs, as well as reprogramming them into tumor-restraining CAFs, are promising strategies for advancing pancreatic cancer therapy [128]. Targeting specific CAF subtypes as well as reprogramming and deactivating fibroblasts at early stages of pancreatic carcinogenesis holds potential for significantly enhancing treatment efficacy. Such early interventions may pave the way for more effective therapeutic approaches, potentially disrupting the progression of pancreatic cancer precursors in clinical settings (Figure 5).

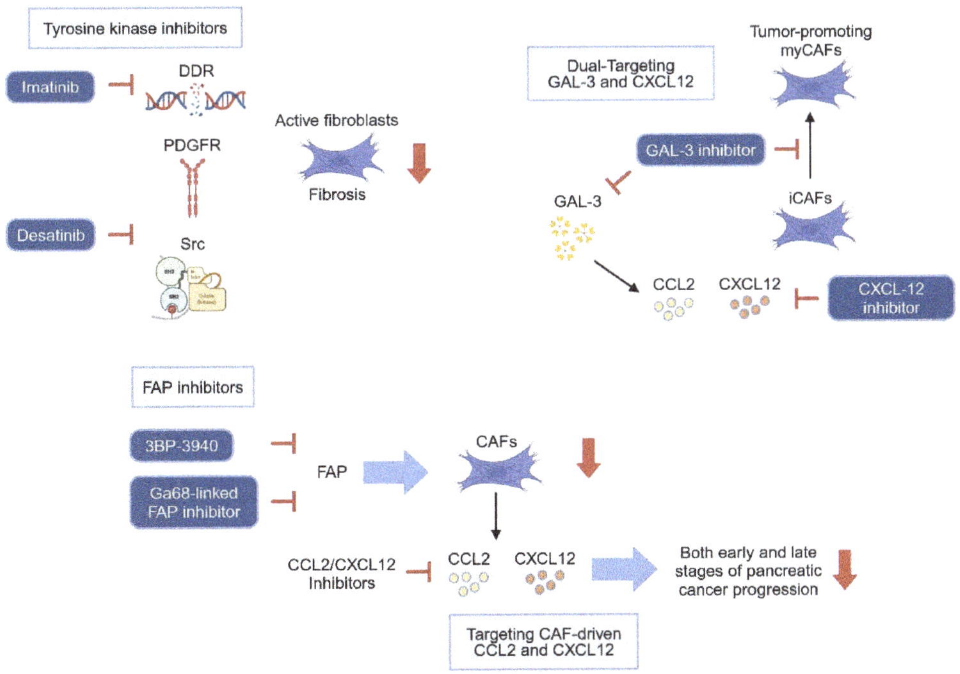

Figure 5. Therapeutic strategies to target stroma in inflammation-driven pancreatic carcinogenesis. Tyrosine kinase inhibitors such as Imatinib and Dasatinib inhibit PDGFR and Src signaling, reducing fibroblast activation and fibrosis. FAP inhibitors, including 3BP-3940 and Ga68-linked FAP inhibitors, selectively deplete tumor-promoting fibroblasts. Strategies targeting CAF-driven chemokines like CCL2 and CXCL12 aim to disrupt tumor-stromal interactions at both early and late stages of pancreatic cancer progression. Additionally, dual inhibition of Galectin-3 (GAL-3) and CXCL12 is proposed to modulate iCAFs and tumor-promoting myCAFs. These interventions have potential for reprogramming the tumor microenvironment and improving therapeutic efficacy in pancreatic cancer. Inhibition symbols are colored red. Created in https://BioRender.com.

5.1. Targeting Stroma Cells to Prevent Precursor Progression

As previously mentioned, activated fibroblasts upregulate several proteins including α-SMA, DDR2, desmin, FAP, vimentin, and PDGF receptors, and depletion of these factors could be considered as a therapeutic strategy. However, in preclinical pancreatic cancer mouse models, the deletion of α-SMA-positive cells promotes the development of hypoxic, invasive, undifferentiated tumors, and decreases animal survival [87]. Especially in the precursor stage, active fibroblasts could play important roles for tissue regeneration, thereby depletion of fibroblasts may enhance tissue injury leading to pancreatic cancer precursor progression. Interestingly, pharmacological targeting of DDR1 and DDR2 by Imatinib, which is also an inhibitor for Bcr-Abl, c-Kit, and PDGFR [129,130], attenuates pancreatic fibrosis by inhibiting activation of PSCs via TGFβ/SMAD signaling in a cerulein-induced chronic pancreatitis mouse model [34]. Another tyrosine kinase inhibitor Dasatinib also attenuates inflammation and fibrosis by inhibiting various tyrosine kinases such as PDGFR and Src in a cerulein-induced chronic pancreatitis mouse model [131]. Additionally, the PARP-inhibitor Olaparib has shown beneficial effects in the same chronic pancreatitis model, reducing tissue injury, inflammation markers (*Il1b*, *Tnfa*, and *Il6*) and fibrosis markers (*Tgf1b*, α-SMA and *Col1a1*), suggesting direct or indirect fibroblast deactivation through PARP-inhibition [132]. These findings indicate that inhibiting fibroblast activation may help curb precursor lesion progression. However, further clarification is needed to determine whether these anti-fibrosis effects stem from the direct targeting of activated fibroblasts or from broader effects on tissue injury and inflammation.

Another promising target for preventing precursor progression is FAP, as deletion of FAP-positive CAFs has been associated with increased survival in contrast to the depletion of α-SMA-positive CAF in a PDAC mouse model [133]. Recently, novel selective FAP inhibitors have been developed and paired with radiotracers for use in positron emission tomography/computer tomography (PET/CT) [134] and have been tested in patients with IPMN and pancreatic cancer [135,136]. Interestingly, cumulative FAP expression in both CAFs and epithelial cells is upregulated at the stage of high-grade dysplasia and persists throughout the progression of pancreatic cancer [137]. These findings suggest that FAP could serve as a valuable target for both CAFs and neoplastic cells. Inhibiting FAP combined with radiotracer technology may ultimately aid in the early diagnosis and treatment of pancreatic cancer precursors.

5.2. *Targeting Paracrine Communication Between Stroma and Precancerous Cells*

FAP-positive CAFs are key sources of the chemokine CCL2, which plays a central role in recruiting monocyte-derived suppressor cells (MDSCs) and promoting tumor progression. This recruitment function is significantly reduced in conventional *Ccr2* knockout mice, indicating the importance of CCL2 in the tumor-supporting microenvironment created by FAP-positive CAFs [138]. CCL2 production is not limited to FAP-positive CAFs—TGF-β, for example, stimulates pancreatic cancer cells to secrete CCL2 and recruit macrophages [139]. However, targeting the CCL2/CCR2 signaling axis remains a promising therapeutic approach. In experimental models of acute pancreatitis, treatment with the CCL2 synthesis blocker Bindarit reduced macrophage infiltration and alleviated pancreatic injury and inflammation, suggesting its potential utility in early pancreatic carcinogenesis [140,141]. Additionally, FAP-positive CAFs express CXCL12 [142], a chemokine that interacts with receptors CXCR4 and CXCR7 [143], both commonly co-expressed in pancreatic cancer tissues [144]. Studies have shown that in early pancreatic cancer cell lines, knockdown of CXCR7 inhibits CXCL12-driven proliferation, while in more advanced cell lines, silencing CXCR4 effectively reduces proliferation [144]. This suggests that targeting CAF-driven CXCL12 signaling could offer therapeutic benefits across both early and late stages of pancreatic cancer progression.

Targeting the reciprocal communication between CAFs and tumor cells, wherein paracrine factors from precancerous cells induce CAFs to produce additional tumor-promoting signals, represents another promising strategy. Galectin-3 (GAL3), a beta-galactoside-binding lectin, is associated with chronic inflammation, fibrosis, and cancer [145] and has been shown to activate pancreatic stellate cells (PSCs) while stimulating

IL-8 and CCL2 production [146]. In a pancreatic cancer mouse model, genetic deletion of Galectin-3 (*Pdx1-Cre; LSL-Kras*$^{G12D/+}$; *Trp53*$^{lox/lox}$; *Lgals3*$^{-/-}$) effectively inhibited tumor progression [147]. Interestingly, this deletion also preserved an early-stage CAF subtype composition, with a high proportion of iCAFs expressing elevated levels of CXCL12 and a reduced myCAF subtype, contrasting with the CAF composition observed in late-stage pancreatic cancer, where myCAFs predominate [147]. This CAF profile in early-stage pancreatic cancer suggests that targeting both Galectin-3 and CXCL12 could reinforce therapeutic efficacy, especially when tailored to tumor stage [147].

In summary, selective targeting of chemokine pathways like CCL2/CCR2 and CXCL12/CXCR4-CXCR7, alongside key mediators such as Galectin-3, presents a multifaceted approach to intercepting CAF-driven tumorigenesis. These strategies hold potential to disrupt the tumor-promoting microenvironment in early pancreatic carcinogenesis, laying the groundwork for more effective and stage-specific therapeutic interventions.

6. Conclusions

PDAC remains one of the most lethal malignancies largely due to its complex and highly desmoplastic tumor microenvironment. The emerging evidence suggests that pancreatic stroma cells, like PSCs, MSCs, and CAFs, play a pivotal role in early-stage pancreatic carcinogenesis, from ADM and PanIN progression to invasive PDAC. The interactions between these and immune cells, neural components, and pre-invasive epithelial lesions collectively create an environment that fosters tumor progression while simultaneously suppressing antitumor immunity. Notably, pancreatic stroma cell heterogeneity presents a significant challenge, with subpopulations exerting either tumor-promoting or tumor-restraining functions. Understanding the precise mechanisms of pancreatic stroma cell activation and differentiation as well as function remains essential for developing effective therapeutic strategies. Further, recent findings highlight the metabolic reprogramming of fibroblasts as well as the intricate crosstalk between fibroblasts and neural components in pancreatic carcinogenesis. Despite substantial progress in understanding the role of inflammation-driven stromal remodeling, targeting pancreatic stroma remains a double-edged sword. Strategies such as reprogramming tumor-supportive stroma cells into tumor-restraining phenotypes or modulating key paracrine interactions hold promise for future therapeutic interventions. Moreover, emerging diagnostic approaches may offer novel opportunities for early detection and intervention in pancreatic cancer precursors. In conclusion, the interplay between stroma and the epithelium undergoing malignant transformation represents a critical yet underexplored dimension of early-stage pancreatic carcinogenesis. Future studies should focus on refining our understanding of pancreatic stroma cell plasticity, identifying actionable targets for therapeutic intervention, and integrating stromal-targeting strategies into multimodal treatment approaches. In doing so, we may enhance early detection and improve outcomes for patients with PDAC.

Author Contributions: Conceptualization, T.S., N.O., Y.S., L.P.M. and J.K.; Writing-creation of original draft, T.S. and N.O.; Writing-review and editing, M.G., Y.S., L.P.M. and J.K.; Visualization, T.S. and N.O. All authors have read and agreed to the published version of the manuscript.

Funding: The work was conducted within the Research Training Group 2751 (InCuPanc), funded by the Deutsche Forschungsgemeinschaft (DFG, German Research Foundation), grant number 449501615.

Conflicts of Interest: The authors declare no conflicts of interest.

References

1. Moir, J.A.G.; Mann, J.; White, S.A. The role of pancreatic stellate cells in pancreatic cancer. *Surg. Oncol.* **2015**, *24*, 232–238. [CrossRef]
2. Herreros-Villanueva, M. Mouse models of pancreatic cancer. *World J. Gastroenterol.* **2012**, *18*, 1286. [CrossRef] [PubMed]
3. Kirkegård, J.; Mortensen, F.V.; Cronin-Fenton, D. Chronic Pancreatitis and Pancreatic Cancer Risk: A Systematic Review and Meta-analysis. *Am. J. Gastroenterol.* **2017**, *112*, 1366–1372. [CrossRef]
4. Manohar, M.; Verma, A.K.; Venkateshaiah, S.U.; Sanders, N.L.; Mishra, A. Pathogenic mechanisms of pancreatitis. *World J. Gastrointest. Pharmacol. Ther.* **2017**, *8*, 10. [CrossRef]
5. Garcia, P.E.; Scales, M.K.; Allen, B.L.; Pasca di Magliano, M. Pancreatic Fibroblast Heterogeneity: From Development to Cancer. *Cells* **2020**, *9*, 2464. [CrossRef]
6. Han, L.; Wu, Y.; Fang, K.; Sweeney, S.; Roesner, U.K.; Parrish, M.; Patel, K.; Walter, T.; Piermattei, J.; Trimboli, A.; et al. The splanchnic mesenchyme is the tissue of origin for pancreatic fibroblasts during homeostasis and tumorigenesis. *Nat. Commun.* **2023**, *14*, 1. [CrossRef] [PubMed]
7. Oñate, M.K.; Oon, C.; Bhattacharyya, S.; Low, V.; Chen, C.; Zhao, X.; Yan, Z.; Hang, Y.; Kim, S.K.; Xia, Z.; et al. Stromal KITL/SCF promotes pancreas tissue homeostasis and restrains tumor progression. *bioRxiv* **2024**. [CrossRef]
8. Kalluri, R. The biology and function of fibroblasts in cancer. *Nat. Rev. Cancer* **2016**, *16*, 582–598. [CrossRef]
9. Kalluri, R.; Zeisberg, M. Fibroblasts in cancer. *Nat. Rev. Cancer* **2006**, *6*, 392–401. [CrossRef]
10. Desmouliere, A.; Darby, I.A.; Laverdet, B.; Bonté, F. Fibroblasts and myofibroblasts in wound healing. *Clin. Cosmet. Investig. Dermatol.* **2014**, *7*, 301–311. [CrossRef]
11. Rønnov-Jessen, L.; Petersen, O.W. Induction of alpha-smooth muscle actin by transforming growth factor-beta 1 in quiescent human breast gland fibroblasts. Implications for myofibroblast generation in breast neoplasia. *Lab. Investig.* **1993**, *68*, 696–707. [PubMed]
12. Micallef, L.; Vedrenne, N.; Billet, F.; Coulomb, B.; Darby, I.A.; Desmoulière, A. The myofibroblast, multiple origins for major roles in normal and pathological tissue repair. *Fibrogenesis Tissue Repair* **2012**, *5*, S5. [CrossRef]
13. Gabbiani, G.; Ryan, G.B.; Majne, G. Presence of modified fibroblasts in granulation tissue and their possible role in wound contraction. *Experientia* **1971**, *27*, 549–550. [CrossRef]
14. Strutz, F.; Okada, H.; Lo, C.W.; Danoff, T.; Carone, R.L.; Tomaszewski, J.E.; Neilson, E.G. Identification and characterization of a fibroblast marker: FSP1. *J. Cell Biol.* **1995**, *130*, 393–405. [CrossRef]
15. Sugimoto, H.; Mundel, T.M.; Kieran, M.W.; Kalluri, R. Identification of fibroblast heterogeneity in the tumor microenvironment. *Cancer Biol. Ther.* **2006**, *5*, 1640–1646. [CrossRef] [PubMed]
16. Österreicher, C.H.; Penz-Österreicher, M.; Grivennikov, S.I.; Guma, M.; Koltsova, E.K.; Datz, C.; Sasik, R.; Hardiman, G.; Karin, M.; Brenner, D.A. Fibroblast-specific protein 1 identifies an inflammatory subpopulation of macrophages in the liver. *Proc. Natl. Acad. Sci. USA* **2011**, *108*, 308–313. [CrossRef] [PubMed]
17. Arnold, J.N.; Magiera, L.; Kraman, M.; Fearon, D.T. Tumoral immune suppression by macrophages expressing fibroblast activation protein-α and heme oxygenase-1. *Cancer Immunol. Res.* **2014**, *2*, 121–126. [CrossRef]
18. Lau, J.; Kawahira, H.; Hebrok, M. Hedgehog signaling in pancreas development and disease. *Cell. Mol. Life Sci. CMLS* **2006**, *63*, 642–652. [CrossRef]
19. Hui, C.; Angers, S. Gli Proteins in Development and Disease. *Annu. Rev. Cell Dev. Biol.* **2011**, *27*, 513–537. [CrossRef]
20. Garcia, P.E.; Adoumie, M.; Kim, E.C.; Zhang, Y.; Scales, M.K.; El-Tawil, Y.S.; Shaikh, A.Z.; Wen, H.-J.; Bednar, F.; Allen, B.L.; et al. Differential Contribution of Pancreatic Fibroblast Subsets to the Pancreatic Cancer Stroma. *Cell. Mol. Gastroenterol. Hepatol.* **2020**, *10*, 581–599. [CrossRef]
21. Larsen, B.M.; Hrycaj, S.M.; Newman, M.; Li, Y.; Wellik, D.M. Mesenchymal Hox6 function is required for pancreatic endocrine cell differentiation. *Development* **2015**, *142*, 3859–3868. [CrossRef] [PubMed]
22. Asahina, K.; Tsai, S.Y.; Li, P.; Ishii, M.; Maxson, R.E.; Sucov, H.M.; Tsukamoto, H. Mesenchymal origin of hepatic stellate cells, submesothelial cells, and perivascular mesenchymal cells during mouse liver development. *Hepatology* **2009**, *49*, 998–1011. [CrossRef] [PubMed]
23. Apte, M.V.; Haber, P.S.; Applegate, T.L.; Norton, I.D.; McCaughan, G.W.; Korsten, M.A.; Pirola, R.C.; Wilson, J.S. Periacinar stellate shaped cells in rat pancreas: Identification, isolation, and culture. *Gut* **1998**, *43*, 128–133. [CrossRef]
24. Cassiman, D.; Barlow, A.; Vander Borght, S.; Libbrecht, L.; Pachnis, V. Hepatic stellate cells do not derive from the neural crest. *J. Hepatol.* **2006**, *44*, 1098–1104. [CrossRef]
25. Chan, K.; Fu, Y.; Wu, T.; Hsu, P.; Lee, W. Hepatic stellate cells promote the differentiation of embryonic stem cell-derived definitive endodermal cells into hepatic progenitor cells. *Hepatol. Res.* **2013**, *43*, 648–657. [CrossRef] [PubMed]
26. Niki, T.; Pekny, M.; Hellemans, K.; De Bleser, P.; Van Den Berg, K.; Vaeyens, F.; Quartier, E.; Schuit, F.; Geerts, A. Class Vi Intermediate Filament Protein Nestin Is Induced During Activation of Rat Hepatic Stellate Cells. *Hepatology* **1999**, *29*, 520–527. [CrossRef]

27. Bachem, M.G.; Schneider, E.; Groß, H.; Weidenbach, H.; Schmid, R.M.; Menke, A.; Siech, M.; Beger, H.; Grünert, A.; Adler, G. Identification, culture, and characterization of pancreatic stellate cells in rats and humans. *Gastroenterology* **1998**, *115*, 421–432. [CrossRef]
28. Masamune, A.; Watanabe, T.; Kikuta, K.; Shimosegawa, T. Roles of Pancreatic Stellate Cells in Pancreatic Inflammation and Fibrosis. *Clin. Gastroenterol. Hepatol.* **2009**, *7*, S48–S54. [CrossRef]
29. Walther, T.C.; Farese, R.V. Lipid Droplets and Cellular Lipid Metabolism. *Annu. Rev. Biochem.* **2012**, *81*, 687–714. [CrossRef]
30. Sunami, Y.; Rebelo, A.; Kleeff, J. Lipid Metabolism and Lipid Droplets in Pancreatic Cancer and Stellate Cells. *Cancers* **2017**, *10*, 3. [CrossRef]
31. Molenaar, M.R.; Haaker, M.W.; Vaandrager, A.B.; Houweling, M.; Helms, J.B. Lipidomic profiling of rat hepatic stellate cells during activation reveals a two-stage process accompanied by increased levels of lysosomal lipids. *J. Biol. Chem.* **2023**, *299*, 103042. [CrossRef]
32. Birtolo, C.; Pham, H.; Morvaridi, S.; Chheda, C.; Go, V.L.W.; Ptasznik, A.; Edderkaoui, M.; Weisman, M.H.; Noss, E.; Brenner, M.B.; et al. Cadherin-11 Is a Cell Surface Marker Up-Regulated in Activated Pancreatic Stellate Cells and Is Involved in Pancreatic Cancer Cell Migration. *Am. J. Pathol.* **2017**, *187*, 146–155. [CrossRef] [PubMed]
33. Haber, P.S.; Keogh, G.W.; Apte, M.V.; Moran, C.S.; Stewart, N.L.; Crawford, D.H.G.; Pirola, R.C.; McCaughan, G.W.; Ramm, G.A.; Wilson, J.S. Activation of Pancreatic Stellate Cells in Human and Experimental Pancreatic Fibrosis. *Am. J. Pathol.* **1999**, *155*, 1087–1095. [CrossRef]
34. Bansod, S.; Saifi, M.A.; Godugu, C. Inhibition of discoidin domain receptors by imatinib prevented pancreatic fibrosis demonstrated in experimental chronic pancreatitis model. *Sci. Rep.* **2021**, *11*, 12894. [CrossRef] [PubMed]
35. DeLeon-Pennell, K.Y.; Barker, T.H.; Lindsey, M.L. Fibroblasts: The arbiters of extracellular matrix remodeling. *Matrix Biol.* **2020**, *91–92*, 1–7. [CrossRef] [PubMed]
36. Phillips, P.A.; Yang, L.; Shulkes, A.; Vonlaufen, A.; Poljak, A.; Bustamante, S.; Warren, A.; Xu, Z.; Guilhaus, M.; Pirola, R.; et al. Pancreatic stellate cells produce acetylcholine and may play a role in pancreatic exocrine secretion. *Proc. Natl. Acad. Sci. USA* **2010**, *107*, 17397–17402. [CrossRef]
37. Omary, M.B.; Lugea, A.; Lowe, A.W.; Pandol, S.J. The pancreatic stellate cell: A star on the rise in pancreatic diseases. *J. Clin. Investig.* **2007**, *117*, 50–59. [CrossRef]
38. Qin, A.; Shi, K.; Tindall, R.R.; Li, J.; Cheng, B.; Li, J.; Yang, B.; Yu, Q.; Zhang, Y.; Hong, B.; et al. Characterization of Pancreatic Collagen-Expressing Fibroblasts in Mouse Acute Pancreatitis. *Gastro Hep Adv.* **2025**, *4*, 100557. [CrossRef]
39. Erkan, M.; Adler, G.; Apte, M.V.; Bachem, M.G.; Buchholz, M.; Detlefsen, S.; Esposito, I.; Friess, H.; Gress, T.M.; Habisch, H.-J.; et al. StellaTUM: Current consensus and discussion on pancreatic stellate cell research. *Gut* **2012**, *61*, 172–178. [CrossRef]
40. Lu, P.; Takai, K.; Weaver, V.M.; Werb, Z. Extracellular matrix degradation and remodeling in development and disease. *Cold Spring Harb. Perspect. Biol.* **2011**, *3*, a005058. [CrossRef]
41. Tomasek, J.J.; Gabbiani, G.; Hinz, B.; Chaponnier, C.; Brown, R.A. Myofibroblasts and mechano-regulation of connective tissue remodelling. *Nat. Rev. Mol. Cell Biol.* **2002**, *3*, 349–363. [CrossRef]
42. Powell, D.W.; Mifflin, R.C.; Valentich, J.D.; Crowe, S.E.; Saada, J.I.; West, A.B. Myofibroblasts. I. Paracrine cells important in health and disease. *Am. J. Physiol.* **1999**, *277*, C1–C19. [CrossRef] [PubMed]
43. Masamune, A.; Sakai, Y.; Kikuta, K.; Satoh, M.; Satoh, A.; Shimosegawa, T. Activated Rat Pancreatic Stellate Cells Express Intercellular Adhesion Molecule-1 (ICAM-1) in Vitro. *Pancreas* **2002**, *25*, 78–85. [CrossRef] [PubMed]
44. Masamune, A.; Kikuta, K.; Watanabe, T.; Satoh, K.; Satoh, A.; Shimosegawa, T. Pancreatic stellate cells express Toll-like receptors. *J. Gastroenterol.* **2008**, *43*, 352–362. [CrossRef]
45. Shimizu, K.; Kobayashi, M.; Tahara, J.; Shiratori, K. Cytokines and Peroxisome Proliferator-Activated Receptor γ Ligand Regulate Phagocytosis by Pancreatic Stellate Cells. *Gastroenterology* **2005**, *128*, 2105–2118. [CrossRef] [PubMed]
46. Dominici, M.; Le Blanc, K.; Mueller, I.; Slaper-Cortenbach, I.; Marini, F.; Krause, D.S.; Deans, R.J.; Keating, A.; Prockop, D.J.; Horwitz, E.M. Minimal criteria for defining multipotent mesenchymal stromal cells. The International Society for Cellular Therapy position statement. *Cytotherapy* **2006**, *8*, 315–317. [CrossRef]
47. Gao, Q.; Wang, L.; Wang, S.; Huang, B.; Jing, Y.; Su, J. Bone Marrow Mesenchymal Stromal Cells: Identification, Classification, and Differentiation. *Front. Cell Dev. Biol.* **2022**, *9*, 787118. [CrossRef]
48. Soliman, H.; Theret, M.; Scott, W.; Hill, L.; Underhill, T.M.; Hinz, B.; Rossi, F.M.V. Multipotent stromal cells: One name, multiple identities. *Cell Stem Cell* **2021**, *28*, 1690–1707. [CrossRef]
49. Katzerke, C.; Schaffrath, J.; Lützkendorf, J.; Janssen, M.; Merbach, A.-K.; Nerger, K.; Binder, M.; Baum, C.; Lauer, K.; Rohde, C.; et al. Reduced proliferation of bone marrow MSC after allogeneic stem cell transplantation is associated with clinical outcome. *Blood Adv.* **2023**, *7*, 2811–2824. [CrossRef]
50. Zhang, Y.; Ravikumar, M.; Ling, L.; Nurcombe, V.; Cool, S.M. Age-Related Changes in the Inflammatory Status of Human Mesenchymal Stem Cells: Implications for Cell Therapy. *Stem Cell Rep.* **2021**, *16*, 694–707. [CrossRef]

51. Li, C.; Wang, B. Mesenchymal Stem/Stromal Cells in Progressive Fibrogenic Involvement and Anti-Fibrosis Therapeutic Properties. *Front. Cell Dev. Biol.* **2022**, *10*, 902677. [CrossRef] [PubMed]
52. Qin, L.; Liu, N.; Bao, C.; Yang, D.; Ma, G.; Yi, W.; Xiao, G.; Cao, H. Mesenchymal stem cells in fibrotic diseases—The two sides of the same coin. *Acta Pharmacol. Sin.* **2023**, *44*, 268–287. [CrossRef]
53. Weiss, A.R.R.; Dahlke, M.H. Immunomodulation by Mesenchymal Stem Cells (MSCs): Mechanisms of Action of Living, Apoptotic and Dead MSCs. *Front. Immunol.* **2019**, *10*, 1191. [CrossRef]
54. Glenn, J.D. Mesenchymal stem cells: Emerging mechanisms of immunomodulation and therapy. *World J. Stem Cells* **2014**, *6*, 526. [CrossRef]
55. Cooper, T.T.; Sherman, S.E.; Bell, G.I.; Ma, J.; Kuljanin, M.; Jose, S.E.; Lajoie, G.A.; Hess, D.A. Characterization of a Vimentinhigh /Nestinhigh proteome and tissue regenerative secretome generated by human pancreas-derived mesenchymal stromal cells. *Stem Cells* **2020**, *38*, 666–682. [CrossRef]
56. Epshtein, A.; Sakhneny, L.; Landsman, L. Isolating and Analyzing Cells of the Pancreas Mesenchyme by Flow Cytometry. *J. Vis Exp.* **2017**, *119*, 55344. [CrossRef]
57. Gopurappilly, R.; Bhat, V.; Bhonde, R. Pancreatic tissue resident mesenchymal stromal cell (MSC)-like cells as a source of in vitro islet neogenesis. *J. Cell. Biochem.* **2013**, *114*, 2240–2247. [CrossRef] [PubMed]
58. Boland, L.K.; Burand, A.J.; Boyt, D.T.; Dobroski, H.; Di, L.; Liszewski, J.N.; Schrodt, M.V.; Frazer, M.K.; Santillan, D.A.; Ankrum J.A. Nature vs. Nurture: Defining the Effects of Mesenchymal Stromal Cell Isolation and Culture Conditions on Resiliency to Palmitate Challenge. *Front. Immunol.* **2019**, *10*, 1080. [CrossRef]
59. Thirlwell, K.L.; Colligan, D.; Mountford, J.C.; Samuel, K.; Bailey, L.; Cuesta-Gomez, N.; Hewit, K.D.; Kelly, C.J.; West, C.C.; McGowan, N.W.A.; et al. Pancreas-derived mesenchymal stromal cells share immune response-modulating and angiogenic potential with bone marrow mesenchymal stromal cells and can be grown to therapeutic scale under Good Manufacturing Practice conditions. *Cytotherapy* **2020**, *22*, 762–771. [CrossRef]
60. Wang, Y.; Fang, J.; Liu, B.; Shao, C.; Shi, Y. Reciprocal regulation of mesenchymal stem cells and immune responses. *Cell Stem Cell* **2022**, *29*, 1515–1530. [CrossRef]
61. Cao, H.; Chu, Y.; Zhu, H.; Sun, J.; Pu, Y.; Gao, Z.; Yang, C.; Peng, S.; Dou, Z.; Hua, J. Characterization of immortalized mesenchymal stem cells derived from foetal porcine pancreas. *Cell Prolif.* **2011**, *44*, 19–32. [CrossRef] [PubMed]
62. Seeberger, K.L.; Eshpeter, A.; Rajotte, R.V.; Korbutt, G.S. Epithelial cells within the human pancreas do not coexpress mesenchymal antigens: Epithelial-mesenchymal transition is an artifact of cell culture. *Lab. Investig.* **2009**, *89*, 110–121. [CrossRef] [PubMed]
63. Habtezion, A.; Gukovskaya, A.S.; Pandol, S.J. Acute Pancreatitis: A Multifaceted Set of Organelle and Cellular Interactions *Gastroenterology* **2019**, *156*, 1941–1950. [CrossRef]
64. Thierens, N.D.E.; Verdonk, R.C.; Löhr, J.M.; van Santvoort, H.C.; Bouwense, S.A.; van Hooft, J.E. Chronic pancreatitis. *Lancet* **2025**, *404*, 2605–2618. [CrossRef]
65. Kong, X.; Sun, T.; Kong, F.; Du, Y.; Li, Z. Chronic Pancreatitis and Pancreatic Cancer. *Gastrointest. Tumors* **2014**, *1*, 123–134. [CrossRef]
66. Liot, S.; Balas, J.; Aubert, A.; Prigent, L.; Mercier-Gouy, P.; Verrier, B.; Bertolino, P.; Hennino, A.; Valcourt, U.; Lambert, E. Stroma Involvement in Pancreatic Ductal Adenocarcinoma: An Overview Focusing on Extracellular Matrix Proteins. *Front. Immunol.* **2021**, *12*, 612271. [CrossRef]
67. Hingorani, S.R. Epithelial and stromal co-evolution and complicity in pancreatic cancer. *Nat. Rev. Cancer* **2023**, *23*, 57–77. [CrossRef] [PubMed]
68. Habtezion, A. Inflammation in acute and chronic pancreatitis. *Curr. Opin. Gastroenterol.* **2015**, *31*, 395–399. [CrossRef]
69. Bachem, M.G.; Zhou, Z.; Zhou, S.; Siech, M. Role of stellate cells in pancreatic fibrogenesis associated with acute and chronic pancreatitis. *J. Gastroenterol. Hepatol.* **2006**, *21* (Suppl. S3), S92–S96. [CrossRef]
70. Murtaugh, L.C.; Keefe, M.D. Regeneration and repair of the exocrine pancreas. *Annu. Rev. Physiol.* **2015**, *77*, 229–249. [CrossRef]
71. Munir, F.; Jamshed, M.B.; Shahid, N.; Muhammad, S.A.; Ghanem, N.B.; Qiyu, Z. Current status of diagnosis and Mesenchymal stem cells therapy for acute pancreatitis. *Physiol. Rep.* **2019**, *7*, e14170. [CrossRef] [PubMed]
72. Kleeff, J.; Whitcomb, D.C.; Shimosegawa, T.; Esposito, I.; Lerch, M.M.; Gress, T.; Mayerle, J.; Drewes, A.M.; Rebours, V.; Akisik, F.; et al. Chronic pancreatitis. *Nat. Rev. Dis. Prim.* **2017**, *3*, 17060. [CrossRef]
73. Kirkegård, J.; Cronin-Fenton, D.; Heide-Jørgensen, U.; Mortensen, F.V. Acute Pancreatitis and Pancreatic Cancer Risk: A Nationwide Matched-Cohort Study in Denmark. *Gastroenterology* **2018**, *154*, 1729–1736. [CrossRef]
74. Xue, J.; Sharma, V.; Hsieh, M.H.; Chawla, A.; Murali, R.; Pandol, S.J.; Habtezion, A. Alternatively activated macrophages promote pancreatic fibrosis in chronic pancreatitis. *Nat. Commun.* **2015**, *6*, 7158. [CrossRef] [PubMed]
75. Hah, N.; Sherman, M.H.; Yu, R.T.; Downes, M.; Evans, R.M. Targeting Transcriptional and Epigenetic Reprogramming in Stromal Cells in Fibrosis and Cancer. *Cold Spring Harb. Symp. Quant. Biol.* **2015**, *80*, 249–255. [CrossRef] [PubMed]
76. Zambirinis, C.P.; Levie, E.; Nguy, S.; Avanzi, A.; Barilla, R.; Xu, Y.; Seifert, L.; Daley, D.; Greco, S.H.; Deutsch, M.; et al. TLR9 ligation in pancreatic stellate cells promotes tumorigenesis. *J. Exp. Med.* **2015**, *212*, 2077–2094. [CrossRef]

77. Koliaraki, V.; Prados, A.; Armaka, M.; Kollias, G. The mesenchymal context in inflammation, immunity and cancer. *Nat. Immunol.* **2020**, *21*, 974–982. [CrossRef]
78. Caligiuri, G.; Tuveson, D.A. Activated fibroblasts in cancer: Perspectives and challenges. *Cancer Cell* **2023**, *41*, 434–449. [CrossRef]
79. Öhlund, D.; Elyada, E.; Tuveson, D. Fibroblast heterogeneity in the cancer wound. *J. Exp. Med.* **2014**, *211*, 1503–1523. [CrossRef]
80. Lavie, D.; Ben-Shmuel, A.; Erez, N.; Scherz-Shouval, R. Cancer-associated fibroblasts in the single-cell era. *Nat. Cancer* **2022**, *3*, 793–807. [CrossRef]
81. Hu, Z.-Y.; Ding, D.; Song, Y.; Deng, Y.-F.; Zhang, C.-M.; Yu, T. Molecular mechanism of pancreatic ductal adenocarcinoma: The heterogeneity of cancer-associated fibroblasts and key signaling pathways. *World J. Clin. Oncol.* **2025**, *16*, 97007. [CrossRef] [PubMed]
82. Öhlund, D.; Handly-Santana, A.; Biffi, G.; Elyada, E.; Almeida, A.S.; Ponz-Sarvise, M.; Corbo, V.; Oni, T.E.; Hearn, S.A.; Lee, E.J.; et al. Distinct populations of inflammatory fibroblasts and myofibroblasts in pancreatic cancer. *J. Exp. Med.* **2017**, *214*, 579–596. [CrossRef] [PubMed]
83. Elyada, E.; Bolisetty, M.; Laise, P.; Flynn, W.F.; Courtois, E.T.; Burkhart, R.A.; Teinor, J.A.; Belleau, P.; Biffi, G.; Lucito, M.S.; et al. Cross-species single-cell analysis of pancreatic ductal adenocarcinoma reveals antigen-presenting cancer-associated fibroblasts. *Cancer Discov.* **2019**, *9*, 1102–1123. [CrossRef] [PubMed]
84. Neuzillet, C.; Tijeras-Raballand, A.; Ragulan, C.; Cros, J.; Patil, Y.; Martinet, M.; Erkan, M.; Kleeff, J.; Wilson, J.; Apte, M.; et al. Inter- and intra-tumoural heterogeneity in cancer-associated fibroblasts of human pancreatic ductal adenocarcinoma. *J. Pathol.* **2019**, *248*, 51–65. [CrossRef]
85. Brichkina, A.; Polo, P.; Sharma, S.D.; Visestamkul, N.; Lauth, M. A Quick Guide to CAF Subtypes in Pancreatic Cancer. *Cancers* **2023**, *15*, 2614. [CrossRef]
86. Peiffer, R.; Boumahd, Y.; Gullo, C.; Crake, R.; Letellier, E.; Bellahcène, A.; Peulen, O. Cancer-Associated Fibroblast Diversity Shapes Tumor Metabolism in Pancreatic Cancer. *Cancers* **2022**, *15*, 61. [CrossRef]
87. Özdemir, B.C.; Pentcheva-Hoang, T.; Carstens, J.L.; Zheng, X.; Wu, C.-C.; Simpson, T.R.; Laklai, H.; Sugimoto, H.; Kahlert, C.; Novitskiy, S.V.; et al. Depletion of Carcinoma-Associated Fibroblasts and Fibrosis Induces Immunosuppression and Accelerates Pancreas Cancer with Reduced Survival. *Cancer Cell* **2015**, *28*, 831–833. [CrossRef]
88. Sunami, Y.; Häußler, J.; Kleeff, J. Cellular Heterogeneity of Pancreatic Stellate Cells, Mesenchymal Stem Cells, and Cancer-Associated Fibroblasts in Pancreatic Cancer. *Cancers* **2020**, *12*, 3770. [CrossRef]
89. Rhim, A.D.; Oberstein, P.E.; Thomas, D.H.; Mirek, E.T.; Palermo, C.F.; Sastra, S.A.; Dekleva, E.N.; Saunders, T.; Becerra, C.P.; Tattersall, I.W.; et al. Stromal elements act to restrain, rather than support, pancreatic ductal adenocarcinoma. *Cancer Cell* **2014**, *25*, 735–747. [CrossRef]
90. Ho, W.J.; Jaffee, E.M.; Zheng, L. The tumour microenvironment in pancreatic cancer—Clinical challenges and opportunities. *Nat. Rev. Clin. Oncol.* **2020**, *17*, 527–540. [CrossRef]
91. de La, O.J.-P.; Emerson, L.L.; Goodman, J.L.; Froebe, S.C.; Illum, B.E.; Curtis, A.B.; Murtaugh, L.C. Notch and Kras reprogram pancreatic acinar cells to ductal intraepithelial neoplasia. *Proc. Natl. Acad. Sci. USA* **2008**, *105*, 18907–18912. [CrossRef]
92. Kopp, J.L.; von Figura, G.; Mayes, E.; Liu, F.-F.; Dubois, C.L.; Morris, J.P.; Pan, F.C.; Akiyama, H.; Wright, C.V.E.; Jensen, K.; et al. Identification of Sox9-Dependent Acinar-to-Ductal Reprogramming as the Principal Mechanism for Initiation of Pancreatic Ductal Adenocarcinoma. *Cancer Cell* **2012**, *22*, 737–750. [CrossRef]
93. Helms, E.J.; Berry, M.W.; Chaw, R.C.; DuFort, C.C.; Sun, D.; Onate, M.K.; Oon, C.; Bhattacharyya, S.; Sanford-Crane, H.; Horton, W.; et al. Mesenchymal Lineage Heterogeneity Underlies Nonredundant Functions of Pancreatic Cancer–Associated Fibroblasts. *Cancer Discov.* **2022**, *12*, 484–501. [CrossRef] [PubMed]
94. Bhatia, R.; Siddiqui, J.A.; Ganguly, K.; Thompson, C.M.; Cannon, A.; Aithal, A.; Perumal, N.; Maurya, S.K.; Li, X.; Cox, J.L.; et al. Muc4 loss mitigates epidermal growth factor receptor activity essential for PDAC tumorigenesis. *Oncogene* **2023**, *42*, 759–770. [CrossRef]
95. Nimmakayala, R.K.; Ogunleye, A.O.; Parte, S.; Krishna Kumar, N.; Raut, P.; Varadharaj, V.; Perumal, N.K.; Nallasamy, P.; Rauth, S.; Cox, J.L.; et al. PAF1 cooperates with YAP1 in metaplastic ducts to promote pancreatic cancer. *Cell Death Dis.* **2022**, *13*, 839. [CrossRef] [PubMed]
96. Ji, B.; Tsou, L.; Wang, H.; Gaiser, S.; Chang, D.Z.; Daniluk, J.; Bi, Y.; Grote, T.; Longnecker, D.S.; Logsdon, C.D. Ras Activity Levels Control the Development of Pancreatic Diseases. *Gastroenterology* **2009**, *137*, 1072–1082.e6. [CrossRef]
97. Liou, G.-Y.; Döppler, H.; Necela, B.; Krishna, M.; Crawford, H.C.; Raimondo, M.; Storz, P. Macrophage-secreted cytokines drive pancreatic acinar-to-ductal metaplasia through NF-κB and MMPs. *J. Cell Biol.* **2013**, *202*, 563–577. [CrossRef]
98. Corcoran, R.B.; Contino, G.; Deshpande, V.; Tzatsos, A.; Conrad, C.; Benes, C.H.; Levy, D.E.; Settleman, J.; Engelman, J.A.; Bardeesy, N. STAT3 Plays a Critical Role in KRAS -Induced Pancreatic Tumorigenesis. *Cancer Res.* **2011**, *71*, 5020–5029. [CrossRef] [PubMed]
99. Means, A.L.; Logsdon, C.D. Acinar Ductal Metaplasia: Yap Fills a Gap. *Gastroenterology* **2016**, *151*, 393–395. [CrossRef]

100. Velez-Delgado, A.; Donahue, K.L.; Brown, K.L.; Du, W.; Irizarry-Negron, V.; Menjivar, R.E.; Lasse Opsahl, E.L.; Steele, N.G.; The, S.; Lazarus, J.; et al. Extrinsic KRAS Signaling Shapes the Pancreatic Microenvironment Through Fibroblast Reprogramming. *Cell. Mol. Gastroenterol. Hepatol.* **2022**, *13*, 1673–1699. [CrossRef]
101. Parte, S.; Kaur, A.B.; Nimmakayala, R.K.; Ogunleye, A.O.; Chirravuri, R.; Vengoji, R.; Leon, F.; Nallasamy, P.; Rauth, S.; Alsafwani, Z.W.; et al. Cancer-Associated Fibroblast Induces Acinar-to-Ductal Cell Transdifferentiation and Pancreatic Cancer Initiation Via LAMA5/ITGA4 Axis. *Gastroenterology* **2024**, *166*, 842–858.e5. [CrossRef] [PubMed]
102. Bell, A.T.F.; Mitchell, J.T.; Kiemen, A.L.; Lyman, M.; Fujikura, K.; Lee, J.W.; Coyne, E.; Shin, S.M.; Nagaraj, S.; Deshpande, A.; et al. PanIN and CAF transitions in pancreatic carcinogenesis revealed with spatial data integration. *Cell Syst.* **2024**, *15*, 753–769.e5. [CrossRef] [PubMed]
103. Hosein, A.N.; Huang, H.; Wang, Z.; Parmar, K.; Du, W.; Huang, J.; Maitra, A.; Olson, E.; Verma, U.; Brekken, R.A. Cellular heterogeneity during mouse pancreatic ductal adenocarcinoma progression at single-cell resolution. *JCI Insight* **2019**, *4*, e129212. [CrossRef] [PubMed]
104. Cui Zhou, D.; Jayasinghe, R.G.; Chen, S.; Herndon, J.M.; Iglesia, M.D.; Navale, P.; Wendl, M.C.; Caravan, W.; Sato, K.; Storrs, E.; et al. Spatially restricted drivers and transitional cell populations cooperate with the microenvironment in untreated and chemo-resistant pancreatic cancer. *Nat. Genet.* **2022**, *54*, 1390–1405. [CrossRef]
105. Sousa, C.M.; Biancur, D.E.; Wang, X.; Halbrook, C.J.; Sherman, M.H.; Zhang, L.; Kremer, D.; Hwang, R.F.; Witkiewicz, A.K.; Ying, H.; et al. Pancreatic stellate cells support tumour metabolism through autophagic alanine secretion. *Nature* **2016**, *536*, 479–483. [CrossRef]
106. Niu, N.; Shen, X.; Wang, Z.; Chen, Y.; Weng, Y.; Yu, F.; Tang, Y.; Lu, P.; Liu, M.; Wang, L.; et al. Tumor cell-intrinsic epigenetic dysregulation shapes cancer-associated fibroblasts heterogeneity to metabolically support pancreatic cancer. *Cancer Cell* **2024**, *42*, 869–884.e9. [CrossRef]
107. Ohri, N.; Häußler, J.; Javakhishvili, N.; Vieweg, D.; Zourelidis, A.; Trojanowicz, B.; Haemmerle, M.; Esposito, I.; Glaß, M.; Sunami, Y.; et al. Gene expression dynamics in fibroblasts during early-stage murine pancreatic carcinogenesis. *iScience* **2024**, *28*, 111572. [CrossRef]
108. Zińczuk, J.; Zaręba, K.; Romaniuk, W.; Kamińska, D.; Nizioł, M.; Baszun, M.; Kędra, B.; Guzińska-Ustymowicz, K.; Pryczynicz, A. Expression of Chosen Carcinoembryonic-Related Cell Adhesion Molecules in Pancreatic Intraepithelial Neoplasia (PanIN) Associated with Chronic Pancreatitis and Pancreatic Ductal Adenocarcinoma (PDAC). *Int. J. Med. Sci.* **2019**, *16*, 583–592. [CrossRef]
109. Criscimanna, A.; Duan, L.-J.; Rhodes, J.A.; Fendrich, V.; Wickline, E.; Hartman, D.J.; Monga, S.P.S.; Lotze, M.T.; Gittes, G.K.; Fong, G.-H.; et al. PanIN-Specific Regulation of Wnt Signaling by HIF2α during Early Pancreatic Tumorigenesis. *Cancer Res.* **2013**, *73*, 4781–4790. [CrossRef]
110. Cheng, M.-F.; Tsai, W.-C.; Hsia, K.-T.; Yang, Y.-S.; Jin, J.-S. Expression of urocortin in pancreatic ductal adenocarcinoma and pancreatic intraepithelial neoplasia. *APMIS* **2014**, *122*, 147–154. [CrossRef]
111. Waldmann, J.; Fendrich, V.; Reichert, M.; Hecker, A.; Bartsch, D.K.; Padberg, W.; Holler, J.P.N. Expression of neuropeptide Y and its receptors Y1 and Y2 in pancreatic intraepithelial neoplasia and invasive pancreatic cancer in a transgenic mouse model and human samples of pancreatic cancer. *J. Surg. Res.* **2018**, *223*, 230–236. [CrossRef] [PubMed]
112. Nan, P.; Dong, X.; Bai, X.; Lu, H.; Liu, F.; Sun, Y.; Zhao, X. Tumor-stroma TGF-β1-THBS2 feedback circuit drives pancreatic ductal adenocarcinoma progression via integrin $\alpha v\beta 3$/CD36-mediated activation of the MAPK pathway. *Cancer Lett.* **2022**, *528*, 59–75. [CrossRef]
113. Yauch, R.L.; Gould, S.E.; Scales, S.J.; Tang, T.; Tian, H.; Ahn, C.P.; Marshall, D.; Fu, L.; Januario, T.; Kallop, D.; et al. A paracrine requirement for hedgehog signalling in cancer. *Nature* **2008**, *455*, 406–410. [CrossRef]
114. Mathew, E.; Zhang, Y.; Holtz, A.M.; Kane, K.T.; Song, J.Y.; Allen, B.L.; Pasca di Magliano, M. Dosage-Dependent Regulation of Pancreatic Cancer Growth and Angiogenesis by Hedgehog Signaling. *Cell Rep.* **2014**, *9*, 484–494. [CrossRef]
115. Hampton, R.F.; Jimenez-Gonzalez, M.; Stanley, S.A. Unravelling innervation of pancreatic islets. *Diabetologia* **2022**, *65*, 1069–1084. [CrossRef]
116. Nathan, J.D.; Peng, R.Y.; Wang, Y.; McVey, D.C.; Vigna, S.R.; Liddle, R.A. Primary sensory neurons: A common final pathway for inflammation in experimental pancreatitis in rats. *Am. J. Physiol. Liver Physiol.* **2002**, *283*, G938–G946. [CrossRef]
117. Saloman, J.L.; Albers, K.M.; Li, D.; Hartman, D.J.; Crawford, H.C.; Muha, E.A.; Rhim, A.D.; Davis, B.M. Ablation of sensory neurons in a genetic model of pancreatic ductal adenocarcinoma slows initiation and progression of cancer. *Proc. Natl. Acad. Sci. USA* **2016**, *113*, 3078–3083. [CrossRef]
118. Demir, I.E.; Boldis, A.; Pfitzinger, P.L.; Teller, S.; Brunner, E.; Klose, N.; Kehl, T.; Maak, M.; Lesina, M.; Laschinger, M.; et al. Investigation of Schwann Cells at Neoplastic Cell Sites Before the Onset of Cancer Invasion. *JNCI J. Natl. Cancer Inst.* **2014**, *106*, dju184. [CrossRef] [PubMed]

119. Demir, I.E.; Kujundzic, K.; Pfitzinger, P.L.; Saricaoglu, Ö.C.; Teller, S.; Kehl, T.; Reyes, C.M.; Ertl, L.S.; Miao, Z.; Schall, T.J.; et al. Early pancreatic cancer lesions suppress pain through CXCL12-mediated chemoattraction of Schwann cells. *Proc. Natl. Acad. Sci. USA* **2017**, *114*, E85–E94. [CrossRef]
120. Harari, N.; Sakhneny, L.; Khalifa-Malka, L.; Busch, A.; Hertel, K.J.; Hebrok, M.; Landsman, L. Pancreatic pericytes originate from the embryonic pancreatic mesenchyme. *Dev. Biol.* **2019**, *449*, 14–20. [CrossRef]
121. Natarajan, V.; Ha, S.; Delgado, A.; Jacobson, R.; Alhalhooly, L.; Choi, Y.; Kim, J. Acquired αSMA Expression in Pericytes Coincides with Aberrant Vascular Structure and Function in Pancreatic Ductal Adenocarcinoma. *Cancers* **2022**, *14*, 2448. [CrossRef] [PubMed]
122. Lin, P.-Y.; Peng, S.-J.; Shen, C.-N.; Pasricha, P.J.; Tang, S.-C. PanIN-associated pericyte, glial, and islet remodeling in mice revealed by 3D pancreatic duct lesion histology. *Am. J. Physiol. Liver Physiol.* **2016**, *311*, G412–G422. [CrossRef]
123. Liang, J.; Li, H.; Han, J.; Jiang, J.; Wang, J.; Li, Y.; Feng, Z.; Zhao, R.; Sun, Z.; Lv, B.; et al. Mex3a interacts with LAMA2 to promote lung adenocarcinoma metastasis via PI3K/AKT pathway. *Cell Death Dis.* **2020**, *11*, 614. [CrossRef] [PubMed]
124. Clark, C.E.; Hingorani, S.R.; Mick, R.; Combs, C.; Tuveson, D.A.; Vonderheide, R.H. Dynamics of the Immune Reaction to Pancreatic Cancer from Inception to Invasion. *Cancer Res.* **2007**, *67*, 9518–9527. [CrossRef] [PubMed]
125. Zhang, Y.; Lazarus, J.; Steele, N.G.; Yan, W.; Lee, H.-J.; Nwosu, Z.C.; Halbrook, C.J.; Menjivar, R.E.; Kemp, S.B.; Sirihorachai, V.R.; et al. Regulatory T-cell Depletion Alters the Tumor Microenvironment and Accelerates Pancreatic Carcinogenesis. *Cancer Discov.* **2020**, *10*, 422–439. [CrossRef]
126. Bernard, V.; Semaan, A.; Huang, J.; San Lucas, F.A.; Mulu, F.C.; Stephens, B.M.; Guerrero, P.A.; Huang, Y.; Zhao, J.; Kamyabi, N.; et al. Single-Cell Transcriptomics of Pancreatic Cancer Precursors Demonstrates Epithelial and Microenvironmental Heterogeneity as an Early Event in Neoplastic Progression. *Clin. Cancer Res.* **2019**, *25*, 2194–2205. [CrossRef]
127. Mucciolo, G.; Curcio, C.; Roux, C.; Li, W.Y.; Capello, M.; Curto, R.; Chiarle, R.; Giordano, D.; Satolli, M.A.; Lawlor, R.; et al. IL17A critically shapes the transcriptional program of fibroblasts in pancreatic cancer and switches on their protumorigenic functions. *Proc. Natl. Acad. Sci. USA* **2021**, *118*, e2020395118. [CrossRef]
128. Sunami, Y.; Böker, V.; Kleeff, J. Targeting and Reprograming Cancer-Associated Fibroblasts and the Tumor Microenvironment in Pancreatic Cancer. *Cancers* **2021**, *13*, 697. [CrossRef]
129. Kim, H.-G.; Tan, L.; Weisberg, E.L.; Liu, F.; Canning, P.; Choi, H.G.; Ezell, S.A.; Wu, H.; Zhao, Z.; Wang, J.; et al. Discovery of a potent and selective DDR1 receptor tyrosine kinase inhibitor. *ACS Chem. Biol.* **2013**, *8*, 2145–2150. [CrossRef]
130. Berestjuk, I.; Lecacheur, M.; Carminati, A.; Diazzi, S.; Rovera, C.; Prod'homme, V.; Ohanna, M.; Popovic, A.; Mallavialle, A.; Larbret, F.; et al. Targeting Discoidin Domain Receptors DDR1 and DDR2 overcomes matrix-mediated tumor cell adaptation and tolerance to BRAF-targeted therapy in melanoma. *EMBO Mol. Med.* **2022**, *14*, e11814. [CrossRef]
131. Zeng, X.-P.; Wang, L.-J.; Guo, H.-L.; He, L.; Bi, Y.-W.; Xu, Z.-L.; Li, Z.-S.; Hu, L.-H. Dasatinib ameliorates chronic pancreatitis induced by caerulein via anti-fibrotic and anti-inflammatory mechanism. *Pharmacol. Res.* **2019**, *147*, 104357. [CrossRef] [PubMed]
132. El-Hamoly, T.; Hajnády, Z.; Nagy-Pénzes, M.; Bakondi, E.; Regdon, Z.; Demény, M.A.; Kovács, K.; Hegedűs, C.; Abd El-Rahman, S.S.; Szabó, É.; et al. Poly(ADP-Ribose) Polymerase 1 Promotes Inflammation and Fibrosis in a Mouse Model of Chronic Pancreatitis. *Int. J. Mol. Sci.* **2021**, *22*, 3593. [CrossRef]
133. McAndrews, K.M.; Chen, Y.; Darpolor, J.K.; Zheng, X.; Yang, S.; Carstens, J.L.; Li, B.; Wang, H.; Miyake, T.; Correa de Sampaio, P.; et al. Identification of Functional Heterogeneity of Carcinoma-Associated Fibroblasts with Distinct IL6-Mediated Therapy Resistance in Pancreatic Cancer. *Cancer Discov.* **2022**, *12*, 1580–1597. [CrossRef] [PubMed]
134. Chandekar, K.R.; Prashanth, A.; Vinjamuri, S.; Kumar, R. FAPI PET/CT Imaging-An Updated Review. *Diagnostics* **2023**, *13*, 2018. [CrossRef]
135. Greifenstein, L.; Gunkel, A.; Hoehne, A.; Osterkamp, F.; Smerling, C.; Landvogt, C.; Mueller, C.; Baum, R.P. 3BP-3940, a highly potent FAP-targeting peptide for theranostics—Production, validation and first in human experience with Ga-68 and Lu-177. *iScience* **2023**, *26*, 108541. [CrossRef] [PubMed]
136. Lang, M.; Spektor, A.-M.; Hielscher, T.; Hoppner, J.; Glatting, F.M.; Bicu, F.; Hackert, T.; Heger, U.; Pausch, T.; Gutjahr, E.; et al. Static and Dynamic 68Ga-FAPI PET/CT for the Detection of Malignant Transformation of Intraductal Papillary Mucinous Neoplasia of the Pancreas. *J. Nucl. Med.* **2023**, *64*, 244–251. [CrossRef]
137. McGahan, W.; Gough, M.; Liu, C.; Hoyte, S.; Gill, A.J.; Cavallucci, D. Fibroblast Activation Protein Is Overexpressed on Both Stromal and Epithelial Cells Before Pancreatic Ductal Adenocarcinoma: Implications for Early Diagnosis on 68Ga-FAPI-PET/CT. *Gastroenterology* **2024**, *167*, 1217–1220. [CrossRef]
138. Yang, X.; Lin, Y.; Shi, Y.; Li, B.; Liu, W.; Yin, W.; Dang, Y.; Chu, Y.; Fan, J.; He, R. FAP Promotes Immunosuppression by Cancer-Associated Fibroblasts in the Tumor Microenvironment via STAT3-CCL2 Signaling. *Cancer Res.* **2016**, *76*, 4124–4135. [CrossRef]
139. Deng, D.; Begum, H.; Liu, T.; Zhang, J.; Zhang, Q.; Chu, T.-Y.; Li, H.; Lemenze, A.; Hoque, M.; Soteropoulos, P.; et al. NFAT5 governs cellular plasticity-driven resistance to KRAS-targeted therapy in pancreatic cancer. *J. Exp. Med.* **2024**, *221*, e20240766. [CrossRef]

140. Bhatia, M.; Ramnath, R.D.; Chevali, L.; Guglielmotti, A. Treatment with bindarit, a blocker of MCP-1 synthesis, protects mice against acute pancreatitis. *Am. J. Physiol. Gastrointest. Liver Physiol.* **2005**, *288*, G1259–G1265. [CrossRef]
141. Hu, F.; Lou, N.; Jiao, J.; Guo, F.; Xiang, H.; Shang, D. Macrophages in pancreatitis: Mechanisms and therapeutic potential. *Biomed. Pharmacother.* **2020**, *131*, 110693. [CrossRef] [PubMed]
142. Feig, C.; Jones, J.O.; Kraman, M.; Wells, R.J.B.; Deonarine, A.; Chan, D.S.; Connell, C.M.; Roberts, E.W.; Zhao, Q.; Caballero, O.L.; et al. Targeting CXCL12 from FAP-expressing carcinoma-associated fibroblasts synergizes with anti-PD-L1 immunotherapy in pancreatic cancer. *Proc. Natl. Acad. Sci. USA* **2013**, *110*, 20212–20217. [CrossRef] [PubMed]
143. Khare, T.; Bissonnette, M.; Khare, S. CXCL12-CXCR4/CXCR7 Axis in Colorectal Cancer: Therapeutic Target in Preclinical and Clinical Studies. *Int. J. Mol. Sci.* **2021**, *22*, 7371. [CrossRef]
144. Roberto, M.; Arrivi, G.; Di Civita, M.A.; Barchiesi, G.; Pilozzi, E.; Marchetti, P.; Santini, D.; Mazzuca, F.; Tomao, S. The role of CXCL12 axis in pancreatic cancer: New biomarkers and potential targets. *Front. Oncol.* **2023**, *13*, 1154581. [CrossRef] [PubMed]
145. Ahmed, R.; Anam, K.; Ahmed, H. Development of Galectin-3 Targeting Drugs for Therapeutic Applications in Various Diseases. *Int. J. Mol. Sci.* **2023**, *24*, 8116. [CrossRef]
146. Zhao, W.; Ajani, J.A.; Sushovan, G.; Ochi, N.; Hwang, R.; Hafley, M.; Johnson, R.L.; Bresalier, R.S.; Logsdon, C.D.; Zhang, Z.; et al. Galectin-3 Mediates Tumor Cell-Stroma Interactions by Activating Pancreatic Stellate Cells to Produce Cytokines via Integrin Signaling. *Gastroenterology* **2018**, *154*, 1524–1537.e6. [CrossRef]
147. Yang, D.; Sun, X.; Moniruzzaman, R.; Wang, H.; Citu, C.; Zhao, Z.; Wistuba, I.I.; Wang, H.; Maitra, A.; Chen, Y. Genetic Deletion of Galectin-3 Inhibits Pancreatic Cancer Progression and Enhances the Efficacy of Immunotherapy. *Gastroenterology* **2024**, *167*, 298–314. [CrossRef]

cancers

MDPI

Review

Exploring the Horizon: Anti-Fibroblast Growth Factor Receptor Therapy in Pancreatic Cancer with Aberrant Fibroblast Growth Factor Receptor Expression—A Scoping Review

Elena Orlandi [1,*], Massimo Guasconi [2,3], Stefano Vecchia [4], Serena Trubini [1], Mario Giuffrida [5], Manuela Proietto [1], Elisa Anselmi [1], Patrizio Capelli [5] and Andrea Romboli [5]

1 Department of Oncology-Hematology, Azienda USL of Piacenza, 29121 Piacenza, Italy; s.trubini@ausl.pc.it (S.T.); m.proietto@ausl.pc.it (M.P.); e.anselmi@ausl.pc.it (E.A.)
2 Department of Medicine and Surgery, University of Parma, 43121 Parma, Italy; massimo.guasconi@unipr.it
3 Department of Health Professions Management, Azienda USL of Piacenza, 29121 Piacenza, Italy
4 Department of Pharmacy, Azienda USL of Piacenza, 29121 Piacenza, Italy; s.vecchia@ausl.pc.it
5 Department of General Surgery, Azienda USL of Piacenza, 29121 Piacenza, Italy; m.giuffrida@ausl.pc.it (M.G.); p.capelli@ausl.pc.it (P.C.); a.romboli@ausl.pc.it (A.R.)
* Correspondence: elena.orlandi1987@gmail.com

Simple Summary: Pancreatic cancer is one of the deadliest cancers due to its subtle onset and advanced stage at diagnosis. With most patients having inoperable cancer at diagnosis, survival rates remain low despite existing treatments. Our review aims to map and summarize current studies on FGFR inhibitors, a promising new treatment targeting specific cancer pathways. We found that while there are many preclinical studies, clinical research is still emerging, focusing mainly on the efficacy and safety of these treatments. Although FGFR alterations are relatively rare in pancreatic cancer, the few available real-life data are promising. Future research should aim to better identify the genetic drivers of this cancer and gather more data on long-term outcomes. This could lead to improved treatments and better survival rates for patients with pancreatic cancer.

Abstract: Pancreatic cancer is a highly lethal disease, often diagnosed at advanced stages, with a 5-year overall survival rate of around 10%. Current treatments have limited effectiveness, underscoring the need for new therapeutic options. This scoping review aims to identify and summarize preclinical and clinical studies on FGFR (Fibroblast Growth Factor Receptor) inhibitors, including tyrosine kinase inhibitors (TKIs) and FGFR-specific inhibitors, in pancreatic cancer with FGFR alterations. We included studies analyzing efficacy, safety, and survival outcomes in various populations. A comprehensive search across major databases identified 73 relevant studies: 32 preclinical, 16 clinical, and 25 from gray literature. The clinical trials focused primarily on efficacy (20 studies) and safety (14 studies), with fewer studies addressing survival outcomes. FGFR1 was the most studied alteration, followed by FGFR2 and FGFR4. Although FGFR alterations are relatively rare in pancreatic cancer, the available data, including promising real-life outcomes, suggest significant potential for FGFR inhibitors. However, more extensive research is needed to identify the correct genetic drivers and gather robust survival data. Ongoing and future trials are expected to provide more comprehensive insights, potentially leading to improved targeted therapies for pancreatic cancer patients with FGFR alterations.

Keywords: FGFR; target therapy; pancreatic cancer; FGFR alteration; scoping review

1. Introduction

Pancreatic cancer (PC) stands out as one of the deadliest forms of cancer, characterized by a subtle onset, aggressive behavior, and a 5-year overall survival rate hovering around 10%, primarily due to the majority of cases being diagnosed at an advanced stage, owing to the clinical characteristics of the disease and its often asymptomatic nature [1]. As a result, 80–90% of patients have unresectable cancer at the time of diagnosis [2]. PC represents a substantial challenge in the management of oncological diseases, ranking as the 12th most prevalent malignancy and the 7th leading cause of cancer-related mortality (accounting for 4.7% of all cancers) [1]. Chemotherapeutic regimens currently represent the standard of care, with median survival rates that seldom exceed one year from the initiation of first-line treatment [3]. Although some promising results have been observed with the use of the poly (ADP-ribose) polymerase (PARP) inhibitor olaparib in patients with germline BRCA mutations [4], the results of phase II/III trials investigating both targeted therapies and their combinations have failed to demonstrate a significant advantage [5–8].

The role of FGFR (Fibroblast Growth Factor Receptor) in tumor carcinogenesis pathways is integral to the regulation of key cellular processes. FGFR actively participates in signaling cascades governing cell growth, survival, and differentiation, positioning itself as a pivotal factor in the initiation and progression of tumorigenesis [9]. Dysregulation of FGFR signaling, often associated with genetic alterations such as mutations, amplifications, or overexpression, can instigate uncontrolled cell proliferation and contribute significantly to the pathogenesis of various cancers [10]. This aberrant activation of FGFR pathways leads to downstream effects on critical signaling pathways, including MAPK (Mitogen-Activated Protein Kinase) and PI3K/Akt (Phosphoinositide 3-Kinase/Protein Kinase B), resulting in enhanced cell survival, angiogenesis, and metastatic potential [11]. The pivotal role of FGFR in pancreatic cancer (PC) has been extensively explored. Elevated levels of FGFR expression have been associated with an advanced tumor stage, while lower FGFR expression has been significantly correlated with extended post-operative survival; compared to basic FGF expression in patients with PC, the overexpression of FGFR demonstrates itself as a more valuable prognostic indicator [12].

FGFR1, identified over two decades ago as abnormally expressed in PC, has been associated with aberrant autocrine and paracrine pathways [13]. In up to 10% of patients with advanced pancreatic ductal adenocarcinoma (PDAC), there is a description of amplification and overexpression of FGFR1 [14]. However, this occurrence is less common in cohorts of patients with resectable PDAC [15]. FGFR1 exhibited a broader expression pattern in both healthy and diseased pancreatic tissues; it demonstrated a robust correlation with the epithelial-to-mesenchymal transition (EMT) phenotype but did not show a significant association with the epithelial subtypes of PDAC, whether classical or basal-like [16]. Nuclear FGFR1 also regulates Neuregulin transcription, which acts in an autocrine fashion in pancreatic stellate cells, promoting invasion [17]. Distinct isoforms of FGFR1, such as FGFR1 IIIb and FGFR1 IIIc, exert varying influences on tumorigenesis, with IIIb suppressing tumor formation and growth in mice and IIIc promoting cell growth through mitogenic signaling via the FRS2-MAPK pathway, with the potential to increase the transformation of pancreatic ductal cells [18,19]. In only 0.54% of PDAC cases, FGFR2 is amplified, yet it does not exhibit mutations [20], while FGFR2 fusion has been identified in 6.7% of patients [21]. FGFR-2 and its isoforms clinically contribute to aggressiveness in PDAC [22]; previous studies demonstrated the correlation between the level of FGFR-2 IIIb and venous invasion and VEGF-A expression [23]; FGFR2 IIIc overexpression promoted cell proliferation and enhanced tumor growth and liver metastases in vivo [24].

Regarding the limited data showing that FGFR3 can exhibit both tumor-suppressive and oncogenic properties, it may be prudent to consider this information when evaluating the targeting of a TKI [25]. FGFR4 expression is exclusively detected in epithelial cells, significantly elevated in the classical/epithelial phenotype, and is associated with better outcomes [16]. It is substantially increased in high-grade pancreatic intraepithelial neoplasia (PanIN) and PDAC compared with normal and low-grade PanIN [26]. The stimulation of PDAC cells with FGFR4 significantly enhanced cell adhesion to laminin and fibronectin while concurrently reducing cell migration, with the upregulation of the integrin $\alpha 4$ family as the underlying cause of these effects, suggesting a potential tumor-suppressive function. Conversely, cell morphology and proliferation in PDAC cells remained unaffected [26].

Endogenous FGFR4 levels limit the malignant phenotype of PDAC, primarily by restraining mTORC1 pathway activity [16]. FGFR4-deficient cells showed increased activity in the MAPK and mTORC1 pathways. Downregulation of FGFR4 correlated with enriched PI3K/Akt/mTOR signatures and increased phosphorylation of 4E-BP1, a known mTORC1 substrate linked to cell proliferation [27]. Currently available therapeutic options targeting the FGF/FGFR-induced signaling cascade mainly include non-selective tyrosine kinase inhibitors (TKIs), selective TKIs (pan-FGFR, FGFR1/2/3, and FGFR4 inhibitors), monoclonal antibodies, and FGF ligand traps [28]. Even considering that the high heterogeneity of different tumor types significantly influences the efficacy of these drug classes, non-selective TKIs have generally shown non-significant effects in clinical trials for tumors with altered FGFR, despite dose-limiting toxicities such as hypertension [28]. Among selective TKIs, several drugs are in the early stages of trials for solid tumors with FGFR alterations. AZD4547, Debio-1347, and E7090 are FGFR1/2/3 inhibitors that have shown promising results in phase I and II studies [29–31]. Robitinib is an FGFR4 inhibitor with available phase I/II study results [32]. FP-1039 is an FGF ligand trap that has completed phase I trials [33]. The effectiveness of these drugs varies widely across different types of tumors, potentially due to tumor heterogeneity.

The identification of potential treatments for patients exhibiting FGFR pathway alterations in metastatic pancreatic cancer is of significant importance, given the limited therapeutic options available and the poor prognosis associated with this disease. In order to provide a comprehensive picture of treatment against pancreatic cancer with FGFR alteration, this scoping review aims to identify and present the available information concerning preclinical or clinical study and the results of anti-FGFR (TKI or FGFR-specific inhibitors) in pancreatic cancer harboring FGFR alterations, and regarding clinical study in terms of population analyzed, toxicity, and efficacy.

2. Materials and Methods

We prepared and elaborated this document according to the latest review process proposed in 2022 by the JBI [34], and the preferred reporting items for systematic reviews and meta-analyses extension for scoping reviews (PRISMA-ScR) checklist for reporting was used [35]. This scoping was registered prospectively with Figshare as suggested by JBI [34]: https://doi.org/10.6084/m9.figshare.26001772.

2.1. Research Question

The aim of this research was to identify the presence of available information concerning preclinical or clinical studies and the results of anti-FGFR (TKI or FGFR-specific inhibitor) in pancreatic cancer harboring FGFR alterations, and regarding clinical studies in terms of the population analyzed, toxicity, and efficacy.

2.2. Inclusion Criteria

Studies were included if they met the following population, concept, and context criteria:

Type of participants: We focused on patients with a diagnosis of pancreatic cancer disease with proven FGFR alteration. Regarding clinical studies, we included patients of any age and both genders who received various anti-FGFR treatments. We considered oncological outcomes such as progression-free survival (PFS), overall survival (OS), and recurrence rates. Articles were also eligible for inclusion if they performed a subgroup analysis considering the specific population with "FGFR mutation in pancreatic cancer". Preclinical studies both in vivo and in vitro focusing on the targeted therapy against FGFR aberrations in pancreatic cancer were also included.

Concept: We considered any studies that included anti-FGFR treatment, both tyrosine kinase inhibitors (TKI), or FGFR-specific inhibitors.

Context: The studies focused on a target therapy directed toward dysregulation of FGFR signaling with aberrant activation of FGFR pathways.

Type of evidence source: This scoping review systematically considered randomized controlled trials, non-randomized controlled trials, before and after studies, and interrupted time-series studies. In addition, analytical observational studies, including prospective and retrospective cohort studies, case–control studies, and analytical cross-sectional studies, were considered for inclusion. This review also considered descriptive observational study designs, including case series, individual case reports, and descriptive cross-sectional studies, for inclusion. Text and opinion papers were also considered for inclusion in this scoping review. Gray literature was included as long as the research design was clearly recognizable. There were no date limitations or language restrictions. The reference lists of retrieved studies were reviewed to identify additional reports of relevant trials.

2.3. Exclusion Criteria

Studies that did not meet the specific above-stated inclusion criteria were excluded.

2.4. Search Strategy

A search was carried out on the online databases PubMed, Embase, Cochrane, Scopus, Web of Science, EBSCO, Open Dissertation databases, and the CENTRAL registry. An initial search strategy was launched in PubMed, then the strategy was supplemented and modified based on the initial results obtained. The search strategy used for PubMed is reported in the Supplementary Materials, and the strategies used for the other databases were derived from that for PubMed. Additionally, we included ongoing studies, as well as studies listed on ClinicalTrials.gov, even if a full publication was not available; the keyword selected for the conditions was "FGFR". The search was initially conducted in September 2023 and was updated periodically to ensure the inclusion of the most recent literature. The most recent search was executed on 1 June 2024.

2.5. Study Selection

After removing duplicates, two researchers independently reviewed the titles and abstracts of the studies to determine which ones to include. The review process consisted of two levels of screening using Rayyan QCRI online software: (1) a title and abstract review and (2) a full-text review. For both levels, two authors independently screened the articles, with conflicts resolved by a third author. The reasons for exclusion were recorded and presented in the PRISMA flow diagram (Figure 1).

2.6. Data Extraction

For each outcome, the information from the included texts was extracted into a dedicated data form. The data form was reviewed by the research team and pretested by all reviewers before implementation to ensure accuracy. The collected data included the following information: title; authors; publication year; country in which the study was performed for the clinical trial; study design; baseline characteristics of enrolled patients, including performance status, type of anti-FGFR drugs, type of FGFR, concept and context; and key findings relevant to the scoping review research questions.

2.7. Data Synthesis

The analysis and presentation of results followed the JBI guidelines for scoping reviews. The results were also displayed using charts and figures. The most effective method for presenting data was determined based on the findings at the conclusion of the study.

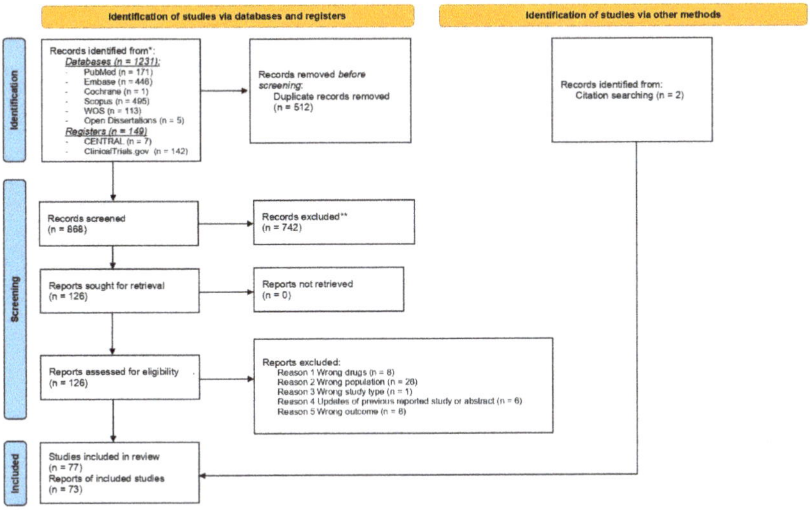

Figure 1. PRISMA 2020 flow diagram. * Consider, if feasible to do so, reporting the number of records identified from each database or register searched (rather than the total number across all databases/registers). ** If automation tools were used, indicate how many records were excluded by a human and how many were excluded by automation tools [36].

3. Results

Out of the 1380 studies found during the initial literature search, 73 were included in the final analysis. The primary reasons for excluding the 742 papers during the screening phase were the wrong population, wrong drug, wrong publication type, and wrong outcomes, as detailed in Supplementary Material Table S2 (reason for exclusion). The details of the excluded studies, along with their references, are also specified in the Supplementary Materials. A summary of the study selection process is illustrated in the PRISMA flow diagram (Figure 1).

The majority of studies reported in the literature were preclinical (n = 32): 16 were clinical studies and 25 were studies from gray literature (Table 1).

Table 1. Population characteristics: (total number of studies = 73).

Variables	Numbers of Studies
Type of studies	
Preclinical	32
Clinical	16
Gray literature	25
Abstract [a]	4
Sample size	
Only one case	7
1–10 patients	7
>10	2
Included only patients with pancreatic cancer [b]	5
FGFR alterations	
FGFR alteration generic	9
FGFR2 fusion [c]	4
FGFR 2 amplification/rearrangement	3
Type of drugs	
Selective inhibitors pan-FGFR	
Erdafinitinib	3

Table 1. *Cont.*

Variables	Numbers of Studies
Pemigatinib	4
Futibatinib	2
Selective inhibitors FGFR 1/2/3	
Lirafugratinib	1
Fexagratinib	2
Monoclonal antibodies	
Aprutumab ixadotin	1
FGF ligand traps	
FB-1039	1
Non-selective TKIs	
Pazopanib	1
Ponatinib	1
Dovitinib	1
Clinical outcomes (primary)	
Safety	8
Survival outcomes	1
Efficacy	5

[a] included in clinical studies; [b] 2 abstract congress presentation and 3 case reports; [c] 2 studies reporting cases of fusion and rearrangement.

Regarding the trials (n = 12), five were phase I studies, two were phase II studies, one was a phase I/II basket trial, and four were phase II basket trials (references in Tables S3 and S4 in Supplementary Materials).

The studies selected from clinicaltrial.gov included 25 trials, of which 4 were phase I studies, 1 was a phase I/II study, 17 were phase II studies, 1 was a phase III study, and 1 was defined as a post-market study (expanding access program) (NCT numbers in Supplementary Materials).

3.1. Study Distribution Over Time

The studies were published over a span of 25 years, with an increasing trend in the number of publications over time. The periods of publication are detailed in Figure 2, with the majority of studies (18) being published between 2018 and 2022.

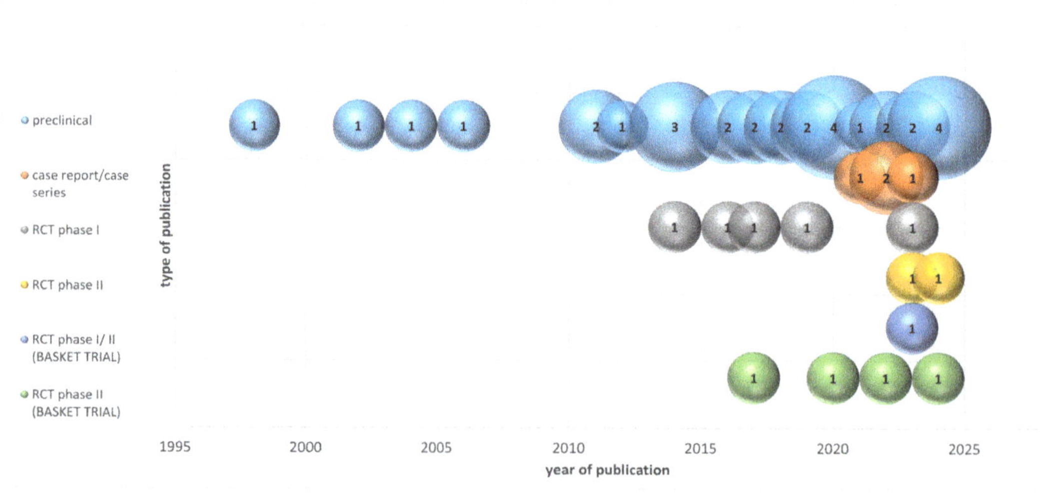

Figure 2. Distribution of studies by type of publication and year of publication.

3.2. Preclinical Studies

In the preclinical setting, 32 studies focused on various FGFR alterations in pancreatic cancer. FGFR1 was the most frequently studied alteration, being the focus of 16 studies, followed by FGFR2 (8 studies), FGFR3 (1 study), FGFR4 (3 studies), and combinations of FGFR alterations (4 studies) (references in Table S5 in Supplementary Materials, Table 2, Figure 3).

Table 2. Numbers of studies dealing in preclinical setting (numbers of total studies = 32).

Variables	Numbers of Studies
Period of publication	
1998–2002	1
2003–2007	2
2008–2012	3
2013–2017	7
2018–2022	13
Up to 2023	6
Type of FGFR alteration	
FGFR1	16
FGFR2	8
FGFR3	1
FGFR4	3
FGFR1-2-3	3
FGFR1-2-3-4	1

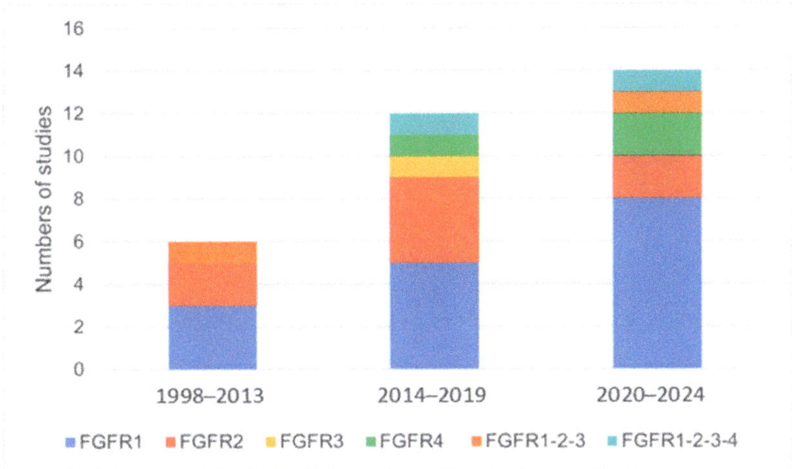

Figure 3. Classification of preclinical studies on specific FGFR alteration, based on the years of publication.

3.3. Clinical Studies

The clinical studies included 16 studies examining FGFR alterations and their impact on pancreatic cancer treatment. Various selective FGFR inhibitors were investigated, including Erdafitinib (three studies), Pemigatinib (four studies), and Futibatinib (two studies), as well as non-selective TKIs like Pazopanib, Ponatinib, and Dovitinib (one study each). The studies primarily focused on the efficacy (five studies) and safety (eight studies) of these treatments, with a smaller subset examining survival outcomes (one study) (references in Tables S3 and S4 in Supplementary Materials, Table 1).

3.4. Gray Literature

A total of 25 studies were identified from gray literature, primarily sourced from clinicaltrial.gov. These studies often included both adult (22 studies) and pediatric populations (3 studies). The status of these studies varied, with 15 being active but not recruiting, 9 closed or terminated, and 1 approved for marketing (Table 3).

Table 3. Total of studies dealing in gray literature (total studies = 25).

Variables *	Numbers of Studies
Gray literature (clinicaltrial.gov)	25
Included patients	
Only adult	22
Adult and child	3
Status of Study	
Closed, terminated, withdrawn, or unknown	9
Active but not recruiting; recruiting	15
Approved for marketing	1
FGFR alterations	
FGFR alteration (generic)	21
FGFR2 expression or overexpression	3
Type of drugs	
Selective inhibitors pan-FGFR	11
Non-selective TKIs	1
Phase of study	
Phase I	4
Phase I/II	1
Phase II	17
Phase III	1
Post-market	1
Clinical outcomes (primary)	
Safety [a]	6
Survival outcomes [b]	2
Efficacy [a]	20

* Source clinicaltrial.gov; [a] four studies with mixed outcomes with efficacy/safety or part A and part B studies; [b] only one study with dedicated survival outcomes.

The studies assessed FGFR alterations generically (21 studies) and specifically FGFR2 expression or overexpression (3 studies). The types of drugs investigated included selective inhibitors pan-FGFR (11 studies) and non-selective TKIs (1 study) (NCT numbers in Supplementary Materials).

3.5. Clinical Outcomes

The primary clinical outcomes assessed in the studies included safety, efficacy, and survival. In the gray literature, 20 studies reported on efficacy, 6 on safety, and 2 on survival outcomes. Among the clinical studies, eight reported on safety, five on efficacy, and one on survival outcomes (references in Tables S3 and S4 in Supplementary Materials, Table 1).

3.6. Synthesis of Results

The review identified 73 relevant studies, including 32 preclinical and 41 clinical studies, focusing on FGFR inhibitors in pancreatic cancer with FGFR alterations. Clinical studies primarily assessed efficacy, with 20 studies, and safety, with 14 studies, while only a few focused on survival outcomes. The majority of trials involved adult populations, with manageable toxicity profiles documented. Ongoing trials are expected to provide more comprehensive data on the efficacy and survival outcomes of FGFR-targeted therapies in this patient population.

4. Discussion

In the present scoping review, we mapped and summarized the current literature reporting epidemiological data on FGFR inhibitors against FGFR alterations in pancreatic cancer. Considering the current lack of a comprehensive overview in this field, conducting a scoping review is the most effective and suitable approach to systematically map the existing literature and provide a broad understanding of anti-FGFR therapy in pancreatic cancer with FGFR alterations.

FGFR1 alteration was the most frequently studied FGFR alteration in preclinical studies, followed by FGFR2, with an increase in evaluations of FGFR4 alterations in the past four years (Figure 3). The review highlighted the limited number of studies specifically dedicated to pancreatic cancer, reflecting the relatively low percentage of FGFR alterations in this cancer type [12]. Various FGFR inhibitors have demonstrated promising efficacy in clinical settings. Specific inhibitors such as Erdafitinib, Pemigatinib, and Futibatinib have been evaluated in multiple clinical trials, showcasing significant antitumor activity in patients with advanced pancreatic cancer harboring FGFR alterations [37–40]. These studies have reported the Overall Response Rate (ORR) and PFS benefits in a subset of patients, suggesting that FGFR inhibitors can provide a targeted therapeutic option. Ongoing clinical trials continue to explore the full potential of these inhibitors, including their use in combination with other therapeutic agents, to enhance treatment outcomes and overcome resistance mechanisms.

The safety profiles of FGFR inhibitors have been well documented across several clinical studies. Common adverse events associated with these agents include hyperphosphatemia, stomatitis, fatigue, and gastrointestinal disturbances [33,38,39,41–44]. These side effects are generally manageable with dose adjustments and supportive care. However, while the safety data are robust, there is a need for more extensive studies to fully understand the long-term impact of FGFR inhibitors on survival outcomes. Current evidence suggests that while these agents can provide disease control, their effect on OS remains to be conclusively determined. The ongoing clinical trials primarily emphasize evaluating the efficacy of FGFR inhibitors, with a significant number of studies focusing on this aspect. Notably, two studies have designated survival as the primary outcome, highlighting a crucial interest in understanding the long-term benefits of these treatments. Therefore, we anticipate that future results from these trials will provide more comprehensive and robust data on both the efficacy of FGFR inhibitors and their impact on survival outcomes in patients with pancreatic cancer.

The promising real-life data from the case reports and case series identified underscore the potential of FGFR inhibitors in treating pancreatic cancer, despite the relatively low frequency of FGFR alterations in this disease.

The preclinical studies provided further insights into the significance of FGFR alterations in pancreatic cancer. FGFR1 was the most frequently studied receptor alteration, being the focus of 16 preclinical studies, followed by FGFR2 (8 studies), FGFR3 (1 study), and FGFR4 (3 studies). Additionally, combinations of FGFR alterations were investigated in four studies. These preclinical findings underline the critical role of FGFR1 and FGFR2 in the pathophysiology of pancreatic cancer.

4.1. Research Implications

Given the current landscape of research, our scoping review highlights significant gaps and challenges in the literature concerning anti-FGFR therapy for pancreatic cancer with FGFR alterations. While numerous preclinical studies exist, there is a notable scarcity of clinical trials, most of which have been conducted in recent years. This trend is further supported by the increasing number of ongoing trials.

Many of these trials have been withdrawn or terminated, often due to issues such as low enrollment rates or the termination of agreements with drug suppliers. Additionally, the majority of trials are basket trials, which lack a specific focus on pancreatic cancer, thereby limiting the generalizability of their findings to this particular patient population.

Despite the generally unremarkable ORR observed, the few available real-life observational data indicate significantly promising outcomes. To advance the field, future research should aim to address these gaps by conducting more targeted trials specifically on pancreatic cancer, ensuring adequate enrollment, and fostering collaborations to maintain continuity with drug suppliers. Such efforts will be crucial in enhancing the applicability and impact of anti-FGFR therapies for patients with pancreatic cancer.

4.2. Strengths and Limitations

This is the first scoping review to encompass such a wide range of studies reporting on anti-FGFR therapies for pancreatic cancer with FGFR alterations. This review includes both preclinical and clinical studies, identifying the volume and distribution of the existing evidence base. We have also mapped the key concepts and research priorities within this literature.

The strength of this study lies in its methodology. To capture the highest possible number of relevant studies, we employed a comprehensive search strategy incorporating various terms. Additionally, the search was conducted across major databases without any restrictions. In line with the objectives of scoping reviews, the inclusion criteria were intentionally broad, allowing us to gather findings from diverse sources. Moreover, to ensure completeness and transparency in reporting, the PRISMA-ScR checklist was utilized.

However, there are some limitations to consider. Firstly, many trials were withdrawn or terminated, often due to low enrollment or discontinued partnerships with drug suppliers. Additionally, most of the trials were basket trials, which do not focus specifically on pancreatic cancer, thus limiting the generalizability of the results to this specific population. Although we followed a rigorous approach and included various types of publications, this strategy may have excluded findings from studies addressing other research questions.

5. Conclusions

This scoping review provides a comprehensive overview of the available preclinical and clinical studies on FGFR inhibitors in pancreatic cancer harboring FGFR alterations. The results indicate that while there are a substantial number of preclinical studies (32) exploring the underlying mechanisms and potential therapeutic targets, clinical studies (41) are still emerging, with a significant focus on drug efficacy (20 studies) and safety (14 studies). Only a few studies have thus far reported on survival outcomes, highlighting a gap in long-term efficacy data. These findings underscore the potential of FGFR inhibitors as a targeted therapy for pancreatic cancer patients with FGFR alterations, despite the relatively low incidence of these alterations in this cancer type. More extensive research is needed to better identify the correct genetic drivers and to gather robust data on survival outcomes. Future studies should focus on optimizing FGFR-targeted therapies, exploring combination treatments, and validating biomarkers for patient selection to maximize therapeutic benefits.

In summary, while the current data are encouraging, continued efforts in clinical research are essential to fully understand and harness the potential of FGFR inhibitors in pancreatic cancer treatment.

Supplementary Materials: The following supporting information can be downloaded at: https://www.mdpi.com/article/10.3390/cancers16162912/s1, Table S1: Search strategy; Table S2: Reason and round of exclusion; Table S3: Characteristics of primary research; Table S4: Primary research; population characteristics; Table S5: FGFR receptor alteration characteristics in preclinical studies; Table S6: Included gray literature characteristics from clinicaltrial.gov.

Author Contributions: E.O. assessed the conception and design of the manuscript. M.G. (Massimo Guasconi), A.R. and E.O. contributed to the investigation and data curation. M.G. (Mario Giuffrida) and S.T. drafted the article. E.O., A.R. and S.V. critically revised it for important intellectual content. E.O. and A.R. reviewed and edited the final version of the manuscript. E.A., P.C. and M.P. supervised and mentored the research team. S.V. and S.T. revised the English language. All authors have read and agreed to the published version of the manuscript.

Funding: This research received no external funding.

Acknowledgments: This work was supported by Associazione Malato Oncologico Piacentino (AMOP).

Conflicts of Interest: The authors declare no conflicts of interest.

References

1. Ilic, I.; Ilic, M. International Patterns in Incidence and Mortality Trends of Pancreatic Cancer in the Last Three Decades: A Joinpoint Regression Analysis. *World J. Gastroenterol.* **2022**, *28*, 4698–4715. [CrossRef] [PubMed] [PubMed Central]
2. Rawla, P.; Sunkara, T.; Gaduputi, V. Epidemiology of Pancreatic Cancer: Global Trends, Etiology and Risk Factors. *World J. Oncol.* **2019**, *10*, 10–27. [CrossRef] [PubMed] [PubMed Central]
3. Di Costanzo, F.; Antonuzzo, L.; Mazza, E.; Giommoni, E. Optimizing First-Line Chemotherapy in Metastatic Pancreatic Cancer: Efficacy of FOLFIRINOX versus Nab-Paclitaxel Plus Gemcitabine. *Cancers* **2023**, *15*, 416. [CrossRef] [PubMed] [PubMed Central]
4. Golan, T.; Hammel, P.; Reni, M.; Van Cutsem, E.; Macarulla, T.; Hall, M.J.; Park, J.O.; Hochhauser, D.; Arnold, D.; Oh, D.Y.; et al. Maintenance Olaparib for Germline BRCA-Mutated Metastatic Pancreatic Cancer. *N. Engl. J. Med.* **2019**, *381*, 317–327. [CrossRef] [PubMed] [PubMed Central]
5. Philip, P.A.; Benedetti, J.; Corless, C.L.; Wong, R.; O'Reilly, E.M.; Flynn, P.J.; Rowland, K.M.; Atkins, J.N.; Mirtsching, B.C.; Rivkin, S.E.; et al. Phase III Study Comparing Gemcitabine Plus Cetuximab versus Gemcitabine in Patients with Advanced Pancreatic Adenocarcinoma: Southwest Oncology Group-Directed Intergroup Trial S0205. *J. Clin. Oncol.* **2010**, *28*, 3605–3610. [CrossRef] [PubMed] [PubMed Central]
6. Infante, J.R.; Somer, B.G.; Park, J.O.; Li, C.P.; Scheulen, M.E.; Kasubhai, S.M.; Oh, D.Y.; Liu, Y.; Redhu, S.; Steplewski, K.; et al. A Randomised, Double-Blind, Placebo-Controlled Trial of Trametinib, an Oral MEK Inhibitor, in Combination with Gemcitabine for Patients with Untreated Metastatic Adenocarcinoma of the Pancreas. *Eur. J. Cancer* **2014**, *50*, 2072–2081. [CrossRef] [PubMed]
7. Bodoky, G.; Timcheva, C.; Spigel, D.R.; La Stella, P.J.; Ciuleanu, T.E.; Pover, G.; Tebbutt, N.C. A Phase II Open-Label Randomized Study to Assess the Efficacy and Safety of Selumetinib (AZD6244 [ARRY-142886]) versus Capecitabine in Patients with Advanced or Metastatic Pancreatic Cancer Who Have Failed First-Line Gemcitabine Therapy. *Investig. New Drugs* **2012**, *30*, 1216–1223. [CrossRef] [PubMed]
8. Moore, M.J.; Goldstein, D.; Hamm, J.; Figer, A.; Hecht, J.R.; Gallinger, S.; Au, H.J.; Murawa, P.; Walde, D.; Wolff, R.A.; et al. National Cancer Institute of Canada Clinical Trials Group. Erlotinib Plus Gemcitabine Compared with Gemcitabine Alone in Patients with Advanced Pancreatic Cancer: A Phase III Trial of the National Cancer Institute of Canada Clinical Trials Group. *J. Clin. Oncol.* **2007**, *25*, 1960–1966. [CrossRef] [PubMed]
9. Johnson, D.E.; Williams, L.T. Structural and Functional Diversity in the FGF Receptor Multigene Family. *Adv. Cancer Res.* **1993**, *60*, 1–41.
10. Helsten, T.; Elkin, S.; Arthur, E.; Tomson, B.N.; Carter, J.; Kurzrock, R. The FGFR Landscape in Cancer: Analysis of 4853 Tumors by Next-Generation Sequencing. *Clin. Cancer Res.* **2016**, *22*, 259–267. [CrossRef]
11. Turner, N.; Grose, R. Fibroblast Growth Factor Signalling: From Development to Cancer. *Nat. Rev. Cancer* **2010**, *10*, 116–129. [CrossRef]
12. Ohta, T.; Yamamoto, M.; Numata, M.; Iseki, S.; Tsukioka, Y.; Miyashita, T.; Kayahara, M.; Nagakawa, T.; Miyazaki, I.; Nishikawa, K.; et al. Expression of Basic Fibroblast Growth Factor and its Receptor in Human Pancreatic Carcinomas. *Br. J. Cancer* **1995**, *72*, 824–831. [CrossRef] [PubMed] [PubMed Central]
13. Kobrin, M.S.; Yamanaka, Y.; Friess, H.; Lopez, M.E.; Korc, M. Aberrant Expression of Type I Fibroblast Growth Factor Receptor in Human Pancreatic Adenocarcinomas. *Cancer Res.* **1993**, *53*, 4741–4744.
14. Aguirre, A.J.; Nowak, J.A.; Camarda, N.D.; Moffitt, R.A.; Ghazani, A.A.; Hazar-Rethinam, M. Real-Time Genomic Characterization of Advanced Pancreatic Cancer to Enable Precision Medicine. *Cancer Discov.* **2018**, *8*, 1096–1111. [CrossRef]
15. Cancer Genome Atlas Research Network. Integrated Genomic Characterization of Pancreatic Ductal Adenocarcinoma. *Cancer Cell* **2017**, *32*, 185–203.e13. [CrossRef]
16. D'Agosto, S.; Pezzini, F.; Veghini, L.; Delfino, P.; Fiorini, C.; Temgue Tane, G.D.; Del Curatolo, A.; Vicentini, C.; Ferrari, G.; Pasini, D.; et al. Loss of FGFR4 Promotes the Malignant Phenotype of PDAC. *Oncogene* **2022**, *41*, 4371–4384. [CrossRef] [PubMed] [PubMed Central]
17. Coetzee, A.S.; Carter, E.P.; Rodríguez-Fernández, L. Nuclear FGFR1 Promotes Pancreatic Stellate Cell-Driven Invasion through Up-Regulation of Neuregulin 1. *Oncogene* **2023**, *42*, 491–500. [CrossRef]
18. Liu, Z.; Neiss, N.; Zhou, S.; Henne-Bruns, D.; Korc, M.; Bachem, M.; Kornmann, M. Identification of a Fibroblast Growth Factor Receptor 1 Splice Variant that Inhibits Pancreatic Cancer Cell Growth. *Cancer Res.* **2007**, *67*, 2712–2719. [CrossRef] [PubMed]
19. Kornmann, M.; Ishiwata, T.; Matsuda, K.; Lopez, M.E.; Fukahi, K.; Asano, G.; Beger, H.G.; Korc, M. IIIc Isoform of Fibroblast Growth Factor Receptor 1 is Overexpressed in Human Pancreatic Cancer and Enhances Tumorigenicity of Hamster Ductal Cells. *Gastroenterology* **2002**, *123*, 301–313. [CrossRef] [PubMed]

20. Li, J.; Hu, K.; Huang, J.; Zhou, L.; Yan, Y.; Xu, Z. A Pan-Cancer Analysis of the Expression Landscape and Clinical Relevance of Fibroblast Growth Factor Receptor 2 in Human Cancers. *Front. Oncol.* **2021**, *11*, 644854. [CrossRef] [PubMed] [PubMed Central]
21. Helal, C.; Valéry, M.; Ducreux, M.; Hollebecque, A.; Smolenschi, C. FGFR2 Fusion in Metastatic Pancreatic Ductal Adenocarcinoma: Is There Hope? *Eur. J. Cancer* **2022**, *176*, 168–170. [CrossRef] [PubMed]
22. Matsuda, Y.; Yoshimura, H.; Suzuki, T.; Uchida, E.; Naito, Z.; Ishiwata, T. Inhibition of Fibroblast Growth Factor Receptor 2 Attenuates Proliferation and Invasion of Pancreatic Cancer. *Cancer Sci.* **2014**, *105*, 1212–1219. [CrossRef] [PubMed] [PubMed Central]
23. Cho, K.; Ishiwata, T.; Uchida, E. Enhanced Expression of Keratinocyte Growth Factor and its Receptor Correlates with Venous Invasion in Pancreatic Cancer. *Am. J. Pathol.* **2007**, *170*, 1964–1974. [CrossRef]
24. Ishiwata, T.; Matsuda, Y.; Yamamoto, T.; Uchida, E.; Korc, M.; Naito, Z. Enhanced Expression of Fibroblast Growth Factor Receptor 2 IIIc Promotes Human Pancreatic Cancer Cell Proliferation. *Am. J. Pathol.* **2012**, *180*, 1928–1941. [CrossRef]
25. Lafitte, M.; Moranvillier, I.; Garcia, S.; Peuchant, E.; Iovanna, J.; Rousseau, B.; Dubus, P.; Guyonnet-Dupérat, V.; Belleannée, G.; Ramos, J.; et al. FGFR3 Has Tumor Suppressor Properties in Cells with Epithelial Phenotype. *Mol. Cancer* **2013**, *12*, 83. [CrossRef] [PubMed] [PubMed Central]
26. Motoda, N.; Matsuda, Y.; Onda, M.; Ishiwata, T.; Uchida, E.; Naito, Z. Overexpression of Fibroblast Growth Factor Receptor 4 in High-Grade Pancreatic Intraepithelial Neoplasia and Pancreatic Ductal Adenocarcinoma. *Int. J. Oncol.* **2011**, *38*, 133–143. [PubMed]
27. Dowling, R.J.; Topisirovic, I.; Alain, T.; Bidinosti, M.; Fonseca, B.D.; Petroulakis, E. mTORC1-Mediated Cell Proliferation, but Not Cell Growth, Controlled by the 4E-BPs. *Science* **2010**, *328*, 1172–1176. [CrossRef]
28. Du, S.; Zhang, Y.; Xu, J. Current Progress in Cancer Treatment by Targeting FGFR Signaling. *Cancer Biol. Med.* **2023**, *20*, 490–499. [CrossRef] [PubMed] [PubMed Central]
29. Chae, Y.K.; Hong, F.; Vaklavas, C.; Cheng, H.H.; Hammerman, P.; Mitchell, E.P. Phase II Study of AZD4547 in Patients with Tumors Harboring Aberrations in the FGFR Pathway: Results from the NCI-MATCH Trial (EAY131) Subprotocol W. *J. Clin. Oncol.* **2020**, *38*, 2407–2417. [CrossRef]
30. Voss, M.H.; Hierro, C.; Heist, R.S.; Cleary, J.M.; Meric-Bernstam, F.; Tabernero, J. A Phase I, Open-Label, Multicenter, Dose Escalation Study of the Oral Selective FGFR Inhibitor Debio 1347 in Patients with Advanced Solid Tumors Harboring FGFR Gene Alterations. *Clin. Cancer Res.* **2019**, *25*, 2699–2707. [CrossRef]
31. Koyama, T.; Shimizu, T.; Iwasa, S.; Fujiwara, Y.; Kondo, S.; Kitano, S. First-in-Human Phase I Study of E7090, a Novel Selective Fibroblast Growth Factor Receptor Inhibitor, in Patients with Advanced Solid Tumors. *Cancer Sci.* **2020**, *111*, 571–579. [CrossRef]
32. Chan, S.L.; Schuler, M.; Kang, Y.K.; Yen, C.J.; Edeline, J.; Choo, S.P. A First-in-Human Phase 1/2 Study of FGF401 and Combination of FGF401 with Spartalizumab in Patients with Hepatocellular Carcinoma or Biomarker-Selected Solid Tumors. *J. Exp. Clin. Cancer Res.* **2022**, *41*, 189. [CrossRef]
33. Tolcher, A.W.; Papadopoulos, K.P.; Patnaik, A.; Wilson, K.; Thayer, S.; Zanghi, J. A Phase I, First-in-Human Study of FP-1039 (GSK3052230), a Novel FGF Ligand Trap, in Patients with Advanced Solid Tumors. *Ann. Oncol.* **2016**, *27*, 526–532. [CrossRef] [PubMed]
34. Peters, M.D.J.; Godfrey, C.; McInerney, P.; Khalil, H.; Larsen, P.; Marnie, C.; Pollock, D.; Tricco, A.C.; Munn, Z. Best Practice Guidance and Reporting Items for the Development of Scoping Review Protocols. *JBI Evid. Synth.* **2022**, *20*, 953–968. [CrossRef] [PubMed]
35. Tricco, A.C.; Lillie, E.; Zarin, W. PRISMA Extension for Scoping Reviews (PRISMA-ScR): Checklist and Explanation. *Ann. Intern. Med.* **2018**, *169*, 467–473. [CrossRef]
36. Page, M.J.; McKenzie, J.E.; Bossuyt, P.M.; Boutron, I.; Hoffman, T.C.; Mulrow, C.D.; Shamseer, L.; Tetzlaff, J.M.; Akl, E.A.; Brennan, S.E.; et al. The PRISMA 2020 statement an updated guideline for reporting systematic reviews. *BMJ* **2021**, *29*, n71. [CrossRef]
37. Rodon, J.; Damian, S.; Furqan, M.; García-Donas, J.; Imai, H.; Italiano, A.; Spanggaard, I.; Ueno, M.; Yokota, T.; Veronese, M.L.; et al. Pemigatinib in previously treated solid tumors with activating FGFR1-FGFR3 alterations: Phase 2 FIGHT-207 basket trial. *Nat. Med.* **2024**, *30*, 1645–1654. [CrossRef]
38. Subbiah, V.; Iannotti, N.O.; Gutierrez, M.; Smith, D.C.; Féliz, L.; Lihou, C.F.; Tian, C.; Silverman, I.M.; Ji, T.; Saleh, M. FIGHT-101, a first-in-human study of potent and selective FGFR 1-3 inhibitor pemigatinib in pan-cancer patients with FGF/FGFR alterations and advanced malignancies. *Ann. Oncol.* **2022**, *33*, 522–533. [CrossRef]
39. Kuboki, Y.; Matsubara, N.; Bando, H.; Shitara, K.; Yoh, K.; Kojima, T.; Ohno, I.; Takahashi, H.; Harano, K.; Kondo, S.; et al. First-in-human (FIH) study of TAS-120, a highly selective covalent oral fibroblast growth factor receptor (FGFR) inhibitor, in patients (pts) with advanced solid tumors. *Ann. Oncol.* **2017**, *28*, v124. [CrossRef]
40. Pant, S.; Schuler, M.; Iyer, G.; Witt, O.; Doi, T.; Qin, S.; Tabernero, J.; Reardon, D.A.; Massard, C.; Minchon, A.; et al. Erdafitinib in patients with advanced solid tumours with FGFR alterations (RAGNAR): An international, single-arm, phase 2 study. *Lancet Oncol.* **2023**, *24*, 925–935. [CrossRef] [PubMed]
41. Saka, H.; Kitagawa, C.; Kogure, Y.; Takahashi, Y.; Fujikawa, K.; Sagawa, T.; Iwasa, S.; Takahashi, N.; Fukao, T.; Tchinou, C.; et al. Safety, tolerability and pharmacokinetics of the fibroblast growth factor receptor inhibitor AZD4547 in Japanese patients with advanced solid tumours: A Phase I study. *Investig. New Drugs* **2017**, *30*, 451–462. [CrossRef]

42. Quintela-Fandino, M.; Bueno, M.J.; Lombardia, L.; Gil, M.; Gonzalez-Martin, A.; Marquez, R.; Bratos, R.; Guerra, J.; Tan, E.; Lopez, A.; et al. Elective activity over a constitutively active RET-variant of the oral multikinase inhibitor dovitinib: Results of the CNIO-BR002 phase I-trial. *Mol. Oncol.* **2014**, *8*, 1719–1728. [CrossRef] [PubMed]
43. Doi, T.; Shitara, K.; Kojima, T.; Kuboki, Y.; Matsubara, N.; Bando, H.; Yoh, K.; Naito, Y.; Hirai, H.; Kurokawa, Y.; et al. Phase I study of the irreversible fibroblast growth factor receptor 1–4 inhibitor futibatinib in Japanese patients with advanced solid tumors. *Cancer Sci.* **2023**, *114*, 574–585. [CrossRef]
44. Kim, S.B.; Meric-Bernstam, F.; Kalyan, A.; Babich, A.; Liu, R.; Tanigawa, T.; Sommer, A.; Osada, M.; Reetz, F.; Laurent, D.; et al. First-in-Human Phase I Study of Aprutumab Ixadotin, a Fibroblast Growth Factor Receptor 2 Antibody Drug Conjugate (BAY 1187982) in Patients with Advanced Cancer. *Target Oncol.* **2019**, *14*, 591–601. [CrossRef]

cancers

MDPI

Review

Gaps and Opportunities in the Diagnosis and Treatment of Pancreatic Cancer

Miłosz Caban * and Ewa Małecka-Wojciesko

Department of Digestive Tract Diseases, Medical University of Lodz, 90-153 Lodz, Poland; ewa.malecka-panas@umed.lodz.pl
* Correspondence: milosz.caban@stud.umed.lodz.pl

Simple Summary: Pancreatic cancer, including primarily pancreatic ductal adenocarcinoma (PDAC), represents a highly lethal disease and an increasingly common cause of cancer mortality worldwide. Diagnostics and treatment of PDAC represent a great challenge for modern medicine. PDAC is a highly malignant diagnosis, characterised by rapid local progression and distant metastasis formation. The screening of disease in general population is not cost effective but may be considered in high-risk groups. Recently, there has been great interest in developing new PDAC serum biomarkers: diagnostic, prognostic, and predictive. The most common management of early stage PDAC is radical surgery, which is rarely possible upon diagnosis. There is a strong need for further research to improve PDAC early detection and management.

Abstract: Pancreatic cancer is one of the leading causes off cancer-related deaths globally. In Europe, this type of cancer has the lowest survival rate of all cancers. A majority of patients have unresectable or even metastatic disease. In addition, actual therapeutic options are not curative, and surgical treatment is associated with high post-operative morbidity and a lack of uniform translation of surgical success into long-term survival. Moreover, there is no screening for the general population which is recommended, and the overall poor prognosis in pancreatic cancer is related to late clinical detection. Therefore, early diagnosis and early treatment of pancreatic cancer are particularly critical. In this review, we summarize the most significant gaps and opportunities in the diagnosis and treatment of pancreatic cancer to emphasize need for improvement of early detection and the therapeutic efficacy of the available treatment for this cancer. Novel, inclusive, and intentional research is needed to produce improvements in pancreatic cancer in mm the world.

Keywords: early detection; morbidity; mortality; pancreatic cancer; pancreatic ductal adenocarcinoma; screening

1. Introduction

Pancreatic cancer (PC) is a lethal disorder characterized by poor prognosis and response to treatment. In the past three decades, a more than 2.5-fold increase in the global annual number of PC cases has been reported. In the years 2020 and 2017, there were approximately 495,773 and 441,000 new identified PCs worldwide, respectively, in comparison to 196,000 subjects in the year 1990 [1,2]. Globally, PC has been identified as the leading cause of cancer-related deaths [3]. In 2019, PC was the fourth cause of cancer-related death in Japan [4]. It is estimated that PC will be the second-leading cause of death associated with cancer in the United States by the year 2030, surpassing prostate, breast, and colorectal cancers [5]. It results from the biology, high malignancy, late diagnosis, inefficient therapy and the lack of screening possibilities in the general population. In addition, PC is associated with an insidious clinical course and unspecific symptoms at the initial stages of the disease [6,7]. It may be incidentally detected at the advanced stage when still asymptomatic [8]. It must be emphasized that surgical resection is the only therapeutic option giving a chance for longer survival. Nevertheless, surgical resection and standard chemotherapy result in a 5-year survival rate lower than 30% [9]. In addition, only 20–30% of patients with PC are diagnosed at the resectable stage of the disease [10]. In consequence, the general 5-years survival rate of PC is significantly lower and is estimated at only about 10% [11]. Despite such unfavourable data, screening of the asymptomatic adult population is not viable or recommended with current modalities due mainly to the low incidence of the disease, the lack of simple diagnostic tests or treatment not being cost-effective About 90% of all cases with PC are sporadic, while 10% of cases develop in patients with hereditary syndromes or familial predisposition. The screening of individuals in high-risk groups is recommended, but its efficacy is not satisfactory and there are no detailed schedules elaborated [12,13]. New biomarkers of PC are constantly being searched for. Due to the fact that pancreatic ductal adenocarcinoma (PDAC) is the most common among patients with PC, we focused on data in the context of PDAC in this article.

This article discusses major gaps and opportunities in the diagnosis and treatment of PDAC. Also, the review was prepared to highlight the necessity of devoting more attention to PC that requires improvement of therapeutic efficacy and early detection.

2. Gaps in the Diagnosis of PDAC

2.1. Unspecific Symptoms

Generally, typical symptoms of PDAC, such as jaundice, weight loss, main pancreatic duct obstruction, or cholangitis associated with PDAC, appear at the advanced, non-resectable stage of the disease. At the early stage, the disease is usually asymptomatic or accompanied by nonspecific symptoms, such as epigastric or back pain, nausea, fatigue, bloating, abdominal fullness or change in stool consistency. In consequence, they are often understandably attributed to alternative, more frequent causes, causing a delay of adequate diagnosis. In turn, data show that the clinical symptoms occurring with the highest frequency at the time of diagnosis include abdominal pain, abnormal liver function tests, jaundice, new-onset diabetes, dyspepsia, nausea, vomiting, back pain and weight loss. It is worth emphasizing that clinical presentation of the disease depends on the location of the tumour within the pancreas. Biliary obstruction and the ensuing jaundice are typical for the cancer of pancreas head. Cancers of the pancreatic body are characterized by the tendency to invasion of local vascular structures including the celiac, hepatic, and superior mesenteric vessels and the portal vein. In addition, they are more likely to cause back pain. In turn, pancreatic tail cancers are often advanced at the time of diagnosis, may often grow unimpeded due to fewer anatomical barriers, and symptoms often result from metastases. It should be mentioned that cancer causing obstruction of the main pancreatic duct may induce symptoms of pancreatic enzyme insufficiency, or malabsorption of fat, contributing to post-prandial abdominal pain, flatulence, steatorrhea and deficiency of fat-soluble vitamins [14]. In a prospective cohort study, Walter et al. proved that symptoms, such as indigestion, back pain, diabetes, self-reported anxiety or depression, were associated with long total diagnostic interval (time between the occurrence of the symptom and diagnosis). It indicates that special vigilance should be maintained when these symptoms occur [15]. Primarily, proton pump inhibitor-resistant pain and back pain not associated with a disease of the musculoskeletal system may suggest pain related to PDAC. Interestingly, the chronic use of proton pump inhibitors is a risk factor for PDAC occurrence and may contribute to the development of the cancer by, among other factors, hypergastrinemia or low secretion of gastric acid promoting bacterial growth and secretion of nitrosamine stimulating pancreatic cell overgrowth [16].

2.2. Inadequacy of Radiological and Endoscopic Diagnosis

Radiological imaging (US, CT, MRI) and EUS play a key role in detection, staging, differential diagnosis or follow-up of PC. EUS and MRI are suggested as methods useful for screening high-risk individuals. EUS is characterized by higher sensitivity for PDAC tumour detection of less than 2 cm diameter compared to CT (95.2% vs. 42.8%) [17,18]. In turn, EUS may not distinguish malignant from benign lesions without biopsy (EUS-FNA). It results from the fact that the majority of pancreatic tumours, even benign, have a hypoechogenic appearance. For differentiating between inflammatory masses and malignancies, endoscopic ultrasound-guided fine-needle biopsy (EUS-FNB) seems to have higher diagnostic accuracy and sensitivity than EUS-FNA (93.0% and 86.6% vs. 83.6% and 69.5%). In consequence, it should be the preferred technique for diagnosis of cancer, especially in the setting of chronic pancreatitis that may simulate PDAC as pseudotumoral masses [19]. It is worth emphasizing that the choice of needle in EUS-FNB significantly affects diagnostic sensitivity. An appropriate needle should enable preservation of the cellular architecture, histological core procurement, and its use should be safe and easy. The end-cutting FNB needles are highly performing, and their use is associated with improved control at the puncture site and stability at the tip, allowing for enhanced penetration. However, their availability is limited [20]. The choice of an adequate needle determines appropriate tissue acquisition that is still impaired by the relatively high rate of false negatives dependent on inadequate tissue samples, representing remarkable gaps in the diagnostic process of PDAC. It is caused mainly by the consistent presence of fibrosis and necrosis inside the pancreatic mass, hindering proper diagnosis [21].

Different methods are characterized by various capabilities for the detection of early PDAC. A multicentre retrospective study conducted by Kanno et al. revealed several key points concerning the diagnosis and management of early-stage PDAC in a group of 200 cases at stages 0 and I, 20% of which were symptomatic. Analysis showed that the diagnostic accuracy of transabdominal ultrasound (TAUS), CT, MRI, and EUS was 67.5%, 98.0%, 86.5%, and 86.5%, respectively. In addition, a dilation and irregular stenosis of the main pancreatic duct (MPD) are main symptoms of early PDAC that may be overlooked and interpreted as not associated with malignancy. Interestingly, Kanno and co-researchers revealed also that local fatty changes of the pancreatic parenchyma occurred in stages 0 and I of PDAC with a frequency of 42% and 41.8%, respectively. Those are not the specific changes, however their detection may be associated with the possibility of PDAC and should suggest an extended diagnostics [22]. The search for new imaging techniques advancements, and their development enabling adequate identification of non-characteristic features of PDAC, including artificial intelligence, may facilitate the diagnosis of the disease. In turn, data demonstrate that contrast-enhanced endoscopic ultrasound (CEH EUS) is characterized by higher efficacy in the detection of PDAC compared to the conventional EUS: a prospective study found that the CEH EUS had a higher sensitivity (94.5% vs. 83.1%) and accuracy (84.1% vs. 78.6%) [23]. Also, the meta-analysis conducted by Yamashita and co-workers confirmed these results. This research group estimated the sensitivity and specificity of CEH EUS for PC diagnosis, at the level of 93% (95% CI = 0.91–0.95) and 80% (95% CI = 0.75–0.85), respectively [24]. It shows that new imagining technologies are necessary to improve detection of PDAC. Nevertheless, the use and operation of EUS and CEH EUS are not easy, and the accuracy of the method is strongly dependent on operator experience and qualifications [25–27].

2.3. Unsatisfactory Screening

PDAC belongs to one of the most common causes of cancer-associated death. Despite this, screening for the general population is not recommended [18,28]. Enriching the population by targeting subgroups at greater risk for PC, including PDAC, could enhance the diagnostic yield of screening. Actually, PDAC surveillance focuses on genetically predisposed subjects. It is estimated that about 10% to 15% of PDAC are due to inherited mutations. High-risk cases may be offered surveillance, depending on genetic mutation. The risk of PC for individual genetic mutations is presented in Table 1. Actually, an accepted threshold to consider PDAC surveillance is a lifetime risk of 5%.The International Cancer of the Pancreas Screening (CAPS) Consortium suggests surveillance for individuals with familial risk, from the age of 50–55 or from 10 years earlier than when the youngest relative with PC was diagnosed. High-risk of PDAC for subjects eligible for surveillance is defined in Table 2. EUS, MRI, MRCP are the recommended surveillance tests [29]. Surveillance programs in both Europe and the United States have showed that surveillance of high-risk individuals, using EUS and MRI/MRCP may be associated with the early detection of PDAC with very high rates of resectability (75–90%) [30,31]. However, it should be emphasized that the relative benefit of surveillance in families with familial pancreatic cancer is not evident. In addition, despite screening, PDAC at the advanced stage is detected too often, and the five-year survival rate is not significantly increased [30,31]. In contrast, for the general population, the screening is not recommended. It results from some facts, such as the lack of cost effectiveness, actually low incidence of PC, lack of simple biomarker or limited availability and invasiveness of EUS [32].

Table 1. The risk of PC for individual genetic syndromes.

Genetic Syndrome	Risk of PC throughout Life
FAMMM	to 17%
Peutz-Jeghers syndrome	to 36%
Lynch syndrome	to 5%
Cystic fibrosis	5%
Hereditary pancreatitis	30–40%
BRCA1/BRCA2 mutation	various

Table 2. Definition of high-risk individuals eligible for PC surveillance. It is worth emphasizing that high-risk individuals eligible for pancreatic cancer surveillance were defined for patients regardless of gene mutation status: if at least three affected relatives on the same side of the family, of whom at least one is a first-degree relative to the individual considered for surveillance or if at least two affected relatives who are first-degree relatives to each other, of whom at least one is a first-degree relative to the individual considered for surveillance or if at least two affected relatives on the same side of the family, of whom at least one is a first-degree relative to the individual considered for surveillance. ATM, ataxia telangiectasia mutated; BRCA2, breast cancer 2; CDKN2A, cyclin-dependent kinase inhibitor 2A; FAMMM, familial atypical multiple mole melanoma; LKB1/STK11, liver kinase B1/serine/threonine kinase 11; MLH1, mutL homolog 1; MSH2, mutS homolog 2; MSH6, mutS homolog 6; PALB2, partner and localizer of BRCA2.

Genetic Syndrome/Gene Mutation	Criteria of PDAC Family History
Peutz-Jeghers syndrome (*LKB1/STK11*)	Regardless of family history
FAMMM (*CDKN2A p16*)	Regardless of family history
Lynch syndrome (*MLH1/MSH2/MSH6*)	If at least one affected first-degree relative
BRCA1	If at least one affected first-degree relative
BRCA2	If at least one affected first-degree relative or at least two affected relatives of any degree
PALB2	If at least one affected first-degree relative
ATM	If at least one affected first-degree relative

So far, the CA 19-9 remains the only approved biomarker for diagnosis and response assessment, but its utility is limited by low sensitivity and specificity. Despite a numerous studies searching for novel biomarkers in single and in panels of PDAC, none of them has been established for use in clinical practice. Interestingly, the combinations of markers, among others CA 19-9 and the ratio of neutrophils to lymphocytes, may turn out to be more effective and accurate compared to single biomarkers in the diagnosis and prognosis of PDAC. It was proven that the panels of biomarkers may be characterized by high levels of sensitivity, specificity and overall accuracy, and represent potential in the early diagnosis of

PDAC. Nevertheless, so far, there is no recommended combination of biomarkers accepted for diagnosis and prognosis of PDAC [33,34].

In addition, differentiation between PDAC and chronic pancreatitis (CP) is also difficult with CT, MRI and MRCP. In consequence, novel biomarkers, especially measurable in easily available biological material, may represent significant diagnostic progress. Actually, there is no single biomarker clearly differentiating PDAC from CP. Nonetheless, some studies demonstrated that particles, such as soluble urokinase-type plasminogen activator receptor, osteopontin or soluble AXL receptor tyrosine kinase, may be considered for this purpose [35–37]. In addition, many cytokine panels together with inflammatory biomarkers have been proposed for discriminating autoimmune pancreatitis (AIP) and PDAC. Significantly higsher levels of IL-1β, IL-7, IL-13, and granulocyte colony-stimulating factor (G-CSF) were observed in patients with AIP in comparison to subjects with PDAC [38].

New-onset diabetes is actually an early symptom of PDAC often overlooked by clinicians. Also, it should be remembered that patients with PDAC may have a higher risk of diabetes. In addition to conventional imaging, annual glucose testing or assessment of HbA1C is recommended to diagnose new-onset diabetes in high-risk individuals. The screening of PDAC in new-onset diabetes was proposed, but not actually introduced [39]. It results from the very high number of new cases of diabetes annually, which are mostly not associated with PDAC. There is a strong need to find the biomarker differentiating PDAC-associated diabetes from type 2 diabetes mellitus.

3. Gaps in the Treatment of PDAC

3.1. Gaps in the Surgical Treatment of PDAC

The surgical treatment may result in numerous complications, both associated with surgery itself and anaesthesia, such as organ space/deep surgical site infection, wound dehiscence, fistulas, sepsis, stroke, coma, myocardial infarction, venous thromboembolism, pneumonia, renal failure or infection. In addition, intra-abdominal abscess, haemorrhage, fistulae of the pancreatointestinal anastomosis, delayed gastric emptying are other surgical complications, more specific for pancreatic resection. Data show that the post-operative mortality in non-specialized centres may amount to 20%, however, it is about 6% or less in specialist centres [40]. It is worth emphasizing that the most recent data indicate that the Whipple procedure is associated with high morbidity that may reach up to even 45% [41]. Comparing data, despite the development of research and surgical techniques and a decrease of mortality rate being approximately 1% in high-volume centres, there continues to be a high morbidity in these centres [42]. Moreover, the risk of complications occurring after pancreatic resection is estimated to be about 50% [43]. Interestingly, the development of postoperative complications contributes to poorer overall survival in patients who underwent curative surgery [44].

The surgical procedure, perioperative care and the surgical strategy should be carefully planned to assess the possibility of tumour resection in detail, decrease the risk of complications occurrence, as well as primarily to avoid unnecessary surgery, impossible due to the advancement of the tumour [44]. In addition, there are data indicating that use of neoadjuvant treatment may improve oncological outcomes and reduce the risk of surgical complications [43]. On the other hand, a retrospective study performed by Zhang and co-workers revealed that laparoscopic pancreaticoduodenectomy may be effective and feasible for managing selected patients with PDAC. This kind of operation is associated with decreased risk of the occurrence of postoperative pneumonia and abdominal infection in comparison to open pancreaticoduodenectomy [45]. Also, it is worth to emphasizing that proper qualification to the surgical treatment and careful choice of potential candidates have significant roles in adequately planning surgery and avoiding the impossibility of performing excision of a tumour due to non-resectability being confirmed during operation. This situation may result from difficult differentiation of necrosis, fibrosis, and oedematous tissue from malignant tumour cells, as well as the lack of reliable assessment of the extent and infiltration of cancer tissue demonstrated in preoperative imaging modalities [46].

3.2. Gaps in the Chemotherapy of PDAC

Over the years, new chemotherapy schemes have been developed. Chemotherapy is associated with a lot of side effects. New chemotherapeutics with low toxicity are still sought after. There are some schemes of chemotherapy for PDAC depending on the advancement of the disease: metastatic disease, resectable PDAC or locally advanced irresectable disease [47]. Barnes and co-researchers identified educational gaps according to the treatment of PDAC among oncologists in the United States. They demonstrated that 44% of oncologists did not select an evidence-based adjuvant chemotherapy regimen in patients with resectable PDAC. In turn, 57% of oncologists did not choose an evidence-based second-line chemotherapy regimen, and 35% selected a regimen containing oxaliplatin, a chemotherapeutic causing neuropathy, in a group of subjects who developed neuropathy after first-line nab-paclitaxel/gemcitabine followed by chemoradiation. In contrast, in the group with metastatic disease, only 34% of oncologists recommended a biopsy, chest imaging, and liver function tests which should be the standard of care assessments with this manifestation [48]. This study revealed significant educational gaps and discrepancies between oncologists' recommendations and standard evidence-based guidelines. Also, Hamad et al. showed disparities in stage-specific guideline-concordant cancer-directed therapy for patients with PDAC. Adherence to stage-specific standard of care treatment occurred in only 45.3% of subjects among the entire cohort and varied by stage of disease. The use of standard therapy resulted in lowered risk of death by about 47% in comparison to subjects who did not receive standard of care treatment. The discrepancies were the most frequent in the group of patients with locally advanced stage disease, and especially with older age, women, African Americans, and patients with comorbidity burden. In contrast, treatment at a high-volume centre and higher education level led to higher likelihood of receiving stage-specific standard of care treatment [49]. Also, Lima and co-researchers presented that the patients with PDAC treated at minority-serving hospitals were less likely to obtain National Comprehensive Cancer Network-compliant care, whose the lack is related to worse overall survival and reduced long-term oncological outcomes [50].

3.3. Pancreatic Exocrine Insufficiency

A lot of patients with PDAC are characterized by malnutrition and weight loss, nutrient deficiencies, and associated-cachexia. It reduces quality of life and limits the effectiveness of anti-cancer treatment. Pancreatic exocrine insufficiency (PEI), resulting from inappropriate secretion of pancreatic enzymes, belongs to the significant causes of malnutrition in PC, including PDAC [51]. Systematic review and meta-analysis from 2020 presented that PEI may affect even 72% patients with advanced PC. It is worth emphasizing that pancreatic head tumours are more likely to coexist with PEI compared to the tumours of body and tail [52]. In addition, surgical treatment may lead to PEI and it is dependent on the type of surgery. Roeyen et al. conducted a prospective cohort study and showed that 64.1% of patients required pancreatic enzyme replacement therapy (PERT) after pancreaticoduodenectomy performed for oncologic indications [53]. By definition, it is important to remember that all patients after total pancreatectomy will have PEI and require PERT. Generally, pancreaticoduodenectomy is related to increased risk of PEI compared to the distal pancreatectomy [54]. Preoperative diameter of the main pancreatic duct greater than 3 mm, hard pancreatic texture, and the use of adjuvant chemotherapy were identified as risk factors for the development of PEI in PDAC [55]. Noteworthy is the fact that the detection of PEI in PDAC is difficult, and the problem is often overlooked.

Generally, the diagnosis of PEI in PDAC is based on faecal elastase-, dietary concentration, and further dietary consultation and the use of PERT is being introduced. Comprehensive nutritional assessment, intake of smaller and more frequent meals, replacement of any deficiencies in fat-soluble vitamins, vitamin B12, iron, and lipoproteins should follow. PERT should be used in adequate dosing: recommended starting dose is approximately 40,000–50,000 units of lipase with meals and 25,000 units of lipase with snacks. Alternative doses are 500–2500 units of lipase/kg/meal, half for snacks, to a maximum of 10,000 units of lipase per kg per day [51]. Nevertheless, even adequate use of PERT cannot lead to the complete alleviation of clinical symptoms of PEI. This is due to the numerous interactions between pancreatic maldigestion, intestinal inflammation or intestinal microbiota [56].

In a retrospective study, Landers and co-researchers revealed that 72% of patients with metastatic PDAC had symptoms of PEI. However, only 21% of them supplemented PERT. This is probably due to the lack of awareness of PEI in PDAC, as well as the benefits of PERT to long-term outcomes, and insufficient screening [57]. It is worth to emphasizing that there are conflicting data about the improvement of nutritional status, quality of life and overall survival in patients with PDAC receiving PERT [51,58–60]. The contradictory evidences is limited by the small study groups, heterogeneity of the PDAC patients population (e.g., tumour localization, the presence of metastatic variant of the disease, tumour resectability), and availability of specialized dietary support for the patients in individual health centre. Generally, PERT in PDAC seems to be useful and improves patients' survival. Nevertheless, the use of PERT in PDAC is too often overlooked by clinicians.

4. Opportunities in the Diagnosis of PC

4.1. Acute Pancreatitis

Acute pancreatitis (AP) is an inflammatory disorder characterized by high mortality. In addition, the disease is one of the leading gastrointestinal causes of hospitalisation [61]. AP may be caused by the underlying PDAC.

It is well established that recurrent AP may lead to chronic pancreatitis which is a well-known PDAC risk factor. Over the past decade, numerous studies evaluated AP as a risk factor for PC. Munigala and co-researchers conducted a retrospective study using a nationwide Veterans Administration database spanning 1999–2015. They revealed that there was increased risk of PDAC 3–10 years after AP irrespective of the aetiology [62]. In addition, in a nationwide, population-based, matched cohort study, Kirkegård et al. demonstrated that subjects with AP had an elevated risk of PDAC compared to the age- and sex-matched general population [63]. Moreover, there are two meta-analyses showing the increased risk of PDAC after AP. However, AP is unlikely to be a causative factor for PDAC [64,65]. Taking into account that the risk of developing PDAC after AP decreases with time (a strong relationship between AP and PDAC occurs in the first two years after AP), it seems that AP has no causal correlation with PDAC. Therefore, AP may be sometimes the first symptom of the cancer causing obstruction of the pancreatic ducts and accompanying inflammation [66]. It is estimated that approximately 1% of AP is caused by PDAC that is usually diagnosed within a few months after the diagnosis of AP [67]. Most cases of AP caused by PDAC have a mild clinical course, which may result in limited diagnostics towards a potential malignancy. Mild AP turned out to be a predictor of PDAC, while severe AP was not associated with PDAC [67,68]. Therefore, in patients with mild AP without an identifiable cause, a possible underlying PDAC may be suspected. Furthermore, dilation of the pancreatic duct, anaemia, age over 50, newly diagnosed diabetes mellitus, evidence of CP features in imaging tests or weight loss may be factors indicating on PDAC as a cause of AP with undetermined aetiology [68–70]. Interestingly, cancers identified in patients with AP tend to be in the early stages, are smaller in size and more often resectable, leading to lower mortality compared to patients without a history of AP. This is caused by the earlier onset of clinical symptoms due to the painful AP episode [67,71–73]. Therefore, in all patients with AP without an identifiable cause, serum measurement of CA 19-9 may be considered. Teng and co-workers proved that significantly increased level of CA 19-9 in patients with AP predicts the presence of PDAC [74]. Nonetheless, the normal levels of this marker do not exclude the cancer disease.

On the other hand, there is also evidence showing AP preceding PDAC resection, especially moderate and severe, as a condition that may reduce the patient survival. It results from severe peripancreatic inflammation causing surgical resection to be difficult with higher rate of postoperative complications [75,76].

4.2. Diabetes Mellitus

Data indicate that there is bidirectional association between diabetes mellitus (DM) and PDAC. In addition, it is proved that DM may be independent risk factor, as well as a complication of PDAC. It is estimated that approximately 85% of the patients with PDAC have impaired glucose tolerance or even diabetes. Type 2 DM occurring in the elderly usually over 65 years, new onset diabetes (less than 30 days) in elderly patients, heavy smoker, low BMI, history of CP, weight loss associated with DM onset are alarming signs and indicators that may suggest PDAC [77,78]. In turn, about 0.8–1% of individuals aged over 50 years with new-onset diabetes generally have diabetes secondary to PDAC [13].

Patients with type 2 DM lasting over 5 years have a 1–1.5-fold elevated risk of PDAC compared to the general population. In contrast, the relative risk of PDAC occurring in subjects with type 2 DM in less than 1 year increases to even 5.4-fold [79]. Also, another meta-analysis demonstrated a 6.69 times increased risk of PDAC in new onset diabetes, particularly within first year of diagnosis [80]. Interestingly, new onset DM associated with PDAC is diagnosed less than 24–36 months before diagnosis of PDAC, and it's course is mitigated by surgical resection of the tumour causing primarily a reduction of fasting blood glucose [81]. Dankner and co-researchers revealed a high risk of PDAC development in both women and men (HR of 15.24 and 13.88 respectively) in the first year after the DM diagnosis in a large cohort of 2.3 million Israelis [82]. Aggarwal et al. observed a very high prevalence of DM (68%) in patients with PDAC compared to age matched other cancers subjects or non-cancer controls [83]. It is worth emphasizing that the occurrence of dysglycaemia in PDAC was detected more frequently with the standard oral glucose tolerance test (OGTT) than fasting glucose levels (78% vs. 45%) [78,83,84]. On the other hand, a significant number of new onset DM in patients with PDAC regressed after tumour resection [85]. Those data may indicate that new onset DM may represent an early biomarker for PDAC. The detailed mechanisms underlying this coincidence remain unclear. However, it is considered that PDAC may lead to DM through releasing cancer cell mediators stimulating hyperglycaemia or β-cell dysfunction and enhancing insulin resistance, such as adrenomedullin, islet amyloid polypeptide. DM is associated with β-cell dysfunction mediated by inflammation, β-cell loss occurring as a consequence of oxidative stress and aberrant activation of the inflammation- and cancer-associated pathways, inducing cell apoptosis [81]. Moreover, elevated levels of glycated haemoglobin (HbA1c) being a mark of deterioration of the existing glycaemic control may be associated with the development of PDAC. Lu and co-workers proved that the level of HbA1c has been rising from the diagnosis of DM to detecting PDAC definitely more severely than in patients without diagnosis of PDAC after detecting DM. It shows that rising HbA1c may be an independent risk factor for PDAC [84].

The routine use of radiological imaging to detect PDAC after the DM diagnosis is not cost-efficient. Imaging in this group of patients does not fulfil the criteria of screening, and the incidence of DM in the general population is too high and in the vast majority of cases, there is no PDAC. Nevertheless, imaging diagnosis, including MRI/CT of the pancreas, can be dedicated to middle age and elderly patients ($\geq$50 years) developing DM, as well as in those with rapidly altered glycaemic indices, body weight loss in the preceding months prior to DM onset, absence of typical signs of the metabolic syndrome or of family history of PDAC [86,87]. Data derived from the next next studies revealed clinical prediction models determining high-risk individuals among those with newly diagnosed DM who might benefit from PDAC screening. Sharma et al. developed a model, including age at diabetes diagnosis and change in weight and blood glucose, and stratified patients into three risk groups. The sensitivity and specificity of the cut-off for the high-risk group was 80% [88]. In contrast, Boursi et al. validated two models. The first of them takes into account inter alia age, BMI, change in BMI, smoking, use of anti-diabetic medications, serum levels of HbA1C. Its sensitivity and specificity were 45% and 94%, respectively [89]. The second model comprised age, BMI, proton pump inhibitor use, total cholesterol, low-density lipoprotein, alanine aminotransferase and alkaline phosphatase and was dedicated to patients with impaired fasting glucose. The model achieved good discrimination (area under the curve 0.71 (95% CI, 0.67–0.75) [90]. Nevertheless, DM may be helpful and suggestive of diagnosis of PDAC. However, further studies are necessary to identify new markers distinguishing PDAC-associated diabetes from typical type 2 DM.

4.3. *New Techniques of Imaging*

Konno et al. proved that intrapancreatic late enhancement of pre-diagnostic contrast-enhanced CT is relevant in the early detection of PDAC. Additionally, it occurred significantly more frequent in PDAC compared to other indirect findings of cancer, such as MPD abnormalities or focal pancreatic parenchymal atrophy. Consequently, intrapancreatic late enhancement without other indirect findings can facilitate detection of PDAC, mainly located in the head of pancreas [91]. Real-time elastography (RTE), a novel method for the assessment of tissue elasticity using ultrasound, is used in the diagnosis of various type of tumours to differentiate malignant from benign lesions. There are two semi-quantitative elastography methods: mean strain histograms (SH) and strain ratio (SR). The mean SH value corresponds to the hardness of the lesion depicted by the colour on the scale from hardest to softest. The novel diagnostic option of PDAC is shear-wave elastography (SWE) that enables quantification of mechanical and elastic tissue properties: tissue of PDAC is stiffer than the healthy parenchyma [92]. Another valuable EUS-related technique for the diagnosis of PDAC is contrast-enhanced EUS (CE-EUS). The use of contrast enhancers could provide additional information about the vascularization of the tissue and facilitate the diagnosis of malignant lesions in the pancreas. CE-EUS is able to differentiate PDAC from neuroendocrine tumours (NET), as well as primary pancreatic tumours from metastases. Generally, NET is characterized by hypervascularization and a low microvessel architecture, whereas PDAC has iso-enhancement or hypo-enhancement, arterial irregularity and absent venous vasculature within a mass. In turn, metastases are mostly hypervascular, however they may be both hypernehanced and hypoenhanced depending on type and localization of the primary tumour. In addition, this method is characterized by higher accuracy for the diagnosis of small PDAC compared to contrast-enhanced multidetector CT [92].

The combination of RTE and EUS-FNA had higher diagnostic accuracy, sensitivity, and specificity compared to EUS-FNA alone [93]. In addition, it was evidenced that pathological assay combined with analysis of KRAS-mutation using allelic discrimination demonstrated higher accuracy (88% vs. 73%) and sensitivity (93% vs. 85%) for PDAC diagnosis compared to cytopathology alone [94]. Also, novel optical system-spatial-domain low-coherence quantitative phase microscopy (SL-QPM) enhanced the accuracy of EUS-FNA cytological diagnosis and elevated the sensitivity of cytology for identifying PC from 72% to 94% [95].

4.4. *Artificial Intelligence*

Artificial intelligence (AI) is a complex integration of a computational machine system, whose aim is the replication of human intelligence to carry out given tasks and improve themselves in accordance with the information they collect. Actually, clinical practice is revolutionized by three main branches of AI, such as machine learning (ML) (including deep learning (DL)), artificial neural networks (ANN) and expert systems (ES). The use of AI may facilitate converting data into functionality perception, increasing diagnostic efficacy and predicting real-time prognosis [96,97]. Most studies concerning AI in the context of PDAC have focused on classifying cancer and healthy pancreas pictures using CT scans or differentiating PDAC from radiological mimickers in AI-assisted EUS. The AI may evaluate thousands of photos on a pixel-by-pixel basis. In addition, it is not vulnerable to human error. The rapid diagnosis is another advantage of AI. It takes less than a minute from the original CT picture being entered to diagnosis. The most recent studies used AI to PDAC diagnosis in CT, however its sensitivity and accuracy were not clearly determined [98–100].

In addition, AI could be applied in the prognosis of PDAC. Research performed by the Alliance of Pancreatic Cancer Consortium Imaging Working Group aimed to extract the pre- and post-diagnosis CT, MRI, and transabdominal ultrasound images from subjects who are eventually diagnosed with PDAC. The images will be used to create repository which may be shared and examined later, and it may contribute to constructing models of AI diagnosing PDAC at the early stages and calculating the advent of the cancer [101]. The analysis of real-world clinical records using ML approaches is another possible platform for introducing ML to the need for early detection of PDAC [102].

In the context of EUS, a lot of studies have been conducted to determine and compare the diagnostic accuracy of non-AI- and AI-enhanced models of EUS for PDAC. For example, a retrospective study performed by Kuwahara and co-researchers revealed that the sensitivity, specificity, and accuracy of the DL algorithm using EUS images as input data for detection of IPMN malignancy were approximately 95.7%, 92.6%, and 94.0%, respectively. It should be emphasized that the accuracy of this AI algorithm for identifying malignant probability was higher than human diagnosis and determination based on the presence of mural nodules in the tumour [103]. In contrast, another retrospective study assessed the utility and ability of support vector machine (SVM) AI-assisted EUS to differentiate PC from normal tissue. All patients underwent EUS-guided FNA and pathologic analysis. The researchers proved that the SVM model was characterized by the accuracy, sensitivity and specificity of 98%, 94.3%, and 99.5%, respectively, suggesting its strong potential for PC screening [104]. Furthermore, a systematic review from 2022 disclosed the general accuracy, sensitivity, and specificity in the ranges of 80–97.5%, 83–100%, and 50–99%, respectively. It indicates the high potential of AI-assisted EUS models as diagnostic tools for the detection of PDAC [105].

It is worth to emphasizing that differentiating PDAC from CP or AIP is the diagnostic challenge. It results from the fact that CP and AIP have characteristic features in sonographic and cross-sectional radiological imaging mimicking PDAC [96]. Nevertheless, there are data suggesting the use of AI-assisted EUS models to improve the sensitivity and specificity of EUS in differentiating CP and AIP from PDAC among other by using ANN, convolutional neural networks (CNN) or extended neural network (ENN) [106–108]. In spite of many advantages, the use of AI has also some limitations, including statistical management, small size of the input data, unsatisfactory quality of the input data, inefficient data handling, inadequate standardization and validation or ethical and legal aspects [97].

4.5. Circulome in PDAC

The "circulome" is described as a collection of circulating cancer cells or various particles, molecules, metabolites, such as growth factors, proteins, fatty acids, characteristic off the disease. For example, the prostate-specific antigen (PSA) is well-established marker for prostate cancer used for screening. In turn, CA 19-9 may be used in the PDAC diagnostics, however it is not useful in the screening of PDAC.

In the blood of patients with PDAC, cell-free nucleic acids (cfNAs), such as DNA, mRNA, and noncoding RNA may also be used to monitor PDAC. Circulating tumour DNA (ctDNA) derives from primary tumour or metastases and occurs in the serum as a consequence of apoptosis, lysis or necrosis of cancer cells. Therefore, ctDNA may be valuable biomarker of cancer and applied for detection of the disease. In addition, profiling ctDNA, including quality assessment of cancer genomes such as mutations, amplifications, deletions and translocations, may facilitate the identification of genetic alterations for patient stratification, and even therapeutic response prediction [109]. Moreover, the amount of ctDNA may correlate with a higher number of liver metastases, the presence of lung and/or peritoneal metastases, tumour burden and higher CA 19-9 levels [110]. In addition, ctDNA may be useful for the identification of cancer relapse: the detection of ctDNA is up to 10 months earlier than the disclosure of circulating tumours cells [111,112]. In the context of PC, a lot of studies were performed to assess the utility of ctDNA as a biomarker in PDAC. Most of them utilized K-RAS mutations to target ctDNA. Nevertheless, the sensitivity and specificity were not satisfactory and ranged between 27–81% and 33–100%, respectively [113–116]. On the other hand, the presence K-RAS mutation in serum cell-free ctDNA is unfavourable and associated with significantly shorter survival than that of patients without mutations [117]. Nevertheless, the association between the presence of K-RAS mutation in ctDNA and poor prognosis of patients with PDAC was confirmed in some studies [113,118]. Besides gene mutation, DNA methylation is an emerged diagnostics in liquid biopsy. Shen and co-researchers demonstrated that the methylation patterns in ctDNA may detect PDAC, even tumours at early stage [119]. The meta-analysis conducted by Guven et al. revealed that positive preoperative or postoperative ctDNA was correlated with lower relapse-free survival/progression-free survival (HR: 2.27, 95% CI: 1.59–3.24, $p < 0.001$) and overall survival (HR: 2.04, 95% CI: 1.29–3.21, $p = 0.002$) in localized PC. Similarly, positive baseline ctDNA was related to lower relapse-free survival/progression-free survival (HR: 2.61, 95% CI: 1.94–3.51, $p < 0.001$) and overall survival (HR: 2.41, 95% CI: 1.74–3.34, $p < 0.001$) in advanced PDAC [120]. Therefore ctDNA analyses may serve a leading role in streamlining candidate biomarkers of PDAC and could be a promising tool to individualize treatment planning and improve outcomes [121]. Unfortunately, this method is actually difficult to access.

In turn, miRNAs are small non-coding RNA molecules of about 18–22 nucleotides regulating gene expression by mRNA degradation or translatory inhibition. In addition, they play significant roles in oncogenesis and tumour metastasis, and the expression pattern of miRNA is unique to cancer type and may be a rich source of data about tumour pathogenesis. Moreover, the most recent data demonstrate that miRNAs may be used as biomarkers or even prognostic factors for many cancers, including pancreatic cancer. It is worth emphasizing that stability in serum and a convenient method of miRNA detection are the main advantages of using miRNA in the context of PDAC [122]. Eun Jo Lee et al. using pancreatic cancer, paired benign pancreatic tissue, a normal pancreas, and pancreatitis tissues along with nine cell lines and revealed miRNA expression profiles in PDAC. They showed that miRNA-345, miRNA-142-P, miRNA-139, miRNA-424, miRNA-100, miRNA-301, miRNA-212, miRNA-125b-1 were aberrantly expressed. The expression of first three was downregulated, whereas the expression of relevant molecules was upregulated in cancer samples compared to normal pancreatic samples [123]. Other data showed the overexpression of miRNA-196a, miRNA-190, miRNA-186, miRNA-221, miRNA-222, miRNA-200b, miRNA-15b, and miRNA-95, miRNA-21, miRNA-26b, miRNA-194, miRNA-200b, miRNA-200c, miRNA-320, miRNA-374 and miRNA-429 in PC tissue or PDAC cells [124]. In contrast, miRNA-96, miRNA-217, miRNA-141, miRNA-20a, and miRNA-29c were characterized by downregulated expression in PDAC samples compared to normal pancreatic tissue [125]. Furthermore, increased expression of miRNA-155 and -21 was also revealed in IPMN, one of the precursor lesions for PDAC [126]. Above data suggest a potential significance of using miRNAs as biomarkers PDAC. Also, there is evidence presenting miRNA as prognostic marker of PDAC. Also, the assessment of miRNA expression may facilitate determination of chemoresistance and responsiveness to different therapeutic options. For example, increased levels of miRNA-200c was associated with higher post-surgery survival rate [127]. In contrast, lowered expression of miRNA-200b, miRNA-200c, let-7b, let-7c, let-7d and let-7e occurred in gemcitabine-resistant cells of PDAC [128]. Described data indicate that miRNA in serum, pancreatic juice, pancreatic tissue or fluid of pancreatic cysts may represent the predictive and prognostic markers for PDAC. However, further studies are needed to establish their utility in PDAC diagnosis and prognosis.

Another component of circulome is circulating tumour cells (CTC) being cells with low abundance in the blood stream. They are detached from the primary tumour and are the main source of metastases [129,130]. Generally, CTC number in PDAC patients was an independent indicator for worse progression-free survival [131]. Unlike ctDNA, CTCs may provide a lot of information, not only genetic variation, but also the expression of genes and cytoplasm proteins, of cellular contents which are preserved and garnered by the cell membrane. In addition, it is possible to conduct ex vivo CTC culture, enabling determination of personalized therapeutic response prediction and drug screening [132,

133]. It was evidenced that the CTC count in PDAC correlated with staging, prognosis, tumour resectability, as well as contributing to an adequate choice of oncological therapy. CTC is an unique opportunity to examine an aggressive population of an individual patient's cancer cells that have achieved the metastatic step of intravasation and may determine response to the treatment [134]. The main limitation of the use of circulating pancreatic epithelial cells in the blood stream is their low amount in blood at PDAC early stages. However, technologies to extract and process large volumes of blood, such as leukapheresis, have being developed [135]. Above findings indicate that cancer cells may be detected in the circulation of patients before the development advanced PDAC, and it might be used in risk assessment and the diagnostic process. Nonetheless, large-scale prospective clinical trials with circulating pancreatic epithelial cells/CTC-guided management are still necessary to assess the clinical potential of these cells.

Despite many advantages, the assessment of circulome is difficult to assess and requires extensive laboratory facilities. The assessment of mi-RNA seems to be the most promising among other components of the circulome. However, it's actual availability is still extremely limited. Meanwhile, simple tests such as serum biomarkers, would be desirable, currently unavailable due to the complex genetic background of PDAC.

5. Opportunities in the Treatment of PDAC

Currently, there are new opportunities in the therapy of PDAC, both in radical and palliative treatment. In the context radical therapies, minimally invasive pancreaticoduodenectomy seems to be the procedure with lower risk of complications, therefore improving the prognosis of patients with PDAC [136]. In addition, mesenteric vascular resections with reconstructions are also possible during laparoscopic pancreaticoduodenectomy, which is challenging and requires advanced skills of both resection and reconstruction compared to the open pancreaticoduodenectomy [136,137]. There are few methods of minimal invasive pancreaticoduodenectomy, including total laparoscopic pancreaticoduodenectomy with both completed laparoscopic resection and digestive reconstruction, hand-assisted laparoscopic pancreaticoduodenectomy, total robotic pancreaticoduodenectomy with both resection and digestive reconstruction using da Vinci surgical system and robotic-assisted pancreaticoduodenectomy with laparoscopic dissection and reconstruction completed by da Vinci surgical system [138]. Randomized clinical trial from 2018 showed that the length of stay and post-operative complication burden were reduced after laparoscopic surgery compared to the open pancreaticoduodenectomy [139]. Interestingly, data from two meta-analyses, did not reveal significant differences in rates off surgical mortality and pancreatic fistulas or overall survival and 5-year survival after laparoscopic and open pancreaticoduodenectomy [140–143]. However, R0 resections and harvested lymph nodes were significantly higher in the group of laparoscopic pancreaticoduodenectomy [142,143]. In addition, robotic pancreaticoduodenectomy was accompanied with decreased blood loss and rate of severe complications as opposed to open surgery, as well as reduced wound infections and earlier activity after surgery. However, robotic pancreaticoduodenectomy was associated with longer operation time, and the number of experienced centres and surgeons is limited [144,145].

In the context of palliative care, there are opportunities in surgical, endoscopic and oncological treatment. Biliary obstruction occurring in non-resectable PDAC requires drainage with endoscopic retrograde cholangiopancreatography (ERCP) with stenting, or percutaneous transhepatic cholangiodrainage (PTCD). In patients with gastroduodenal obstruction, endoscopic therapy should be considered. However, the efficacy is limited due to frequent stent dislocation and recurrent obstruction. Nevertheless, in a lot of cases with PDAC, the failure of ERCP is observed. The most recent studies show high feasibility and effectiveness of EUS-guided biliary drainage (EUS-BD) for the palliation of jaundice resulting from distal malignant biliary obstruction (MBO). Therefore, after lack of success of ERCP, the EUS-BD should be considered as the next options for the treatment of MBO in PDAC. EUS-BD may be achieved through different approaches, depending on the experience and preference of the endoscopist, the availability of specific devices, the localization of the biliary obstruction and the accessibility of the papilla, such as EUS-guided antegrade stenting, EUS-guided choledochoduodenostomy (EUS-CDS) or choledocho-gastrostomy, EUS-guided hepato-gastrostomy (EUS-HGS), Rendez-vous (RV) technique, EUS-guided cholecysto-gastrostomy (as a last resort). Initially, luminal biliary stents dedicated to EUS intervention were used with predictable shortcomings in technical success, outcome and adverse effects. However, the development of new metal stents contributed to significant improvement of the EUS-BD results. Lumen-apposing metal stents (LAMS), new fully covered "dumbbell"-shaped short metal stents specifically constructed for transluminal drainage, have been created available for EUS-guided procedures, primarily intended for the management of fluid collections. In addition, electrocautery-enhanced LAMS (EC-LAMS), newer modification of LAMS, simplification of the classic multi-step procedure of EUS-BD allow direct access to the target lumen. The safety and effectiveness of EUS-BD using LAMS and EC-LAMS were confirmed, and this method seems to be one of the most often performed techniques for EUS-BD. However, adverse events, such as duodenal perforation, bleeding, transient cholangitis, stent obstruction, kinking, spontaneous dislodgement, food impaction, may occur. Further studies are needed to determine newer technical innovation in the design and delivery system, improving LAMS performance by increase the duration of patency and reduction of adverse effects during deployment [146–148].

After failure of endoscopic methods and for the remaining cases, biliary, gastroenteric or double bypass may be introduced, improving the quality of the patient's life. However, the most recent data showed that such proceedings are associated with higher mortality and morbidity compared to explorative surgery only [149]. That is why these methods should be individually implemented with due caution. Irreversible electroporation or Nanoknife ablation being non-thermal ablative techniques are valuable therapeutic methods and associated with induction of high voltage, short pulse electrical fields, leading to local cellular apoptosis [150]. These methods may destroy tumours tissue without compromising adjacent vessels or bile ducts. In consequence, they could be applied as a potential palliative option in unresectable, locally advanced PDAC [151,152]. Martin and co-researchers conducted a pilot study enrolling patients with unresectable locally advanced PDAC and performed either resection of the primary tumour with IRE (NanoKnife®) margin accentuation (n = 8) or IRE alone (n = 19). Their 3 month-observation was associated with complete tumour destruction in all subjects without local recurrence [153]. There is no evidence presenting detailed data about the impact of NanoKnife® on the survival of patients with PDAC. However, clinical trials assessing the safety and efficacy of the NanoKnife® system for the ablation of stage 3 PDAC are in progress (NCT03899636 and NCT03899649).

Palliative chemotherapy is dedicated for unresectable and metastatic PDAC patients to improve overall survival. A lot of schemes of therapies are still assessed. Multidrug schemes have advantage over schemes with one chemotherapeutic. Phase III clinical trials demonstrated that FOLFIRINOX or nab-paclitaxel with gemcitabine improved median overall survival compared to gemcitabine alone [154,155]. Also, research on adjuvant chemotherapy after surgery in PDAC is still in progress. Improvement of overall survival from single agent-adjuvant therapy using 5-FU or gemcitabine been proven [156–158]. The ESPAC-4 study presented longer overall survival after the use of gemcitabine with capecitabine as adjuvant chemotherapy in comparison to gemcitabine monotherapy (28 vs. 25.5 months) [158]. In turn, PRODIGE 24, a large multinational phase III trial, revealed the superiority of a modified FOLFIRINOX regimen (reduced irinotecan and no bolus 5-FU) over gemcitabine in the adjuvant setting, improving overall survival (54.4 months vs. 35 months). Nonetheless, more toxicity was also observed [159]. Generally, patients in good general condition are administered more aggressive treatment strategies which contribute to longer overall survival, such as the FOLFIRINOX programme or gemcitabine in combination with nab-paclitaxel (albumin-bound paclitaxel). This formulation of paclitaxel increases the drug concentration in PDAC cells by 30%. There are also new available drugs.

Olaparib, PARP inhibitor, was accepted by FDA in 2019 for metastatic PDAC treatment in patients with BRCA mutation. In turn, pembrolizumab, programmed cell death protein 1-targeted antibody, may be used for PDAC with microsatellite instability (MSI) as a second line-chemotherapy after detecting high MSI or mismatched repair deficiency. For the PDAC-patients with neurotrophic tropomyosin receptor kinase (NTRK) gene fusion mutation, other targeted drugs, such as larotrectinib and entrectinib (NTRK inhibitors) may be used as second-line therapy based on phase I and case series experience [160–162].

Over the last decade, the development and progression of studies aimed to reveal significant pathways, genes or immunological processes engaged in PDAC contributed to identification of pharmacological targets. Data show that approximately 25% of the patients with PDAC have somatic/germ line mutations in DNA damage repair (DDR) pathway (BRCA 1,2, PALB2) homologous recombination repair (HRR) genes (ATM, BAP1, BARD1, BLM, BRIP1, CHEK2, FAM175A, FANCA, FANCC, NBN, RAD50, RAD51, RAD51C, and RTEL1). The detection of DDR pathway deficiency in PDAC may be key, because these patients respond to platinum-based therapy, and they may benefit from the use of PARP inhibitors, such as olaparib [163]. In contrast, mutations of K-RAS gen, especially codon 12, are detected in about 95% patients with PDAC [164]. K-RAS therapeutics are actually subjects of numerous research. For example, agents, such as sotorasib and adagrasib, K-RAS G12C inhibitors, revealed clinically meaningful benefit and safety [163,165].

PDAC is considered immunologically "cold", and the past studies did not reveal any response to immunotherapy. Nevertheless, studies using immunological mechanisms in the context of PDAC are still in progress. There is some evidence aimed at making tumours immunologically active by stimulation innate lymphocytes or inducing an inflammatory reaction in the tumour microenvironment. Leidner and co-researchers proved the utility of neoantigen T-cell receptor gene therapy in progressive metastatic PDAC. The infusion of genetically engineered autologous T cells led to the regression of visceral metastases [166]. Selvanesan and co-workers administered non-disease-causing Listeria bacteria carrying a gene encoding for tetanus toxin into mice model of PDAC. The tetanus toxin-induced memory T cells stimulated cytotoxic T cells in tumour microenvironment, leading to a reduction of tumour size and then low dose gemcitabine was administered [167]. There is a clinical trial (NCT04999969) assessing the role of AZD 0171 (anti LIF1 monoclonal antibody), durvalumab (PDL-1 inhibitor) in combination with gemcitabine and nabpaclitaxel in an open label phase II study. In turn, antibodies, such as ipilimumab and nivolumab, may prove to be efficient in patients with PDAC concomitant with harbouring germ line HRD genetic mutations, resistant to platinum-based chemotherapy and PARP inhibitors [168]. A lot of novel drugs dedicated to metastatic PDAC targeting metabolism, tumour stroma, oncogenic pathways and immunosuppression are in clinical development [169]. Nevertheless, the development of next-generation sequencing testing, molecular experiments and genetic assays in the context of PDAC are necessary for the development of targeted and personalized therapy in PDAC.

Neoadjuvant radiotherapy should be also developed. The PREOPANC-1 study from 2018 presented evidence of the utility of neoadjuvant chemoradiation in border-line resectable patients. The 246 patients with borderline resectable PDAC into either neoadjuvant gemcitabine with 36 Gy radiation administered between two cycles of gemcitabine or upfront surgery. It is worth emphasizing that both groups received adjuvant chemotherapy. A smaller number of patients in the chemoradiation group underwent surgical resection (62% vs. 72%). However, these subjects achieved significantly better R0 resection rate (65% vs. 31%), disease-free survival (median 11.2 vs. 7.9 months) and overall survival (median 17.1 vs. 13.3 months) [170]. Therefore, neoadjuvant chemoradiation may be an opportunity for some patients with borderline resectable PDAC. In contrast, CivaSheet, an FDA-cleared implantable sheet with a matrix of unidirectional planar low-dose-rate (LDR) Palladium-103 (Pd-103) sources, could be considered and used in the treatment of borderline resectable PDAC. Achievement of negative surgical margins remains technically challenging after pancreatectomy, and positive margins lead to increased local recurrences and worse overall survival. The CivaSheet may easily be implanted at the time of surgical treatment [171]. On the other hand, ablation treatments may be considered in the management of unresectable locally advanced PDAC without metastases. Nevertheless, expertise is required to use this method and to avoid serious or fatal complications [172]. Interestingly, irreversible electroporation has an advantage over radiofrequency ablation after induction chemotherapy for treating locally advanced PC. It is worth emphasizing that the comparable efficacy of these two therapies was presented for tumours larger than 4 cm [173].

The most recent data present photodynamic therapy as a valuable therapeutic method supporting adjuvant therapy of PDAC. It may be implemented in the treatment of a multifocal disease with the least amount of health tissue damage. The use of photodynamic therapy leads to cancer cell apoptosis, the damage of pathological vessels and even enhancement of anti-cancer immune response. However, the desired effect may not be achieved due to resistance mechanisms of PDAC cells or limitations of current photosensitizers, such as restricted penetration depth, poor targeted therapy and inappropriate generation of reactive oxygen species. Photodynamic therapy may be an adjuvant therapeutic option after surgery and combined with chemotherapy to clear residual lesions both locally and systematically. Also, the combination of photodynamic therapy with chemotherapeutics may effectively decrease their doses, resulting in reduced systemic toxicity. Moreover, photodynamic therapy may be applied as supportive therapy in metastatic PDAC and achieve satisfactory outcomes, leading to reduction of patients' suffering. Despite described advantages of the use of photodynamic therapy in PDAC, further clinical trials are necessary to confirm its utility. It seems that the development of novel hypotoxic photosensitizers may have a key role for improvement of the application of photodynamic therapy in multimodality treatment of PDAC [174,175].

On the other hand, the drug resistance is a key factor limiting therapy effectiveness and remains a significant clinical oncology challenge. It seems that the use of nanotechnology may overcome this restriction. Data revealed that the application of nanomedicine in PDAC was related to beneficial effects, such as bypass drug efflux pumps, sensitization to radiotherapy or counteracting immune suppression, which collectively mitigated various mechanisms of tumour resistance. Mainly, in the context of PDAC, nanomedicine is tested using nanoparticles being drug delivery systems. They improve pharmacokinetics of drugs, protect against degradation and regulate controlled release, contributing to precision targeting of drugs to the tumour. So far, two clinically approved nanomedicines, Abraxane (paclitaxel) and Onivyde (irinotecan), are used in the treatment of PDAC, with numerous others demonstrating promise as agents at various stages of development. Therefore, novel bioformulations of drugs may occur important for improvement of the PDAC therapy and change the outlook for PDAC patients. Nevertheless, further clinical trials are needed and they should include co-load multiple cargoes within a single nanoparticle platform, allowing for the aggressive targeting of multiple aspects of PDAC pathophysiology [176].

Noteworthy is microbiome that plays a key role in the development and progression of many cancers. Data showed the association between oral and tumour microbiome, and PDAC. Changes in abundances of some bacteria taxa were observed. For example, McKinley and co-researchers presented translocation of oral microbiota into the PDAC tumour microenvironment. *Veillonella atypica* was the most prevalent and abundant taxon found within both saliva and tumour tissue samples. In addition, it was cultured from patient saliva, sequenced and annotated, identifying genes potentially contributing to tumorigenesis. High sequence similarity was revealed between sequences recovered from patient matched saliva and tumour tissue, indicating that the taxa identified in PDAC tumours may derive from the mouth [177]. In contrast, Kabwe et al. proved that *Porphyromonas* can promote the growth of PC. There is evidence that bacteriophages may access and treat multiantibiotic resistant pancreatic infections. Therefore, the use of bacteriophages may modulate pancreatic microbiome, reducing the development of PDAC [178]. Interestingly, the bacteria most associated with PC are *Gammaproteobacteria*, including *Enterobacter and Pseudomonas*, that may produce cytidine deaminase and stimulate the metabolism of gemcitabine into its inactive form, 2′,2′-difluorodeoxyuridine, contributing to the degradation and resistance of gemcitabine. The combination of gemcitabine and antibiotics is more efficient than gemcitabine alone [179,180]. However, the use of penicillin is closely associated with the occurrence of PDAC, and the association increased with the number of antibiotic courses. This dependence was confirmed by determining adjusted odds-ratios and 95% confidence intervals using conditional logistic regression in a nested case-control study using a large population-based electronic medical record database [181]. In turn, the application of probiotics during chemotherapy of PDAC may enhance the efficacy of chemotherapeutics. It was evidenced that probiotics combined with chemotherapy are able to increase the DNA damage of PDAC cells, inhibit the cancer cells cycle or even stimulate cell apoptosis. In addition, probiotics may restore the number of platelets damaged by gemcitabine [180,182]. On the other hand, probiotics containing *Lactobacillus* and *Bifidobacterium* have a protective effect on radiotherapy-induced intestinal toxicity and may significantly decrease the incidence of severe diarrhoea [183,184]. Interestingly, faecal microbiome transplantation is still tested in the context of PDAC [180]. Nevertheless, there is a need for intensification of studies assessing the role of microbiota, microbiome, antibiotics and probiotics in the development and progression of PDAC

The most recent data show that effectiveness and safety of administration of oncolytic viruses in the treatment of PDAC. Oncolytic viruses created by modified engineering of the oncolytic viruses' genome and insertion of intended transgenes including cytokines or shRNAs may inhibit development of tumours directly and some through activation of immune responses. This treatment caused increased patient survival compared to the control group. However, using oncolytic viruses alone has not been efficient in the inhibition of tumours development [185].

There is no strong evidence of the improvement of overall survival after therapies using oncolytic viruses or microbiome. Surgical treatment, adequate chemotherapy and eventually radiotherapy lengthen the lives of patients with PDAC, however only for several months.

6. Summary

There are some gaps in the diagnosis and treatment of PDAC (Figures 1 and 2), inducing a lot of challenges and problems requiring improvement (Table 3). The early diagnosis of PDAC, which is key and necessary to extend survival, remains challenging. It requires improvements in diagnostic technology and methodologies. Unfortunately, actually there is no role for the use of any routine biomarker in the diagnosis of PDAC.

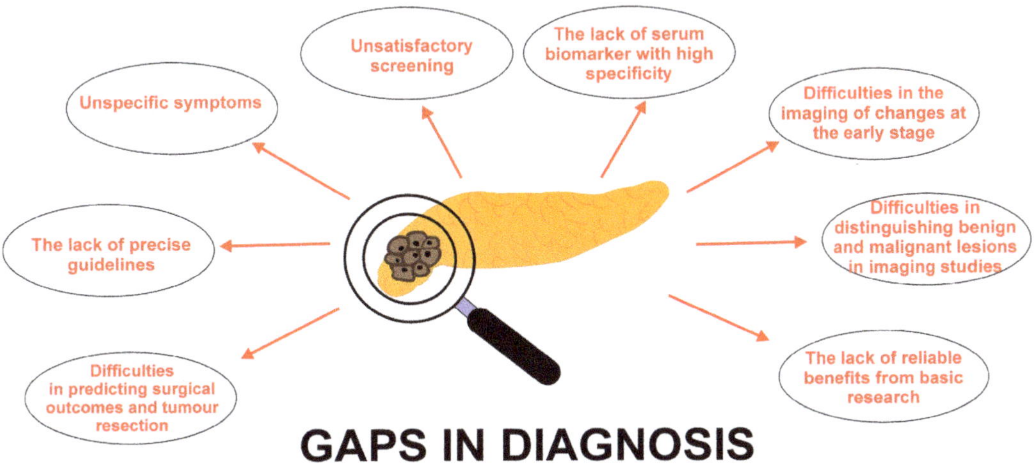

Figure 1. Main gaps of PDAC diagnosis.

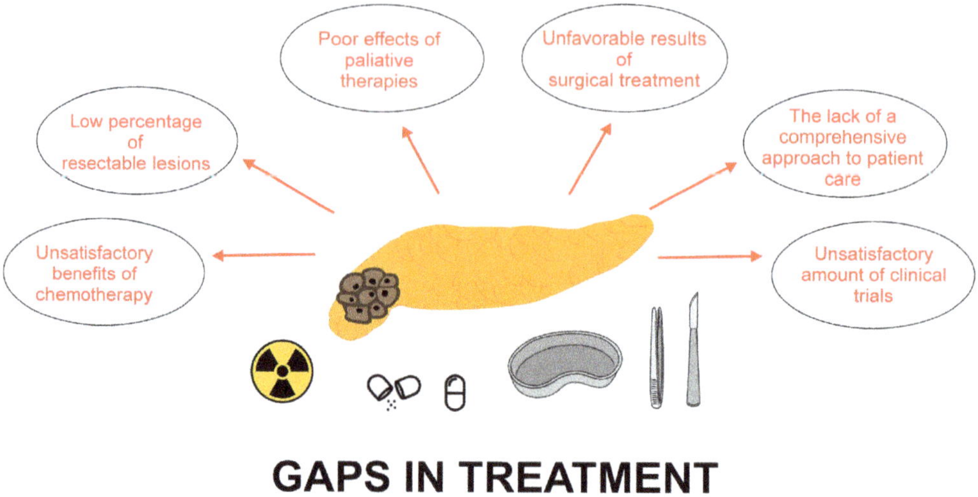

Figure 2. Main gaps of PDAC treatment.

Table 3. Table summarizing the recent challenges faced in treatment and diagnosis of PDAC.

Strategy	Challenges
Awareness	Poor awareness of the early signs and symptoms of PDAC amongst mainly older people and clinicians; Limited awareness of the burden of PDAC on the population with risk factor among clinicians; Poor awareness of the risk factor of PDAC among general population;
Detection and diagnosis	The lack of screening with proven efficacy; Limited capacities and use of comprehensive assessment to help shape of diagnosis pathways for patients with PDAC; Limited efficacy of available diagnostic methods for diagnosis of PDAC; The biology of PDAC hard to understand;
Treatment and care	Limited access to quality care in some regions of the world; Poor national development/integration of guidelines for the assessment and treatment of patients with PDAC; Limited capacities to manage patients with PDAC, especially these with multiple morbidities; Poor therapeutic response; Delays in time to approval of life-saving treatment; Insufficient development of targeted therapy;
Health system integration	Limited integration of training in oncology within core medical and nursing training; Global shortage of specialists to support a multidisciplinary treatment approach; Limited financial and other protection measures for patients with PDAC; Limited availability of oncology clinics; Variable integration of services within national health system and cancer planning; Differences in healthcare and financial outlays in various countries;
Research	Insufficient amount of clinical trials in the context of new therapeutic options with high efficacy in PDAC; Poor integration of patients with PDAC into clinical trials, which reduces their relevance; Limited translational research into the needs of patients with PDAC; Limited data on the investment-case;

Actually, there are some main issues that require repair to improve the diagnosis and treatment of PDAC. Firstly, it is worth enhancing our understanding of this complex disease by the organization of campaigns promoting knowledge and awareness of the disease in the societies of the countries, establishment of management plans with improvement of the role of PDAC in national cancer control programmes or changes in early recognition of PDAC through national campaigns targeting patients and physicians. These actions may contribute to earlier detection of the disease, raising survival. Secondly, it is necessary to pay special attention to symptoms, such as pain not reacting to protein pump inhibitors, back pain not associated with spine diseases. Thirdly, new correct tools for earlier diagnosis are necessary to adequately identify cancer at early stage of disease advancement. The development of novel imaging technologies to detect PDAC at a very early stage and the identification of biomarkers suitable for reliable detection may be critical. New technological solutions supporting currently available radiological and endoscopic imaging, such as artificial intelligence, as well as new imaging technologies should be extensively developed to increase the diagnostic accuracy of imaging. Another important aspect is the evolution of strategies to overcome resistance to systemic therapies by development of molecular treatment approaches targeting both tumour cells and components of the surrounding microenvironment.

7. Conclusions

Further clinical studies are needed to improve the diagnosis and treatment of PDAC by identifying new pharmacological targets, therapeutic options and biomarkers of the disease, as well as novel diagnostic imaging. Actually, it is necessary to develop new preventive, diagnostic and therapeutic strategies that could improve the effectiveness of PDAC treatment. The identification of new diagnostic markers may prove to be key for early diagnosis of PDAC, improving patients' prognosis and their overall survival.

Author Contributions: Conceptualization, E.M.-W. and M.C.; methodology, M.C; validation, E.M.-W.; resources, M.C. and E.M.-W.; writing-original draft preparation, M.C. and E.M.-W.; writing-review and editing, E.M.-W. and M.C.; supervision, E.M.-W. All authors have read and agreed to the published version of the manuscript.

Funding: The study was supported by grant No. 503/1-002-01/503-11-001 from the Medical University of Lodz, Poland.

Conflicts of Interest: The authors declare no conflict of interest.

Abbreviations

AI: artificial intelligence; AP, acute pancreatitis; CP, chronic pancreatitis; CTC, circulating tumour cells; PC, pancreatic cancer; PDAC, pancreatic ductal adenocarcinoma; PEI, pancreatic exocrine insufficiency

References

1. Klein, A.P. Pancreatic cancer epidemiology: Understanding the role of lifestyle and inherited risk factors. *Nat. Rev. Gastroenterol. Hepatol.* **2021**, *18*, 493–502. [CrossRef]
2. Sung, H.; Ferlay, J.; Siegel, R.L.; Laversanne, M.; Soerjomataram, I.; Jemal, A.; Bray, F. Global Cancer Statistics 2020: GLOBOCAN Estimates of Incidence and Mortality Worldwide for 36 Cancers in 185 Countries. *CA Cancer J. Clin.* **2021**, *71*, 209–249. [CrossRef]
3. Siegel, R.L.; Miller, K.D.; Fuchs, H.E.; Jemal, A. Cancer statistics, 2022. *CA Cancer J. Clin.* **2022**, *72*, 7–33. [CrossRef]
4. Okusaka, T.; Furuse, J. Recent advances in chemotherapy for pancreatic cancer: Evidence from Japan and recommendations in guidelines. *J. Gastroenterol.* **2020**, *55*, 369–382. [CrossRef]
5. Rahib, L.; Smith, B.D.; Aizenberg, R.; Rosenzweig, A.B.; Fleshman, J.M.; Matrisian, L.M. Projecting cancer incidence and deaths to 2030: The unexpected burden of thyroid, liver, and pancreas cancers in the united states. *Cancer Res.* **2014**, *74*, 2913–2921. [CrossRef]
6. Moutinho-Ribeiro, P.; Iglesias-Garcia, J.; Gaspar, R.; Macedo, G. Early pancreatic cancer—The role of endoscopic ultrasound with or without tissue acquisition in diagnosis and staging. *Dig. Liver Dis.* **2019**, *51*, 4–9. [CrossRef] [PubMed]
7. Luu, A.M.; Fahlbusch, T.; Munding, J.; Uhl, W.; Braumann, C. The Unusual Suspects of the Pancreas—Understanding Pancreatic Acinar Cell Carcinomas and Adenomas. *J. Gastrointest. Cancer* **2020**, *51*, 172–178. [CrossRef] [PubMed]
8. Caban, M.; Małecka-Wojciesko, E. Pancreatic Incidentaloma. *J. Clin. Med.* **2022**, *11*, 4648. [CrossRef]
9. Roth, M.T.; Berlin, J.D. Current Concepts in the Treatment of Resectable Pancreatic Cancer. *Curr. Oncol. Rep.* **2018**, *20*, 39. [CrossRef] [PubMed]

10. Furuse, J.; Shibahara, J.; Sugiyama, M. Development of chemotherapy and significance of conversion surgery after chemotherapy in unresectable pancreatic cancer. *J. Hepatobiliary Pancreat. Sci.* **2018**, *25*, 261–268. [CrossRef] [PubMed]
11. Liu, S.; Cai, Y.; Changyong, E.; Sheng, J.; Zhang, X. Screening and Validation of Independent Predictors of Poor Survival in Pancreatic Cancer. *Pathol. Oncol. Res.* **2021**, *27*, 1609868. [CrossRef] [PubMed]
12. Ansari, D.; Tingstedt, B.; Andersson, B.; Holmquist, F.; Sturesson, C.; Williamsson, C.; Sasor, A.; Borg, D.; Bauden, M.; Andersson R. Pancreatic cancer: Yesterday, today and tomorrow. *Futur. Oncol.* **2016**, *12*, 1929–1946. [CrossRef] [PubMed]
13. Pereira, S.P.; Oldfield, L.; Ney, A.; Hart, P.A.; Keane, M.G.; Pandol, S.J.; Li, D.; Greenhalf, W.; Jeon, C.Y.; Koay, E.J.; et al. Early detection of pancreatic cancer. *Lancet Gastroenterol. Hepatol.* **2020**, *5*, 698–710. [CrossRef] [PubMed]
14. Mizrahi, J.D.; Surana, R.; Valle, J.W.; Shroff, R.T. Pancreatic cancer. *Lancet* **2020**, *395*, 2008–2020. [CrossRef] [PubMed]
15. Walter, F.M.; Mills, K.; Mendonça, S.C.; Abel, G.A.; Basu, B.; Carroll, N.; Ballard, S.; Lancaster, J.; Hamilton, W.; Rubin, G.P.; et al Symptoms and patient factors associated with diagnostic intervals for pancreatic cancer (SYMPTOM pancreatic study): A prospective cohort study. *Lancet Gastroenterol. Hepatol.* **2016**, *1*, 298–306. [CrossRef] [PubMed]
16. Poly, T.N.; Islam, M.M.; Walther, B.A.; Lin, M.C.; Li, Y.C. Proton Pump Inhibitors Use and the Risk of Pancreatic Cancer: Evidence from Eleven Epidemiological Studies, Comprising 1.5 Million Individuals. *Cancers* **2022**, *14*, 5357. [CrossRef] [PubMed]
17. Maguchi, H.; Takashi, K.; Osanai, M.; Katanuma, A. Small pancreatic lesions: Is there need for EUS-FNA preoperatively? What to do with the incidental lesions? *Endoscopy* **2006**, *38*, 53–56. [CrossRef]
18. Yang, J.; Xu, R.; Wang, C.; Qiu, J.; Ren, B.; You, L. Early screening and diagnosis strategies of pancreatic cancer: A comprehensive review. *Cancer Commun.* **2021**, *41*, 1257–1274. [CrossRef]
19. Grassia, R.; Imperatore, N.; Capone, P.; Cereatti, F.; Forti, E.; Antonini, F.; Tanzi, G.P.; Martinotti, M.; Buffoli, F.; Mutignani, M.; et al EUS-guided tissue acquisition in chronic pancreatitis: Differential diagnosis between pancreatic cancer and pseudotumoral masses using EUS-FNA or core biopsy. *Endosc. Ultrasound* **2020**, *9*, 122–129. [CrossRef]
20. Facciorusso, A.; Singh Bajwa, H.; Menon, K.; Buccino, V.R.; Muscatiello, N. Comparison between 22G aspiration and 22G biopsy needles for EUS-guided sampling of pancreatic lesions: A meta-analysis. *Endosc. Ultrasound* **2020**, *9*, 167–174. [CrossRef]
21. Facciorusso, A.; Mohan, B.P.; Crinò, S.F.; Ofosu, A.; Ramai, D.; Lisotti, A.; Chandan, S.; Fusaroli, P. Contrast-enhanced harmonic endoscopic ultrasound-guided fine-needle aspiration versus standard fine-needle aspiration in pancreatic masses: A meta-analysis. *Expert Rev. Gastroenterol. Hepatol.* **2021**, *15*, 821–828. [CrossRef] [PubMed]
22. Kanno, A.; Masamune, A.; Hanada, K.; Maguchi, H.; Shimizu, Y.; Ueki, T.; Hasebe, O.; Ohtsuka, T.; Nakamura, M.; Takenaka, M.; et al. Multicenter study of early pancreatic cancer in Japan. *Pancreatology* **2018**, *18*, 61–67. [CrossRef]
23. Bunganič, B.; Laclav, M.; Dvořáková, T.; Bradáč, O.; Traboulsi, E.; Suchánek, Š.; Frič, P.; Zavoral, M. Accuracy of EUS and CEH EUS for the diagnosis of pancreatic tumours. *Scand. J. Gastroenterol.* **2018**, *53*, 1411–1417. [CrossRef]
24. Yamashita, Y.; Shimokawa, T.; Napoléon, B.; Fusaroli, P.; Gincul, R.; Kudo, M.; Kitano, M. Value of contrast-enhanced harmonic endoscopic ultrasonography with enhancement pattern for diagnosis of pancreatic cancer: A meta-analysis. *Dig. Endosc.* **2019**, *31*, 125–133. [CrossRef] [PubMed]
25. Shahidi, N.; Ou, G.; Lam, E.; Enns, R.; Telford, J. When trainees reach competency in performing endoscopic ultrasound: A systematic review. *Endosc. Int. Open* **2017**, *5*, E239–E243. [CrossRef] [PubMed]
26. Ang, T.L.; Kwek, A.B.E.; Wang, L.M. Diagnostic endoscopic ultrasound: Technique, current status and future directions. *Gut Liver* **2018**, *12*, 483–496. [CrossRef]
27. Harmsen, F.J.; Domagk, D.; Dietrich, C.F.; Hocke, M. Discriminating chronic pancreatitis from pancreatic cancer: Contrast-enhanced EUS and multidetector computed tomography in direct comparison. *Endosc. Ultrasound* **2018**, *7*, 395–403. [CrossRef]
28. Siegel, R.L.; Miller, K.D.; Wagle, N.S.; Jemal, A. Cancer statistics, 2023. *CA Cancer J. Clin.* **2023**, *73*, 17–48. [CrossRef]
29. Goggins, M.; Overbeek, K.A.; Brand, R.; Syngal, S.; Del Chiaro, M.; Bartsch, D.K.; Bassi, C.; Carrato, A.; Farrell, J.; Fishman, E.K.; et al. Management of patients with increased risk for familial pancreatic cancer: Updated recommendations from the International Cancer of the Pancreas Screening (CAPS) Consortium. *Gut* **2020**, *69*, 7–17. [CrossRef]
30. Vasen, H.; Ibrahim, I.; Robbers, K.; Van Mil, A.M.; Potjer, T.; Bonsing, B.A.; Bergman, W.; Wasser, M.; Morreau, H.; De Vos Tot Nederveen Cappel, W.H.; et al. Benefit of surveillance for pancreatic cancer in high-risk individuals: Outcome of long-term prospective follow-up studies from three European expert centers. *J. Clin. Oncol.* **2016**, *34*, 2010–2019. [CrossRef]
31. Canto, M.I.; Almario, J.A.; Schulick, R.D.; Yeo, C.J.; Klein, A.; Blackford, A.; Shin, E.J.; Sanyal, A.; Yenokyan, G.; Lennon, A.M.; et al. Risk of Neoplastic Progression in Individuals at High Risk for Pancreatic Cancer Undergoing Long-term Surveillance. *Gastroenterology* **2018**, *155*, 740–751.e2. [CrossRef] [PubMed]
32. Cai, J.; Chen, H.; Lu, M.; Zhang, Y.; Lu, B.; You, L.; Zhang, T.; Dai, M.; Zhao, Y. Advances in the epidemiology of pancreatic cancer: Trends, risk factors, screening, and prognosis. *Cancer Lett.* **2021**, *520*, 1–11. [CrossRef] [PubMed]
33. Hasan, S.; Jacob, R.; Manne, U.; Paluri, R. Advances in pancreatic cancer biomarkers. *Oncol. Rev.* **2019**, *13*, 69–76. [CrossRef]
34. Kapszewicz, M.; Małecka-Wojciesko, E. Simple serum pancreatic ductal adenocarcinoma (Pdac) protein biomarkers—Is there anything in sight? *J. Clin. Med.* **2021**, *10*, 5463. [CrossRef] [PubMed]
35. Rychlíková, J.; Vecka, M.; Jáchymová, M.; Macášek, J.; Hrabák, P.; Zeman, M.; Vávrová, L.; Řoupal, J.; Krechler, T.; Ák, A. Osteopontin as a discriminating marker for pancreatic cancer and chronic pancreatitis. *Cancer Biomark.* **2016**, *17*, 55–65. [CrossRef]
36. Aronen, A.; Aittoniemi, J.; Huttunen, R.; Nikkola, A.; Rinta-Kiikka, I.; Nikkola, J.; Limnell, O.; Nordback, I.; Sand, J.; Laukkarinen, J. Plasma suPAR may help to distinguish between chronic pancreatitis and pancreatic cancer. *Scand. J. Gastroenterol.* **2021**, *56*, 81–85. [CrossRef]

37. Martínez-Bosch, N.; Cristóbal, H.; Iglesias, M.; Gironella, M.; Barranco, L.; Visa, L.; Calafato, D.; Jiménez-Parrado, S.; Earl, J.; Carrato, A.; et al. Soluble AXL is a novel blood marker for early detection of pancreatic ductal adenocarcinoma and differential diagnosis from chronic pancreatitis. *eBioMedicine* **2022**, *75*, 103797. [CrossRef]
38. Ghassem-Zadeh, S.; Gaida, M.M.; Szanyi, S.; Acha-Orbea, H.; Frossard, J.L.; Hinz, U.; Hackert, T.; Strobel, O.; Felix, K. Distinct pathophysiological cytokine profiles for discrimination between autoimmune pancreatitis, chronic pancreatitis, and pancreatic ductal adenocarcinoma. *J. Transl. Med.* **2017**, *15*, 126. [CrossRef]
39. Wood, L.D.; Canto, M.I.; Jaffee, E.M.; Simeone, D.M. Pancreatic Cancer: Pathogenesis, Screening, Diagnosis, and Treatment. *Gastroenterology* **2022**, *163*, 386–402.e1. [CrossRef]
40. Halloran, C.M.; Ghaneh, P.; Bosonnet, L.; Hartley, M.N.; Sutton, R.; Neoptolemos, J.P. Complicaions of pancreatic cancer resection. *Dig. Surg.* **2002**, *19*, 138–146. [CrossRef]
41. Robatel, S.; Schenk, M. Current Limitations and Novel Perspectives in Pancreatic Cancer Treatment. *Cancers* **2022**, *14*, 985. [CrossRef]
42. Simon, R. Complications After Pancreaticoduodenectomy. *Surg. Clin. N. Am.* **2021**, *101*, 865–874. [CrossRef] [PubMed]
43. Henry, A.C.; Van Dongen, J.C.; Van Goor, I.W.J.M.; Smits, F.J.; Nagelhout, A.; Besselink, M.G.; Busch, O.R.; Bonsing, B.A.; Bosscha, K.; Van Dam, R.M.; et al. Impact of complications after resection of pancreatic cancer on disease recurrence and survival, and mediation effect of adjuvant chemotherapy: Nationwide, observational cohort study. *BJS Open* **2023**, *7*, zrac174. [CrossRef] [PubMed]
44. Aoyama, T.; Murakawa, M.; Katayama, Y.; Yamaoku, K.; Kanazawa, A.; Higuchi, A.; Shiozawa, M.; Morimoto, M.; Yoshikawa, T.; Yamamoto, N.; et al. Impact of postoperative complications on survival and recurrence in pancreatic cancer. *Anticancer Res.* **2015**, *35*, 2401–2409. [PubMed]
45. Zhang, B.; Xu, Z.; Gu, W.; Zhou, J.; Tang, N.; Zhang, S.; Chen, C.; Zhang, Z. Postoperative complications and short-term prognosis of laparoscopic pancreaticoduodenectomy vs. open pancreaticoduodenectomy for treating pancreatic ductal adenocarcinoma: A retrospective cohort study. *World J. Surg. Oncol.* **2023**, *21*, 26. [CrossRef]
46. Handgraaf, H.J.M.; Boonstra, M.C.; Van Erkel, A.R.; Bonsing, B.A.; Putter, H.; Van De Velde, C.J.H.; Vahrmeijer, A.L.; Mieog, J.S.D. Current and Future Intraoperative Imaging Strategies to Increase Radical Resection Rates in Pancreatic Cancer Surgery. *Biomed Res. Int.* **2014**, *2014*, 890230. [CrossRef]
47. Springfeld, C.; Jäger, D.; Büchler, M.W.; Strobel, O.; Hackert, T.; Palmer, D.H.; Neoptolemos, J.P. Chemotherapy for pancreatic cancer. *Press. Medicale* **2019**, *48*, e159–e174. [CrossRef]
48. Barnes, J.A.; Ellis, M.L.; Hwang, S.; Emarine, J.; Merwin, P.; Salinas, G.D.; Musher, B.L. Identification of Educational Gaps among Oncologists Who Manage Patients with Pancreatic Cancer. *J. Gastrointest. Cancer* **2019**, *50*, 84–90. [CrossRef]
49. Hamad, A.; DePuccio, M.; Reames, B.N.; Dave, A.; Kurien, N.; Cloyd, J.M.; Shen, C.; Pawlik, T.M.; Tsung, A.; McAlearney, A.S.; et al. Disparities in Stage-Specific Guideline-Concordant Cancer-Directed Treatment for Patients with Pancreatic Adenocarcinoma. *J. Gastrointest. Surg.* **2021**, *25*, 2889–2901. [CrossRef]
50. Lima, H.A.; Alaimo, L.; Moazzam, Z.; Endo, Y.; Woldesenbet, S.; Katayama, E.; Munir, M.M.; Shaikh, C.; Ruff, S.M.; Dillhoff, M.; et al. Disparities in NCCN Guideline-Compliant Care for Patients with Early-Stage Pancreatic Adenocarcinoma at Minority-Serving versus Non-Minority-Serving Hospitals. *Ann. Surg. Oncol.* **2023**, *30*, 4363–4372. [CrossRef]
51. Lan, X.; Robin, G.; Kasnik, J.; Wong, G.; Abdel-Rahman, O. Challenges in Diagnosis and Treatment of Pancreatic Exocrine Insufficiency among Patients with Pancreatic Ductal Adenocarcinoma. *Cancers* **2023**, *15*, 1331. [CrossRef]
52. de la Iglesia, D.; Avci, B.; Kiriukova, M.; Panic, N.; Bozhychko, M.; Sandru, V.; de-Madaria, E.; Capurso, G. Pancreatic exocrine insufficiency and pancreatic enzyme replacement therapy in patients with advanced pancreatic cancer: A systematic review and meta-analysis. *United Eur. Gastroenterol. J.* **2020**, *8*, 1115–1125. [CrossRef]
53. Roeyen, G.; Jansen, M.; Hartman, V.; Chapelle, T.; Bracke, B.; Ysebaert, D.; De Block, C. The impact of pancreaticoduodenectomy on endocrine and exocrine pancreatic function: A prospective cohort study based on pre- and postoperative function tests. *Pancreatology* **2017**, *17*, 974–982. [CrossRef] [PubMed]
54. Tseng, D.S.J.; Molenaar, I.Q.; Besselink, M.G.; Van Eijck, C.H.; Rinkes, I.H.B.; Van Santvoort, H.C. Pancreatic exocrine insufficiency in patients with pancreatic or periampullary cancer a systematic review. *Pancreas* **2016**, *45*, 325–330. [CrossRef] [PubMed]
55. Budipramana, V.S.; Witarto, A.P.; Witarto, B.S.; Pramudito, S.L.; Ratri, L.C.; Wairooy, N.A.P.; Putra, A.J.E. Risk factors for exocrine pancreatic insufficiency after pancreatic surgery: A systematic review and meta-analysis. *Can. J. Surg.* **2022**, *65*, E770–E781. [CrossRef]
56. Pezzilli, R.; Caccialanza, R.; Capurso, G.; Brunetti, O.; Milella, M.; Falconi, M. Pancreatic enzyme replacement therapy in pancreatic cancer. *Cancers* **2020**, *12*, 275. [CrossRef]
57. Landers, A.; Muircroft, W.; Brown, H. Pancreatic enzyme replacement therapy (PERT) for malabsorption in patients with metastatic pancreatic cancer. *BMJ Support. Palliat. Care* **2016**, *6*, 75–79. [CrossRef] [PubMed]
58. Woo, S.M.; Joo, J.; Kim, S.Y.; Park, S.J.; Han, S.S.; Kim, T.H.; Koh, Y.H.; Chung, S.H.; Kim, Y.H.; Moon, H.; et al. Efficacy of pancreatic exocrine replacement therapy for patients with unresectable pancreatic cancer in a randomized trial. *Pancreatology* **2016**, *16*, 1099–1105. [CrossRef]
59. Zdenkowski, N.; Radvan, G.; Pugliese, L.; Charlton, J.; Oldmeadow, C.; Fraser, A.; Bonaventura, A. Treatment of pancreatic insufficiency using pancreatic extract in patients with advanced pancreatic cancer: A pilot study (PICNIC). *Support. Care Cancer* **2017**, *25*, 1963–1971. [CrossRef]

60. Saito, T.; Nakai, Y.; Isayama, H.; Hirano, K.; Ishigaki, K.; Hakuta, R.; Takeda, T.; Saito, K.; Umefune, G.; Akiyama, D.; et al. A Multicenter Open-Label Randomized Controlled Trial of Pancreatic Enzyme Replacement Therapy in Unresectable Pancreatic Cancer. *Pancreas* **2018**, *47*, 800–806. [CrossRef]
61. Wos-Wroniewicz, E.; Caban, M.; Malecka-Panas, E. Role of adipokines in the assessment of severity and predicting the clinical course of acute pancreatitis. *J. Physiol. Pharmacol.* **2020**, *71*, 605–614. [CrossRef]
62. Munigala, S.; Almaskeen, S.; Subramaniam, D.S.; Bandi, S.; Bowe, B.; Xian, H.; Sheth, S.G.; Burroughs, T.E.; Agarwal, B. Acute Pancreatitis Recurrences Augment Long-Term Pancreatic Cancer Risk. *Am. J. Gastroenterol.* **2023**, *118*, 727–737. [CrossRef] [PubMed]
63. Kirkegård, J.; Cronin-Fenton, D.; Heide-Jørgensen, U.; Mortensen, F.V. Acute Pancreatitis and Pancreatic Cancer Risk: A Nationwide Matched-Cohort Study in Denmark. *Gastroenterology* **2018**, *154*, 1729–1736. [CrossRef] [PubMed]
64. Zhang, X.; An, R.; Tian, H.; Zhao, J. Increased risk of pancreatic cancer after acute pancreatitis: A meta-analysis of prospective cohort studies. *Clin. Res. Hepatol. Gastroenterol.* **2019**, *43*, e39–e41. [CrossRef]
65. Liu, J.; Wang, Y.; Yu, Y. Meta-analysis reveals an association between acute pancreatitis and the risk of pancreatic cancer. *World J. Clin. Cases* **2020**, *8*, 4416–4430. [CrossRef] [PubMed]
66. Alhobayb, T.; Peravali, R.; Ashkar, M. The Relationship between Acute and Chronic Pancreatitis with Pancreatic Adenocarcinoma: Review. *Diseases* **2021**, *9*, 93. [CrossRef]
67. Kirkegård, J.; Gaber, C.; Lund, J.L.; Hinton, S.P.; Ladekarl, M.; Heide-Jørgensen, U.; Cronin-Fenton, D.; Mortensen, F.V. Acute pancreatitis as an early marker of pancreatic cancer and cancer stage, treatment, and prognosis. *Cancer Epidemiol.* **2020**, *64*, 101647. [CrossRef] [PubMed]
68. Xiong, Y.; Zhao, Y.; Han, X.; Chen, G.; Windsor, J.; Wu, D.; Qian, J. Clinical characteristics and outcome of tumor-associated acute pancreatitis: A single-center cohort study. *Ann. Transl. Med.* **2021**, *9*, 639. [CrossRef]
69. Kirkegård, J.; Mortensen, F.V.; Heide-Jørgensen, U.; Cronin-Fenton, D. Predictors of underlying pancreatic cancer in patients with acute pancreatitis: A Danish nationwide cohort study. *Hpb* **2020**, *22*, 553–562. [CrossRef]
70. Dzeletovic, I.; Harrison, M.E.; Crowell, M.D.; Pannala, R.; Nguyen, C.C.; Wu, Q.; Faigel, D.O. Pancreatitis before pancreatic cancer clinical features and influence on outcome. *J. Clin. Gastroenterol.* **2014**, *48*, 801–805. [CrossRef]
71. Gong, Y.; Fan, Z.; Luo, G.; Huang, Q.; Qian, Y.; Cheng, H.; Jin, K.; Ni, Q.; Yu, X.; Liu, C. Prior history of acute pancreatitis predicts poor survival in patients with resectable pancreatic ductal adenocarcinoma. *Pancreatology* **2020**, *20*, 716–721. [CrossRef]
72. Lupinacci, R.M.; Faron, M.; Bachellier, P.; Sauvanet, A.; Beauchet, A.; Le Treut, Y.P.; Adham, M.; Mabrut, J.Y.; Delpero, J.R.; Paye, F. Acute Pancreatitis as the Initial Presentation of Pancreatic Adenocarcinoma does not Impact Short- and Long-term Outcomes of Curative Intent Surgery: A Study of the French Surgical Association. *World J. Surg.* **2021**, *45*, 3146–3156. [CrossRef] [PubMed]
73. Singh, R.R.; Klein, A.P.; Sharma, N.R.; O'Reilly, E.M. Does acute pancreatitis herald pancreatic ductal adenocarcinoma? A multicenter electronic health research network study. *Cancer Med.* **2023**, *12*, 2505–2513. [CrossRef] [PubMed]
74. Teng, D.; Wu, K.; Sun, Y.; Zhang, M.; Wang, D.; Wu, J.; Yin, T.; Gong, W.; Ding, Y.; Xiao, W.; et al. Significant increased CA199 levels in acute pancreatitis patients predicts the presence of pancreatic cancer. *Oncotarget* **2018**, *9*, 12745–12753. [CrossRef]
75. Feng, Q.; Li, C.; Zhang, S.; Tan, C.L.; Mai, G.; Liu, X.B.; Chen, Y.H. Recurrence and survival after surgery for pancreatic cancer with or without acute pancreatitis. *World J. Gastroenterol.* **2019**, *25*, 6006–6015. [CrossRef]
76. Chen, Y.H.; Xie, S.M.; Zhang, H.; Tan, C.L.; Ke, N.W.; Mai, G.; Liu, X.B. Clinical impact of preoperative acute pancreatitis in patients who undergo pancreaticoduodenectomy for periampullary tumors. *World J. Gastroenterol.* **2015**, *21*, 6937–6943. [CrossRef] [PubMed]
77. Khadka, R.; Tian, W.; Hao, X.; Koirala, R. Risk factor, early diagnosis and overall survival on outcome of association between pancreatic cancer and diabetes mellitus: Changes and advances, a review. *Int. J. Surg.* **2018**, *52*, 342–346. [CrossRef]
78. Roy, A.; Sahoo, J.; Kamalanathan, S.; Naik, D.; Mohan, P.; Kalayarasan, R. Diabetes and pancreatic cancer: Exploring the two-way traffic. *World J. Gastroenterol.* **2021**, *27*, 4939–4962. [CrossRef]
79. Ben, Q.; Xu, M.; Ning, X.; Liu, J.; Hong, S.; Huang, W.; Zhang, H.; Li, Z. Diabetes mellitus and risk of pancreatic cancer: A meta-analysis of cohort studies. *Eur. J. Cancer* **2011**, *47*, 1928–1937. [CrossRef]
80. Batabyal, P.; Vander Hoorn, S.; Christophi, C.; Nikfarjam, M. Association of diabetes mellitus and pancreatic adenocarcinoma: A meta-analysis of 88 studies. *Ann. Surg. Oncol.* **2014**, *21*, 2453–2462. [CrossRef]
81. Hart, P.A.; Bellin, M.D.; Andersen, D.K.; Bradley, D.; Cruz-Monserrate, Z.; Forsmark, C.E.; Goodarzi, M.O.; Habtezion, A.; Korc, M.; Kudva, Y.C.; et al. Type 3c (pancreatogenic) diabetes mellitus secondary to chronic pancreatitis and pancreatic cancer. *Lancet Gastroenterol. Hepatol.* **2016**, *1*, 226–237. [CrossRef]
82. Dankner, R.; Boffetta, P.; Balicer, R.D.; Boker, L.K.; Sadeh, M.; Berlin, A.; Olmer, L.; Goldfracht, M.; Freedman, L.S. Time-dependent risk of cancer after a diabetes diagnosis in a cohort of 2.3 million adults. *Am. J. Epidemiol.* **2016**, *183*, 1098–1106. [CrossRef]
83. Aggarwal, G.; Kamada, P.; Chari, S.T. Prevalence of diabetes mellitus in pancreatic cancer compared to common cancers. *Pancreas* **2013**, *42*, 198–201. [CrossRef] [PubMed]
84. Lu, Y.; Rodríguez, L.A.G.; Malgerud, L.; González-Pérez, A.; Martín-Pérez, M.; Lagergren, J.; Bexelius, T.S. New-onset type 2 diabetes, elevated HbA1c, anti-diabetic medications, and risk of pancreatic cancer. *Br. J. Cancer* **2015**, *113*, 1607–1614. [CrossRef] [PubMed]
85. Pannala, R.; Leirness, J.B.; Bamlet, W.R.; Basu, A.; Petersen, G.M.; Chari, S.T. Prevalence and Clinical Profile of Pancreatic Cancer-Associated Diabetes Mellitus. *Gastroenterology* **2008**, *134*, 981–987. [CrossRef] [PubMed]

86. Singhi, A.D.; Koay, E.J.; Chari, S.T.; Maitra, A. Early Detection of Pancreatic Cancer: Opportunities and Challenges. *Gastroenterology* **2019**, *156*, 2024–2040. [CrossRef]
87. Pizzato, M.; Turati, F.; Rosato, V.; La Vecchia, C. Exploring the link between diabetes and pancreatic cancer. *Expert Rev. Anticancer Ther.* **2019**, *19*, 681–687. [CrossRef]
88. Sharma, A.; Kandlakunta, H.; Nagpal, S.J.S.; Feng, Z.; Hoos, W.; Petersen, G.M.; Chari, S.T. Model to Determine Risk of Pancreatic Cancer in Patients with New-Onset Diabetes. *Gastroenterology* **2018**, *155*, 730–739.e3. [CrossRef]
89. Boursi, B.; Finkelman, B.; Giantonio, B.J.; Haynes, K.; Rustgi, A.K.; Rhim, A.D.; Mamtani, R.; Yang, Y.X. A Clinical Prediction Model to Assess Risk for Pancreatic Cancer among Patients with New-Onset Diabetes. *Gastroenterology* **2017**, *152*, 840–850.e3. [CrossRef]
90. Boursi, B.; Finkelman, B.; Giantonio, B.J.; Haynes, K.; Rustgi, A.K.; Rhim, A.D.; Mamtani, R.; Yang, Y.X. A Clinical Prediction Model to Assess Risk for Pancreatic Cancer among Patients with Prediabetes. *Eur. J. Gastroenterol. Hepatol.* **2022**, *34*, 33–38. [CrossRef]
91. Konno, Y.; Sugai, Y.; Kanoto, M.; Suzuki, K.; Hiraka, T.; Toyoguchi, Y.; Niino, K. A retrospective preliminary study of intrapancreatic late enhancement as a noteworthy imaging finding in the early stages of pancreatic adenocarcinoma. *Eur. Radiol.* **2023**, *33*, 5131–5141. [CrossRef]
92. Rogowska, J.O.; Durko, Ł.; Malecka-Wojciesko, E. The Latest Advancements in Diagnostic Role of Endosonography of Pancreatic Lesions. *J. Clin. Med.* **2023**, *12*, 4630. [CrossRef] [PubMed]
93. Facciorusso, A.; Martina, M.; Buccino, R.V.; Nacchiero, M.C.; Muscatiello, N. Diagnostic accuracy of fine-needle aspiration of solid pancreatic lesions guided by endoscopic ultrasound elastography. *Ann. Gastroenterol.* **2018**, *31*, 513–518. [CrossRef] [PubMed]
94. Bournet, B.; Selves, J.; Grand, D.; Danjoux, M.; Hanoun, N.; Cordelier, P.; Buscail, L. Endoscopic ultrasound-guided fine-needle aspiration biopsy coupled with a KRAS mutation assay using allelic discrimination improves the diagnosis of pancreatic cancer. *J. Clin. Gastroenterol.* **2014**, *49*, 50–56. [CrossRef] [PubMed]
95. Ma, H.; Wang, P.; Shang, D.; Liu, Y. Spatial-domain low-coherence quantitative phase microscopy to improve the cytological diagnosis of pancreatic cancer. *J. Investig. Med.* **2020**, *68*, 60–67. [CrossRef] [PubMed]
96. Dahiya, D.S.; Al-Haddad, M.; Chandan, S.; Gangwani, M.K.; Aziz, M.; Mohan, B.P.; Ramai, D.; Canakis, A.; Bapaye, J.; Sharma, N. Artificial Intelligence in Endoscopic Ultrasound for Pancreatic Cancer: Where Are We Now and What Does the Future Entail? *J. Clin. Med.* **2022**, *11*, 7476. [CrossRef] [PubMed]
97. Katta, M.R.; Kalluru, P.K.R.; Bavishi, D.A.; Hameed, M.; Valisekka, S.S. Artificial intelligence in pancreatic cancer: Diagnosis, limitations, and the future prospects—A narrative review. *J. Cancer Res. Clin. Oncol.* **2023**, *149*, 6743–6751. [CrossRef] [PubMed]
98. Chu, L.C.; Park, S.; Kawamoto, S.; Fouladi, D.F.; Shayesteh, S.; Zinreich, E.S.; Graves, J.S.; Horton, K.M.; Hruban, R.H.; Yuille, A.L.; et al. Utility of CT radiomics features in differentiation of pancreatic ductal adenocarcinoma from normal pancreatic tissue. *Am. J. Roentgenol.* **2019**, *213*, 349–357. [CrossRef]
99. Fu, M.; Wu, W.; Hong, X.; Liu, Q.; Jiang, J.; Ou, Y.; Zhao, Y.; Gong, X. Hierarchical combinatorial deep learning architecture for pancreas segmentation of medical computed tomography cancer images. *BMC Syst. Biol.* **2018**, *12*, 56–127. [CrossRef]
100. Liu, S.L.; Li, S.; Guo, Y.T.; Zhou, Y.P.; Zhang, Z.D.; Li, S.; Lu, Y. Establishment and application of an artificial intelligence diagnosis system for pancreatic cancer with a faster region-based convolutional neural network. *Chin. Med. J.* **2019**, *132*, 2795–2803. [CrossRef]
101. Young, M.R.; Abrams, N.; Ghosh, S.; Rinaudo, J.A.S.; Marquez, G.; Srivastava, S. Prediagnostic Image Data, Artificial Intelligence, and Pancreatic Cancer: A Tell-Tale Sign to Early Detection. *Pancreas* **2020**, *49*, 882–886. [CrossRef] [PubMed]
102. Santus, E.; Schuster, T.; Tahmasebi, A.M.; Li, C.; Yala, A.; Lanahan, C.R.; Prinsen, P.; Thompson, S.F.; Coons, S.; Mynderse, L.; et al. Exploiting Rules to Enhance Machine Learning in Extracting Information From Multi-Institutional Prostate Pathology Reports. *JCO Clin. Cancer Inform.* **2020**, *4*, 865–874. [CrossRef] [PubMed]
103. Kuwahara, T.; Hara, K.; Mizuno, N.; Okuno, N.; Matsumoto, S.; Obata, M.; Kurita, Y.; Koda, H.; Toriyama, K.; Onishi, S.; et al. Usefulness of deep learning analysis for the diagnosis of malignancy in intraductal papillary mucinous neoplasms of the pancreas. *Clin. Transl. Gastroenterol.* **2019**, *10*, e00045. [CrossRef] [PubMed]
104. Zhang, M.M.; Yang, H.; Jin, Z.D.; Yu, J.G.; Cai, Z.Y.; Li, Z.S. Differential diagnosis of pancreatic cancer from normal tissue with digital imaging processing and pattern recognition based on a support vector machine of EUS images. *Gastrointest. Endosc.* **2010**, *72*, 978–985. [CrossRef] [PubMed]
105. Goyal, H.; Sherazi, S.A.A.; Gupta, S.; Perisetti, A.; Achebe, I.; Ali, A.; Tharian, B.; Thosani, N.; Sharma, N.R. Application of artificial intelligence in diagnosis of pancreatic malignancies by endoscopic ultrasound: A systemic review. *Therap. Adv. Gastroenterol.* **2022**, *15*, 1–11. [CrossRef] [PubMed]
106. Das, A.; Nguyen, C.C.; Li, F.; Li, B. Digital image analysis of EUS images accurately differentiates pancreatic cancer from chronic pancreatitis and normal tissue. *Gastrointest. Endosc.* **2008**, *67*, 861–867. [CrossRef] [PubMed]
107. Săftoiu, A.; Vilmann, P.; Gorunescu, F.; Gheonea, D.I.; Gorunescu, M.; Ciurea, T.; Popescu, G.L.; Iordache, A.; Hassan, H.; Iordache, S. Neural network analysis of dynamic sequences of EUS elastography used for the differential diagnosis of chronic pancreatitis and pancreatic cancer. *Gastrointest. Endosc.* **2008**, *68*, 1086–1094. [CrossRef]
108. Marya, N.B.; Powers, P.D.; Chari, S.T.; Gleeson, F.C.; Leggett, C.L.; Abu Dayyeh, B.K.; Chandrasekhara, V.; Iyer, P.G.; Majumder, S.; Pearson, R.K.; et al. Utilisation of artificial intelligence for the development of an EUS-convolutional neural network model trained to enhance the diagnosis of autoimmune pancreatitis. *Gut* **2021**, *70*, 1335–1344. [CrossRef]

109. Hou, J.; Li, X.T.; Xie, K.P. Coupled liquid biopsy and bioinformatics for pancreatic cancer early detection and precision prognosti cation. *Mol. Cancer* **2021**, *20*, 34. [CrossRef]
110. Uesato, Y.; Sasahira, N.; Ozaka, M.; Sasaki, T.; Takatsuki, M.; Zembutsu, H. Evaluation of circulating tumor DNA as a biomarker in pancreatic cancer with liver metastasis. *PLoS ONE* **2020**, *15*, e0235623. [CrossRef]
111. Bettegowda, C.; Sausen, M.; Leary, R.J.; Kinde, I.; Wang, Y.; Agrawal, N.; Bartlett, B.R.; Wang, H.; Luber, B.; Alani, R.M.; et al. Detection of circulating tumor DNA in early- and late-stage human malignancies. *Sci. Transl. Med.* **2014**, *6*, 224. [CrossRef]
112. Tie, J.; Wang, Y.; Tomasetti, C.; Li, L.; Springer, S.; Kinde, I.; Silliman, N.; Tacey, M.; Wong, H.L.; Christie, M.; et al. Circulating tumor DNA analysis detects minimal residual disease and predicts recurrence in patients with stage II colon cancer. *Sci. Transl Med.* **2016**, *8*, 346ra92. [CrossRef] [PubMed]
113. Kim, M.K.; Woo, S.M.; Park, B.; Yoon, K.A.; Kim, Y.H.; Joo, J.; Lee, W.J.; Han, S.S.; Park, S.J.; Kong, S.Y. Prognostic implications of multiplex detection of KRAS mutations in cell-Free DNA from patients with pancreatic ductal adenocarcinoma. *Clin. Chem.* **2018** *64*, 726–734. [CrossRef] [PubMed]
114. Sausen, M.; Phallen, J.; Adleff, V.; Jones, S.; Leary, R.J.; Barrett, M.T.; Anagnostou, V.; Parpart-Li, S.; Murphy, D.; Li, Q.K.; et al. Clinical implications of genomic alterations in the tumour and circulation of pancreatic cancer patients. *Nat. Commun.* **2015** *6*, 7686. [CrossRef]
115. Wu, J.; Zhou, Y.; Zhang, C.Y.; Song, B.B.; Wang, B.L.; Pan, B.S.; Lou, W.H.; Guo, W. Co-amplification at lower denaturation temperature PCR combined with unlabled-probe high-resolution melting to detect KRAS codon 12 and 13 mutations in plasma circulating DNA of pancreatic adenocarcinoma cases. *Asian Pacific J. Cancer Prev.* **2014**, *15*, 10647–10652. [CrossRef] [PubMed]
116. Cohen, J.D.; Javed, A.A.; Thoburn, C.; Wong, F.; Tie, J.; Gibbs, P.; Schmidt, C.M.; Yip-Schneider, M.T.; Allen, P.J.; Schattner, M.; et al. Combined circulating tumor DNA and protein biomarker-based liquid biopsy for the earlier detection of pancreatic cancers. *Proc Natl. Acad. Sci. USA* **2017**, *114*, 10202–10207. [CrossRef]
117. Kinugasa, H.; Nouso, K.; Miyahara, K.; Morimoto, Y.; Dohi, C.; Tsutsumi, K.; Kato, H.; Matsubara, T.; Okada, H.; Yamamoto, K Detection of K-ras gene mutation by liquid biopsy in patients with pancreatic cancer. *Cancer* **2015**, *121*, 2271–2280. [CrossRef]
118. Van Laethem, J.L.; Riess, H.; Jassem, J.; Haas, M.; Martens, U.M.; Weekes, C.; Peeters, M.; Ross, P.; Bridgewater, J.; Melichar, B.; et al Phase I/II Study of Refametinib (BAY 86-9766) in Combination with Gemcitabine in Advanced Pancreatic cancer. *Target. Oncol* **2017**, *12*, 97–109. [CrossRef]
119. Shen, S.Y.; Singhania, R.; Fehringer, G.; Chakravarthy, A.; Roehrl, M.H.A.; Chadwick, D.; Zuzarte, P.C.; Borgida, A.; Wang, T.T. Li, T.; et al. Sensitive tumour detection and classification using plasma cell-free DNA methylomes. *Nature* **2018**, *563*, 579–583 [CrossRef]
120. Guven, D.C.; Sahin, T.K.; Yildirim, H.C.; Aktepe, O.H.; Dizdar, O.; Yalcin, S. A systematic review and meta-analysis of the association between circulating tumor DNA (ctDNA) and prognosis in pancreatic cancer. *Crit. Rev. Oncol. Hematol.* **2021**, *168* 103528. [CrossRef]
121. Sivapalan, L.; Kocher, H.M.; Ross-Adams, H.; Chelala, C. Molecular profiling of ctDNA in pancreatic cancer: Opportunities and challenges for clinical application. *Pancreatology* **2021**, *21*, 363–378. [CrossRef]
122. Li, Y.; Sarkar, F.H. MicroRNA targeted therapeutic approach for pancreatic cancer. *Int. J. Biol. Sci.* **2016**, *12*, 326–337. [CrossRef]
123. Eun, J.L.; Gusev, Y.; Jiang, J.; Nuovo, G.J.; Lerner, M.R.; Frankel, W.L.; Morgan, D.L.; Postier, R.G.; Brackett, D.J.; Schmittgen, T.D Expression profiling identifies microRNA signature in pancreatic cancer. *Int. J. Cancer* **2007**, *120*, 1046–1054. [CrossRef]
124. Zhang, Y.; Li, M.; Wang, H.; Fisher, W.E.; Lin, P.H.; Yao, Q.; Chen, C. Profiling of 95 MicroRNAs in pancreatic cancer cell lines and surgical specimens by real-time PCR analysis. *World J. Surg.* **2009**, *33*, 698–709. [CrossRef]
125. Hong, T.H.; Park, I.Y. MicroRNA expression profiling of diagnostic needle aspirates from surgical pancreatic cancer specimens *Ann. Surg. Treat. Res.* **2014**, *87*, 290–297. [CrossRef]
126. Habbe, N.; Koorstra, J.B.M.; Mendell, J.T.; Offerhaus, G.J.; Ji, K.R.; Feldmann, G.; Mullendore, M.E.; Goggins, M.G.; Hong, S.M. Maitra, A. MicroRNA miR-155 is a biomarker of early pancreatic neoplasia. *Cancer Biol. Ther.* **2009**, *8*, 340–346. [CrossRef]
127. Yu, J.; Ohuchida, K.; Mizumoto, K.; Sato, N.; Kayashima, T.; Fujita, H.; Nakata, K.; Tanaka, M. MicroRNA, hsa-miR-200c, is an independent prognostic factor in pancreatic cancer and its upregulation inhibits pancreatic cancer invasion but increases cell proliferation. *Mol. Cancer* **2010**, *9*, 169. [CrossRef] [PubMed]
128. Li, Y.; Vandenboom, T.G.; Kong, D.; Wang, Z.; Ali, S.; Philip, P.A.; Sarkar, F.H. Up-regulation of miR-200 and let-7 by natural agents leads to the reversal of epithelial-to-mesenchymal transition in gemcitabine-resistant pancreatic cancer cells. *Cancer Res* **2009**, *69*, 6704–6712. [CrossRef] [PubMed]
129. Nguyen, D.X.; Bos, P.D.; Massagué, J. Metastasis: From dissemination to organ-specific colonization. *Nat. Rev. Cancer* **2009**, *9* 274–284. [CrossRef] [PubMed]
130. Pantel, K.; Speicher, M.R. The biology of circulating tumor cells. *Oncogene* **2016**, *35*, 1216–1224. [CrossRef] [PubMed]
131. Xing, Y.; Zhang, X.; Qin, F.; Yang, J.; Ai, L.; Wang, Q.; Zhai, Y. The clinical significance of circulating tumor cells and T lymphocyte subtypes in pancreatic cancer patients. *Bioengineered* **2022**, *13*, 2130–2138. [CrossRef] [PubMed]
132. Yu, M.; Bardia, A.; Aceto, N.; Bersani, F.; Madden, M.W.; Donaldson, M.C.; Desai, R.; Zhu, H.; Comaills, V.; Zheng, Z.; et al Ex vivo culture of circulating breast tumor cells for individualized testing of drug susceptibility. *Science* **2014**, *345*, 216–220 [CrossRef] [PubMed]

133. Antonarakis, E.S.; Lu, C.; Luber, B.; Wang, H.; Chen, Y.; Zhu, Y.; Silberstein, J.L.; Taylor, M.N.; Maughan, B.L.; Denmeade, S.R.; et al. Clinical significance of androgen receptor splice variant-7 mRNA detection in circulating tumor cells of men with metastatic castration-resistant prostate cancer treated with first & second-line Abiraterone & Enzalutamide. *J. Clin. Oncol.* **2017**, *35*, 2149–2156. [CrossRef] [PubMed]
134. DiPardo, B.J.; Winograd, P.; Court, C.M.; Tomlinson, J.S. Pancreatic cancer circulating tumor cells: Applications for personalized oncology. *Expert Rev. Mol. Diagn.* **2018**, *18*, 809–820. [CrossRef] [PubMed]
135. Mishra, A.; Dubash, T.D.; Edd, J.F.; Jewett, M.K.; Garre, S.G.; Karabacak, N.M.; Rabe, D.C.; Mutlu, B.R.; Walsh, J.R.; Kapur, R.; et al. Ultrahigh-throughput magnetic sorting of large blood volumes for epitope-agnostic isolation of circulating tumor cells. *Proc. Natl. Acad. Sci. USA* **2020**, *117*, 16839–16847. [CrossRef] [PubMed]
136. Kendrick, M.L.; Sclabas, G.M. Major venous resection during total laparoscopic pancreaticoduodenectomy. *Hpb* **2011**, *13*, 454–458. [CrossRef] [PubMed]
137. Croome, K.P.; Farnell, M.B.; Que, F.G.; Reid-Lombardo, K.M.; Truty, M.J.; Nagorney, D.M.; Kendrick, M.L. Pancreaticoduodenectomy with Major Vascular Resection: A Comparison of Laparoscopic Versus Open Approaches. *J. Gastrointest. Surg.* **2015**, *19*, 189–194. [CrossRef]
138. Wang, M.; Cai, H.; Meng, L.; Cai, Y.; Wang, X.; Li, Y.; Peng, B. Minimally invasive pancreaticoduodenectomy: A comprehensive review. *Int. J. Surg.* **2016**, *35*, 139–146. [CrossRef]
139. Poves, I.; Burdío, F.; Morató, O.; Iglesias, M.; Radosevic, A.; Ilzarbe, L.; Visa, L.; Grande, L. Comparison of perioperative outcomes between laparoscopic and open approach for pancreatoduodenectomy: The Padulap randomized controlled trial. *Ann. Surg.* **2018**, *268*, 731–739. [CrossRef]
140. Song, K.B.; Kim, S.C.; Hwang, D.W.; Lee, J.H.; Lee, D.J.; Lee, J.W.; Park, K.M.; Lee, Y.J. Matched case-control analysis comparing laparoscopic and open pylorus-preserving pancreaticoduodenectomy in patients with periampullary tumors. *Ann. Surg.* **2015**, *262*, 146–155. [CrossRef]
141. Stauffer, J.A.; Coppola, A.; Villacreses, D.; Mody, K.; Johnson, E.; Li, Z.; Asbun, H.J. Laparoscopic versus open pancreaticoduodenectomy for pancreatic adenocarcinoma: Long-term results at a single institution. *Surg. Endosc.* **2017**, *31*, 2233–2241. [CrossRef] [PubMed]
142. Jiang, Y.L.; Zhang, R.C.; Zhou, Y.C. Comparison of overall survival and perioperative outcomes of laparoscopic pancreaticoduodenectomy and open pancreaticoduodenectomy for pancreatic ductal adenocarcinoma: A systematic review and meta-analysis. *BMC Cancer* **2019**, *19*, 781. [CrossRef] [PubMed]
143. Yin, Z.; Jian, Z.; Hou, B.; Jin, H. Surgical and Oncological Outcomes of Laparoscopic Versus Open Pancreaticoduodenectomy in Patients with Pancreatic Duct Adenocarcinoma. *Pancreas* **2019**, *48*, 861–867. [CrossRef] [PubMed]
144. Zureikat, A.H.; Postlewait, L.M.; Liu, Y.; Gillespie, T.W.; Weber, S.M.; Abbott, D.E.; Ahmad, S.A.; Maithel, S.K.; Hogg, M.E.; Zenati, M.; et al. A multi-institutional comparison of perioperative outcomes of robotic and open pancreaticoduodenectomy. *Ann. Surg.* **2016**, *264*, 640–649. [CrossRef]
145. Chen, K.; Pan, Y.; Liu, X.L.; Jiang, G.; Wu, D.Y.; Maher, H.; Cai, X.J. Minimally invasive pancreaticoduodenectomy for periampullary disease: A comprehensive review of literature and meta-analysis of outcomes compared with open surgery. *BMC Gastroenterol.* **2017**, *17*, 120. [CrossRef] [PubMed]
146. Anderloni, A.; Troncone, E.; Fugazza, A.; Cappello, A.; Del Vecchio Blanco, G.; Monteleone, G.; Repici, A. Lumen-apposing metal stents for malignant biliary obstruction: Is this the ultimate horizon of our experience? *World J. Gastroenterol.* **2019**, *25*, 3857–3869. [CrossRef] [PubMed]
147. Fugazza, A.; Fabbri, C.; Di Mitri, R.; Petrone, M.C.; Colombo, M.; Cugia, L.; Amato, A.; Forti, E.; Binda, C.; Maida, M.; et al. EUS-guided choledochoduodenostomy for malignant distal biliary obstruction after failed ERCP: A retrospective nationwide analysis. *Gastrointest. Endosc.* **2022**, *95*, 896–904. [CrossRef]
148. Waldthaler, A.; Rutkowski, W.; Valente, R.; Arnelo, U.; Löhr, J.-M. Palliative therapy in pancreatic cancer-interventional treatment with stents. *Transl. Gastroenterol. Hepatol.* **2019**, *4*, 7. [CrossRef]
149. Hofmann, F.O.; Miksch, R.C.; Weniger, M.; Keck, T.; Anthuber, M.; Witzigmann, H.; Nuessler, N.C.; Reissfelder, C.; Königer, J.; Ghadimi, M.; et al. Outcomes and risks in palliative pancreatic surgery: An analysis of the German StuDoQ | Pancreas registry. *BMC Surg.* **2022**, *22*, 389. [CrossRef]
150. Rubinsky, B.; Onik, G.; Mikus, P. Irreversible electroporation: A new ablation modality-Clinical implications. *Technol. Cancer Res. Treat.* **2007**, *6*, 37–48. [CrossRef]
151. Maor, E.; Ivorra, A.; Leor, J.; Rubinsky, B. The effect of irreversible electroporation on blood vessels. *Technol. Cancer Res. Treat.* **2007**, *6*, 307–312. [CrossRef]
152. Martin, R.C.G. Irreversible electroporation of stage 3 locally advanced pancreatic cancer: Optimal technique and outcomes. *J. Vis. Surg.* **2015**, *1*, 4. [CrossRef]
153. Martin, R.C.G.; McFarland, K.; Ellis, S.; Velanovich, V. Irreversible electroporation therapy in the management of locally advanced pancreatic adenocarcinoma. *J. Am. Coll. Surg.* **2012**, *215*, 361–369. [CrossRef]
154. Conroy, T.; Desseigne, F.; Ychou, M.; Bouché, O.; Guimbaud, R.; Bécouarn, Y.; Adenis, A.; Raoul, J.-L.; Gourgou-Bourgade, S.; de la Fouchardière, C.; et al. FOLFIRINOX versus Gemcitabine for Metastatic Pancreatic Cancer. *N. Engl. J. Med.* **2011**, *364*, 1817–1825. [CrossRef] [PubMed]

155. Von Hoff, D.D.; Ervin, T.; Arena, F.P.; Chiorean, E.G.; Infante, J.; Moore, M.; Seay, T.; Tjulandin, S.A.; Ma, W.W.; Saleh, M.N.; et al. Increased Survival in Pancreatic Cancer with nab-Paclitaxel plus Gemcitabine. *N. Engl. J. Med.* **2013**, *369*, 1691–1703. [CrossRef] [PubMed]
156. Carrato, A.; Vieitez, J.M.; Benavides, M.; Rodriguez-Garrote, M.; Castillo, A.; Ogalla, G.D.; Bermejo, L.G.; Ruiz de Mena, I.; Guillén-Ponce, C.; Aranda, E.; et al. Phase I/II trial of sequential treatment of nab-paclitaxel in combination with gemcitabine followed by modified FOLFOX chemotherapy in patients with untreated metastatic exocrine pancreatic cancer: Phase I results. *Eur. J. Cancer* **2020**, *139*, 51–58. [CrossRef] [PubMed]
157. Golan, T.; Hammel, P.; Reni, M.; Van Cutsem, E.; Macarulla, T.; Hall, M.J.; Park, J.-O.; Hochhauser, D.; Arnold, D.; Oh, D.-Y.; et al. Maintenance Olaparib for Germline BRCA -Mutated Metastatic Pancreatic Cancer. *N. Engl. J. Med.* **2019**, *381*, 317–327. [CrossRef] [PubMed]
158. Neoptolemos, J.P.; Palmer, D.H.; Ghaneh, P.; Psarelli, E.E.; Valle, J.W.; Halloran, C.M.; Faluyi, O.; O'Reilly, D.A.; Cunningham, D.; Wadsley, J.; et al. Comparison of adjuvant gemcitabine and capecitabine with gemcitabine monotherapy in patients with resected pancreatic cancer (ESPAC-4): A multicentre, open-label, randomised, phase 3 trial. *Lancet* **2017**, *389*, 1011–1024. [CrossRef]
159. Conroy, T.; Hammel, P.; Hebbar, M.; Ben Abdelghani, M.; Wei, A.C.; Raoul, J.-L.; Choné, L.; Francois, E.; Artru, P.; Biagi, J.J.; et al. FOLFIRINOX or Gemcitabine as Adjuvant Therapy for Pancreatic Cancer. *N. Engl. J. Med.* **2018**, *379*, 2395–2406. [CrossRef]
160. Pishvaian, M.J.; Garrido-Laguna, I.; Liu, S.V.; Multani, P.S.; Chow-Maneval, E.; Rolfo, C. Entrectinib in TRK and ROS1 Fusion-Positive Metastatic Pancreatic Cancer. *JCO Precis. Oncol.* **2018**, *2*, 1–7. [CrossRef]
161. Okusaka, T.; Nakamura, M.; Yoshida, M.; Kitano, M.; Uesaka, K.; Ito, Y.; Furuse, J.; Hanada, K.; Okazaki, K. Clinical Practice Guidelines for Pancreatic Cancer 2019 from the Japan Pancreas Society: A Synopsis. *Pancreas* **2020**, *49*, 326–335. [CrossRef] [PubMed]
162. Yin, C.; Alqahtani, A.; Noel, M.S. The Next Frontier in Pancreatic Cancer: Targeting the Tumor Immune Milieu and Molecular Pathways. *Cancers* **2022**, *14*, 2619. [CrossRef] [PubMed]
163. Kolbeinsson, H.M.; Chandana, S.; Wright, G.P.; Chung, M. Pancreatic Cancer: A Review of Current Treatment and Novel Therapies. *J. Investig. Surg.* **2023**, *36*, 2129884. [CrossRef]
164. Casolino, R.; Paiella, S.; Azzolina, D.; Beer, P.A.; Corbo, V.; Lorenzoni, G.; Gregori, D.; Golan, T.; Braconi, C.; Froeling, F.E.; et al. Homologous Recombination Deficiency in Pancreatic Cancer: A Systematic Review and Prevalence Meta-Analysis. *J. Clin. Oncol.* **2021**, *39*, 2617–2632. [CrossRef] [PubMed]
165. Dalmasso, B.; Puccini, A.; Catalano, F.; Borea, R.; Iaia, M.L.; Bruno, W.; Fornarini, G.; Sciallero, S.; Rebuzzi, S.E.; Ghiorzo, P. Beyond BRCA: The Emerging Significance of DNA Damage Response and Personalized Treatment in Pancreatic and Prostate Cancer Patients. *Int. J. Mol. Sci.* **2022**, *23*, 4709. [CrossRef]
166. Leidner, R.; Sanjuan Silva, N.; Huang, H.; Sprott, D.; Zheng, C.; Shih, Y.-P.; Leung, A.; Payne, R.; Sutcliffe, K.; Cramer, J.; et al. Neoantigen T-Cell Receptor Gene Therapy in Pancreatic Cancer. *N. Engl. J. Med.* **2022**, *386*, 2112–2119. [CrossRef] [PubMed]
167. Selvanesan, B.C.; Chandra, D.; Quispe-Tintaya, W.; Jahangir, A.; Patel, A.; Meena, K.; Da Silva, R.A.A.; Friedman, M.; Gabor, L.; Khouri, O.; et al. Listeria delivers tetanus toxoid protein to pancreatic tumors and induces cancer cell death in mice. *Sci. Transl. Med.* **2022**, *14*, eabc1600. [CrossRef]
168. Marabelle, A.; Le, D.T.; Ascierto, P.A.; Di Giacomo, A.M.; De Jesus-Acosta, A.; Delord, J.P.; Geva, R.; Gottfried, M.; Penel, N.; Hansen, A.R.; et al. Efficacy of Pembrolizumab in Patients with Noncolorectal High Microsatellite Instability/Mismatch Repair—Deficient Cancer: Results from the Phase II KEYNOTE-158 Study abstract. *J. Clin. Oncol.* **2020**, *38*, 1–10. [CrossRef]
169. Dorman, K.; Heinemann, V.; Kobold, S.; Bergwelt-Baildon, M.; Boeck, S. Novel systemic treatment approaches for metastatic pancreatic cancer. *Expert Opin. Investig. Drugs* **2022**, *31*, 249–262. [CrossRef]
170. Van Tienhoven, G.; Versteijne, E.; Suker, M.; Groothuis, K.B.C.; Busch, O.R.; Bonsing, B.A.; de Hingh, I.H.J.T.; Festen, S.; Patijn, G.A.; de Vos-Geelen, J.; et al. Preoperative chemoradiotherapy versus immediate surgery for resectable and borderline resectable pancreatic cancer (PREOPANC-1): A ran-domized, controlled, multicenter phase III trial. *J. Clin. Oncol.* **2018**, *36* (Suppl. 18), LBA4002. [CrossRef]
171. Taylor, R.J.; Todor, D.; Kaplan, B.J.; Stover, W.; Fields, E.C. CivaSheet intraoperative radiation therapy for pancreatic cancer. *Brachytherapy* **2022**, *21*, 255–259. [CrossRef] [PubMed]
172. Paiella, S.; De Pastena, M.; Romeo, F.; D'onofrio, M.; Fontana, M.; Pea, A.; De Marchi, G.; Crinò, S.F.; Bassi, C.; Salvia, R. Ablation treatments in unresectable pancreatic cancer. *Minerva Chir.* **2019**, *74*, 263–269. [CrossRef] [PubMed]
173. He, C.; Wang, J.; Zhang, Y.; Cai, Z.; Lin, X.; Li, S. Comparison of combination therapies in the management of locally advanced pancreatic cancer: Induction chemotherapy followed by irreversible electroporation vs radiofrequency ablation. *Cancer Med.* **2020**, *9*, 4699–4710. [CrossRef] [PubMed]
174. Wang, Y.; Wang, H.; Zhou, L.; Lu, J.; Jiang, B.; Liu, C.; Guo, J. Photodynamic therapy of pancreatic cancer: Where have we come from and where are we going? *Photodiagnosis Photodyn. Ther.* **2020**, *31*, 101876. [CrossRef] [PubMed]
175. Bhattacharya, D.; Mukhopadhyay, M.; Shivam, K.; Tripathy, S.; Patra, R.; Pramanik, A. Recent developments in photodynamic therapy and its application against multidrug resistant cancers. *Biomed. Mater.* **2023**, *18*, 062005. [CrossRef] [PubMed]
176. Greene, M.K.; Johnston, M.C.; Scott, C.J. Nanomedicine in Pancreatic Cancer: Current Status and Future Opportunities for Overcoming Therapy Resistance. *Cancers* **2021**, *13*, 6175. [CrossRef] [PubMed]

177. McKinley, K.N.L.; Herremans, K.M.; Riner, A.N.; Vudatha, V.; Freudenberger, D.C.; Hughes, S.J.; Triplett, E.W.; Trevino, J.G. Translocation of Oral Microbiota into the Pancreatic Ductal Adenocarcinoma Tumor Microenvironment. *Microorganisms* **2023**, *11*, 1466. [CrossRef]
178. Kabwe, M.; Dashper, S.; Tucci, J. The Microbiome in Pancreatic Cancer-Implications for Diagnosis and Precision Bacteriophage Therapy for This Low Survival Disease. *Front. Cell. Infect. Microbiol.* **2022**, *12*, 871293. [CrossRef]
179. Geller, L.T.; Barzily-rokni, M.; Danino, T.; Jonas, O.H.; Shental, N.; Nejman, D.; Gavert, N.; Zwang, Y.; Cooper, Z.A.; Shee, K.; et al. Potential role of intratumor bacteria in mediating tumor resistance to the chemotherapeutic drug gemcitabine. *Science* **2017**, *357*, 1156–1160. [CrossRef]
180. Chen, Z.; Zhang, S.; Dong, S.; Xu, H.; Zhou, W. Association of the Microbiota and Pancreatic Cancer: Opportunities and Limitations. *Front. Immunol.* **2022**, *13*, 844401. [CrossRef]
181. Boursi, B.; Mamtani, R.; Haynes, K.; Yang, Y.X. Recurrent antibiotic exposure may promote cancer formation-Another step in understanding the role of the human microbiota? *Eur. J. Cancer* **2015**, *51*, 2655–2664. [CrossRef] [PubMed]
182. Panebianco, C.; Pisati, F.; Ulaszewska, M.; Andolfo, A.; Villani, A.; Federici, F.; Laura, M.; Rizzi, E.; Potenza, A.; Latiano, T.P.; et al. Tuning gut microbiota through a probiotic blend in gemcitabine-treated pancreatic cancer xenografted mice. *Clin. Transl. Med.* **2021**, *11*, e580. [CrossRef] [PubMed]
183. Ciorba, M.A.; Riehl, T.E.; Rao, M.S.; Moon, C.; Ee, X.; Nava, G.M.; Walker, M.R.; Marinshaw, J.M.; Stappenbeck, T.S.; Stenson, W.F. Lactobacillus probiotic protects intestinal epithelium from radiation injury in a TLR-2/cyclo-oxygenase-2-dependent manner. *Gut* **2012**, *61*, 829–838. [CrossRef] [PubMed]
184. Jones, R.M.; Desai, C.; Darby, T.M.; Luo, L.; Wolfarth, A.A.; Scharer, C.D.; Ardita, C.S.; Reedy, A.R.; Keebaugh, E.S.; Neish, A.S. Lactobacilli Modulate Epithelial Cytoprotection through the Nrf2 Pathway. *Cell Rep.* **2015**, *12*, 1217–1225. [CrossRef]
185. Hamidi-Sofiani, V.; Rakhshi, R.; Moradi, N.; Zeynali, P.; Nakhaie, M.; Behboudi, E. Oncolytic viruses and pancreatic cancer. *Cancer Treat. Res. Commun.* **2022**, *31*, 100563. [CrossRef]

cancers

MDPI

Review

Pancreatic Exocrine Insufficiency and the Gut Microbiome in Pancreatic Cancer: A Target for Future Diagnostic Tests and Therapies?

James M. Halle-Smith [1,2,*], Lewis A. Hall [1,3], Sarah F. Powell-Brett [1,3], Nabeel Merali [4,5,6], Adam E. Frampton [4,5,6], Andrew D. Beggs [2,7], Paul Moss [4] and Keith J. Roberts [1,3]

1 Hepatobiliary and Pancreatic Surgery Unit, Queen Elizabeth Hospital Birmingham, University Hospitals Birmingham NHS Foundation Trust, Birmingham B15 2GW, UK; j.k.roberts@bham.ac.uk (K.J.R.)
2 Cancer and Genomic Sciences, University of Birmingham, Birmingham B15 2GW, UK; a.beggs@bham.ac.uk
3 Institute of Immunology and Immunotherapy, University of Birmingham, Birmingham B15 2TT, UK
4 Section of Oncology, Department of Clinical & Experimental Medicine, University of Surrey, Guildford GU2 7WG, UK; adam.frampton@surrey.ac.uk (A.E.F.); p.moss@bham.ac.uk (P.M.)
5 Minimal Access Therapy Training Unit (MATTU), Leggett Building, University of Surrey, Guildford GU2 7WG, UK
6 Department of Hepato-Pancreato-Biliary (HPB) Surgery, Royal Surrey County Hospital, Egerton Road, Guildford GU2 7XX, UK
7 Colorectal Surgery Department, Queen Elizabeth Hospital Birmingham, University Hospitals Birmingham NHS Foundation Trust, Birmingham B15 2GW, UK
* Correspondence: james.hallesmith@doctors.org.uk

Simple Summary: It is now thought that bacteria in the gut and tumour of patients with pancreatic cancer play an important role in the growth of the cancer and its sensitivity to chemotherapy. It has been shown that pancreatic exocrine insufficiency (PEI), common in pancreatic cancer patients, is linked to poorer outcomes. Conversely, it has also been demonstrated that treatment with pancreatic enzyme replacement therapy (PERT) can improve survival in pancreatic cancer patients. The reasons for this are not fully understood, but it is possible that PEI alters the gut and tumour microbiome of pancreatic cancer patients towards a less favourable composition, whereas PERT can reverse these changes and make the gut and tumour microbiome more favourable. If true, this could represent an opportunity for the development of new diagnostic tests and therapies for pancreatic cancer, which remains one of the deadliest cancers.

Abstract: Pancreatic exocrine insufficiency (PEI) is common amongst pancreatic cancer patients and is associated with poorer treatment outcomes. Pancreatic enzyme replacement therapy (PERT) is known to improve outcomes in pancreatic cancer, but the mechanisms are not fully understood. The aim of this narrative literature review is to summarise the current evidence linking PEI with microbiome dysbiosis, assess how microbiome composition may be impacted by PERT treatment, and look towards possible future diagnostic and therapeutic targets in this area. Early evidence in the literature reveals that there are complex mechanisms by which pancreatic secretions modulate the gut microbiome, so when these are disturbed, as in PEI, gut microbiome dysbiosis occurs. PERT has been shown to return the gut microbiome towards normal, so called rebiosis, in animal studies. Gut microbiome dysbiosis has multiple downstream effects in pancreatic cancer such as modulation of the immune response and the response to chemotherapeutic agents. It therefore represents a possible future target for future therapies. In conclusion, it is likely that the gut microbiome of pancreatic cancer patients with PEI exhibits dysbiosis and that this may potentially be reversible with PERT. However, further human studies are required to determine if this is indeed the case.

Keywords: pancreatic cancer; microbiome; pancreatic exocrine insufficiency; pancreatic enzyme replacement therapy

1. Introduction

1.1. The Human Microbiota

The human microbiota is a term used to describe the approximately 100 trillion microorganisms present in each individual [1–3]. With the emergence of more sophisticated bacterial genome sequencing [4–7], there is increasing interest in the interactions between the human microbiota and the human host. Such sequencing techniques include organism-level profiling with 16s rRNA gene sequencing or the more sophisticated gene-level profiling possible with metagenomic and metatranscriptomic sequencing [4–7]. These sequencing techniques have allowed a greater understanding not only of the composition of these microbial communities, but also an insight into their function [4–7], and the role they may play in the wider metabolic and immune function of the host [8].

1.2. The Gut Microbiome

A microbiome is defined as a population of microorganisms in conjunction with their genes in a specific body system; as such the microbial community in the bowel is referred to as the gut microbiome [1–3]. It has been demonstrated that the gut microbiome plays a key role in modulating host metabolic and immune function [9]. Within the gut, it has been demonstrated that the gut microbiome plays an important role in the development and progression of inflammatory bowel disease [10–12] and colorectal cancer [13,14]. Recent evidence highlights a functional role of the gut microbiome not only in cancer development and progression but also in defining the efficacy and toxicity of chemotherapeutic agents [15]. Beyond the gut however, it is thought that the gut microbiome is also linked to the progression of certain conditions such as chronic liver disease [16,17] and pancreatic ductal adenocarcinoma (PDAC) [18,19]. In terms of mechanisms, it is thought that bacteria and their metabolites exert their effects through translocation via the portal circulation, mesenteric lymph nodes or directly through the biliary and pancreatic duct systems [20–22]. All this combined means that the gut microbiome is increasingly viewed as a potential route for future diagnostic tests and a therapeutic target for many different conditions, including PDAC.

1.3. Pancreatic Ductal Adenocarcinoma

Whilst progress has been made in the treatment of other major malignancy types, PDAC remains one of the leading causes of cancer death worldwide, with 5-year survival rates persistently below 10% [23–25]. One reason for this poor survival is the tendency for PDAC to present late, meaning that many patients already have involvement of nearby major vascular structures which can preclude curative resection [26]. Similarly, many PDAC patients have distant metastatic disease at presentation, with the majority being hepatic due to the portal drainage of the pancreas [27–29], and current international practice guidelines advise against resection of PDAC in the setting of liver metastases [30–34]. Should the tumour be resectable and the patient receive systemic therapy, 5-year survival can reach up to 30% [35].

Even when surgical resection is achieved, there is a high likelihood that the patient will experience disease recurrence [36]; 75% of patients who undergo surgical resection and adjuvant therapy for primary PDAC will experience recurrence within 2 years [23,37,38]. As a result, there is an urgent need for new diagnostic and therapeutic targets in this challenging disease. The gut microbiome may represent one of the more promising prospects for future therapies.

1.4. Changes in the Gut Microbiome in PDAC Patients

It is increasingly appreciated that the gut microbiome is linked to the evolution of PDAC, with a recent study identifying changes in the gut microbiome that are present early in the disease process [19]. Further evidence that the gut microbiome may play an active role in the progression of PDAC comes from differences reported in the composition of the gut microbiome between short-term survival (STS) and long-term survival (LTS) PDAC patients, with greater diversity being associated with a more favourable prognosis [39].

1.5. Pancreatic Exocrine Insufficiency in Pancreatic Cancer

Pancreatic exocrine insufficiency (PEI) is defined as insufficient secretion of pancreatic enzymes and bicarbonate to maintain a normal digestion [40]. PEI has been shown to be both prevalent and progressive amongst patients with pancreatic cancer. A recent prospective cohort study used the ^{13}C mixed triglyceride breath test to investigate the prevalence of PEI amongst 254 patients awaiting pancreatoduodenectomy for an oncologic indication [41]. This study reported an incidence of 32.8% in those awaiting resection [41]. In addition, a systematic review in 2016 identified four studies evaluating PEI preoperatively, all using faecal elastase (FE-1), and found a median prevalence of 44% (range 42–47%) [42]. This results from lower enzyme secretion due to tumour burden as well as reduced enzyme delivery and activation as a consequence of pancreatic duct obstruction, which prevents the passage of enzymes and their accompanying bicarbonate-rich fluid into the duodenum [43]. Following pancreatoduodenectomy, there is also significant disruption to the physiological mechanisms by which pancreatic secretion is controlled, with some data indicating that the method of reconstruction may influence the degree of postoperative endocrine and exocrine pancreatic function [44,45].

Untreated PEI has a significant impact on quality of life and leads to a range of mentally and physically distressing symptoms including frequency, urgency, bloating, diarrhoea, fatty stool flatulence, loss of appetite and vomiting [46,47]. A major consequence is maldigestion resulting in malabsorption, malnutrition, and the ensuing nutritional deficiencies (including albumin, pre-albumin, transferrin, lipoproteins, fat soluble vitamins, calcium, magnesium, zinc, thiamine, and folic acid [48,49]). Clinically, PEI is associated with an increased risk of osteoporosis, sarcopenia, and cardiovascular events [50–52]. In pancreatic cancer, sarcopenia has been associated with increased perioperative mortality and reduced overall survival. There are multiple neural and hormonal factors that influence sarcopenia in PC and many of these also have interactions with the gut microbiome [53,54]. PEI has also been shown to increase length of stay, post-operative complications and costs following pancreatic resection [55,56]. It is also likely that PEI associated with PDAC leads to important changes in the gut microbiome which, if more clearly understood, could lead to the identification of new diagnostic and therapeutic targets.

1.6. Pancreatic Enzyme Replacement Therapy

Pancreatic enzyme replacement therapy (PERT) refers to the oral administration of capsules containing commercially produced digestive enzymes, namely lipase, protease and lipase. Treatment of PEI with PERT has been shown to improve quality of life [57,58] and also significantly increases survival in resectable and unresectable pancreatic cancer patients [59,60]. This has led the United Kingdom's National Institute of Health and Care Excellence (NICE) to recommend PERT for pancreatic cancer patients [61,62] without the need for a positive diagnostic test. This was supported by UK specialty consensus guidelines release in 2021 [62]. The underlying basis for the beneficial effects of PERT are not fully understood, but contributing factors appear to be related to the ability to alleviate malabsorption [63,64], which allows patients to tolerate physiologically demanding treatments such as major pancreatic resection and/or chemotherapy. On a micronutrient level, the absorption of fat-soluble vitamins appears crucial. For example, Vitamin D modulates the function of stromal cells (e.g., fibroblasts) in patients with PDAC [65] and deficiency is associated with poorer survival in advanced pancreatic cancer [66]. Recently, interest has been increasing in the intestinal microbiome as a modulator of many diseases (e.g., inflammatory bowel disease) although how PEI may affect this is still being understood.

1.7. Pancreatic Exocrine Insufficiency and the Intestinal Microbiome

PEI is thought to lead to changes in the composition of the gut microbiome, leading to a state of dysbiosis characterised by an imbalance in microbiome diversity [67–70]. Understanding how the microbiome and PEI are interconnected could aid the search for novel diagnostic and therapeutic targets and help improve outcomes in PDAC. Indeed, recent evidence indicates a role for the gut microbiome in the aetiology and progression of PDAC [19] and has also linked changes in the gut microbiome to outcome and treatment response [20,39,71–73]. The aim of this review is to summarise the current evidence linking PEI with microbiome dysbiosis, assess how microbiome composition may be influenced by PERT treatment, and look towards possible future diagnostic and therapeutic targets in this area.

2. The Interaction between Pancreatic Exocrine Function and Gut Microbiome

2.1. Effects of Pancreatic Exocrine Insufficiency on the Gut Microbiome

PEI is prevalent in patients with PC and there is emerging evidence that pancreatic exocrine function is closely linked to the composition of the gut microbiome [67–69]. Differences in the gut microbiome have been reported in patients with PEI, the main changes observed being a reduction in alpha-diversity, small intestine bacterial overgrowth and loss of 'beneficial' bacteria [67–69]. A large population-based study by Frost et al. gives significant insight into the importance of pancreatic exocrine function in regulating the gut microbiome [67]. This study compared the composition of the gut microbiome, via 16S rRNA gene sequencing of stool samples, to pancreatic function, using pancreatic elastase levels in over 1700 patients [67]. Their results showed that changes in the gut microbiome composition were much more closely linked to pancreatic exocrine function, rather than other commonly measured host factors such as age, dietary factors, diabetes or smoking [67]. This led the authors to conclude that pancreatic exocrine function appeared to be the most important host factor involved in shaping the human intestinal microbiome [67]. It is therefore likely that patients with pancreatic cancer, many of whom have PEI [42], will also have a deranged gut microbiome (Figure 1A) [19].

2.2. Pancreatic Regulation of Gut Microbiome

With increasing interest in the role that pancreatic exocrine function plays in the regulation of the gut microbiome, attention has turned towards the exact mechanisms by which pancreatic exocrine products influence gut bacteria. There are three main cell types in the adult pancreas: acinar cells that produce digestive enzymes; duct epithelial cells that produce a bicarbonate rich fluid which functions to carry digestive enzymes into the digestive tract and also to establish an optimal pH for enzyme function, and the cells of the Islets of Langerhans, which have an endocrine function, producing hormones such as glucagon and insulin [74,75]. In one large study, the role of the two main exocrine cell types (acinar and ductal) were investigated separately [67]. Acinar cell function was quantified with an immunochemical faecal elastase assay [76,77], and ductal cell function was assessed using secretin-stimulated magnetic resonance cholangiopancreatography (sMRCP) [67,78]. The results from this study demonstrated that acinar cell function was more closely related to gut microbiome composition than ductal cell function [67].

Acinar cells produce many different products, so determining which of these play a role in the composition of the gut microbiome has also been investigated. It has been shown that pancreatic secretions possess both bacteriostatic activity against common bacterial pathogens and fungistatic activity against Candida albicans [79]. However, this function of canine pancreatic secretions persisted when digestive enzymes were inhibited, which likely indicates that digestive enzymes are not the main factors that regulate the intestinal flora [67,79]. Apart from digestive enzymes, it has been shown that the pancreas produces antimicrobial peptides [67,80–82]. One such example of important antimicrobial peptides produced by the pancreas are cathelicidins, these are small proteolytically activated peptides shown to be active against bacteria, fungi and some viruses [83]. Murine studies have indicated that cathelicidin-related antimicrobial peptide (CRAMP) plays an important role in the regulation of the intestinal microbiome; when genetic modifications were made to reduce levels of CRAMP production in the murine pancreas, fatal bacterial overgrowth in the intestine occurred [81]. In human studies however, cathelicidin antimicrobial peptide (CAMP) levels in faeces have not been shown to be different in patients with PEI compared to healthy controls [67], this does not necessarily mean that this peptide is unimportant and may be due to sampling difficulties [67]. These products and their roles are summarised in Table 1.

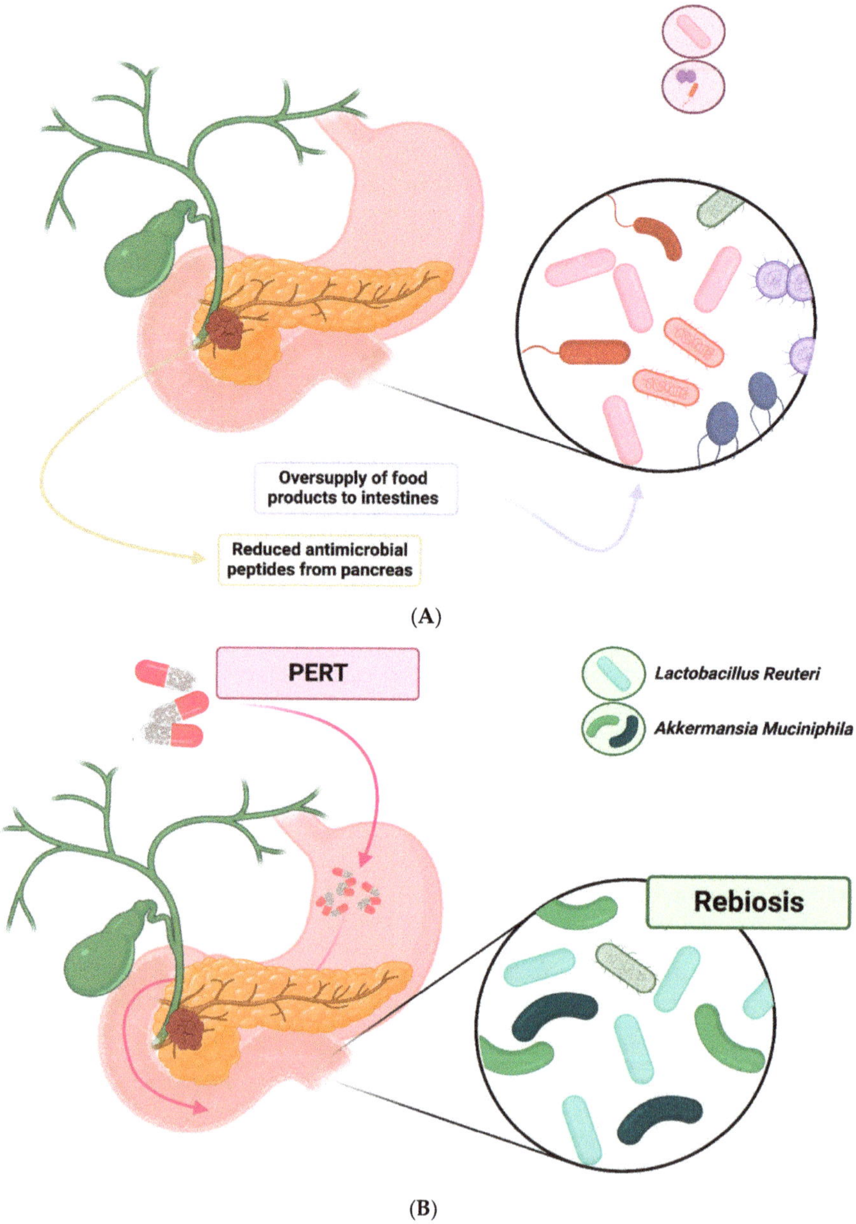

Figure 1. (**A**) mechanisms of dysbiosis in PEI; (**B**) mechanisms of rebiosis in PEI.

Table 1. Summary of exocrine pancreatic products and their effect on the gut microbiome.

Exocrine Pancreatic Product	Example	Source Pancreatic Cell Type	Function	Effect on Gut Microbiome
Bicarbonate rich fluid	-	Duct epithelial cell	Carry pancreatic enzymes into small intestine. Optimise pH for enzyme action.	sMRCP indicates negligible role
Digestive enzymes	Lipase, protease, amylase	Acinar cell	Digest food products	Oversupply of food products leads to significant changes especially complex carbohydrates. Inhibition in canine models did not affect composition of microbiome.
Antimicrobial peptides	CAMP and CRAMP	Acinar cell	Bacteriostatic properties	Murine studies indicate a regulatory role for the gut microbiome. Human studies remain inconclusive due to sampling issues

sMRCP = secretin-stimulated magnetic resonance cholangiopancreatography CAMP = cathelicidin antimicrobial peptide; CRAMP = cathelicidin-related antimicrobial peptide.

Another mechanism by which it is thought PEI may lead to significant changes in the gut microbiome is by the oversupply of food products to the intestine, leading to the overgrowth of dominant bacteria [70]. In particular, it has been suggested that the increased availability of complex carbohydrates, seen in patients with PEI due to reduced digestive activity, may act as a substrate for certain communities within the gut microbiome [67]. Given that acinar cell activity has been closely linked to gut microbiome composition in humans [67], and the main function of these cells is to produce digestive enzymes, this seems like another plausible mechanism by which PEI may influence gut microbiome composition.

2.3. Gut Microbiome Changes from Pancreatic Exocrine Insufficiency in Different Disease States

Whilst there is credible evidence from both animal and human studies to suggest that PEI leads to significant changes in the gut microbiome, it is important to understand the impact that different disease processes leading to PEI in humans may have on the gut microbiome, such as chronic pancreatitis (CP) and pancreatic cancer (PC). For example, chronic pancreatitis (CP) is one of the main causes of PEI in humans and is known to be linked to changes in the gut microbiome [68–70,84], but it is often caused by excessive smoking or alcohol consumption, which in themselves may lead to changes in the gut microbiome. Indeed, a recent study in which the gut microbiome of chronic pancreatitis patients was investigated with 16S rRNA gene sequencing and compared to a matched population of healthy controls described some important findings [68]. The study by Frost et al. reported that not only did CP lead to significant changes in the gut microbiome, namely reduced microbial diversity and increased abundance of pathogenic bacteria, but more importantly these changes were independent of exocrine function (measured with stool elastase) [68]. This suggests that gut microbiome changes in pancreatic disease are not solely related to reduced pancreatic exocrine function.

At present, there is limited data on the changes in the gut microbiome related to PEI in PC patients. It is plausible that, as observed in CP patients [68], there are multiple factors influencing the gut microbiome composition in PC patients, beyond just PEI. For example, many PC patients experience cancer cachexia, characterised by systemic inflammation and nutritional depletion [53]. Links between the state of cancer cachexia and the gut microbiome have been drawn [85,86] and this means that changes in the gut microbiome in PC patients are likely to differ to those in CP patients, even though both experience PEI. As such, further study is required to understand the changes in the gut microbiome changes in different pancreatic disease processes such as CP and PC. Improved understanding of the changes to the gut microbiome in both CP and PC patients will inform future studies investigating therapeutics that aim to return the gut microbiome towards a healthier phenotype in these patients.

2.4. Effects of Pancreatic Enzyme Replacement on the Gut Microbiome

From the evidence outlined above, it appears that PEI is associated with gut microbiome dysbiosis, which in turn is thought to be associated with multiple adverse downstream effects. Therefore, it is desirable to identify strategies by which harmful effects of PEI on the gut microbiome may be mitigated and the microbiome returned towards a healthier state. One logical method in PC patients would be through pancreatic enzyme replacement therapy (PERT), which is frequently under prescribed, despite being recommended for all with pancreatic cancer by national practice guidelines [61,62]. In animal models, PERT has been shown to reverse changes to the microbiome caused by PEI [87,88]. Specifically, an increase in beneficial bacterial species, such as *Akkermansia muciniphila* and *Lactobacillus reuteri* [87,88], and a reduction in species associated with dysbiosis such as *Prevotella* and those of the phylum *Proteobacteria* [87]. This reestablishment of a healthy complex microbiome after dysbiosis has occurred (sometimes referred to as 'rebiosis' [69]) (Figure 1B), reduces intestinal inflammation, improves PEI-associated symptoms and mediates nutritional decline [69,88]. Therefore, it may be a further mechanism by which PERT acts to improve quality of life [57,58] and survival amongst pancreatic cancer patients [59,60] (Figure 2). That said, some animal evidence has suggested that the gut microbiome of animals treated with PERT still exhibits important differences to healthy controls [89]. As a result, further study is required to evaluate to what degree PERT can return the gut microbiome of PC patients with PEI towards a healthier composition and whether this translates into improved outcomes.

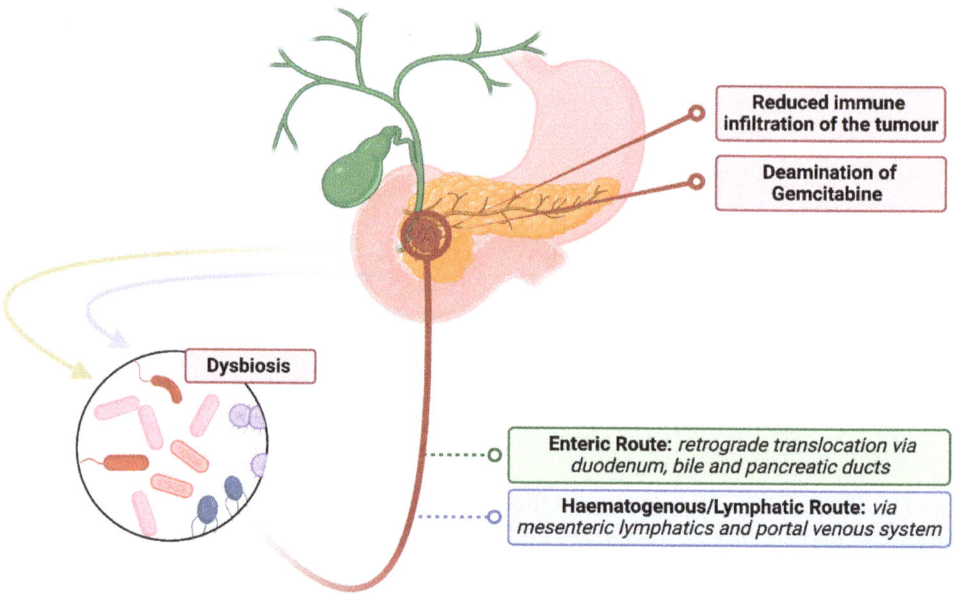

Figure 2. Links between gut microbiome and pancreatic tumour microbiome.

3. Effects of the Intestinal Microbiome in Pancreatic Cancer Patients

3.1. Intestinal Microbiome and Clinical Outcomes in Pancreatic Cancer

Associations between microbiome composition and clinical outcome for patients with PDAC are now being observed. Differences in intestinal microbiome composition between patients with short-term survival (STS) and long-term survival (LTS) have been demonstrated with 16S rRNA gene sequencing [21,39]. An increasing abundance of *Acinetobacter* was identified in the highly aggressive 'basal-like' subtype of pancreatic ductal adenocarcinoma (PDAC) using metagenomic sequencing of resected tumours [90]. However, in the absence of mechanistic insights, these findings remain associative rather than causative.

3.2. Extraintestinal Effects of the Gut Microbiome in Pancreatic Disease

The effects of intestinal microbiome dysbiosis have been shown to extend beyond the intestinal tract in patients with pancreatic disease. In acute and chronic pancreatitis, a frequent clinical issue is the colonisation of pancreatic necrosis and fluid collections with pathogenic bacteria. Evidence suggests that numbers of beneficial bacterial species such as *Faecalibacterium* [91,92] and *Fusicatenibacter* [93] are reduced in patients with CP [68]. These bacterial species are thought to play an anti-inflammatory role in the colon and preserve the intestinal barrier through the production of short-chain fatty acids and lactate [91,92], reducing the chance of extraintestinal translocation of pathogenic bacteria [93,94]. As a result, gut microbiome changes can be directly related to the severity of the disease [68,95].

Importantly, for pancreatic cancer patients, it is now appreciated that pancreatic tumours themselves harbour a population of bacteria, referred to as the tumour microbiome [21,73,96,97], which has been shown to influence the prognosis of PDAC [21,39,98]. Relevant to this article, it has been shown that the gut microbiome influences the composition of this tumour microbiome in pancreatic cancer [39]. The exact mechanism for this remains debated, but possible routes include retrograde translocation from the gut, via the duodenum and bile/pancreatic ducts, spread from the portal circulation or mesenteric lymph nodes (Figure 2) [20–22]. The importance of the tumour microbiome is attracting increasing interest [96,99] and has been shown to differentiate between different phenotypes of pancreatic cancer, as well as influencing clinical outcome [39,90]. For example, some human pancreatic tumours are colonised by *Gammaproteobacteria*, a subset of which possess an isoform of cytidine deaminase, which is capable of metabolising gemcitabine into an inactive form [21] and, in so doing, increases the tumour's chemoresistance and therefore reduces treatment efficacy [100,101]. Evidence of clinical benefit in modulating the tumour microbiome has also been demonstrated in a recent large cohort study which showed that peri-chemotherapy antibiotics in metastatic PDAC patients improved cancer-specific survival [102]. Interestingly, a survival benefit was seen only in patients receiving gemcitabine, not fluorouracil, adding to the growing body of evidence that bacteria-mediated gemcitabine resistance is prevalent in PDAC patients [20] and could represent a target for future therapies.

3.3. Tumour Microbiome and Immune Infiltration

A further route by which it is thought that the tumour microbiome influences the prognosis of PDAC includes local immunosuppression and subsequent accelerated oncogenesis [103–106]. A relationship between the tumour microbiome and tumour immune infiltration has been demonstrated [103] with an increase in infiltration of CD8+ T cells reported following ablation of the tumour microbiome with antibiotics [103]. Furthermore, transfer of selected bacteria from PDAC tissue accelerated tumorigenesis [103]. This highlights a possible mechanism by which a more favourable gut microbiome, which is observed through appropriate treatment of PEI with PERT, may influence cancer-related outcomes in PDAC patients. Future studies should therefore seek to compare the gut and tumour microbiome composition to immune infiltration of tumours, for example via immunohistochemistry, to further investigate this relationship.

4. Diagnostic and Therapeutic Applications for Greater Understanding of the Gut Microbiome in Pancreatic Cancer Patients

4.1. Use of Intestinal Microbiome Testing for Diagnosis of Pancreatic Exocrine Insufficiency

If changes in the microbiome are observed in PEI, then it may also be possible to diagnose this using intestinal microbiome sequencing from stool samples. The incidence of PEI preoperatively is challenging to assess, and no ideal diagnostic test currently exists. The secretin test and coefficient of fat absorption (CFA) are accurate but expensive and unpleasant, whilst faecal elastase (FE-1), although suitable for routine use, has poor sensitivity in mild PEI [107]. Traditionally, a combination of patient reported symptoms, such as steatorrhoea, and faecal elastase (FE-1) have been used to diagnose PEI. However, the diagnostic accuracy of FE-1 has been questioned, especially amongst those who have undergone surgical resection where the increased ratio of faecal fat to FE-1 reduces the sensitivity of the test [107,108]. The ^{13}C mixed triglyceride breath test is emerging as a promising diagnostic tool [109], but expense and time limit its use to specialist or research centres only [109,110]. Therefore, if changes in the microbiome in patients with PEI are further understood, these could be measured and quantified to be used as a new diagnostic test.

4.2. Titration of Pancreatic Enzyme Replacement Therapy

Given the difficulties in diagnosing PEI in routine clinical practice, monitoring the response to PERT is arguably even more challenging. Whilst UK NICE recommend consideration of PERT treatment for all patients following pancreatic resection [61,62] without the need for a positive diagnostic test, it can be challenging to ensure that each patient is taking the correct dose. If changes in the intestinal microbiome with PERT treatment in PEI patients are quantifiable, then it may be possible to monitor long-term trends with PERT treatment and make dose changes accordingly using stool sample sequencing.

4.3. Positive Effects of Pancreatic Enzyme Replacement Therapies on the Intestinal Microbiome

As described above, early evidence suggests that by modulating the gut microbiome it may be possible to alter the composition of the tumour microbiome. This has been demonstrated in animal studies using faecal microbiota transplantation (FMT) [39,73]. Using the knowledge that differences in intestinal microbiome composition between short-term survival (STS) and long-term survival (LTS) patients have been demonstrated with 16S rRNA gene sequencing [21,39]; researchers sought to modulate the intestinal microbiome with FMT. Interestingly, it has been shown that via FMT from STS and LTS patients into mice, it is possible to modulate the tumour microbiome and thus affect tumour growth [39]. This could also link to some possible benefits of PERT as, if treatment is able to return the intestinal microbiome of pancreatic cancer patients towards a healthy composition, this may positively influence the tumour microbiome. Given that *Acinetobacter* abundance has been associated with aggressive 'basal-like' tumours [90], it is noteworthy that this can be reduced in the gut microbiome of a porcine PEI model reduced after administration of PERT [87]. The potential ability of PERT to modulate the intestinal microbiome, and consequently the tumour microbiome, may be an important determinant of clinical outcome and is worthy of more thorough investigation.

5. Conclusions and Future Directions

It is likely that the gut microbiome of pancreatic cancer patients with PEI exhibits profound dysbiosis and that this may potentially be reversible with PERT. However, further research is needed to conclude if this is indeed the case. Future research should seek to elucidate the specific changes that occur in PC patients with PEI as these are likely to be different to gut microbiome changes in patients with other, benign causes of PEI such as cystic fibrosis or CP. It would also be important to investigate whether the gut microbiome of PC patients who have PEI treated with PERT experience a return of gut microbiome towards that of healthy controls. It is also important to acknowledge that supplements, such as probiotics as well as faecal microbiota transplantation, can influence the composition of the gut microbiome and therefore may also be beneficial in PC [111].

In addition, the downstream effects of gut microbiome dysbiosis in PC patients with PEI need to be further explored and understood. For example, future studies should seek to compare the gut microbiome with the tumour microbiome in PC patients with and without PEI. Similarly, the interaction between the gut microbiome and the immune system in this cohort should be further investigated. This could be achieved by measuring the peripheral immune state in PC patients with and without PEI, or before and after PERT treatment. Equally, the immune infiltration of resected tumours could be compared to the gut microbiome of PC patients and their degree of exocrine function and/or PERT treatment.

It is also important to investigate the extent to which the gut microbiome influences chemosensitivity in PC patients, and whether this is influenced by the degree of PEI or PERT. This may be achieved by monitoring treatment response to neoadjuvant chemotherapy via Ca19-9 levels, radiological response or tumour regression grading of resected specimens, and correlating this to exocrine function and PERT treatment.

In summary, it has been recognised that untreated PEI is harmful in PC patients and that PERT treatment leads to improved outcomes. It has been proposed that this is likely due to improved nutritional status, thus allowing more patients to undergo physiologically demanding treatments, but it is possible that treatment of PEI with PERT in PC patients leads to a more favourable gut microbiome. This in turn may modulate the tumour microbiome, thereby directly influencing tumour growth and the quality of the tumour-specific immune response. The effect of PEI and PERT on the gut microbiome of pancreatic cancer patients is a vital area for future study and may open the door to much needed new diagnostic and therapeutic options for this challenging condition.

Author Contributions: Conceptualization, J.M.H.-S., L.A.H., S.F.P.-B. and K.J.R.; methodology, J.M.H.-S., L.A.H., S.F.P.-B. and K.J.R.; writing—original draft preparation, J.M.H.-S., L.A.H., S.F.P.-B. and K.J.R.; writing—review and editing, N.M., A.E.F., A.D.B., P.M. and K.J.R.; supervision, A.E.F., A.D.B., P.M. and K.J.R. All authors have read and agreed to the published version of the manuscript.

Funding: A.D.B. is funded by an MRC Senior Clinical Fellowship (ref MR/X006433/1).

Institutional Review Board Statement: Not applicable.

Informed Consent Statement: Not applicable.

Data Availability Statement: Not applicable.

Conflicts of Interest: The authors declare no conflict of interest.

References

1. Lederberg, J.; Mccray, A.T. COMMENTARY 'Ome Sweet' Omics-A Genealogical Treasury of Words. *Science* **2001**, *15*, 8.
2. Marchesi, J.R.; Ravel, J. The vocabulary of microbiome research: A proposal. *Microbiome* **2015**, *3*, 31. [CrossRef] [PubMed]
3. Mullish, B.H.; Quraishi, M.N.; Segal, J.P.; Ianiro, G.; Iqbal, T.H. The gut microbiome: What every gastroenterologist needs to know. *Frontline Gastroenterol.* **2021**, *12*, 118–127. [CrossRef] [PubMed]
4. Song, S.; Jarvie, T.; Hattori, M. Our second genome-human metagenome: How next-generation sequencer changes our life through microbiology. *Adv. Microb. Physiol.* **2013**, *62*, 119–144. [CrossRef] [PubMed]
5. Zhang, W.; Li, F.; Nie, L. Integrating multiple "omics" analysis for microbial biology: Application and methodologies. *Microbiology* **2010**, *156*, 287–301. [CrossRef] [PubMed]
6. Medini, D.; Serruto, D.; Parkhill, J.; Relman, D.A.; Donati, C.; Moxon, R.; Falkow, S.; Rappuoli, R. Microbiology in the post-genomic era. *Nat. Rev. Microbiol.* **2008**, *6*, 419–430. [CrossRef] [PubMed]
7. Kyrpides, N.C. Fifteen years of microbial genomics: Meeting the challenges and fulfilling the dream. *Nat. Biotechnol.* **2009**, *27*, 627–632. [CrossRef]
8. Fan, Y.; Pedersen, O. Gut microbiota in human metabolic health and disease. *Nat. Rev. Microbiol.* **2020**, *19*, 55–71. [CrossRef]
9. Durack, J.; Lynch, S.V. The gut microbiome: Relationships with disease and opportunities for therapy. *J. Exp. Med.* **2019**, *216*, 20. [CrossRef]
10. Lepage, P.; Hösler, R.; Spehlmann, M.E.; Rehman, A.; Zvirbliene, A.; Begun, A.; Ott, S.; Kupcinskas, L.; Doré, J.; Raedler, A.; et al. Twin study indicates loss of interaction between microbiota and mucosa of patients with ulcerative colitis. *Gastroenterology* **2011**, *141*, 227–236. [CrossRef]

11. Dicksved, J.; Halfvarson, J.; Rosenquist, M.; Järnerot, G.; Tysk, C.; Apajalahti, J.; Engstrand, L.; Jansson, J.K. Molecular analysis of the gut microbiota of identical twins with Crohn's disease. *ISME J.* **2008**, *2*, 716–727. [CrossRef] [PubMed]
12. Segal, J.P.; Mullish, B.H.; Quraishi, M.N.; Acharjee, A.; Williams, H.R.T.; Iqbal, T.; Hart, A.L.; Marchesi, J.R. The application of omics techniques to understand the role of the gut microbiota in inflammatory bowel disease. *Ther. Adv. Gastroenterol.* **2019**, *12*, 1756284818822250. [CrossRef] [PubMed]
13. Mullish, B.H.; Osborne, L.S.; Marchesi, J.R.; Mcdonald, J.A. The implementation of omics technologies in cancer microbiome research. *Ecancermedicalscience* **2018**, *12*, 864. [CrossRef] [PubMed]
14. Shi, F.; Liu, G.; Lin, Y.; Guo, C.L.; Han, J.; Chu, E.S.H.; Shi, C.; Li, Y.; Zhang, H.; Hu, C.; et al. Altered gut microbiome composition by appendectomy contributes to colorectal cancer. *Oncogene* **2022**, *42*, 530–540. [CrossRef] [PubMed]
15. Chrysostomou, D.; Roberts, L.A.; Marchesi, J.R.; Kinross, J.M. Gut Microbiota Modulation of Efficacy and Toxicity of Cancer Chemotherapy and Immunotherapy. *Gastroenterology* **2022**, *164*, 198–213. [CrossRef] [PubMed]
16. Schwenger, K.J.; Clermont-Dejean, N.; Allard, J.P. The role of the gut microbiome in chronic liver disease: The clinical evidence revised. *JHEP Rep.* **2019**, *1*, 214. [CrossRef]
17. Tilg, H.; Cani, P.D.; Mayer, E.A. Gut microbiome and liver diseases. *Gut* **2016**, *65*, 2035–2044. [CrossRef]
18. Nagata, N.; Nishijima, S.; Kojima, Y.; Hisada, Y.; Imbe, K.; Miyoshi-Akiyama, T.; Suda, W.; Kimura, M.; Aoki, R.; Sekine, K.; et al. Metagenomic Identification of Microbial Signatures Predicting Pancreatic Cancer from a Multinational Study. *Gastroenterology* **2022**, *163*, 222–238. [CrossRef]
19. Kartal, E.; Schmidt, T.S.B.; Molina-Montes, E.; Rodríguez-Perales, S.; Wirbel, J.; Maistrenko, O.M.; Akanni, W.A.; Alashkar Alhamwe, B.; Alves, R.J.; Carrato, A.; et al. A faecal microbiota signature with high specificity for pancreatic cancer. *Gut* **2022**, *71*, 1359–1372. [CrossRef]
20. Thomas, R.M.; Jobin, C. Microbiota in pancreatic health and disease: The next frontier in microbiome research. *Nat. Rev. Gastroenterol. Hepatol.* **2019**, *17*, 53–64. [CrossRef]
21. Geller, L.T.; Barzily-Rokni, M.; Danino, T.; Jonas, O.H.; Shental, N.; Nejman, D.; Gavert, N.; Zwang, Y.; Cooper, Z.A.; Shee, K.; et al. Potential role of intratumor bacteria in mediating tumor resistance to the chemotherapeutic drug gemcitabine. *Science* **2017**, *357*, 1156–1160. [CrossRef] [PubMed]
22. Langheinrich, M.; Wirtz, S.; Kneis, B.; Gittler, M.M.; Tyc, O.; Schierwagen, R.; Brunner, M.; Krautz, C.; Weber, G.F.; Pilarsky, C.; et al. Microbiome Patterns in Matched Bile, Duodenal, Pancreatic Tumor Tissue, Drainage, and Stool Samples: Association with Preoperative Stenting and Postoperative Pancreatic Fistula Development. *J. Clin. Med.* **2020**, *9*, 2785. [CrossRef] [PubMed]
23. Oettle, H.; Neuhaus, P.; Hochhaus, A.; Hartmann, J.T.; Gellert, K.; Ridwelski, K.; Niedergethmann, M.; Zülke, C.; Fahlke, J.; Arning, M.B.; et al. Adjuvant chemotherapy with gemcitabine and long-term outcomes among patients with resected pancreatic cancer: The CONKO-001 randomized trial. *JAMA* **2013**, *310*, 1473–1481. [CrossRef]
24. Neoptolemos, J.P.; Palmer, D.H.; Ghaneh, P.; Psarelli, E.E.; Valle, J.W.; Halloran, C.M.; Faluyi, O.; O'Reilly, D.A.; Cunningham, D.; Wadsley, J.; et al. Comparison of adjuvant gemcitabine and capecitabine with gemcitabine monotherapy in patients with resected pancreatic cancer (ESPAC-4): A multicentre, open-label, randomised, phase 3 trial. *Lancet* **2017**, *389*, 1011–1024. [CrossRef] [PubMed]
25. Kleeff, J.; Korc, M.; Apte, M.; La Vecchia, C.; Johnson, C.D.; Biankin, A.V.; Neale, R.E.; Tempero, M.; Tuveson, D.A.; Hruban, R.H.; et al. Pancreatic cancer. *Nat. Rev. Dis. Prim.* **2016**, *2*, 16022. [CrossRef] [PubMed]
26. Isaji, S.; Mizuno, S.; Windsor, J.A.; Bassi, C.; Fernández-del Castillo, C.; Hackert, T.; Hayasaki, A.; Katz, M.H.G.; Kim, S.W.; Kishiwada, M.; et al. International consensus on definition and criteria of borderline resectable pancreatic ductal adenocarcinoma 2017. *Pancreatology* **2018**, *18*, 2–11. [CrossRef]
27. Matsuda, Y.; Hagio, M.; Naito, Z.; Ishiwata, T. Clinicopathological features of 30 autopsy cases of pancreatic carcinoma. *J. Nippon Med. Sch.* **2012**, *79*, 459–467. [CrossRef]
28. Mierke, F.; Hempel, S.; Distler, M.; Aust, D.E.; Saeger, H.D.; Weitz, J.; Welsch, T. Impact of Portal Vein Involvement from Pancreatic Cancer on Metastatic Pattern After Surgical Resection. *Ann. Surg. Oncol.* **2016**, *23*, 730–736. [CrossRef]
29. Bissolati, M.; Sandri, M.T.; Burtulo, G.; Zorzino, L.; Balzano, G.; Braga, M. Portal vein-circulating tumor cells predict liver metastases in patients with resectable pancreatic cancer. *Tumour Biol.* **2015**, *36*, 991–996. [CrossRef]
30. Conroy, T.; Galais, M.-P.; Raoul, J.-L.; Bouché, O.; Gourgou-Bourgade, S.; Douillard, J.-Y.; Etienne, P.-L.; Boige, V.; Martel-Lafay, I.; Michel, P.; et al. Definitive chemoradiotherapy with FOLFOX versus fluorouracil and cisplatin in patients with oesophageal cancer (PRODIGE5/ACCORD17): Final results of a randomised, phase 2/3 trial. *Lancet Oncol.* **2014**, *15*, 305–314. [CrossRef]
31. Von Hoff, D.D.; Ervin, T.; Arena, F.P.; Chiorean, E.G.; Infante, J.; Moore, M.; Seay, T.; Tjulandin, S.A.; Ma, W.W.; Saleh, M.N.; et al. Increased Survival in Pancreatic Cancer with nab-Paclitaxel plus Gemcitabine. *N. Engl. J. Med.* **2013**, *369*, 1691–1703. [CrossRef]
32. Tempero, M.A.; Malafa, M.P.; Behrman, S.W.; Benson, A.B.; Casper, E.S.; Chiorean, E.G.; Chung, V.; Cohen, S.J.; Czito, B.; Engebretson, A.; et al. Pancreatic adenocarcinoma, version 2.2014: Featured updates to the NCCN guidelines. *J. Natl. Compr. Cancer Netw.* **2014**, *12*, 1083–1093. [CrossRef]
33. Bellon, E.; Gebauer, F.; Tachezy, M.; Izbicki, J.R.; Bockhorn, M. Pancreatic cancer and liver metastases: State of the art. *Updates Surg.* **2016**, *68*, 247–251. [CrossRef]
34. Seufferlein, T.; Bachet, J.B.; Van cutsem, E.; Rougier, P. Pancreatic adenocarcinoma: ESMO-ESDO Clinical Practice Guidelines for diagnosis, treatment and follow-up. *Ann. Oncol.* **2012**, *23* (Suppl. 7), vii33–vii40. [CrossRef] [PubMed]

35. Merz, V.; Mangiameli, D.; Zecchetto, C.; Quinzii, A.; Pietrobono, S.; Messina, C.; Casalino, S.; Gaule, M.; Pesoni, C.; Vitale, P.; et al. Predictive Biomarkers for a Personalized Approach in Resectable Pancreatic Cancer. *Front. Surg.* **2022**, *9*, 866173. [CrossRef] [PubMed]
36. Daamen, L.A.; Groot, V.P.; Besselink, M.G.; Bosscha, K.; Busch, O.R.; Cirkel, G.A.; van Dam, R.M.; Festen, S.; Groot Koerkamp, B.; Haj Mohammad, N.; et al. Detection, Treatment, and Survival of Pancreatic Cancer Recurrence in the Netherlands. *Ann. Surg.* **2020**, *275*, 769–775. [CrossRef] [PubMed]
37. Sinn, M.; Bahra, M.; Liersch, T.; Gellert, K.; Messmann, H.; Bechstein, W.; Waldschmidt, D.; Jacobasch, L.; Wilhelm, M.; Rau, B.M.; et al. CONKO-005: Adjuvant Chemotherapy with Gemcitabine Plus Erlotinib Versus Gemcitabine Alone in Patients After R0 Resection of Pancreatic Cancer: A Multicenter Randomized Phase III Trial. *J. Clin. Oncol.* **2017**, *35*, 3330–3337. [CrossRef] [PubMed]
38. Neoptolemos, J.P.; Stocken, D.D.; Bassi, C.; Ghaneh, P.; Cunningham, D.; Goldstein, D.; Padbury, R.; Moore, M.J.; Gallinger, S.; Mariette, C.; et al. Adjuvant chemotherapy with fluorouracil plus folinic acid vs gemcitabine following pancreatic cancer resection: A randomized controlled trial. *JAMA* **2010**, *304*, 1073–1081. [CrossRef]
39. Riquelme, E.; Zhang, Y.; Zhang, L.; Montiel, M.; Zoltan, M.; Dong, W.; Quesada, P.; Sahin, I.; Chandra, V.; San Lucas, A.; et al. Tumor Microbiome Diversity and Composition Influence Pancreatic Cancer Outcomes. *Cell* **2019**, *178*, 795–806.e12. [CrossRef]
40. Dominguez-Muñoz, J.E. Diagnosis and treatment of pancreatic exocrine insufficiency. *Curr. Opin. Gastroenterol.* **2018**, *34*, 349–354. [CrossRef]
41. Hartman, V.; Roeyen, E.; Bracke, B.; Huysentruyt, F.; De Gendt, S.; Chapelle, T.; Ysebaert, D.; Hendrikx, B.; Roeyen, G. Prevalence of pancreatic exocrine insufficiency after pancreatic surgery measured by 13C mixed triglyceride breath test: A prospective cohort study. *Pancreatology* **2023**, *23*, 563–568. [CrossRef] [PubMed]
42. Tseng, D.S.J.; Molenaar, I.Q.; Besselink, M.G.; Van Eijck, C.H.; Rinkes, I.H.B.; Van Santvoort, H.C. Pancreatic exocrine insufficiency in patients with pancreatic or periampullary cancer a systematic review. *Pancreas* **2016**, *45*, 325–330. [CrossRef] [PubMed]
43. Powell-Brett, S.; de Liguori Carino, N.; Roberts, K. Understanding pancreatic exocrine insufficiency and replacement therapy in pancreatic cancer. *Eur. J. Surg. Oncol.* **2021**, *47*, 539–544. [CrossRef] [PubMed]
44. Chirletti Professor, P.; Peparini, N.; Caronna, R.; Papini, F.; Vietri Professor, F.; Gualdi, G. Monitoring Fibrosis of the Pancreatic Remnant after a Pancreaticoduodenectomy with Dynamic MRI: Are the Results Independent of the Adopted Reconstructive Technique? *J. Surg. Res.* **2010**, *164*, e49–e52. [CrossRef]
45. Zaccari, P.; Ribichini, E.; Stigliano, S.; Serrao, G.; Scalese, G.; Caronna, R.; Chirletti, P.; Severi, C. Occurrence of Pathological Abdominal Fat Distribution After Pancreaticoduodenectomy at Long-term Follow-up: A Single-Center Experience. *Pancreas* **2021**, *50*, E15–E16. [CrossRef]
46. Johnson, C.D.; Arbuckle, R.; Bonner, N.; Connett, G.; Dominguez-Munoz, E.; Levy, P.; Staab, D.; Williamson, N.; Lerch, M.M. Qualitative Assessment of the Symptoms and Impact of Pancreatic Exocrine Insufficiency (PEI) to Inform the Development of a Patient-Reported Outcome (PRO) Instrument. *Patient* **2017**, *10*, 615–628. [CrossRef]
47. Johnson, C.D.; Williamson, N.; Janssen-van Solingen, G.; Arbuckle, R.; Johnson, C.; Simpson, S.; Staab, D.; Dominguez-Munoz, E.; Levy, P.; Connett, G.; et al. Psychometric evaluation of a patient-reported outcome measure in pancreatic exocrine insufficiency (PEI). *Pancreatology* **2019**, *19*, 182–190. [CrossRef]
48. Gilliland, T.M.; Villafane-Ferriol, N.; Shah, K.P.; Shah, R.M.; Tran Cao, H.S.; Massarweh, N.N.; Silberfein, E.J.; Choi, E.A.; Hsu, C.; McElhany, A.L.; et al. Nutritional and Metabolic Derangements in Pancreatic Cancer and Pancreatic Resection. *Nutrients* **2017**, *9*, 243. [CrossRef]
49. Lindkvist, B.; Phillips, M.E.; Domínguez-Muñoz, J.E. Clinical, anthropometric and laboratory nutritional markers of pancreatic exocrine insufficiency: Prevalence and diagnostic use. *Pancreatology* **2015**, *15*, 589–597. [CrossRef]
50. Shintakuya, R.; Uemura, K.; Murakami, Y.; Kondo, N.; Nakagawa, N.; Urabe, K.; Okano, K.; Awai, K.; Higaki, T.; Sueda, T. Sarcopenia is closely associated with pancreatic exocrine insufficiency in patients with pancreatic disease. *Pancreatology* **2017**, *17*, 70–75. [CrossRef]
51. de la Iglesia, D.; Vallejo-Senra, N.; López-López, A.; Iglesias-Garcia, J.; Lariño-Noia, J.; Nieto-García, L.; Domínguez-Muñoz, J.E. Pancreatic exocrine insufficiency and cardiovascular risk in patients with chronic pancreatitis: A prospective, longitudinal cohort study. *J. Gastroenterol. Hepatol.* **2019**, *34*, 277–283. [CrossRef] [PubMed]
52. Sikkens, E.C.M.; Cahen, D.L.; Koch, A.D.; Braat, H.; Poley, J.W.; Kuipers, E.J.; Bruno, M.J. The prevalence of fat-soluble vitamin deficiencies and a decreased bone mass in patients with chronic pancreatitis. *Pancreatology* **2013**, *13*, 238–242. [CrossRef] [PubMed]
53. Skipworth, R.J.E.; Stewart, G.D.; Dejong, C.H.C.; Preston, T.; Fearon, K.C.H. Pathophysiology of cancer cachexia: Much more than host-tumour interaction? *Clin. Nutr.* **2007**, *26*, 667–676. [CrossRef] [PubMed]
54. Fearon, K.C.H.; Baracos, V.E. Cachexia in pancreatic cancer: New treatment options and measures of success. *HPB* **2010**, *12*, 323. [CrossRef]
55. Partelli, S.; Frulloni, L.; Minniti, C.; Bassi, C.; Barugola, G.; D'Onofrio, M.; Crippa, S.; Falconi, M. Faecal elastase-1 is an independent predictor of survival in advanced pancreatic cancer. *Dig. Liver Dis.* **2012**, *44*, 945–951. [CrossRef] [PubMed]
56. Heerkens, H.D.; van Berkel, L.; Tseng, D.S.J.; Monninkhof, E.M.; van Santvoort, H.C.; Hagendoorn, J.; Borel Rinkes, I.H.M.; Lips, I.M.; Intven, M.; Molenaar, I.Q. Long-term health-related quality of life after pancreatic resection for malignancy in patients with and without severe postoperative complications. *HPB* **2018**, *20*, 188–195. [CrossRef]

57. Landers, A.; Brown, H.; Strother, M. The effectiveness of pancreatic enzyme replacement therapy for malabsorption in advanced pancreatic cancer, a pilot study. *Palliat. Care Res. Treat.* **2019**, *12*, 1178224218825270. [CrossRef]
58. Seiler, C.M.; Izbicki, J.; Varga-Szabõ, L.; Czakõ, L.; Fiõk, J.; Sperti, C.; Lerch, M.M.; Pezzilli, R.; Vasileva, G.; Pap, Á.; et al. Randomised clinical trial: A 1-week, double-blind, placebo-controlled study of pancreatin 25 000 Ph. Eur. minimicrospheres (Creon 25000 MMS) for pancreatic exocrine insufficiency after pancreatic surgery, with a 1-year open-label extension. *Aliment. Pharmacol. Ther.* **2013**, *37*, 691–702. [CrossRef]
59. Roberts, K.J.; Bannister, C.A.; Schrem, H. Enzyme replacement improves survival among patients with pancreatic cancer: Results of a population based study. *Pancreatology* **2019**, *19*, 114–121. [CrossRef]
60. Roberts, K.J.; Schrem, H.; Hodson, J.; Angelico, R.; Dasari, B.V.M.; Coldham, C.A.; Marudanayagam, R.; Sutcliffe, R.P.; Muiesan, P.; Isaac, J.; et al. Pancreas exocrine replacement therapy is associated with increased survival following pancreatoduodenectomy for periampullary malignancy. *HPB* **2017**, *19*, 859–867. [CrossRef]
61. Pancreatic Cancer in Adults: Diagnosis and Management NICE Guideline. 2018. Available online: www.nice.org.uk/guidance/ng85 (accessed on 3 January 2023).
62. Phillips, M.E.; Hopper, A.D.; Leeds, J.S.; Roberts, K.J.; McGeeney, L.; Duggan, S.N.; Kumar, R. Consensus for the management of pancreatic exocrine insufficiency: UK practical guidelines. *BMJ Open Gastroenterol.* **2021**, *8*, e000643. [CrossRef] [PubMed]
63. Kim, H.; Yoon, Y.S.; Han, Y.; Kwon, W.; Kim, S.W.; Han, H.S.; Yoon, D.S.; Park, J.S.; Park, S.J.; Han, S.S.; et al. Effects of pancreatic enzyme replacement therapy on body weight and nutritional assessments after pancreatoduodenectomy in a randomized trial. *Clin. Gastroenterol. Hepatol.* **2020**, *18*, 926–934. [CrossRef] [PubMed]
64. Bruno, M.J.; Haverkort, E.B.; Tijssen, G.P.; Tytgat, G.N.J.; Van Leeuwen, D.J. Placebo controlled trial of enteric coated pancreatin microsphere treatment in patients with unresectable cancer of the pancreatic head region. *Gut* **1998**, *42*, 92–96. [CrossRef] [PubMed]
65. Sherman, M.H.; Yu, R.T.; Engle, D.D.; Ding, N.; Atkins, A.R.; Tiriac, H.; Collisson, E.A.; Connor, F.; Van Dyke, T.; Kozlov, S.; et al. Vitamin D Receptor-Mediated Stromal Reprogramming Suppresses Pancreatitis and Enhances Pancreatic Cancer Therapy. *Cell* **2014**, *159*, 80. [CrossRef] [PubMed]
66. Cho, M.; Peddi, P.F.; Ding, K.; Chen, L.; Thomas, D.; Wang, J.; Lockhart, A.C.; Tan, B.; Wang-Gillam, A. Vitamin D deficiency and prognostics among patients with pancreatic adenocarcinoma. *J. Transl. Med.* **2013**, *11*, 1–6. [CrossRef] [PubMed]
67. Frost, F.; Kacprowski, T.; Rühlemann, M.; Bülow, R.; Kühn, J.P.; Franke, A.; Heinsen, F.A.; Pietzner, M.; Nauck, M.; Völker, U.; et al. Impaired Exocrine Pancreatic Function Associates With Changes in Intestinal Microbiota Composition and Diversity. *Gastroenterology* **2019**, *156*, 1010–1015. [CrossRef]
68. Frost, F.; Weiss, F.U.; Sendler, M.; Kacprowski, T.; Rühlemann, M.; Bang, C.; Franke, A.; Völker, U.; Völzke, H.; Lamprecht, G.; et al. The Gut Microbiome in Patients With Chronic Pancreatitis Is Characterized by Significant Dysbiosis and Overgrowth by Opportunistic Pathogens. *Clin. Transl. Gastroenterol.* **2020**, *11*, e00232. [CrossRef]
69. Petersen, C.; Round, J.L. Defining dysbiosis and its influence on host immunity and disease. *Cell. Microbiol.* **2014**, *16*, 1024–1033. [CrossRef]
70. Trespi, E.; Ferrieri, A. Intestinal bacterial overgrowth during chronic pancreatitis. *Curr. Med. Res. Opin.* **1999**, *15*, 47–52. [CrossRef]
71. Li, J.J.; Zhu, M.; Kashyap, P.C.; Chia, N.; Tran, N.H.; McWilliams, R.R.; Bekaii-Saab, T.S.; Ma, W.W. The role of microbiome in pancreatic cancer. *Cancer Metastasis Rev.* **2021**, *40*, 777. [CrossRef]
72. Sammallahti, H.; Kokkola, A.; Rezasoltani, S.; Ghanbari, R.; Aghdaei, H.A.; Knuutila, S.; Puolakkainen, P.; Sarhadi, V.K. Microbiota Alterations and Their Association with Oncogenomic Changes in Pancreatic Cancer Patients. *Int. J. Mol. Sci.* **2021**, *22*, 12978. [CrossRef] [PubMed]
73. Merali, N.; Chouari, T.; Kayani, K.; Rayner, C.J.; Jiménez, J.I.; Krell, J.; Giovannetti, E.; Bagwan, I.; Relph, K.; Rockall, T.A.; et al. A Comprehensive Review of the Current and Future Role of the Microbiome in Pancreatic Ductal Adenocarcinoma. *Cancers* **2022**, *14*, 1020. [CrossRef] [PubMed]
74. Pandol, S. *The Exocrine Pancreas*; Morgan & Claypool Life Sciences: San Rafael, CA, USA, 2010.
75. Nicetto, D.; McCarthy, R.L.; Zaret, K.S. Epigenetic Mechanisms in Liver and Pancreas Generation and Regeneration. *Epigenetics Regen.* **2019**, *11*, 231–257. [CrossRef]
76. Struyvenberg, M.R.; Martin, C.R.; Freedman, S.D. Practical guide to exocrine pancreatic insufficiency—Breaking the myths. *BMC Med.* **2017**, *15*, 29. [CrossRef] [PubMed]
77. Dominici, R.; Franzini, C. Fecal elastase-1 as a test for pancreatic function: A review. *Clin. Chem. Lab. Med.* **2002**, *40*, 325–332. [CrossRef]
78. Anaizi, A.; Hart, P.A.; Conwell, D.L. Diagnosing Chronic Pancreatitis. *Dig. Dis. Sci.* **2017**, *62*, 1713. [CrossRef] [PubMed]
79. Rubinstein, E.; Mark, Z.; Haspel, J.; Ben-Ari, G.; Dreznik, Z.; Mirelman, D.; Tadmor, A. Antibacterial Activity of the Pancreatic Fluid. *Gastroenterology* **1985**, *88*, 927–932. [CrossRef]
80. Pierzynowski, S.G.; Sharma, P.; Sobczyk, J.; Garwacki, S.; Barej, W.; Westrom, B. Comparative study of antibacterial activity of pancreatic juice in six mammalian species. *Pancreas* **1993**, *8*, 546–550. [CrossRef]
81. Ahuja, M.; Schwartz, D.M.; Tandon, M.; Son, A.; Zeng, M.; Swaim, W.; Eckhaus, M.; Hoffman, V.; Cui, Y.; Xiao, B.; et al. Orai1-Mediated Antimicrobial Secretion from Pancreatic Acini Shapes the Gut Microbiome and Regulates Gut Innate Immunity. *Cell Metab.* **2017**, *25*, 635–646. [CrossRef]

82. Bassi, C.; Fontana, R.; Vesentini, S.; Cavallini, G.; Marchiori, L.; Falconi, M.; Corra, S.; Pederzoli, P. Antibacterial and mezlocillin-enhancing activity of pure human pancreatic fluid. *Int. J. Pancreatol.* **1991**, *10*, 293–297. [CrossRef]
83. Kościuczuk, E.M.; Lisowski, P.; Jarczak, J.; Strzałkowska, N.; Jóźwik, A.; Horbańczuk, J.; Krzyżewski, J.; Zwierzchowski, L.; Bagnicka, E. Cathelicidins: Family of antimicrobial peptides. A review. *Mol. Biol. Rep.* **2012**, *39*, 10957–10970. [CrossRef] [PubMed]
84. Zhou, C.H.; Meng, Y.T.; Xu, J.J.; Fang, X.; Zhao, J.L.; Zhou, W.; Zhao, J.; Han, J.C.; Zhang, L.; Wang, K.X.; et al. Altered diversity and composition of gut microbiota in Chinese patients with chronic pancreatitis. *Pancreatology* **2020**, *20*, 16–24. [CrossRef] [PubMed]
85. Herremans, K.M.; Riner, A.N.; Cameron, M.E.; Trevino, J.G. The Microbiota and Cancer Cachexia. *Int. J. Mol. Sci.* **2019**, *20*, 6267. [CrossRef] [PubMed]
86. Panebianco, C.; Villani, A.; Potenza, A.; Favaro, E.; Finocchiaro, C.; Perri, F.; Pazienza, V. Targeting Gut Microbiota in Cancer Cachexia: Towards New Treatment Options. *Int. J. Mol. Sci.* **2023**, *24*, 1849. [CrossRef]
87. Ritz, S.; Hahn, D.; Wami, H.T.; Tegelkamp, K.; Dobrindt, U.; Schnekenburger, J. Gut microbiome as a response marker for pancreatic enzyme replacement therapy in a porcine model of exocrine pancreas insufficiency. *Microb. Cell Fact.* **2020**, *19*, 221. [CrossRef]
88. Nishiyama, H.; Nagai, T.; Kudo, M.; Okazaki, Y.; Azuma, Y.; Watanabe, T.; Goto, S.; Ogata, H.; Sakurai, T. Supplementation of pancreatic digestive enzymes alters the composition of intestinal microbiota in mice. *Biochem. Biophys. Res. Commun.* **2017**, *495*, 273–279. [CrossRef]
89. Isaiah, A.; Parambeth, J.C.; Steiner, J.M.; Lidbury, J.A.; Suchodolski, J.S. The fecal microbiome of dogs with exocrine pancreatic insufficiency. *Anaerobe* **2017**, *45*, 50–58. [CrossRef]
90. Guo, W.; Zhang, Y.; Guo, S.; Mei, Z.; Liao, H.; Dong, H.; Wu, K.; Ye, H.; Zhang, Y.; Zhu, Y.; et al. Tumor microbiome contributes to an aggressive phenotype in the basal-like subtype of pancreatic cancer. *Commun. Biol.* **2021**, *4*, 1019. [CrossRef]
91. Polansky, O.; Sekelova, Z.; Faldynova, M.; Sebkova, A.; Sisak, F.; Rychlik, I. Important Metabolic Pathways and Biological Processes Expressed by Chicken Cecal Microbiota. *Appl. Environ. Microbiol.* **2015**, *82*, 1569–1576. [CrossRef]
92. Topping, D.L.; Clifton, P.M. Short-chain fatty acids and human colonic function: Roles of resistant starch and nonstarch polysaccharides. *Physiol. Rev.* **2001**, *81*, 1031–1064. [CrossRef]
93. Takada, T.; Kurakawa, T.; Tsuji, H.; Nomoto, K. *Fusicatenibacter saccharivorans* gen. nov., sp. nov., isolated from human faeces. *Int. J. Syst. Evol. Microbiol.* **2013**, *63*, 3691–3696. [CrossRef] [PubMed]
94. Ménard, S.; Candalh, C.; Bambou, J.C.; Terpend, K.; Cerf-Bensussan, N.; Heyman, M. Lactic acid bacteria secrete metabolites retaining anti-inflammatory properties after intestinal transport. *Gut* **2004**, *53*, 821–828. [CrossRef] [PubMed]
95. Hoque, R.; Farooq, A.; Ghani, A.; Gorelick, F.; Mehal, W.Z. Lactate reduces liver and pancreatic injury in Toll-like receptor- and inflammasome-mediated inflammation via GPR81-mediated suppression of innate immunity. *Gastroenterology* **2014**, *146*, 1763–1774. [CrossRef] [PubMed]
96. Johnston, C.D.; Bullman, S. The tumour-associated microbiome. *Nat. Rev. Gastroenterol. Hepatol.* **2022**, *19*, 347–348. [CrossRef]
97. Liu, J.; Zhang, Y. Intratumor microbiome in cancer progression: Current developments, challenges and future trends. *Biomark. Res.* **2022**, *10*, 1–18. [CrossRef] [PubMed]
98. Balachandran, V.P.; Łuksza, M.; Zhao, J.N.; Makarov, V.; Moral, J.A.; Remark, R.; Herbst, B.; Askan, G.; Bhanot, U.; Senbabaoglu, Y.; et al. Identification of unique neoantigen qualities in long-term survivors of pancreatic cancer. *Nature* **2017**, *551*, S12–S16. [CrossRef]
99. Nejman, D.; Livyatan, I.; Fuks, G.; Gavert, N.; Zwang, Y.; Geller, L.T.; Rotter-Maskowitz, A.; Weiser, R.; Mallel, G.; Gigi, E.; et al. The human tumor microbiome is composed of tumor type-specific intracellular bacteria. *Science* **2020**, *368*, 973–980. [CrossRef]
100. Sayin, S.; Rosener, B.; Li, C.G.; Ho, B.; Ponomarova, O.; Ward, D.V.; Walhout, A.J.M.; Mitchell, A. Evolved bacterial resistance to the chemotherapy gemcitabine modulates its efficacy in co-cultured cancer cells. *Elife* **2023**, *12*, 1–23. [CrossRef]
101. Tintelnot, J.; Xu, Y.; Lesker, T.R.; Schönlein, M.; Konczalla, L.; Giannou, A.D.; Pelczar, P.; Kylies, D.; Puelles, V.G.; Bielecka, A.A.; et al. Microbiota-derived 3-IAA influences chemotherapy efficacy in pancreatic cancer. *Nature* **2023**, *615*, 168–174. [CrossRef]
102. Fulop, D.J.; Zylberberg, H.M.; Wu, Y.L.; Aronson, A.; Labiner, A.J.; Wisnivesky, J.; Cohen, D.J.; Sigel, K.M.; Lucas, A.L. Association of Antibiotic Receipt with Survival Among Patients with Metastatic Pancreatic Ductal Adenocarcinoma Receiving Chemotherapy. *JAMA Netw. Open* **2023**, *6*, e234254. [CrossRef]
103. Pushalkar, S.; Hundeyin, M.; Daley, D.; Zambirinis, C.P.; Kurz, E.; Mishra, A.; Mohan, N.; Aykut, B.; Usyk, M.; Torres, L.E.; et al. The Pancreatic Cancer Microbiome Promotes Oncogenesis by Induction of Innate and Adaptive Immune Suppression. *Cancer Discov.* **2018**, *8*, 403–416. [CrossRef]
104. Thomas, R.M.; Gharaibeh, R.Z.; Gauthier, J.; Beveridge, M.; Pope, J.L.; Guijarro, M.V.; Yu, Q.; He, Z.; Ohland, C.; Newsome, R.; et al. Intestinal microbiota enhances pancreatic carcinogenesis in preclinical models. *Carcinogenesis* **2018**, *39*, 1068–1078. [CrossRef]
105. Sethi, V.; Kurtom, S.; Tarique, M.; Lavania, S.; Malchiodi, Z.; Hellmund, L.; Zhang, L.; Sharma, U.; Giri, B.; Garg, B.; et al. Gut Microbiota Promotes Tumor Growth in Mice by Modulating Immune Response. *Gastroenterology* **2018**, *155*, 33–37.e6. [CrossRef]
106. Daley, D. The role of the microbiome in pancreatic oncogenesis. *Int. Immunol.* **2022**, *34*, 447–454. [CrossRef]
107. Benini, L.; Amodio, A.; Campagnola, P.; Agugiaro, F.; Cristofori, C.; Micciolo, R.; Magro, A.; Gabbrielli, A.; Cabrini, G.; Moser, L.; et al. Fecal elastase-1 is useful in the detection of steatorrhea in patients with pancreatic diseases but not after pancreatic resection. *Pancreatology* **2013**, *13*, 38–42. [CrossRef]

108. Halloran, C.M.; Cox, T.F.; Chauhan, S.; Raraty, M.G.T.; Sutton, R.; Neoptolemos, J.P.; Ghaneh, P. Partial Pancreatic Resection for Pancreatic Malignancy Is Associated with Sustained Pancreatic Exocrine Failure and Reduced Quality of Life: A Prospective Study. *Pancreatology* **2011**, *11*, 535–545. [CrossRef]
109. Domínguez-Muñoz, J.; Nieto, L.; Pancreas, M.V. Development and diagnostic accuracy of a breath test for pancreatic exocrine insufficiency in chronic pancreatitis. *Pancreas* **2016**, *45*, 241–247. [CrossRef]
110. Powell-Brett, S.; Hall, L.; Edwards, M.; Roberts, K. A systematic review and meta-analysis of the accuracy and methodology of the 13C mixed triglyceride breath test for the evaluation of pancreatic function. *Pancreatology* **2023**, *23*, 283–293. [CrossRef]
111. Halle-Smith, J.M.; Hall, L.A.; Powell-Brett, S.F.; Merali, N.; Frampton, A.; Roberts, K.J. Realising the therapeutic potential of the human microbiota in metastatic pancreatic ductal adenocarcinoma. *Clin. Surg. Oncol.* **2023**, *2*, 100020. [CrossRef]

cancers

MDPI

Perspective

Neoadjuvant Therapy in Pancreatic Ductal Adenocarcinoma: Aligning Guideline Recommendations with Real-World Evidence

Roberto Cammarata [1], Alberto Catamerò [1,*], Vincenzo La Vaccara [1], Roberto Coppola [1] and Damiano Caputo [1,2]

1 Operative Research Unit of General Surgery, Fondazione Policlinico Universitario Campus Bio-Medico, 00128 Rome, Italy; roberto.cammarata@policlinicocampus.it (R.C.); v.lavaccara@policlinicocampus.it (V.L.V.); r.coppola@policlinicocampus.it (R.C.); d.caputo@policlinicocampus.it (D.C.)

2 Research Unit of General Surgery, Università Campus Bio-Medico di Roma, 00128 Rome, Italy

* Correspondence: alberto.catamero@unicampus.it; Tel.: +39-06225418856

Simple Summary: Pancreatic ductal adenocarcinoma (PDAC) remains one of the most lethal malignancies, with limited long-term survival even after radical surgery. The historical "surgery-first" approach is challenged by two consistent observations: the frequent presence of micrometastatic disease at diagnosis and the difficulty of completing postoperative treatment due to surgical complications or early relapse. Neoadjuvant therapy, delivered before surgery, provides systemic control at an earlier stage, allows biological selection of patients who will benefit from resection, and increases the probability of achieving complete tumor clearance. Randomized trials in borderline resectable disease have demonstrated improvements in surgical margins and survival, while evidence in resectable disease is more heterogeneous but increasingly supportive. Real-world series confirm feasibility and safety, though with substantial variability in regimens and sequencing. Future perspectives focus on integrating molecular profiling, circulating tumor DNA dynamics, and advanced imaging to refine patient selection and guide personalized multimodal strategies.

Abstract: Pancreatic ductal adenocarcinoma (PDAC) remains one of the most lethal malignancies, with a 5-year overall survival below 12% and high recurrence rates even after R0 resection. Traditionally managed with a "surgery-first" approach, two consistent observations—the near-universal presence of micrometastatic disease at diagnosis and the frequent inability to complete adjuvant therapy—have driven the integration of neoadjuvant therapy (NAT) into clinical practice. NAT offers several theoretical and practical advantages: early systemic control of occult disease, improved delivery and completion of multimodal treatment, biological selection of surgical candidates, and increased R0 resection rates. While in borderline resectable PDAC, randomized trials have consistently demonstrated improved margin-negative resection rates and early survival benefits compared with upfront surgery, in resectable PDAC, evidence is more heterogeneous. Real-world studies corroborate trial findings, reporting higher R0 rates and reduced lymph node positivity without increased perioperative risk, but also highlight substantial heterogeneity in regimens, duration, and radiotherapy use. Limitations to universal NAT adoption include reliance on anatomy-based resectability criteria, absence of validated predictive biomarkers, challenges in response assessment, and concerns over disease progression during preoperative treatment. Future developments will focus on integrating molecular profiling, circulating tumor DNA dynamics, and advanced imaging into patient selection and treatment adaptation, supported by biomarker-enriched and adaptive trial designs. NAT is thus evolving from a selective strategy for borderline disease to an innovative framework to optimize multimodal treatment delivery and refine patient selection in PDAC, with the potential to improve surgical outcomes and inform systemic therapy decisions in both resectable and borderline resectable settings.

Cancers 2025, 17, 3085 https://doi.org/10.3390/cancers17183085

Keywords: pancreatic ductal adenocarcinoma; neoadjuvant therapy; borderline resectable; resectable pancreatic cancer; FOLFIRINOX; gemcitabine; chemoradiotherapy; R0 resection; circulating tumor DNA; precision oncology

1. Introduction: Challenging the "Surgery-First" Paradigm

Pancreatic ductal adenocarcinoma (PDAC) accounts for more than 90% of exocrine pancreatic malignancies and, according to epidemiological projections, is expected to become the second leading cause of cancer-related mortality by 2040 [1,2]. Despite advances in surgical technique and systemic therapies, prognosis remains dismal, with a 5-year overall survival (OS) rate below 12% [3]. Only 15–20% of patients present with anatomically resectable disease at diagnosis [4], and even in this subgroup recurrence rates exceed 70% after R0 resection followed by adjuvant chemotherapy [5].

Two consistent observations have increasingly challenged the traditional "surgery-first" paradigm. The first is the near-universal presence of micrometastatic disease even in apparently localized tumors [6]. The second is that up to half of patients never receive planned adjuvant therapy due to postoperative complications or early disease progression [7]. These realities have created fertile ground for the development of neoadjuvant therapy (NAT) strategies not only in borderline resectable tumors, where NAT is now endorsed by major guidelines, but also in selected anatomically resectable PDAC.

2. Biological and Clinical Rationale for NAT

The rationale for incorporating NAT into the management of PDAC is grounded in both biological principles and pragmatic clinical considerations [8]. From a biological standpoint, PDAC is characterized by an early propensity for systemic spread; autopsy series and molecular studies have shown that micrometastatic deposits can be present at the time of diagnosis even in patients whose disease appears localized on imaging [9]. Administering systemic therapy before surgery provides an opportunity to target these occult lesions at a stage when the tumor burden is lower and the likelihood of chemoresistance may be reduced [10].

Clinically, preoperative delivery of chemotherapy may increase the likelihood that patients receive intended systemic treatment while still in a better physiological state, avoiding the attrition seen with postoperative regimens where surgical complications, delayed recovery, or rapid progression often prevent the completion of adjuvant therapy [10]. This sequencing also acts as a biological filter: patients whose disease remains stable or regresses are more likely to derive benefit from surgery, whereas those who progress are spared the morbidity of an extensive pancreatic resection that would not alter their prognosis [11].

There are additional surgical benefits. NAT can induce tumor shrinkage or fibrosis, facilitating dissection and increasing the likelihood of achieving an R0 resection, an independent predictor of long-term survival [12]. Several studies have reported lower rates of pathological lymph node involvement after NAT, which may translate into reduced locoregional recurrence risk. Moreover, some reports suggest a potential reduction in postoperative pancreatic fistula rates, possibly due to therapy-induced changes in pancreatic texture, although this remains to be confirmed in prospective trials [13].

Historically, radiotherapy was often incorporated into neoadjuvant regimens with the aim of enhancing local control. Retrospective analyses indicate that chemo-radiotherapy may achieve better locoregional disease control compared with chemotherapy alone, particularly in borderline resectable tumors where vessel involvement makes complete clearance challenging [13]. However, the survival benefit of adding radiotherapy remains inconsistent across studies, and its role in the era of highly active systemic regimens such as FOLFIRINOX or gemcitabine/nab-paclitaxel is under active investigation.

Finally, NAT allows for an extended preoperative period during which multidisciplinary teams can perform comprehensive patient optimization, addressing nutrition, biliary drainage, comorbidity control, and psychosocial preparation, all of which may improve perioperative outcomes. Taken together, these factors illustrate why NAT is increasingly viewed not merely as a treatment option, but as a strategic platform for integrating systemic, local, and supportive care interventions in PDAC.

3. Evidence from Borderline Resectable PDAC

In borderline resectable PDAC, the evidence supporting a neoadjuvant approach has become increasingly robust over the past decade. Multiple randomized and prospective studies have demonstrated that delivering systemic therapy, often in combination with radiotherapy—before surgery can increase the likelihood of achieving an R0 resection, improve pathological staging, and potentially translate into longer survival.

Among the pivotal trials, the Dutch PREOPANC-1 randomized controlled trial enrolled both resectable (54%) and borderline resectable (46%) patients, comparing gemcitabine-based chemoradiotherapy (36 Gy) followed by surgery with an upfront surgery strategy, both arms receiving adjuvant gemcitabine [14]. While the overall OS difference in the entire cohort was modest (15.7 vs. 14.3 months), NAT significantly improved the R0 resection rate (71% vs. 40%) and disease-free survival, with the magnitude of benefit particularly notable in the borderline subgroup.

The ESPAC-5F trial adopted a more pragmatic design, randomizing patients with borderline resectable PDAC to four different neoadjuvant options—including FOLFIRINOX, gemcitabine/capecitabine (GemCap), and short-course chemoradiotherapy, versus upfront surgery [15]. Despite its relatively small size, the trial reported a striking one-year OS advantage for patients receiving any form of NAT (77%) compared with immediate surgery (39%), corresponding to a hazard ratio of 0.29. Importantly, these results were achieved without a significant increase in perioperative morbidity, underscoring the feasibility of preoperative treatment in this higher-risk population.

The Alliance A021101 pilot study provided additional support for intensive combination therapy in this setting, testing a sequence of mFOLFIRINOX followed by capecitabine-based chemoradiotherapy in borderline resectable patients [16]. Of the patients who proceeded to resection, 93% achieved margin-negative status, and two patients achieved a pathological complete response, a rare event in PDAC. Although this was not a randomized trial and included only 22 patients, it demonstrated the logistical feasibility and potential oncologic benefit of aggressive, multimodality NAT.

Across different regimens and study designs, a consistent pattern has emerged suggesting that NAT may improve R0 resection rates and early survival outcomes in borderline resectable PDAC compared with surgery-first strategies. However, differences in inclusion criteria, chemotherapy backbones, and the use of radiotherapy limit direct cross-trial comparisons.

4. Evidence from Resectable PDAC

In anatomically resectable PDAC, the case for neoadjuvant therapy is more nuanced and the evidence base considerably more heterogeneous than in borderline disease. While the theoretical advantages of NAT, early micrometastatic control, improved completion of multimodal therapy, and biological selection-apply equally, the potential benefit must be weighed against the risk of delaying surgery in patients who might already have a curative opportunity.

The Prep-02/JSAP-05 trial from Japan is one of the few phases III randomized studies conducted exclusively in a predominantly resectable population. This multicenter trial compared two cycles of gemcitabine plus S-1 followed by surgery with upfront surgery, both arms receiving adjuvant S-1 [17]. NAT was associated with a clear OS advantage (median 36.7 vs. 26.6 months; HR 0.72), without excess perioperative mortality. This study provided high-level evidence that a short-course neoadjuvant regimen could yield survival gains even in anatomically resectable PDAC, particularly in a population where S-1 is widely used and well tolerated.

In contrast, the SWOG S1505 trial adopted a perioperative approach, randomizing patients with resectable PDAC to either mFOLFIRINOX or gemcitabine/nab-paclitaxel for 3 months before and after surgery [18]. While the median OS was approximately 23 months in both arms, not substantially different from historical surgery-first series—the trial was not powered for direct comparison with an upfront surgery control. Nevertheless, S1505 demonstrated that complex multi-agent chemotherapy can be delivered preoperatively in a high proportion of resectable patients, offering proof-of-concept for NAT feasibility in this setting.

More recently, the NORPACT-1 phase II randomized trial directly compared two months of neoadjuvant mFOLFIRINOX followed by surgery with immediate surgery in resectable PDAC [19]. The study found no OS superiority for the NAT arm and reported a lower rate of patients reaching surgery after randomization, highlighting a key practical challenge: attrition between diagnosis and resection. This drop-off underscores the importance of patient selection and treatment coordination if NAT is to be successfully implemented in resectable disease.

Taken together, and as summarized with relevant studies also for borderline PDAC in Table 1, these studies show that while NAT can be delivered safely and may improve outcomes in certain contexts, the survival advantage in resectable PDAC is not as consistently demonstrated as in borderline disease. Differences in chemotherapy backbone, duration, and trial design make direct comparison difficult, and ongoing phase III trials will be crucial to defining the true role of NAT in this population. At the same time, it should be emphasized that attrition before surgery remains a major limitation of the neoadjuvant approach: in randomized trials, only 60–75% of patients ultimately underwent resection (61% in PREOPANC-1 [14], ~77% in SWOG S1505 [18], and 60% in NORPACT-1 [19]), and less than half completed the entire multimodality pathway including postoperative therapy. These findings highlight that, despite the potential oncologic advantages of NAT, curative-intent surgery remains the most eligible and decisive therapeutic step in the management of resectable PDAC.

Table 1. Summary of key trials evaluating NAT in resectable and borderline PDAC.

Study (Year)	Population	NAT Regimen	Control	Primary Endpoint	Main Results
PREOPANC-1 (2020)	Resectable (54%), borderline (46%)	Gem + RT (36 Gy) → surgery → Gem	Surgery → Gem	OS	OS 15.7 vs. 14.3 mo; ↑ R0, ↑ DFS
Prep-02/JSAP-05 (2019)	Resectable (80%), borderline (20%)	Gem + S-1 → surgery → S-1	Surgery → S-1	OS	OS 36.7 vs. 26.6 mo (HR 0.72)
ESPAC-5F (2020)	Borderline	FOLFIRINOX or GemCap ± RT	Upfront surgery	1-year OS	77% vs. 39% (HR 0.29)
SWOG S1505 (2021)	Resectable	mFOLFIRINOX vs. Gem/nab-P	–	OS	~23 mo both arms
NORPACT-1 (2023)	Resectable	mFOLFIRINOX (2 mo) → surgery	Upfront surgery	OS	No OS benefit
Alliance A021101 (2016)	Borderline	mFOLFIRINOX → Cap-RT	–	Safety/Efficacy	Resection 68%, R0 93%

5. Real-World Evidence: Heterogeneity Behind the Numbers

Beyond the controlled environment of randomized clinical trials, multicenter observational studies from high-volume institutions provide an essential perspective on the actual implementation NAT. Large-scale analyses have confirmed that the advantages seen in experimental settings can be reproduced in routine practice [20]. In these cohorts, NAT has been associated with higher rates of margin-negative (R0) resection—often exceeding 80% compared with around two-thirds in surgery-first patients—and a marked reduction in pathological lymph node involvement [21,22]. Importantly, these improvements have been achieved without an increase in perioperative mortality, suggesting that NAT does not compromise short-term surgical safety when delivered in experienced centers [7]. However, such real-world datasets also reveal a striking degree of heterogeneity in how NAT is applied. Regimen selection varies widely, ranging from intensive multi-agent chemotherapy to gemcitabine-based combinations [23]; treatment duration can differ by several weeks; radiotherapy is used selectively, often without a unified rationale [24]; and the timing between completion of therapy and surgery is far from consistent [25]. This variability underscores the current lack of standardized protocols and complicates cross-center comparisons. Furthermore, survival comparisons between NAT and upfront surgery in retrospective or observational cohorts are inherently subject to immortal time bias (ITB), a statistical distortion that can overestimate the benefit of neoadjuvant strategies.

For clinicians, these findings carry a dual message. On one hand, they validate the oncologic and perioperative benefits of NAT outside of clinical trials [18]. On the other hand, they highlight the urgent need for harmonized treatment pathways, ideally grounded in consensus guidelines but adaptable to individual patient and tumor biology, to ensure that NAT's potential is realized consistently across diverse practice settings [10,26].

6. Limitations and Remaining Controversies

Despite encouraging data from both randomized trials and high-quality observational studies, the implementation of NAT in PDAC continues to face significant conceptual and practical hurdles.

A fundamental limitation lies in the current anatomical definition of resectability, which does not account for tumor biology. Clinical experience and population studies have shown that some anatomically "resectable" PDACs recur within months of surgery despite complete (R0) resection, while certain borderline resectable cases achieve durable survival after NAT and surgery [27]. This discrepancy suggests that the anatomical classification, largely based on vascular involvement, is an incomplete surrogate for true biological resectability.

Equally problematic is the lack of robust predictive biomarkers. Carbohydrate antigen (CA) 19-9 remains the most widely used marker, and its weaknesses are inherently linked to the marker itself: poor specificity, elevation in benign conditions, and lack of expression in approximately 10% of patients due to Lewis antigen-negative phenotype. Nevertheless, CA19-9 retains clinical value when interpreted in the appropriate context, supporting both preoperative risk stratification and monitoring of treatment response during NAT. Recent evidence has further expanded its potential utility: Newhook et al. demonstrated that CA19-9 normalization during NAT was independently associated with improved survival, and that distinct dynamic trajectories of CA19-9 levels provided even more refined prognostic stratification than normalization alone. These findings indicate that, despite intrinsic shortcomings, CA19-9 remains a relevant and context-dependent tool in the neoadjuvant setting [28]. More sophisticated tools such as circulating tumor DNA (ctDNA) analysis and radiomics-based imaging signatures have shown promise in early studies for predicting response to NAT and long-term outcomes [29,30], but neither has yet been validated in prospective, multicenter trials.

Assessment of treatment response poses another challenge. Radiographic evaluation after NAT frequently underestimates residual tumor due to therapy-induced desmoplastic fibrosis, making it difficult to distinguish true response from non-viable tissue [31]. Similarly, pathologic complete responses (pCR) remain rare in PDAC, occurring in fewer than 5% of resected cases even after intensive multi-agent NAT [32]. This limits the use of pCR as a reliable surrogate endpoint, in contrast to other malignancies such as breast or rectal cancer.

Treatment heterogeneity, in the choice of chemotherapy backbone, total duration of preoperative treatment, and selective or routine inclusion of radiotherapy, further complicates evidence synthesis. In real-world series, regimens range from short-course gemcitabine-based therapy to prolonged multi-agent protocols such as mFOLFIRINOX, with or without chemoradiotherapy, and there is no consensus on optimal sequencing [23,24].

Finally, the risk of progression during NAT, although relatively uncommon in experienced centers, remains a key psychological barrier to wider adoption, particularly among surgeons accustomed to a surgery-first approach. Importantly, data suggest that progression during NAT usually reflects aggressive tumor biology rather than therapy-induced delay [7], but the perception of "missing the surgical window" continues to influence decision-making in multidisciplinary settings.

Taken together, these limitations highlight the need for a paradigm shift from purely anatomical selection criteria toward a multifactorial, biology-informed framework, integrating molecular, serological, and radiological data to guide NAT decisions and assess treatment benefit. Until such precision tools are available and validated, variability in practice and uncertainty in patient selection will continue to temper the enthusiasm for universal adoption of NAT in all resectable PDAC cases.

7. Future Perspectives: From Anatomy to Biology-Driven NAT

Looking ahead, the most transformative shift will come from advances in systemic therapy and deeper understanding of PDAC biology, such as the development of effective targeted strategies and identification of resistance mechanisms. Radiographic criteria will therefore remain essential for defining surgical resectability and planning, while biological and biochemical insights will complement rather than replace imaging in refining patient selection and treatment sequencing. Molecular profiling has already revealed distinct transcriptional subtypes of PDAC, such as classical and basal-like, with differing prognoses and [33]. Integrating this information into NAT decision-making could allow clinicians to match regimens to tumor biology, improving response rates and long-term outcomes.

Liquid biopsy technologies, particularly ctDNA analysis, offer an additional dimension by enabling real-time monitoring of tumor burden and treatment effect. Dynamic changes in ctDNA during NAT could serve as early predictors of response or progression, guiding escalation, de-escalation, or a switch in therapy before surgery. Likewise, advanced imaging modalities, including functional MRI and PET/MRI, may help distinguish viable tumor from post-treatment fibrosis, improving surgical planning and potentially avoiding non-beneficial resections.

Trial methodology is also evolving. Adaptive trial designs that incorporate early biomarker read-outs, along with biomarker-enriched basket trials, are already underway (e.g., NCT03983057, NCT03322995). These approaches allow for treatment modification in real time and for testing targeted agents in molecularly selected populations. Promising avenues include immunotherapy combinations in tumors with immunogenic phenotypes, targeted therapy in biomarker-defined subsets such as BRCA-mutated PDAC, and perioperative strategies tailored to genomic and transcriptomic profiles.

While these innovations are still in early phases, their convergence with NAT has the potential to redefine the treatment pathway for PDAC, moving from a "one-size-fits-all" approach to a precision, response-adapted strategy that maximizes benefit while avoiding unnecessary toxicity or delay.

8. Conclusions

NAT has progressed from a controversial, selectively applied option to the standard of care for borderline resectable PDAC, and it is now being increasingly considered for anatomically resectable cases with high-risk or biologically aggressive features. This evolution has been driven by the convergence of guideline recommendations, supportive evidence from randomized controlled trials, and corroborating real-world data from high-volume centers. Collectively, these data support the view that NAT may improve rates of R0 resection, reduce lymph node positivity, and maintain perioperative safety, while offering the unique advantage of delivering systemic therapy to all eligible patients prior to surgery.

The challenge now is to refine NAT into a precision oncology tool rather than a uniform preoperative step. This will require integrating biological markers, including genomic and transcriptomic profiles, ctDNA kinetics, and advanced imaging signatures, into patient selection and treatment adaptation. The shift from anatomy-only to anatomy-plus-biology selection will enable more accurate identification of patients most likely to benefit, while sparing others the toxicity and potential delays associated with ineffective therapy.

Standardization of regimens, treatment duration, and the role of radiotherapy will also be essential to reduce the heterogeneity currently observed in real-world practice and to facilitate meaningful comparison across centers and trials. As illustrated by the active clinical trials summarized in Table 2, current research is exploring multiple strategies, from optimized chemotherapy combinations to integrated chemo-immunotherapy and multimodal approaches, across both resectable and borderline resectable disease. These studies not only reflect the rapid diversification of NAT but also provide the framework for evidence-based refinement of patient selection and treatment sequencing.

Table 2. Active trials (neoadjuvant therapy for resectable/borderline resectable PDAC).

NCT	Short Title	Population	Design/Regimens	Phase	Status
NCT04927780 (PREOPANC-3)	Peri-op mFOLFIRINOX vs. adjuvant mFOLFIRINOX	Resectable	Randomized: 8 cycles neo mFOLFIRINOX → surgery → 4 cycles adj vs. surgery → 12 cycles adj	III	Active (ongoing)
NCT06210360	Perioperative vs adjuvant chemotherapy in high-risk resectable	High-risk resectable	Randomized: neo CT + surgery + adj CT vs. surgery + adj CT	III	Recruiting
NCT06423326	Gemcitabine + Cisplatin + nab-paclitaxel neoadjuvant	Resectable/BR	Single arm: Gem/Cis/nab-P before surgery	II	Recruiting
NCT05562297	Sintilimab + Gem/nab-paclitaxel neoadjuvant	Resectable/BR	Chemo-immunotherapy combination pre-op	II	Active (ongoing)
NCT06384560	Triple: chemo + immuno + RT neoadjuvant	Borderline resectable	Integrated pre-op scheme → surgery	II	Recruiting
NCT04617821	AG (Gem/nab-P) vs. mFOLFIRINOX neoadjuvant	BR (includes LA)	Randomized 1:1	III	Recruiting (includes BR; note: also includes LA)
NCT05679050	Sequential AG → FOLFIRINOX neoadjuvant	Resectable/BR	Single arm sequential pre-op	II	Recruiting
NCT06816914	NALIRIFOX perioperative	Resectable	Safety/activity peri-op study	II	Recruiting
NCT07034703 (PANACHE02-screening)	Prospective cohort treated with neoadjuvant	Resectable	Observational/prospective neo-pathway	—	Recruiting

At the same time, adaptive trial designs and biomarker-enriched studies will accelerate the translation of emerging targeted and immunotherapeutic strategies into the neoadjuvant space. As these elements coalesce, NAT has the potential to move beyond its current role as a bridge to surgery. It could become a central platform for precision oncology in PDAC—one that not only optimizes surgical outcomes but also serves as an in vivo testbed for systemic therapy efficacy, informs postoperative treatment strategies, and ultimately contributes to improved long-term survival in this highly lethal disease.

Author Contributions: Conceptualization, R.C. (Roberto Cammarata) and D.C.; methodology, R.C. (Roberto Cammarata), A.C. and V.L.V.; investigation, R.C. (Roberto Cammarata), A.C. and V.L.V.; resources, R.C. (Roberto Cammarata) and R.C. (Roberto Coppola); data curation, A.C. and V.L.V.; writing—original draft preparation, R.C. (Roberto Cammarata); writing—review and editing, A.C., V.L.V., R.C. (Roberto Coppola) and D.C.; supervision, R.C. (Roberto Coppola) and D.C. All authors have read and agreed to the published version of the manuscript.

Funding: This research received no external funding.

Conflicts of Interest: The authors declare no conflicts of interest.

References

1. Rahib, L.; Wehner, M.R.; Matrisian, L.M.; Nead, K.T. Estimated projection of US cancer incidence and death to 2040. *JAMA Netw. Open* **2021**, *4*, e214708. [CrossRef] [PubMed]
2. Quagliarini, E.; Caputo, D.; Cammarata, R.; Caracciolo, G.; Pozzi, D. Coupling magnetic levitation of graphene oxide–protein complexes with blood levels of glucose for early detection of pancreatic adenocarcinoma. *Cancer Nano* **2023**, *14*, 16. [CrossRef]
3. Siegel, R.L.; Kratzer, T.B.; Giaquinto, A.N.; Sung, H.; Jemal, A. Cancer statistics, 2025. *CA Cancer J. Clin.* **2025**, *75*, 10–45. [CrossRef]
4. Neoptolemos, J.P.; Palmer, D.H.; Ghaneh, P.; Psarelli, E.E.; Valle, J.W.; Halloran, C.M.; Faluyi, O.; O'Reilly, D.A.; Cunningham, D.; Wadsley, J.; et al. Comparison of adjuvant gemcitabine and capecitabine with gemcitabine monotherapy in patients with resected pancreatic cancer (ESPAC-4): A multicentre, open-label, randomised, phase 3 trial. *Lancet* **2017**, *389*, 1011–1024. [CrossRef]
5. Conroy, T.; Hammel, P.; Hebbar, M.; Ben Abdelghani, M.; Wei, A.C.; Raoul, J.-L.; Choné, L.; Francois, E.; Artru, P.; Biagi, J.J.; et al. FOLFIRINOX or gemcitabine as adjuvant therapy for pancreatic cancer. *N. Engl. J. Med.* **2018**, *379*, 2395–23406. [CrossRef] [PubMed]
6. Valle, J.W.; Palmer, D.H.; Jackson, R.; Cox, T.; Neoptolemos, J.P.; Ghaneh, P. Optimal duration and timing of adjuvant chemotherapy after definitive surgery for PDAC. *Ann. Oncol.* **2019**, *30*, 1395–1397. [CrossRef]
7. Reni, M.; Balzano, G.; Zanon, S.; Zerbi, A.; Rimassa, L.; Castoldi, R.; Pinelli, D.; Mosconi, S.; Doglioni, C.; Chiaravalli, M.; et al. Safety and efficacy of preoperative or postoperative chemotherapy in resectable pancreatic adenocarcinoma (phase 2 PACT-15 trial). *JAMA Oncol.* **2018**, *4*, 767–774. [CrossRef]
8. Coppola, A.; La Vaccara, V.; Fiore, M.; Farolfi, T.; Ramella, S.; Angeletti, S.; Coppola, R.; Caputo, D. CA19.9 Serum Level Predicts Lymph-Nodes Status in Resectable Pancreatic Ductal Adenocarcinoma: A Retrospective Single-Center Analysis. *Front. Oncol.* **2021**, *11*, 690580. [CrossRef]
9. Wang, S.; Zheng, Y.; Yang, F.; Zhu, L.; Zhu, X.Q.; Wang, Z.F.; Wu, X.L.; Zhou, C.H.; Yan, J.Y.; Hu, B.Y.; et al. The molecular biology of pancreatic adenocarcinoma: Translational challenges and clinical perspectives. *Signal Transduct. Target. Ther.* **2021**, *6*, 249. [CrossRef]
10. Gillen, S.; Schuster, T.; Meyer zum Büschenfelde, C.; Friess, H.; Kleeff, J. Preoperative/neoadjuvant therapy in pancreatic cancer: A systematic review and meta-analysis of response and resection percentages. *PLoS Med.* **2010**, *7*, e1000267. [CrossRef] [PubMed]
11. Katz, M.H.; Marsh, R.; Herman, J.M.; Shi, Q.; Collison, E.; Venook, A.P.; Kindler, H.L.; Alberts, S.R.; Philip, P.; Lowy, A.M.; et al. Borderline resectable pancreatic cancer: Need for standardization and methods for optimal clinical trial design. *Ann. Surg. Oncol.* **2013**, *20*, 2787–2795. [CrossRef] [PubMed]
12. Isaji, S.; Mizuno, S.; Windsor, J.A.; Bassi, C.; Castillo, C.F.-D.; Hackert, T.; Hayasaki, A.; Katz, M.H.; Kim, S.-W.; Kishiwada, M.; et al. International consensus on definition and criteria of borderline resectable pancreatic ductal adenocarcinoma 2017. *Pancreatology* **2018**, *18*, 2–11. [CrossRef]
13. Jang, J.Y.; Han, Y.; Lee, H.; Kim, S.-W.; Kwon, W.; Lee, K.-H.; Oh, D.-Y.; Chie, E.K.; Lee, J.M.; Heo, J.S.; et al. Oncological benefits of neoadjuvant chemoradiation with gemcitabine versus upfront surgery in borderline resectable pancreatic cancer (Prep-02/JSAP-05): A phase 2/3 trial. *Ann. Surg.* **2018**, *268*, 215–222. [CrossRef]
14. Versteijne, E.; Suker, M.; Groothuis, K.; Akkermans-Vogelaar, J.M.; Besselink, M.G.; Bonsing, B.A.; Buijsen, J.; Busch, O.R.; Creemers, G.-J.M.; van Dam, R.M.; et al. Preoperative chemoradiotherapy versus immediate surgery for resectable and borderline resectable pancreatic cancer (PREOPANC trial). *J. Clin. Oncol.* **2020**, *38*, 1763–1773. [CrossRef] [PubMed]

15. Ghaneh, P.; Palmer, D.H.; Cicconi, S.; Halloran, C.; Psarelli, E.E.; Rawcliffe, C.L.; Sripadam, R.; Mukherjee, S.; Wadsley, J.; Al-Mukhtar, A.; et al. ESPAC-5F: Four-arm phase II trial of immediate surgery versus neoadjuvant therapy in borderline resectable pancreatic cancer. *J. Clin. Oncol.* **2020**, *38* (Suppl. S15), 4505. [CrossRef]
16. Katz, M.H.; Shi, Q.; Ahmad, S.A.; Herman, J.M.; Marsh, R.d.W.; Collisson, E.; Schwartz, L.; Frankel, W.; Martin, R.; Conway, W.; et al. Preoperative Modified FOLFIRINOX Treatment Followed by Capecitabine-Based Chemoradiation for Borderline Resectable Pancreatic Cancer: Alliance for Clinical Trials in Oncology Trial A021101. *JAMA Surg.* **2016**, *151*, e161137. [CrossRef]
17. Unno, M.; Motoi, F.; Matsuyama, Y.; Satoi, S.; Toyama, H.; Matsumoto, I.; Aosasa, S.; Shirakawa, H.; Wada, K.; Fujii, T.; et al. Neoadjuvant Chemotherapy with Gemcitabine and S-1 versus Upfront Surgery for Resectable Pancreatic Cancer: Results of the Randomized Phase II/III Prep-02/JSAP05 Trial. *Ann. Surg.* **2025**, *10*, 1097/SLA.0000000000006730. [CrossRef]
18. Sohal, D.P.S.; Duong, M.; Ahmad, S.A.; Gandhi, N.S.; Beg, M.S.; Wang-Gillam, A.; Wade, J.L.; Chiorean, E.G.; Guthrie, K.A.; Lowy, A.M.; et al. Perioperative mFOLFIRINOX vs gemcitabine/nab-paclitaxel in resectable pancreatic cancer (SWOG S1505): A randomized phase 2 trial. *JAMA Oncol.* **2021**, *7*, 421–427. [CrossRef] [PubMed]
19. Labori, K.J.; Bratlie, S.O.; Andersson, B.; Angelsen, J.-H.; Biörserud, C.; Björnsson, B.; Bringeland, E.A.; Elander, N.; Garresori, H.; Grønbech, J.E.; et al. Neoadjuvant FOLFIRINOX versus upfront surgery for resectable pancreatic head cancer (NORPACT-1): A randomized phase 2 trial. *Lancet Gastroenterol. Hepatol.* **2024**, *9*, 205–217. [CrossRef]
20. Aliseda, D.; Martí-Cruchaga, P.; Zozaya, G.; Blanco, N.; Ponz, M.; Chopitea, A.; Rodríguez, J.; Castañón, E.; Pardo, F.; Rotellar, F. Neoadjuvant therapy versus upfront surgery in resectable pancreatic cancer: Reconstructed patient-level meta-analysis of randomized clinical trials. *BJS Open* **2024**, *8*, zrae087. [CrossRef]
21. Truty, M.J.; Kendrick, M.L.; Nagorney, D.M.; Smoot, R.L.; Cleary, S.P.; Graham, R.P.; Goenka, A.H.; Hallemeier, C.L.; Haddock, M.G.; Harmsen, W.S.; et al. Factors predicting response, perioperative outcomes, and survival following total neoadjuvant therapy for borderline/locally advanced PDAC. *Ann. Surg.* **2021**, *273*, 341–349. [CrossRef]
22. Coppola, A.; La Vaccara, V.; Farolfi, T.; Asbun, H.J.; Boggi, U.; Conlon, K.; Edwin, B.; Ferrone, C.; Jonas, E.; Kokudo, N.; et al. Preoperative carbohydrate antigen 19.9 level predicts lymph node metastasis in resectable adenocarcinoma of the head of the pancreas: A further plea for biological resectability criteria. *Int. J. Surg.* **2024**, *110*, 6092–6099. [CrossRef]
23. Hackert, T.; Sachsenmaier, M.; Hinz, U.; Schneider, L.; Michalski, C.W.; Springfeld, C.; Strobel, O.; Jäger, D.; Ulrich, A.; Büchler, M.W. Locally advanced pancreatic cancer: Neoadjuvant therapy with FOLFIRINOX results in resectability in 60% of patients. *Ann. Surg.* **2016**, *264*, 457–463. [CrossRef] [PubMed]
24. Villano, A.M.; O'Halloran, E.; Goel, N.; Ruth, K.; Barrak, D.; Lefton, M.; Reddy, S.S. Total neoadjuvant therapy is associated with improved overall survival and pathologic response in pancreatic adenocarcinoma. *J. Surg. Oncol.* **2022**, *126*, 502–512. [CrossRef]
25. Michelakos, T.; Pergolini, I.; Castillo, C.F.; Honselmann, K.C.; Cai, L.; Deshpande, V.; Wo, J.Y.; Ryan, D.P.; Allen, J.N.; Blaszkowsky, L.S.; et al. Predictors of Resectability and Survival in Patients With Borderline and Locally Advanced Pancreatic Cancer who Underwent Neoadjuvant Treatment With FOLFIRINOX. *Ann. Surg.* **2019**, *269*, 733–740. [CrossRef]
26. Caputo, D.; Pozzi, D.; Farolfi, T.; Passa, R.; Coppola, R.; Caracciolo, G. Nanotechnology and pancreatic cancer management: State of the art and further perspectives. *World J. Gastrointest. Oncol.* **2021**, *13*, 231–237. [CrossRef] [PubMed]
27. Mokdad, A.A.; Minter, R.M.; Zhu, H.; Augustine, M.M.; Porembka, M.R.; Wang, S.C.; Yopp, A.C.; Mansour, J.C.; Choti, M.A.; Polanco, P.M. Neoadjuvant therapy followed by resection vs upfront resection for resectable pancreatic cancer: A propensity score–matched analysis. *J. Clin. Oncol.* **2017**, *35*, 515–522. [CrossRef] [PubMed]
28. Humphris, J.L.; Chang, D.K.; Johns, A.L.; Scarlett, C.J.; Pajic, M.; Jones, M.D.; Colvin, E.K.; Nagrial, A.; Chin, V.T.; Chantrill, L.A.; et al. The prognostic and predictive value of serum CA19-9 in pancreatic cancer. *Ann. Oncol.* **2012**, *23*, 1713–1722. [CrossRef]
29. Lin, Z.; Adeniran, E.A.; Cai, Y.; Qureshi, T.A.; Li, D.; Gong, J.; Li, J.; Pandol, S.J.; Jiang, Y. Early Detection of Pancreatic Cancer: Current Advances and Future Opportunities. *Biomedicines* **2025**, *13*, 1733. [CrossRef]
30. Somers, I.; Bipat, S. Contrast-enhanced CT in determining resectability in patients with pancreatic carcinoma: A meta-analysis of the positive predictive values of CT. *Eur. Radiol.* **2017**, *27*, 3408–3435. [CrossRef]
31. Christofilis, I.; Triantopoulou, C.; Delis, S. Pancreatic Cancer Resectability After Neoadjuvant Treatment: An Imaging Challenge. *Diagnostics* **2025**, *15*, 1810. [CrossRef] [PubMed]
32. Murphy, J.E.; Wo, J.Y.; Ryan, D.P.; Jiang, W.; Yeap, B.Y.; Drapek, L.C.; Blaszkowsky, L.S.; Kwak, E.L.; Allen, J.N.; Clark, J.W.; et al. Total Neoadjuvant Therapy With FOLFIRINOX Followed by Individualized Chemoradiotherapy for Borderline Resectable Pancreatic Adenocarcinoma: A Phase 2 Clinical Trial. *JAMA Oncol.* **2018**, *4*, 963–969. [CrossRef] [PubMed]
33. Collisson, E.A.; Bailey, P.; Chang, D.K.; Biankin, A.V. Molecular subtypes of pancreatic cancer. *Nat. Rev. Gastroenterol. Hepatol.* **2019**, *16*, 207–220. [CrossRef] [PubMed]

cancers

MDPI

Perspective

Exercise Guidelines in Pancreatic Cancer Based on the Dietz Model

Philip J. Chang [1,*], Andrew E. Hendifar [1], Gillian Gresham [1], An Ngo-Huang [2], Paul E. Oberstein [3], Nathan Parker [4] and Andrew L. Coveler [5]

1 Cedars-Sinai Medical Center, Los Angeles, CA 90211, USA
2 MD Anderson Cancer Center, Houston, TX 77030, USA
3 New York University, New York, NY 10012, USA; paul.oberstein@nyulangone.org
4 Moffitt Cancer Center, Tampa, FL 33612, USA
5 University of Washington, Seattle, WA 98105, USA; acoveler@uw.edu
* Correspondence: philip.chang@cshs.org; Tel.: +1-424-315-0250

Simple Summary: Pancreatic and gastrointestinal cancers commonly occur in the elderly and in patients with lower levels of physical function. Physical activity and exercise are one of the primary interventions in combating frailty and disability; however, guidelines are lacking in this patient population. Here, we propose practical exercise guidelines for every phase of disease in these cancers based on the Dietz model. During the prehabilitation phase, patients may optimize their physical abilities before undergoing surgery. Restorative rehabilitation often given through skilled therapies can help patients to recover any function lost from chemotherapy, radiation therapy, and surgery. Supportive rehabilitation can allow patients to continue with regular physical activity during stable or ongoing disease and palliative rehabilitation can help patients maintain the highest possible quality of life when they enter the end stage of life. No matter the stage of disease or phase of treatment, physical activity and exercise have important roles in maintaining well-being.

Abstract: Pancreatic and gastrointestinal cancers are associated with debility, frailty, and chemotherapy regiments with significant toxicity. Practical exercise guidelines to combat these ailments and optimize functional status are lacking. We present a model for exercise for these cancers based on the Dietz framework for rehabilitation in cancer. The Dietz framework for rehabilitation describes four phases of rehabilitation including preventative (prehabilitation), restorative, supportive, and palliative. We present practical guidelines for exercise at each phase. Prehabilitation seeks to optimize functional performance typically prior to surgical resection and may occur concurrently with neoadjuvant therapy. Restorative rehabilitation occurs following the development of a physical deficit such as after surgery and may utilize skilled therapies in the inpatient, subacute, outpatient, and home settings to address functional impairments. Supportive rehabilitation occurs during stable disease or remission and depends on the frequent monitoring of functional status and particularly the development of chemotherapy-induced neuropathy to ensure timely exercise interventions. Palliative rehabilitation occurs at the end stage of life and shifts to a focus on patient comfort and safety. Exercise is a critical component of treatment in cancer demonstrating numerous quality-of-life benefits. The customization of exercise recommendations to individual patients based on their functional status and phase in treatment is essential for safety and adherence.

Keywords: gastrointestinal cancer; pancreatic cancer; exercise guidelines; exercise

1. Introduction

Despite advances in therapy, the mortality associated with gastrointestinal cancers, particularly pancreatic ductal adenocarcinoma (PDAC), continues to be substantial. PDAC is currently projected to be the second leading cause of cancer deaths by 2040 [1], and colorectal cancers have shown increasing incidence of early onset [2]. These malignancies are associated with a disproportionate rate of weight loss, pain, and debility [3]. In addition, chemotherapy, comprised of combinatorial cytotoxic regimens, is the mainstay of therapy and associated with significant toxicities [4].

Weight loss, sarcopenia, and frailty are highly prevalent among patients with gastrointestinal cancers [5]. Up to 80% of PDAC patients have significant weight loss on diagnosis and meet criteria for cancer cachexia [6]. Frailty syndrome, a state of extreme vulnerability to stressors that leads to adverse health outcomes, is also highly prevalent in this population. These features are associated with significant declines in physical activity and performance, therapeutic toxicity, and perioperative complications [3,4,7–9]. They also correlate with shorter progression-free survival (PFS), shorter overall survival (OS), and lower quality of life (QOL) [10].

Physical activity has been associated with decreased cancer incidence and improved outcomes, specifically concerning quality of life [11–15]. In addition, preclinical studies have shown that aerobic exercise reduced PDAC and colon tumor growth by modulating systemic and intra-tumoral immunity [3,16,17]. However, recommendations for the incorporation of physical activity into the care of these cancers to combat weight loss, frailty, and sarcopenia are lacking [18]. Here, we briefly discuss the benefits of exercise in gastrointestinal cancers followed by a practical approach to physical activity based on the Dietz model of rehabilitation in cancer.

2. Review of Preclinical and Clinical Exercise Benefits

Preclinical and some clinical evidence suggests that exercise is useful as an adjuvant to chemotherapy by improving chemotherapy delivery and anti-tumor efficacy. Tumor vasculature is highly disorganized, with a dense stromal component that compresses vasculature, resulting in disrupted blood flow that impedes drug delivery. Moderate-intensity aerobic exercise has been shown to induce vascular normalization in mouse models and humans [19].

One mechanism by which exercise mediates vascular normalization is by shear stress, the mechanical stimuli exerted on endothelial cells by increased blood flow. In a mouse model utilizing moderate-intensity treadmill running to increase blood flow in mice with PDAC tumors, tumor growth was significantly inhibited in mice treated with chemotherapy and aerobic exercise compared to mice treated with chemotherapy alone [20]. In another study, mice bearing patient-derived xenograft tumors were treated with moderate-intensity treadmill exercise, gemcitabine, a combination of exercise plus gemcitabine, or phosphate-buffered saline [21]. Exercise alone had no effect on tumor growth; however, exercise plus gemcitabine caused faster tumor regression and delay in tumor regrowth. In a human study with 70 participants undergoing neoadjuvant therapy for resectable PDAC, patients were prescribed at least 120 min of moderate-intensity, home-based exercise (60 min of aerobic and 60 min of strengthening) per week [21]. Of the 70 patients, 33 underwent resection and 23 had tissue and activity data. Of these 23 patients, the mean time of exercise was 15 weeks (±6.5), with an average of 170 ± 80 min per week of exercise. There was no change in TNM stage or regression, despite seeing an increase in micro-vessel density [21].

In addition to vascular changes, there is a growing awareness that exercise may modulate tumor growth by impacting the immune microenvironment [22,23]. Kurz and colleagues employed a low-intensity treadmill running exercise regimen in several mouse models and demonstrated that this intervention delayed the onset of pancreatic cancer and enhanced the impact of chemotherapy and immunotherapy in controlling tumors [16]. They identified alterations in anti-tumor immunity that were mediated by interleukin-15 signaling [16]. Exercise has also been shown to control tumor growth through the mobilization of natural killer cells [24].

In the small, randomized SUPPORT study, patients assigned to a supervised resistance training program had improved muscle strength in some muscle groups compared to those in a home-based resistance training or control (no training) group [25]. Interestingly, those in the supervised resistance group also had alterations in the tryptophan/kynurenine pathway that may have been associated with improved immune response to tumors [26].

3. Exercise Guidelines

The Dietz framework for rehabilitation in cancer was first described in the 1980s and describes four phases of rehabilitation including preventative rehabilitation, restorative rehabilitation, supportive rehabilitation, and palliative rehabilitation (Box 1). We describe physical activity guidelines in the context of these phases, with a focus on the specific challenges of gastrointestinal cancers. Table 1 highlights relevant clinical trials in pancreatic cancer demonstrating the benefits of exercise programming.

Box 1. Key exercise points

Prehabilitation

- Provide education on prehab benefits
- Goal of 150 min of moderate-intensity aerobic exercise per week
- Goal of 2–3 days per week of resistance training

Restorative Rehab

- Encourage early postoperative mobilization
- Utilize PT (inpatient, home, or outpatient) for gait difficulties and decon-ditioning
- Utilize OT (inpatient, home, or outpatient) for ADL deficits

Supportive Rehab

- Assess for functional deficits at regular intervals
- Routinely discuss fine motor function, gait, balance, and falls, which may occur secondary to chemotherapy neuropathy

End of Life

- Focus should transition to comfort while trying to maximize functional independence

-Consider use of home PT/OT for caregiver training

Table 1. EX (exercise); CON (control).

Study	Design	Sample Size	Intervention	Outcome Measures	Results
Florez et al., 2019 [21]	Prospective single arm with historical control	23 EX, 13 historical CON	Home-based: 60 min aerobic; 60 min strength per week	Tumor vascularity	Twice as many vessels per field in EX group on pathology
Ausania et al., 2019 [15]	RCT	18 EX, 22 CON	Nutritional support: 60 min supervised exercise × 5 days then unsupervised home exercises	Post-op complication rate (Dindo–Clavien classification)	Reduction in delayed gastric emptying in EX group

Table 1. *Cont.*

Study	Design	Sample Size	Intervention	Outcome Measures	Results
Nakajima et al., 2019 [27]	Prospective single arm with historical control	76 EX, 142 historical CON	Home-based unsupervised: 60 min aerobic and resistance 3× per week	Length of hospital stay	Median 23 days vs. 30 days in EX vs. CON groups, respectively
Ngo-Huang et al., 2023 [28]	2-arm RCT	76 EX, 76 CON	Home-based: ≥30 min aerobic 5× per week; ≥2× per week resistance exercise sessions	6 min walking distance	Mean change 28.3 ± 68.2 m in EX vs. 17.8 ± 56.7 m in CON
Okada et al., 2022 [29]	Prospective single arm	43 EX	Inpatient immediate post-operative training with aerobic and resistance exercise	Completion rate of S-1 therapy	93% completion rate, which exceeded the threshold rate of 53%
Streckmann et al., 2024 [30]	3-arm RCT	55 EX, 53 VT, 50 CON	Sensorimotor Training	Development of chemotherapy neuropathy	Decreased incidence of neuropathy in EX and VT groups

4. Prehabilitation (Preventative Rehab)

Pretreatment exercise training, or exercise prehabilitation, is an increasingly adopted strategy to improve the physiologic status of individuals with cancer. Given the importance of maintaining aerobic and muscular fitness and physical functioning throughout cancer survivorship, prehabilitation can be applied as patients approach various therapeutic contexts including chemotherapy, radiation therapy, immunotherapy, targeted therapy, and surgery.

The concept of prehabilitation in medicine emanates primarily from surgical literature. Surgery can have profound and deleterious effects on quality of life through unintended consequences including increased fatigue, reduced physical activity and energy intake, altered sleep, and impaired physical functioning [31]. Suboptimal fitness has been associated with an increased risk of surgical complications, hospital readmissions, nutritional challenges, and requirements for intensive care that can prolong post-operative bed rest and slow recovery [31].

To date, the preoperative context has been the most frequent target for exercise intervention in pancreatic cancer, including interventions delivered concurrently with neoadjuvant therapy. As with other cancer diagnoses, preoperative exercise training capitalizes on a convenient and important window for patients with gastrointestinal cancers. A recent systematic review reported median wait times between workup and surgical resection ranging from 14 to 42 days among patients undergoing upfront operations for resectable pancreatic cancer [32]. These lead times generally align with durations of cancer prehabilitation programs with favorable outcomes involving postoperative functional recovery [33]. Exercise training concurrent with neoadjuvant therapies may be particularly important to improve treatment tolerance and mitigate potential declines in physical functioning and fitness prior to surgery. A new cancer diagnosis represents a major life event and patients may be particularly motivated to make lifestyle changes (e.g., increasing physical activity) that can improve their trajectory and help them maintain an improved quality of life.

An increasing evidence base demonstrates the feasibility, safety, and potential benefits of gastrointestinal cancer prehabilitation. In a randomized trial of a hybrid (in-person supervised and home-based unsupervised) exercise program including both aerobic and resistance training, Ausania et al. (2019) reported a lower rate of delayed gastric emptying in prehabilitation participants compared to those receiving usual care, but no other significant differences in other complications or length of postoperative stay [15]. Nakajima and colleagues (2019) demonstrated improvements in 6 min walking distance and body composition (muscle-to-fat ratio) among participants in a home-based, unsupervised aerobic and resistance training program prior to major abdominal surgeries for hepato-pancreato-biliary malignancies [27]. Comparing outcomes to a propensity score-matched historical group, the study found reduced length of postoperative stay but no difference in surgical complications [27]. A multicenter, randomized, controlled trial found that participants in a multimodal prehabilitation program experienced fewer severe complications postoperatively compared to standard care in patients undergoing colorectal surgery [34]. In a prospective, single-arm study of home-based aerobic and resistance training concurrent with neoadjuvant chemotherapy and chemoradiation therapy, Parker et al. (2019) demonstrated strong aerobic exercise adherence and favorable outcomes involving physical functioning, health-related quality of life, and tumor vascularity [35]. In comparison to a retrospectively identified, non-prehabilitation group, Parker et al. (2020) also found the mitigation of skeletal muscle loss among prehabilitation participants [36]. This group followed the single-arm prehabilitation trial with a randomized trial comparing outcomes among participants in a home-based, unsupervised aerobic and resistance training program to those among patients encouraged to engage in aerobic exercise. Prehabilitation participants engaged in more weekly strength training sessions than enhanced usual care participants, but the two groups engaged in similar levels of Fitbit-measured physical activity. Both groups demonstrated significant improvements in aerobic fitness, as measured by 6 min walk tests. In pooled analyses, higher levels of self-reported exercise and Fitbit-measured physical activity were predictive of better outcomes including physical functioning and fitness [28]. Of particular note, a recent study demonstrated that sensorimotor training consisting of progressive balance exercises during chemotherapy with vinca alkaloids or oxaliplatin reduced the incidence of chemotherapy neuropathy to 30% compared to 70% in the control group [30].

Despite its documented benefits, exercise training for prehabilitation is not yet included in routine clinical practice. There exist no consensus guidelines regarding exercise modalities or program delivery strategies in cancer prehabilitation [31,33], but programs tend to follow the American College of Sports Medicine (ACSM) Exercise Guidelines for Cancer Survivors and incorporate both aerobic training and resistance training [25].

5. Restorative Rehabilitation

Restorative rehabilitation occurs after a decline in function secondary to disease or treatment. There are similar benefits for physical activity postoperatively, during adjuvant therapy, and in survivorship for patients with gastrointestinal cancers. Postoperatively, progressive mobilization on the same day of surgery compared to the day after surgery showed benefits in oxygenation [37]. Postoperative activity has been shown to improve recovery of gastrointestinal function, length of stay, functional recovery, pain [38], risk of readmission, and health-related quality of life. After surgery, mobilization should be initiated as soon as is safe. Ambulation can be accomplished by having nurses, nursing aides, and/or therapy technicians supervise the ambulation if no significant functional concerns are noted. Strategies to enhance postoperative mobility may include posting ambulation goals (via signs and/or activity log) in the patient's room, providing portable cyclers in the room, and, if there is significant postoperative abdominal pain, providing an abdominal binder (if not contraindicated). One study showed that the use of activity trackers after laparoscopic surgery resulted in increased step counts and activity minutes [39]. If there is concern about gait instability and fall risk, an early referral for acute care physical therapy (PT) should be initiated. If the patient has difficulty with activities of daily living (ADL), occupational therapy (OT) should be consulted to evaluate the patient's ability to complete ADL (feeding, grooming, upper and lower body dressing, transfers for self-care, toileting, bathing). OT trains patients and caregivers for mobility-related ADL, provides breathing and energy conservation recommendations, and may provide adaptive equipment (grabber, long-handed sponges, sock aides). Both OT and PT may assess durable medical equipment needs (wheelchair, rollator, standard walker, cane, bedside commode, shower chair, hospital bed) to support a safe discharge to home.

Once patients are medically stable for discharge, if mobility concerns persist, additional rehabilitation options may include prescriptions for outpatient PT/OT and home health services (including home PT/OT) or referrals to an inpatient facility for rehabilitation (skilled nursing facility, acute inpatient rehabilitation, and/or long-term acute care hospital). Improving postoperative mobilization, including physical activity recommendations after discharge from the hospital leading to starting adjuvant chemotherapy, is essential for functional recovery. Supervised exercise during adjuvant chemotherapy resulted in improved rates of S-1 adjuvant chemotherapy completion and reduced frailty [29]. When supervised exercise programs are not readily accessible, patients are encouraged to ambulate at home multiple times per day for the goal of 30 min of mobility per day for six to eight weeks after surgery and refrain from any lifting greater than 10 pounds. A systematic review of exercise for patients with PDAC found that during adjuvant treatment, exercise is safe and effective in mitigating impaired physical function, quality of life, and fatigue [40].

6. Supportive Rehabilitation

Supportive rehabilitation occurs during stable residual disease or remission. This scenario is frequent in advanced gastrointestinal cancers, where patients may be on indefinite treatment. In this survivorship stage, the primary goals of physical activity should be to optimize quality of life and re-integrate into recreational and valued roles.

This stage may not be distinct from the restorative phase and continual reassessment is paramount. During supportive rehabilitation, declines in functional status may occur with worsening liver function, uncontrolled pain, worsening chemotherapy side effects, neuropathy, infections, and prolonged hospitalizations. To assess for such declines, assessment of balance, proprioception, gait, muscle strength, and sensation should occur at regular intervals.

Chemotherapy-induced peripheral neuropathy (CIPN) is a common side effect of oxaliplatin (a component of FOLFIRINOX). In patients with PDAC receiving FOLFIRINOX, 61% had any-grade CIPN and 9% had high-grade CIPN [41,42]. Symptoms include numbness, paresthesia, dysesthesias, or loss of sensation in the distal extremities. CIPN can lead to the loss of balance and falls so early diagnosis and intervention is vital to minimize complications. There is limited strong evidence for CIPN treatments. Patients with peripheral CIPN symptoms are encouraged to wear cotton socks and gloves and avoid extreme heat or cold temperatures. For patients where CIPN has affected their gait and balance, physical therapy and occupational therapy interventions may include gait training; fall recovery training; modalities such as Kinesio taping of the hands, feet, and ankles;

hand therapy to preserve or restore manual dexterity; sensory feedback treatments; and transcutaneous electrical neurostimulation (TENS) treatments to treat pain. Other physical modalities to consider include acupuncture and massage therapy. Pharmacologic treatment for pain/discomfort may include anti-neuropathic agents, with the strongest evidence for duloxetine [43]. There is also emerging evidence for cryotherapy and acupuncture. In one trial, patients receiving oxaliplatin for malignancies of the GI system were randomized to continuous cooling of the hands and feet during their chemotherapy infusion versus usual care (no cooling). Patients in the intervention group had less numbness or tingling in the fingers and toes, pain, and cold sensitivity [44]. Currently pending or in-progress clinical trials include the use of riluzole to prevent CIPN [45]; a multi-site, randomized trial of donepezil to treat oxaliplatin-induced CIPN [46]; and the use of acupuncture with acupressure along with cryotherapy [47].

To maintain mobility and quality of life during treatment, patients should be encouraged to meet ACSM exercise guidelines. Any level of tolerable physical activity, even if small, should be encouraged. Equally important is having patients try to return to their valued roles and identifying gaps where patients functionally are versus where they want to be. Occupational therapists are an indispensable resource in this area and there should be a low threshold for referral. While the effects of exercise on outcomes for long-term pancreatic cancer survivors is currently limited, multiple studies have shown associations with increased survival and increased levels of physical activity [48,49].

7. Hospice and the End of Life

Although palliative care should not be confused with hospice and end-of-life care, in the context of the Dietz framework, palliative rehabilitation applies to those at the end stage of life. For patients who no longer wish to pursue disease-modifying treatment but want to improve their performance status, the guidelines for restorative and supportive rehabilitation apply. However, for patients who are significantly debilitated with poorly controlled symptoms, the goal of rehabilitation should focus on comfort.

Closer to the end of life, functional impairments may become more global, encompassing difficulty with transfers, sitting, standing, ambulation, and the completion of ADL [50–52]. These deficits may further be compounded by side effects from treatment including peripheral neuropathy, cancer-related pain, and sedation from opioid therapy. Despite these impairments, studies have shown that patients in hospice settings and palliative care units may improve functional performance with ADL and transfers [53–55]. While maximizing functional independence is important, the primary goals should be to avoid falls, alleviate symptoms, and reduce caregiver burden.

One of the primary ways these goals can be achieved is through caregiver training to properly and safely assist patients with transfers, ambulation, and ADL, which can be completed through inpatient acute care or inpatient rehabilitation, at a skilled nursing facility, or in the home setting. A case study demonstrated that proper training improves caregiver confidence in assisting with transfers [56], and a short, palliative inpatient rehabilitation program for deconditioning led to a safe home discharge with caregiver assistance [57]. While some hospices may not offer skilled rehabilitation, many may allot 1–2 sessions for caregiver functional training. Additionally, if skilled therapists are available in hospices, physical modalities such as electrical stimulation and compression bandaging may provide symptom relief [58,59]. Patients and caregivers should be educated on the availability of these services so that they can advocate for themselves. They should also be educated that the goal is not for functional recovery but for symptomatic relief and caregiver training. For patients already receiving home hospice care, discussion with the hospice social worker, nurse, or physician on the benefits of a skilled therapy referral may be helpful.

8. Role of Wearable Technology

The majority of cancer patients do not meet exercise guidelines and adherence to activity remains low [60,61]. Furthermore, it is difficult to obtain accurate estimates of a patient's daily activity as patients can experience dynamic changes in their activity patterns throughout their cancer experience. The use of wearable activity monitors can play an important role in motivating physical activity while allowing for the passive collection of objective, continuous measures of physical activity (physical activity duration and intensity, time spent sedentary, steps per day, sleep, heart rate, and other metrics), providing a more complete picture of the patient's activity in their free-living environment [62].

There is growing interest in including daily stepping recommendations in exercise guidelines as step counts are easily interpretable and widely available through wearables and other activity-tracking devices [63]. However, challenges including the lack of standardization across devices and metrics and variability across populations have made it difficult to identify and recommend specific activity targets and stepping dosages to cancer survivors. As more research emerges supporting the role of activity monitoring in promoting physical activity, more data informing guideline recommendations will also become available [63].

Studies that have used wearables and report on daily activity metrics have focused on postoperative outcomes in patients undergoing surgery [28,64–67], while few have evaluated the use of wearables in advanced cancer patients and those undergoing active treatment [62,68]. These studies have reported a range of approximately 3700–6000 steps per day, depending on disease stage and treatment, although significant heterogeneity exists across populations (e.g., stage and treatment), device types, and wear time. To date, no studies have provided tailored recommendations or daily activity targets based on wearable activity monitors for pancreatic cancer patients. While future guidelines should consider the incorporation of wearable activity metrics to provide activity targets, tracking step counts can be helpful in allowing patients to assess their progress (Box 2).

Box 2. Tips for exercise counseling

Tips

- Avoid reciting exercise guidelines and create customized programs based on individual needs
- Start with small, achievable goals (i.e., walking 5 min twice a day) and gradually increase them
- Utilize existing web-based or Electronic Medical Record (EMR)-embedded tools when creating resistance programs for patients
- Track step counts with smartphones and wearable technology to assess progress

9. Conclusions

Patients with gastrointestinal cancers become debilitated secondary to chemotherapy-induced fatigue and muscle loss and due to post-surgical deconditioning and primary cancer effects. Here, we have outlined practical exercise goals and interventions at every phase of illness (Table 2). Exercise training concurrent with neoadjuvant therapies is particularly important to improve treatment tolerance and mitigate potential declines in physical functioning and fitness prior to surgery. Prehabilitation has demonstrated lower rates of delayed gastric emptying, the mitigation of skeletal muscle loss, and reduced lengths of postoperative stay. In postoperative and/or post-adjuvant therapy, there is time for restorative and supportive rehabilitation. We should not assume that patients will automatically exercise and recover to their baseline functional levels without assistance. This time is opportune to build strength back regardless if patients remain cancer-free or relapse. Finally, during and after therapy, assessments of balance, proprioception, gait, muscle strength, and sensation should occur at regular intervals and ideally by a trained professional.

Table 2. ADL (activities of daily living); ECOG (Eastern Cooperative Oncology Group Performance Status); QOL (quality of life); ACSM (American College of Sports Medicine); SMT (sensorimotor training); VT (vibration training).

	Aims/Goals	Screening	Monitoring	Education	Intervention	Issues
Prehabilitation	Optimize functional status prior to surgery	Examine gait, balance, independence with ADL, ECOG score	Continue to monitor gait, ADL, balance, ADL function, and ECOG during routine follow-ups	Discuss with patients the risk of falls and injury; advise to "start low and go slow"; discuss QOL benefits of exercise	If ECOG 0/1 trial, home-based program per ACSM 2019 guidelines; if ECOG 1-3, may refer to home or outpatient physical therapy	May not be feasible in patients planned for upfront surgery depending on lead times; consider implementing SMT or VT to prevent neuropathy during neoadjuvant treatment
Restorative Rehab	Identify and rehabilitate functional deficits occurring during treatment	Examine proximal/distal muscle strength, fine motor coordination, gait, and balance (tandem stance and single leg)	Continue to monitor strength, fine motor coordination, gait, and balance and conduct routine follow-ups	Discuss with patients that the effects of chemotherapy may be cumulative so continued exercise is essential	If deficits in strength, gait, or balance are detected, then refer to skilled therapy; if no deficits, may continue on home program—recommend ambulatory assistive devices when applicable	Start to monitor for chemotherapy-induced peripheral neuropathy (balance, proprioception, fine motor skills); consider implementing SMT or VT to prevent neuropathy during adjuvant treatment
Supportive Rehab	Maintain functional status during ongoing treatments	Examine proximal/distal muscle strength, fine motor coordination, gait, and balance (tandem stance and single leg)	Continue to monitor strength, fine motor coordination, gait, and balance and conduct routine follow-ups	Encourage the maintenance of a physically active lifestyle within functional limits	Continued home-based programming vs. continued physical therapy or institutional or community programs when available—recommend ambulatory assistive devices when applicable	Continue to monitor for chemotherapy-induced peripheral neuropathy
End of Life	Transition focus of care to comfort while maintaining physical function within goals of care	Examine gait, sit-to-stand transfers, and ECOG	Continue to monitor gait, sit-to-stand transfers, and ECOG at routine follow-ups	Discuss with patients the transition of goals and what their goals for care are; discuss a change of goal to comfort as opposed to functional independence	Home-based or outpatient skilled therapies; consider need for durable medical equipment including hospital bed, assistive device, shower chair, raised toilet seat, and grab bars	Consider transition to hospice care where skilled therapy services may still be available

Author Contributions: Conception and Design: all authors; Provision of Study Materials or Patients: N/A; Collection and Assembly of Data: N/A; Data Analysis and Interpretation: N/A; Manuscript Writing: all authors; Final Approval of Manuscript: all authors. All authors have read and agreed to the published version of the manuscript.

Funding: This research received no external funding.

Institutional Review Board Statement: The authors are accountable for all aspects of this work in ensuring that questions related to the accuracy or integrity of any part of this work are appropriately investigated and resolved.

Data Availability Statement: Not applicable.

Conflicts of Interest: All authors have completed the ICMJE uniform disclosure form. The authors have no conflicts of interest to declare.

References

1. Rahib, L.; Wehner, M.R.; Matrisian, L.M.; Nead, K.T. Estimated Projection of US Cancer Incidence and Death to 2040. *JAMA Netw. Open* **2021**, *4*, e214708. [CrossRef] [PubMed]
2. Patel, S.G.; Karlitz, J.J.; Yen, T.; Lieu, C.H.; Boland, C.R. The Rising Tide of Early-Onset Colorectal Cancer: A Comprehensive Review of Epidemiology, Clinical Features, Biology, Risk Factors, Prevention, and Early Detection. *Lancet Gastroenterol. Hepatol.* **2022**, *7*, 262–274. [CrossRef]
3. Arora, S.; Fowler, M.E.; Harmon, C.; Al-Obaidi, M.; Outlaw, D.; Hollis, R.; Gbolahan, O.; Khushman, M.; Giri, S.; Williams, G.R. Differences in Pretreatment Frailty Across Gastrointestinal Cancers in Older Adults: Results from the Cancer and Aging Resilience Evaluation Registry. *JCO Oncol. Pract.* **2022**, *18*, e1796–e1806. [CrossRef]
4. Prado, C.M.M.; Baracos, V.E.; McCargar, L.J.; Mourtzakis, M.; Mulder, K.E.; Reiman, T.; Butts, C.A.; Scarfe, A.G.; Sawyer, M.B. Body Composition as an Independent Determinant of 5-Fluorouracil-Based Chemotherapy Toxicity. *Clin. Cancer Res.* **2007**, *13*, 3264–3268. [CrossRef]
5. Patel, I.; Winer, A. Assessing Frailty in Gastrointestinal Cancer: Two Diseases in One? *Curr. Oncol. Rep.* **2024**, *26*, 90–102. [CrossRef]
6. Hendifar, A.E.; Chang, J.I.; Huang, B.Z.; Tuli, R.; Wu, B.U. Cachexia, and Not Obesity, Prior to Pancreatic Cancer Diagnosis Worsens Survival and Is Negated by Chemotherapy. *J. Gastrointest. Oncol.* **2018**, *9*, 17–23. [CrossRef]
7. Tan, B.H.L.; Birdsell, L.A.; Martin, L.; Baracos, V.E.; Fearon, K.C.H. Sarcopenia in an Overweight or Obese Patient Is an Adverse Prognostic Factor in Pancreatic Cancer. *Clin. Cancer Res.* **2009**, *15*, 6973–6979. [CrossRef]
8. Cousin, S.; Hollebecque, A.; Koscielny, S.; Mir, O.; Varga, A.; Baracos, V.E.; Soria, J.C.; Antoun, S. Low Skeletal Muscle Is Associated with Toxicity in Patients Included in Phase I Trials. *Investig. New Drugs* **2014**, *32*, 382–387. [CrossRef]
9. Ali, R.; Baracos, V.E.; Sawyer, M.B.; Bianchi, L.; Roberts, S.; Assenat, E.; Mollevi, C.; Senesse, P. Lean Body Mass as an Independent Determinant of Dose-Limiting Toxicity and Neuropathy in Patients with Colon Cancer Treated with FOLFOX Regimens. *Cancer Med.* **2016**, *5*, 607–616. [CrossRef]
10. Bachmann, J.; Heiligensetzer, M.; Krakowski-Roosen, H.; Büchler, M.W.; Friess, H.; Martignoni, M.E. Cachexia Worsens Prognosis in Patients with Resectable Pancreatic Cancer. *J. Gastrointest. Surg.* **2008**, *12*, 1193–1201. [CrossRef]
11. Rittberg, R.; Zhang, H.; Lambert, P.; Kudlovich, R.; Kim, C.A.; Dawe, D.E. Utility of the Modified Frailty Index in Predicting Toxicity and Cancer Outcomes for Older Adults with Advanced Pancreatic Cancer Receiving First-Line Palliative Chemotherapy. *J. Geriatr. Oncol.* **2021**, *12*, 112–117. [CrossRef] [PubMed]
12. Steindorf, K.; Clauss, D.; Tjaden, C.; Hackert, T.; Herbolsheimer, F.; Bruckner, T.; Schneider, L.; Ulrich, C.M.; Wiskemann, J. Quality of Life, Fatigue, and Sleep Problems in Pancreatic Cancer Patients—A Randomized Trial on the Effects of Exercise. *Dtsch. Arztebl. Int.* **2019**, *116*, 471–478. [CrossRef] [PubMed]
13. Mima, K.; Nakagawa, S.; Miyata, T.; Yamashita, Y.-I.; Baba, H. Frailty and Surgical Outcomes in Gastrointestinal Cancer: Integration of Geriatric Assessment and Prehabilitation into Surgical Practice for Vulnerable Patients. *Ann. Gastroenterol. Surg.* **2023**, *7*, 27–41. [CrossRef] [PubMed]
14. Negrete-Najar, J.-P.; Sehovic, M.; Rodriquenz, M.G.; Garcia-Martinez, J.; Extermann, M. Development of a Health Data Derived Frailty Index as a Predictor of Adverse Outcomes in Older Patients with Pancreatic Cancer. *J. Geriatr. Oncol.* **2022**, *13*, 308–314. [CrossRef]
15. Ausania, F.; Senra, P.; Meléndez, R.; Caballeiro, R.; Ouviña, R.; Casal-Núñez, E. Prehabilitation in Patients Undergoing Pancreaticoduodenectomy: A Randomized Controlled Trial. *Rev. Esp. Enferm. Dig.* **2019**, *111*, 603–608. [CrossRef]

16. Kurz, E.; Hirsch, C.A.; Dalton, T.; Shadaloey, S.A.; Khodadadi-Jamayran, A.; Miller, G.; Pareek, S.; Rajaei, H.; Mohindroo, C.; Baydogan, S.; et al. Exercise-Induced Engagement of the IL-15/IL-15Rα Axis Promotes Anti-Tumor Immunity in Pancreatic Cancer. *Cancer Cell* **2022**, *40*, 720–737.e5. [CrossRef]
17. Tobias, G.C.; Gomes, J.L.P.; Fernandes, L.G.; Voltarelli, V.A.; de Almeida, N.R.; Jannig, P.R.; de Souza, R.W.A.; Negrão, C.E.; Oliveira, E.M.; Chammas, R.; et al. Aerobic Exercise Training Mitigates Tumor Growth and Cancer-Induced Splenomegaly through Modulation of Non-Platelet Platelet Factor 4 Expression. *Sci. Rep.* **2023**, *13*, 21970. [CrossRef]
18. Hendifar, A.E.; Petzel, M.Q.B.; Zimmers, T.A.; Denlinger, C.S.; Matrisian, L.M.; Picozzi, V.J.; Rahib, L. Precision Promise Consortium Pancreas Cancer-Associated Weight Loss. *Oncologist* **2019**, *24*, 691–701. [CrossRef]
19. Zlotecki, R.A.; Baxter, L.T.; Boucher, Y.; Jain, R.K. Pharmacologic Modification of Tumor Blood Flow and Interstitial Fluid Pressure in a Human Tumor Xenograft: Network Analysis and Mechanistic Interpretation. *Microvasc. Res.* **1995**, *50*, 429–443. [CrossRef]
20. Schadler, K.L.; Thomas, N.J.; Galie, P.A.; Bhang, D.H.; Roby, K.C.; Addai, P.; Till, J.E.; Sturgeon, K.; Zaslavsky, A.; Chen, C.S.; et al. Tumor Vessel Normalization after Aerobic Exercise Enhances Chemotherapeutic Efficacy. *Oncotarget* **2016**, *7*, 65429–65440. [CrossRef]
21. Florez Bedoya, C.A.; Cardoso, A.C.F.; Parker, N.; Ngo-Huang, A.; Petzel, M.Q.; Kim, M.P.; Fogelman, D.; Romero, S.G.; Wang, H.; Park, M.; et al. Exercise during Preoperative Therapy Increases Tumor Vascularity in Pancreatic Tumor Patients. *Sci. Rep.* **2019**, *9*, 13966. [CrossRef] [PubMed]
22. Gomes-Santos, I.L.; Amoozgar, Z.; Kumar, A.S.; Ho, W.W.; Roh, K.; Talele, N.P.; Curtis, H.; Kawaguchi, K.; Jain, R.K.; Fukumura, D. Exercise Training Improves Tumor Control by Increasing CD8+ T-Cell Infiltration via CXCR3 Signaling and Sensitizes Breast Cancer to Immune Checkpoint Blockade. *Cancer Immunol. Res.* **2021**, *9*, 765–778. [CrossRef] [PubMed]
23. Pedersen, L.; Idorn, M.; Olofsson, G.H.; Lauenborg, B.; Nookaew, I.; Hansen, R.H.; Johannesen, H.H.; Becker, J.C.; Pedersen, K.S.; Dethlefsen, C.; et al. Voluntary Running Suppresses Tumor Growth through Epinephrine- and IL-6-Dependent NK Cell Mobilization and Redistribution. *Cell Metab.* **2016**, *23*, 554–562. [CrossRef]
24. Idorn, M.; Hojman, P. Exercise-Dependent Regulation of NK Cells in Cancer Protection. *Trends Mol. Med.* **2016**, *22*, 565–577. [CrossRef]
25. Campbell, K.L.; Winters-Stone, K.M.; May, A.M.; Schwartz, A.L.; Courneya, K.S.; Zucker, D.S.; Matthews, C.E.; Ligibel, J.A.; Gerber, L.H.; Morris, G.S.; et al. Exercise Guidelines for Cancer Survivors: Consensus Statement from International Multidisciplinary Roundtable. *Med. Sci. Sports Exerc.* **2019**, *51*, 2375–2390. [CrossRef]
26. Pal, A.; Zimmer, P.; Clauss, D.; Schmidt, M.E.; Ulrich, C.M.; Wiskemann, J.; Steindorf, K. Resistance Exercise Modulates Kynurenine Pathway in Pancreatic Cancer Patients. *Int. J. Sports Med.* **2021**, *42*, 33–40. [CrossRef]
27. Nakajima, H.; Yokoyama, Y.; Inoue, T.; Nagaya, M.; Mizuno, Y.; Kadono, I.; Nishiwaki, K.; Nishida, Y.; Nagino, M. Clinical Benefit of Preoperative Exercise and Nutritional Therapy for Patients Undergoing Hepato-Pancreato-Biliary Surgeries for Malignancy. *Ann. Surg. Oncol.* **2019**, *26*, 264–272. [CrossRef]
28. Ngo-Huang, A.T.; Parker, N.H.; Xiao, L.; Schadler, K.L.; Petzel, M.Q.B.; Prakash, L.R.; Kim, M.P.; Tzeng, C.-W.D.; Lee, J.E.; Ikoma, N.; et al. Effects of a Pragmatic Home-Based Exercise Program Concurrent with Neoadjuvant Therapy on Physical Function of Patients With Pancreatic Cancer: The PancFit Randomized Clinical Trial. *Ann. Surg.* **2023**, *278*, 22–30. [CrossRef]
29. Okada, K.-I.; Kouda, K.; Kawai, M.; Hirono, S.; Miyazawa, M.; Kitahata, Y.; Kawanishi, M.; Natsume, Y.; Wan, K.; Yamaue, H. Supervised Exercise Therapy and Adjuvant Chemotherapy for Pancreatic Cancer: A Prospective, Single-Arm, Phase II Open-Label, Nonrandomized, Historically Controlled Study. *J. Am. Coll. Surg.* **2022**, *235*, 848–858. [CrossRef]
30. Streckmann, F.; Elter, T.; Lehmann, H.C.; Baurecht, H.; Nazarenus, T.; Oschwald, V.; Koliamitra, C.; Otten, S.; Draube, A.; Heinen, P.; et al. Preventive Effect of Neuromuscular Training on Chemotherapy-Induced Neuropathy: A Randomized Clinical Trial. *JAMA Intern. Med.* **2024**, *184*, 1046–1053. [CrossRef]
31. Scheede-Bergdahl, C.; Minnella, E.M.; Carli, F. Multi-modal Prehabilitation: Addressing the Why, When, What, How, Who and Where Next? *Anaesthesia* **2019**, *74*, 20–26. [CrossRef] [PubMed]
32. Frountzas, M.; Liatsou, E.; Schizas, D.; Pergialiotis, V.; Vailas, M.; Kritikos, N.; Toutouzas, K.G. The Impact of Surgery Delay on Survival of Resectable Pancreatic Cancer: A Systematic Review of Observational Studies. *Surg. Oncol.* **2022**, *45*, 101855. [CrossRef] [PubMed]
33. Michael, C.M.; Lehrer, E.J.; Schmitz, K.H.; Zaorsky, N.G. Prehabilitation Exercise Therapy for Cancer: A Systematic Review and Meta-analysis. *Cancer Med.* **2021**, *10*, 4195–4205. [CrossRef] [PubMed]
34. Molenaar, C.J.L.; Minnella, E.M.; Coca-Martinez, M.; Ten Cate, D.W.G.; Regis, M.; Awasthi, R.; Martínez-Palli, G.; López-Baamonde, M.; Sebio-Garcia, R.; Feo, C.V.; et al. Effect of Multimodal Prehabilitation on Reducing Postoperative Complications and Enhancing Functional Capacity Following Colorectal Cancer Surgery: The PREHAB Randomized Clinical Trial. *JAMA Surg.* **2023**, *158*, 572–581. [CrossRef]
35. Parker, N.H.; Ngo-Huang, A.; Lee, R.E.; O'Connor, D.P.; Basen-Engquist, K.M.; Petzel, M.Q.B.; Wang, X.; Xiao, L.; Fogelman, D.R.; Schadler, K.L.; et al. Physical Activity and Exercise during Preoperative Pancreatic Cancer Treatment. *Support. Care Cancer* **2019**, *27*, 2275–2284. [CrossRef] [PubMed]

36. Parker, N.H.; Gorzelitz, J.; Ngo-Huang, A.; Caan, B.J.; Prakash, L.; Garg, N.; Petzel, M.Q.B.; Schadler, K.; Basen-Engquist, K.; Katz, M.H.G. The Role of Home-Based Exercise in Maintaining Skeletal Muscle During Preoperative Pancreatic Cancer Treatment. *Integr. Cancer Ther.* **2021**, *20*, 1534735420986615. [CrossRef]
37. Fagevik Olsén, M.; Becovic, S.; Dean, E. Short-Term Effects of Mobilization on Oxygenation in Patients after Open Surgery for Pancreatic Cancer: A Randomized Controlled Trial. *BMC Surg.* **2021**, *21*, 185. [CrossRef]
38. Low, C.A.; Bovbjerg, D.H.; Ahrendt, S.; Choudry, M.H.; Holtzman, M.; Jones, H.L.; Pingpank, J.F.; Ramalingam, L.; Zeh, H.J.; Zureikat, A.H.; et al. Fitbit Step Counts during Inpatient Recovery from Cancer Surgery as a Predictor of Readmission. *Ann. Behav. Med.* **2018**, *52*, 88–92. [CrossRef]
39. Wolk, S.; Linke, S.; Bogner, A.; Sturm, D.; Meißner, T.; Müssle, B.; Rahbari, N.N.; Distler, M.; Weitz, J.; Welsch, T. Use of Activity Tracking in Major Visceral Surgery-the Enhanced Perioperative Mobilization Trial: A Randomized Controlled Trial. *J. Gastrointest. Surg.* **2019**, *23*, 1218–1226. [CrossRef]
40. O'Connor, D.; Brown, M.; Eatock, M.; Turkington, R.C.; Prue, G. Exercise Efficacy and Prescription during Treatment for Pancreatic Ductal Adenocarcinoma: A Systematic Review. *BMC Cancer* **2021**, *21*, 43. [CrossRef]
41. Conroy, T.; Hammel, P.; Hebbar, M.; Ben Abdelghani, M.; Wei, A.C.; Raoul, J.-L.; Choné, L.; Francois, E.; Artru, P.; Biagi, J.J.; et al. FOLFIRINOX or Gemcitabine as Adjuvant Therapy for Pancreatic Cancer. *N. Engl. J. Med.* **2018**, *379*, 2395–2406. [CrossRef] [PubMed]
42. Conroy, T.; Desseigne, F.; Ychou, M.; Bouché, O.; Guimbaud, R.; Bécouarn, Y.; Adenis, A.; Raoul, J.-L.; Gourgou-Bourgade, S.; de la Fouchardière, C.; et al. FOLFIRINOX versus Gemcitabine for Metastatic Pancreatic Cancer. *N. Engl. J. Med.* **2011**, *364*, 1817–1825. [CrossRef] [PubMed]
43. Loprinzi, C.L.; Lacchetti, C.; Bleeker, J.; Cavaletti, G.; Chauhan, C.; Hertz, D.L.; Kelley, M.R.; Lavino, A.; Lustberg, M.B.; Paice, J.A.; et al. Prevention and Management of Chemotherapy-Induced Peripheral Neuropathy in Survivors of Adult Cancers: ASCO Guideline Update. *J. Clin. Oncol.* **2020**, *38*, 3325–3348. [CrossRef]
44. Coolbrandt, A.; Tobback, H.; Govaerts, R.; Vandezande, L.; Vinckx, M.; Laenen, A.; Wildiers, H.; Verslype, C.; Dekervel, J.; Van Herpe, F.; et al. A Randomized Controlled Trial of Hand/Foot-Cooling by Hilotherapy to Prevent Oxaliplatin-Related Peripheral Neuropathy in Patients with Malignancies of the Digestive System. *ESMO Open* **2023**, *8*, 101205. [CrossRef]
45. Kerckhove, N.; Busserolles, J.; Stanbury, T.; Pereira, B.; Plence, V.; Bonnetain, F.; Krakowski, I.; Eschalier, A.; Pezet, D.; Balayssac, D. Effectiveness Assessment of Riluzole in the Prevention of Oxaliplatin-Induced Peripheral Neuropathy: RILUZOX-01: Protocol of a Randomised, Parallel, Controlled, Double-Blind and Multicentre Study by the UNICANCER-AFSOS Supportive Care Intergroup. *BMJ Open* **2019**, *9*, e027770. [CrossRef]
46. Kerckhove, N.; Tougeron, D.; Lepage, C.; Pezet, D.; Le Malicot, K.; Pelkowski, M.; Pereira, B.; Balayssac, D. Efficacy of Donepezil for the Treatment of Oxaliplatin-Induced Peripheral Neuropathy: DONEPEZOX, a Protocol of a Proof of Concept, Randomised, Triple-Blinded and Multicentre Trial. *BMC Cancer* **2022**, *22*, 742. [CrossRef]
47. Cohen, S.A.; Veleber, S.; Siman, J.; Guthrie, K.A.; McMillen, K.; Heit, M.; Wadhera, S.; Daniels, J.; Hansen, K.; Jacoby, M.; et al. Use of Acupuncture with Acupressure in Addition to Standard-of-Care Cryotherapy to Decrease Chemotherapy-Associated Neuropathy in Patients with Gastrointestinal Malignancies Receiving Oxaliplatin-Based Chemotherapy: Study Protocol for a Randomized, Controlled Pilot and Feasibility Study. *Contemp. Clin. Trials* **2023**, *131*, 107273. [CrossRef]
48. Dos Santos, M.; Ferrari, G.; Lee, D.H.; Rey-López, J.P.; Aune, D.; Liao, B.; Huang, W.; Nie, J.; Wang, Y.; Giovannucci, E.; et al. Association of the "Weekend Warrior" and Other Leisure-Time Physical Activity Patterns with All-Cause and Cause-Specific Mortality: A Nationwide Cohort Study. *JAMA Intern. Med.* **2022**, *182*, 840–848. [CrossRef]
49. Stamatakis, E.; Ahmadi, M.N.; Gill, J.M.R.; Thøgersen-Ntoumani, C.; Gibala, M.J.; Doherty, A.; Hamer, M. Association of Wearable Device-Measured Vigorous Intermittent Lifestyle Physical Activity with Mortality. *Nat. Med.* **2022**, *28*, 2521–2529. [CrossRef]
50. Brennan, M.J.; Warfel, B.S. Musculoskeletal Complications of CancerA Survey of 50 Patients. *J. Back Musculoskelet. Rehabil.* **1993**, *3*, 1–6. [CrossRef]
51. Cheville, A.L.; Mustian, K.; Winters-Stone, K.; Zucker, D.S.; Gamble, G.L.; Alfano, C.M. Cancer Rehabilitation: An Overview of Current Need, Delivery Models, and Levels of Care. *Phys. Med. Rehabil. Clin. N. Am.* **2017**, *28*, 1–17. [CrossRef] [PubMed]
52. Marciniak, C.M.; Sliwa, J.A.; Spill, G.; Heinemann, A.W.; Semik, P.E. Functional Outcome Following Rehabilitation of the Cancer Patient. *Arch. Phys. Med. Rehabil.* **1996**, *77*, 54–57. [CrossRef] [PubMed]
53. Cobbe, S.; Kennedy, N. Physical Function in Hospice Patients and Physiotherapy Interventions: A Profile of Hospice Physiotherapy. *J. Palliat. Med.* **2012**, *15*, 760–767. [CrossRef]
54. Montagnini, M.; Lodhi, M.; Born, W. The Utilization of Physical Therapy in a Palliative Care Unit. *J. Palliat. Med.* **2003**, *6*, 11–17. [CrossRef]
55. Mueller, K.; Decker, I. Impact of Physical Therapy Intervention on Patient-Centered Outcomes in a Community Hospice. *Top. Geriatr. Rehabil.* **2011**, *27*, 2–9. [CrossRef]
56. Turner, F.; Seiger, C.; Devine, N. Impact of Patient and Caregiver Transfer Training Provided by a Physical Therapist in the Hospice Setting: A Case Study. *Am. J. Hosp. Palliat. Care* **2013**, *30*, 204–209. [CrossRef]

57. Smith, S.; Wilson, C.M.; Lipple, C.; Avromov, M.; Maltese, J.; Siwa, E.; Colombo, R.; Seidell, J.W. Managing Palliative Patients in Inpatient Rehabilitation Through a Short Stay Family Training Program. *Am. J. Hosp. Palliat. Care* **2020**, *37*, 172–178. [CrossRef]
58. Buss, T.; de Walden-Gałuszko, K.; Modlińska, A.; Osowicka, M.; Lichodziejewska-Niemierko, M.; Janiszewska, J. Kinesitherapy Alleviates Fatigue in Terminal Hospice Cancer Patients-an Experimental, Controlled Study. *Support. Care Cancer* **2010**, *18*, 743–749. [CrossRef]
59. Vira, P.; Samuel, S.R.; Amaravadi, S.K.; Saxena, P.P.; Rai Pv, S.; Kurian, J.R.; Gururaj, R. Role of Physiotherapy in Hospice Care of Patients with Advanced Cancer: A Systematic Review. *Am. J. Hosp. Palliat. Care* **2021**, *38*, 503–511. [CrossRef]
60. Smith, W.A.; Nolan, V.G.; Robison, L.L.; Hudson, M.M.; Ness, K.K. Physical Activity among Cancer Survivors and Those with No History of Cancer- a Report from the National Health and Nutrition Examination Survey 2003–2006. *Am. J. Transl. Res.* **2011**, 3, 342–350.
61. Kohler, L.N.; Garcia, D.O.; Harris, R.B.; Oren, E.; Roe, D.J.; Jacobs, E.T. Adherence to Diet and Physical Activity Cancer Prevention Guidelines and Cancer Outcomes: A Systematic Review. *Cancer Epidemiol. Biomark. Prev.* **2016**, *25*, 1018–1028. [CrossRef] [PubMed]
62. Gresham, G.; Schrack, J.; Gresham, L.M.; Shinde, A.M.; Hendifar, A.E.; Tuli, R.; Rimel, B.J.; Figlin, R.; Meinert, C.L.; Piantadosi, S. Wearable Activity Monitors in Oncology Trials: Current Use of an Emerging Technology. *Contemp. Clin. Trials* **2018**, *64*, 13–21. [CrossRef] [PubMed]
63. Stamatakis, E.; Ahmadi, M.; Murphy, M.H.; Chico, T.J.; Milton, K.; Del Pozo Cruz, B.; Katzmarzyk, P.T.; Lee, I.-M.; Gill, J. Journey of a Thousand Miles: From "Manpo-Kei" to the First Steps-Based Physical Activity Recommendations. *Br. J. Sports Med.* **2023**, *57*, 1227–1228. [CrossRef] [PubMed]
64. Cos, H.; Li, D.; Williams, G.; Chininis, J.; Dai, R.; Zhang, J.; Srivastava, R.; Raper, L.; Sanford, D.; Hawkins, W.; et al. Predicting Outcomes in Patients Undergoing Pancreatectomy Using Wearable Technology and Machine Learning: Prospective Cohort Study. *J. Med. Internet Res.* **2021**, *23*, e23595. [CrossRef]
65. Nakajima, H.; Yokoyama, Y.; Inoue, T.; Nagaya, M.; Mizuno, Y.; Kayamoto, A.; Nishida, Y.; Nagino, M. How Many Steps Per Day Are Necessary to Prevent Postoperative Complications Following Hepato-Pancreato-Biliary Surgeries for Malignancy? *Ann. Surg. Oncol.* **2020**, *27*, 1387–1397. [CrossRef]
66. Low, C.A.; Li, M.; Vega, J.; Durica, K.C.; Ferreira, D.; Tam, V.; Hogg, M.; Zeh Iii, H.; Doryab, A.; Dey, A.K. Digital Biomarkers of Symptom Burden Self-Reported by Perioperative Patients Undergoing Pancreatic Surgery: Prospective Longitudinal Study. *JMIR Cancer* **2021**, *7*, e27975. [CrossRef]
67. Steffens, D.; Solomon, M.J.; Beckenkamp, P.R.; Koh, C.E.; Yeo, D.; Sandroussi, C.; Fit-4-Home Collaborators; Hancock, M.J. Individualised, Targeted Step Count Intervention Following Gastrointestinal Cancer Surgery: The Fit-4-Home Randomised Clinical Trial. *ANZ J. Surg.* **2022**, *92*, 703–711. [CrossRef]
68. Gresham, G.; Liu, E.; Diniz, M.A.; Barnhill, K.; Nikravesh, N.; Welborn, A.; Shirazipour, C.; Asher, A.; Osipov, A.; Hendifar, A.E. Association between Remotely-Monitored Activity, Patient-Reported Outcomes, and Physical Function in Patients with Advanced Pancreatic Cancer. *JCO* **2022**, *40*, 1572. [CrossRef]

cancers

MDPI

Systematic Review

Gestational Diabetes Mellitus and Its Correlation in the Development of Pancreatic Cancer: A 10-Year Systematic Review

Sophia Tsokkou [1,2], Ioannis Konstantinidis [1], Maria-Nefeli Georgaki [1,3], Dimitrios Kavvadas [1,2], Kyriaki Papadopoulou [1,2], Antonios Keramas [1,2], Antonia Sioga [1,2], Theodora Papamitsou [1,2] and Sofia Karachrysafi [1,2,*]

1 Research Team "Histologistas", Interinstitutional Postgraduate Program "Health and Environmental Factors", Department of Medicine, Faculty of Health Sciences, Aristotle University of Thessaloniki, 54124 Thessaloniki, Greece; stsokkou@auth.gr (S.T.); ikonsc@auth.gr (I.K.); mgeorgaki@cheng.auth.gr (M.-N.G.); kavvadas@auth.gr (D.K.); kyriakinp@auth.gr (K.P.); antonios@auth.gr (A.K.); sioga@auth.gr (A.S.); thpapami@auth.gr (T.P.)

2 Laboratory of Histology-Embryology, Department of Medicine, Faculty of Health Sciences, Aristotle University of Thessaloniki, 54124 Thessaloniki, Greece

3 Environmental Engineering Laboratory, Department of Chemical Engineering, Aristotle University of Thessaloniki, 54124 Thessaloniki, Greece

* Correspondence: sofia_karachrysafi@outlook.com; Tel.: +30-6949414452

Simple Summary: The purpose of this systematic review was to investigate the correlation between gestational diabetes mellitus—the diabetes women experience during pregnancy—and the development of pancreatic cancer. Thus, for this research a 10-year literature review was conducted using the keywords "gestational diabetes mellitus", "pancreatic cancer" and "adenocarcinoma" in research databases such as PubMed, Scopus and ScienceDirect. After the exclusion criteria were added and the duplicates were removed, the articles were examined for their eligibility, and those suited for the study based on the degree of relevance were included. From the articles selected, the necessary data were extracted into tables, and the necessary information was summarized. Furthermore, a quality assessment was performed based on the type of study found, which revealed a high level of eligibility and related content, making the articles sufficient for us to conclude that gestational diabetes mellitus and pancreatic cancer are correlated.

Abstract: Purpose: Pancreatic cancer (PC) is a fatal malignancy with an aggressive course derived from the cells of pancreatic tissue. Gestational diabetes mellitus (GDM) is a state of spontaneous hyperglycemia occurring during gestation and has been suggested as a risk factor PC. Women with a history of GDM revealed a risk rate of 7.1% for the development of PC. The current systematic review aims to investigate the correlation between GDM and the degree to the prevalence of PC. Methodology: For this systematic review, the PICO model was prepared to construct and outline the exact questions of the study, a PRISMA flow diagram was prepared and quality assessment was conducted using the Newcastle Ottawa Scale (NOS) for Cohort Studies, the NIH Quality Assessment Tool-Criteria for Case Reports and the Cochrane quality assessment tool for Systematic Reviews and Meta-analysis studies. Result: A total of eight articles were retrieved from the main databases, and a table was created to summarize the information found. Even though the data found were limited, the quality assessment performed revealed that the articles were of high validity. Conclusions: It can be concluded that GDM has an association with the development of PC and can be considered as a risk factor.

Keywords: gestational diabetes mellitus; pancreatic cancer; adenocarcinoma

1. Introduction

Recent studies have shown high rates of development of pancreatic cancer (PC), especially in European countries, where its rise is predicted to be the second highest cause of mortality by 2030 [1]. Gestational diabetes mellitus (GDM) has been suggested as a risk factor for the development of PC. Women with a history of GDM revealed a risk rate of 7.1% for PC [2]. The current systematic review aims to investigate the correlation between GDM and the degree of the prevalence of PC.

1.1. Definition and Epidemiology of Pancreatic Cancer

Pancreatic cancer (PC) is a fatal malignancy with an aggressive course derived from cells of pancreatic tissue, mainly of the exocrine cells. PC is the tenth most common type of cancer and the third most common cause of cancer-related death in the United States, with an estimated 64,050 new diagnoses in the United States each year, accounting for 50,550 deaths in 2023 [3]. PC's mortality rate in Europe reached 17 per 100,000 women in 2022 and 22.3 per 100,000 in men, revealing a greater prevalence in the male population [4]. PC is more common with increasing age and has a median age at death at 72 years old based on 2016–2020 cases [3,5]. Approximately 1.7% of men and women are diagnosed with PC at some point during their lifetime, based on 2017–2019 data [3,5]. The most common type of pancreatic cancer is pancreatic duct adenocarcinoma (PDAC), which is responsible for 90% of cases worldwide [6]. PC's high mortality rate is attributed both to late diagnosis, since most patients do not develop symptoms until the disease reaches a more advanced stage, and to limited available responses to existing treatments [7].

Risk Factors of Pancreatic Cancer

Risk factors that are proved to be correlated with PC include both modifiable factors, such as heavy smoking, alcohol consumption, obesity, gut microbiome and Helicobacter pylori infection, and non-modifiable, such as age over 55 years, male sex, blood group, family history of diabetes, chronic pancreatitis cirrhosis of the liver, family history of PC and genetic susceptibility, which accounts for 5–10% of newly-diagnosed cases [8,9]. Diabetes mellitus of recent onset has been found to be one of the clinical manifestations of PC in 68% of the patients in a recent study [10] (Figure 1).

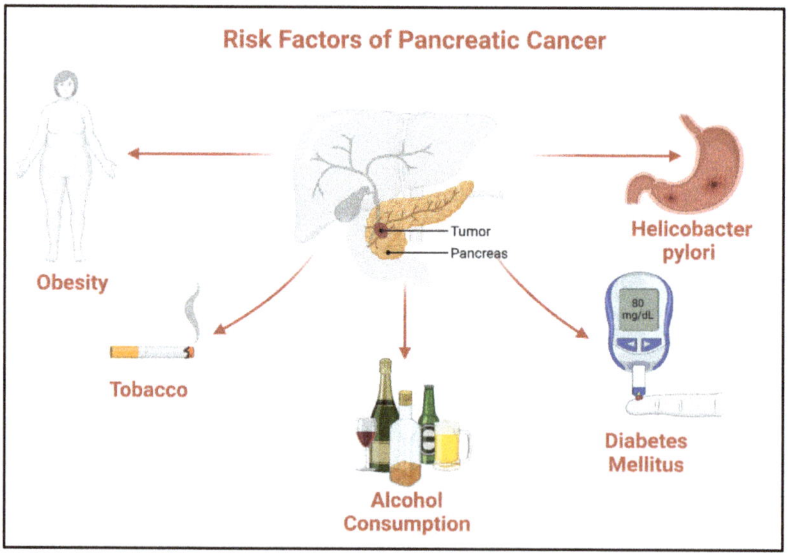

Figure 1. Risk factors of pancreatic cancer; created with BioRender.com [11].

1.2. Diabetes Mellitus

1.2.1. Diabetes Mellitus and Its Classification

By definition, diabetes mellitus (DM) is characterized as a "metabolic disease with highly elevated glucose levels in the bloodstream" [12]. In other words, it is a heterogeneous group of metabolic disturbances in the processes of the glucose metabolism with the key finding being chronic elevated blood glucose concentration (hyperglycemia) as a result of impaired secretion of insulin from pancreatic β-cells, impaired mechanisms of insulin action or both [13]. There are many classifications of DM including type 1 diabetes mellitus (T1DM), type 2 diabetes mellitus (T2DM), gestational diabetes mellitus (GDM), maturity-onset diabetes of the young (MODY), neonatal diabetes mellitus, Wolfram syndrome, type 3c diabetes, steroids-induced diabetes, cystic fibrosis diabetes, Alström Syndrome and latent autoimmune diabetes in adults (LADA) [14]. The three most common types are T1DM, T2DM and GDM. Firstly, T1DM is classified as an autoimmune disease caused by the destruction of β-cells that are responsible for the production of insulin, resulting in the long-term administration of insulin through daily injections, insulin pump therapy and automated insulin delivery systems [15]. Secondly, T2DM is considered the most common type of DM, and it accounts for 90% of cases. It is based on insulin resistance, especially in individuals of age greater than 45. However, in recent years, T2DM has become an increasing issue in children, adolescents and young adults. Thirdly, GDM is the state of spontaneous hyperglycemia occurring during gestation, commonly during the second and third trimesters of pregnancy [16]. It is referred to as a transient state of impaired glucose tolerance solely affecting women throughout pregnancy. Based on the American Diabetes Association (ADA), 10% of pregnancies are affected by GDM annually [17], but according to the most recent (2021) International Diabetes Federation (IDF) Diabetes Atlas, GDM affects approximately 21.1 million live births or 16.7% pregnancies worldwide annually [18].

1.2.2. Pathophysiology of Gestational Diabetes Mellitus

The cause of GDM is the result of various components including genetic and environmental factors, as well as hormonal contributors. During the gestational period, the increased concentration of progestins and estrogens—pregnancy-related hormones—results in slower gastric emptying and lower fasting glucose concentration. Thus, the tissues start to become less sensitive to insulin, leading to an increase in the postprandial glucose concentration (ideal values for women with GDM are fasting glucose $\leq$5–5.3 mmol/L (90–95 mg/dL) and either one-hour post-meal $\leq$ 7.8 mmol/L (140 mg/dL) or 2 h post-meal $\leq$ 6.7 mmol/L (120 mg/dL)) [19,20]. Under normal circumstances, pregnant women should secrete adequate insulin through pancreatic β-cells to make up for the difference in sensitivity of tissues, resulting in an equilibrium of a normoglycemic state; however, women with GDM are not able to secrete adequate insulin to compensate for the resistance, and thus insulin B receptors are unable to undergo tyrosine phosphitylation [21] (Figure 2).

1.2.3. Gestational Diabetes Mellitus Diagnosis

Testing for GDM is a standard screening procedure during the gestational period aiming for the early detection and regulation of affected women [22]. The American Diabetes Association (ADA) suggests that women should be screened between the 24th and 28th weeks of gestation unless they are in a low-risk category [17,22]—women age 25 and younger, of a low-risk race, with normal weight gain and no history of macrosomia [23]. There are two recommended approaches for screening during pregnancy during the 24th to 28th weeks. In the first approach, women are screened in a two-step process by measuring the plasma glucose levels 1 h after administration of 50 g of glucose. Women with a glucose concentration greater or equal to 130 and 140 undergo a 100 gm glucose tolerance test (OGTT) on another day. In the second approach, women are directly tested with 100 gm OGTT. The diagnosis is established by the Carpenter and Coustan criteria (Table 1). Firstly, venous blood is drawn when women are still in the fasting period; after glucose is provided to the women, venous blood is drawn every 1 h consecutively until 3 h are reached [23,24].

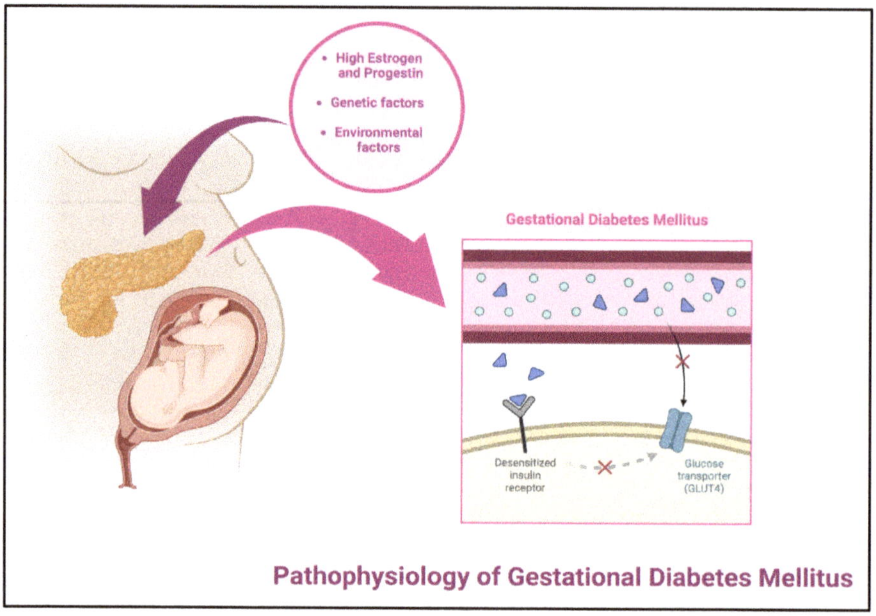

Figure 2. Pathophysiology of gestational diabetes mellitus; created with BioRender.com [11].

Table 1. Carpenter and Coustan criteria. If any 2 values are abnormal, then the patient is diagnosed as GDM.

Plasma Glucose Values (mg/dL)	
Fasting	95
1 h	180
2 h	150
3 h	140

1.2.4. Gestational Diabetes Mellitus—Maternal and Fetal Complications

GDM can have potential short- and long-term complications for both the mother and the infant. GDM can result in preterm births, leading, mainly, to respiratory distress syndrome due to insufficient or absent surfactant from the improper type II pneumonocytes and large for gestational age infants—fetal weight greater than 4000 gr, which increases the risk of proceeding with a C-section to avoid complications caused during vaginal birth, such as shoulder dystocia [25,26]. Other fetal complications include hyperbilirubinemia, neonatal hypoglycemia and hypocalcemia, polycythemia and increased perinatal mortality [27]. Regarding the mother, GDM increases the risk for high blood pressure, which, as a result, increases the likelihood for pre-eclampsia—a life-threatening complication for both the mother and the infant [26]. Studies suggest that women with a history of GDM have a greater risk in developing T2DM compared to women with normoglycemic pregnancies [19]. The risks for the transition from GDM to T2DM ranges between 3% and 70%; however the likelihood rises with women giving birth after the age of 30, birth weight of babies delivered being greater than 3.5 kg and undergoing insulin treatments throughout the gestational period [19,22]. Both T1DM and T2DM have been found to be highly associated with the development of various cancer types, with PC being one of them; however not a lot of studies have addressed the extent of the correlation between GDM and PC. In the current systematic review, the correlation between GDM and PC is examined, Figure 3.

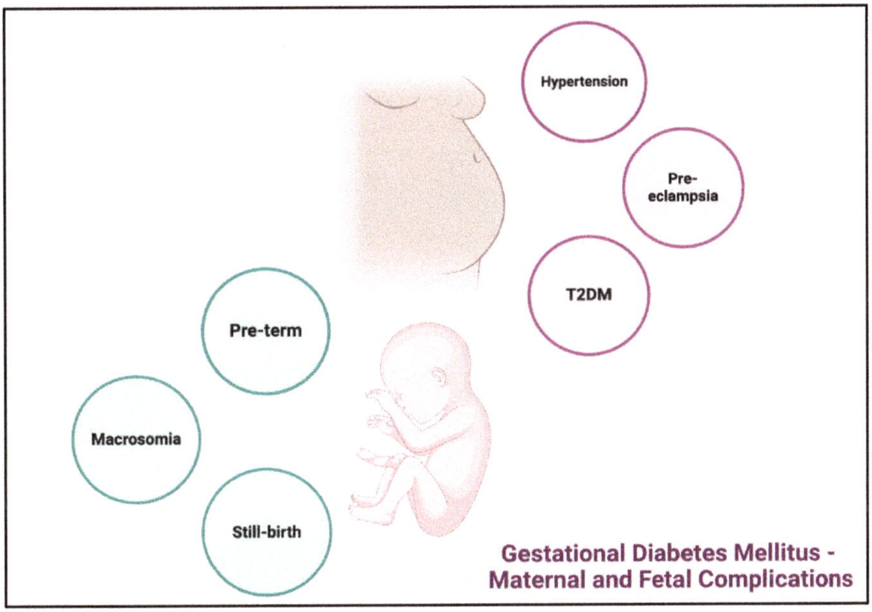

Figure 3. Maternal and fetal complications caused by gestational diabetes mellitus; created with BioRender.com [11].

2. Materials and Methods

2.1. PICO Model

For this systematic review, the PICO model was used to construct and outline the exact question of the study (Table 2), and the Preferred Reporting Items for Systematic Reviews and Meta-Analysis (PRISMA) guidelines were used for the extraction, screening and assessment of the relevant articles found. Additionally, quality assessment tables were prepared depending on the type of studies found, including, the Newcastle Ottawa Scale (NOS) for Cohort Studies, the NIH Quality Assessment Tool-Criteria for Case Reports and the Cochrane quality assessment tool for Systematic Reviews and Meta-analysis studies. The study has not been registered in PROSPERO.

Table 2. PICO table outlining Population (P), Intervention (I), Comparator (C) and Outcome (O).

PICO	
P	Pregnant women of no specific age or number of past pregnancies
I	Gestational diabetes mellitus
C	Pancreatic cancer
O	Gestational diabetes mellitus as a risk factor for the development of pancreatic cancer

2.2. PRISMA Flow Diagram

A PRISMA flow diagram was prepared using the code based on the keywords "((“pancreatic” OR “pancreas”) AND (“adenocarcinoma” OR “carcinoma” OR “adenocarcinomas” OR “carcinomas” OR “cancer” OR “cancers”)) AND ((“gestational diabetes mellitus”) OR (“GDM”))". The inclusion criteria included articles published within a 10-year duration (2014–2024), and review articles of the categories in the literature, both systematic reviews and meta-analyses, as well as case reports were chosen. The articles had to be written in

English and be available in the form of open access. The databases used were PubMed, Scopus and ScienceDirect. Initially, the total number of all articles found without the inclusion criteria were recorded. After the criteria were applied, the automation tools excluded the irrelevant articles, and the remaining articles were screened. Duplicated articles were excluded, and the articles were assessed and retrieved based on the degree of relevance from their titles, abstract and main-text information (Figure 4). A table was then prepared, including all relevant articles that were assessed and accepted as appropriate for this systematic review (Table 3).

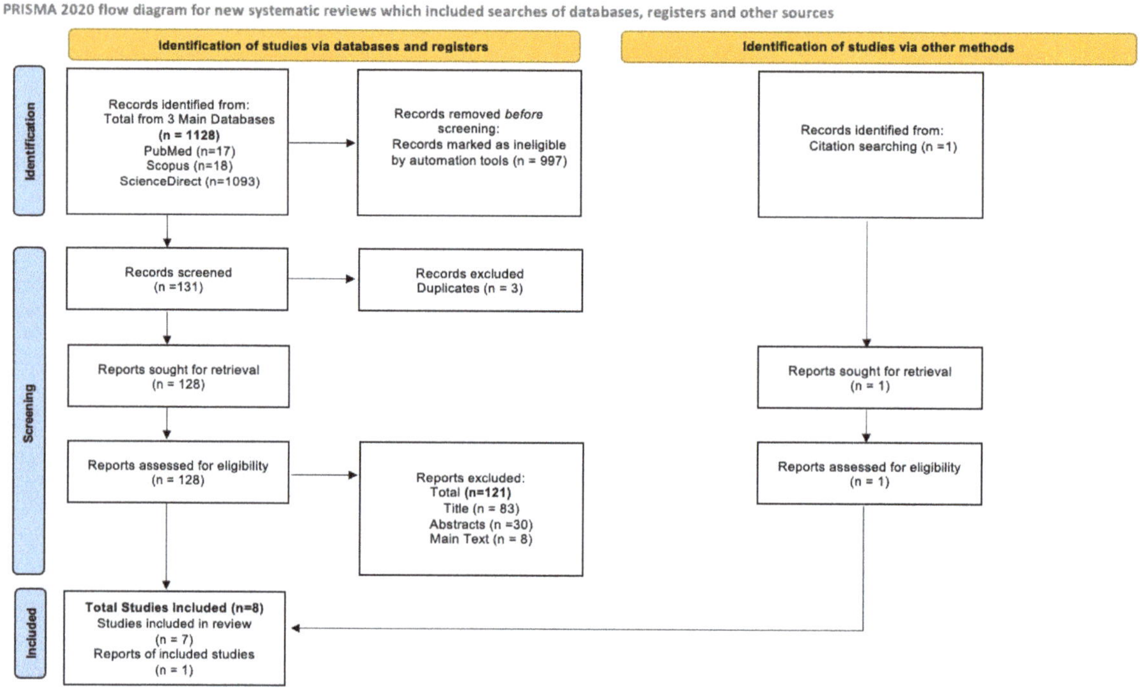

Figure 4. PRISMA Flow Diagram [28].

Table 3. Table summarizing the articles retrieved based on the PRISMA flow diagram. Abbreviations: gestational diabetes mellitus (GDM), pancreatic cancer (PC), type 2 diabetes mellitus (T2DM), diabetes mellitus (DM), polycystic ovarian syndrome (PCOS).

#	Authors	Type of Study	Risk Factor for GDM	Risk Factor for PC	Identification of GDM	Association between PC and GDM
1	Tong, G.-X., 2014 [29]	Systematic Review	Obesity	-	The unexpectedly high prevalence of hyperglycemia among cancer patients led investigators to suggest the use of blood glucose measurements as a new screening or diagnostic method for cancer.	Similar to DM, GDM seems to be related to pancreatic cancer. Five new pancreatic cancer cases were found in women with GDM history and forty-nine without history; the hazard ratio of GDM history was 7.1. Similar results observed in two studies.
2	Shi AW, 2018 [30]	Case report	GDM is reported to be increasing and is more common among African Americans, Hispanics, Asians and Native Americans than among non-Hispanic whites	GDM, HELLP syndrome, pulmonary hypertension and DIC in late pregnancy.	Known GDM before admitted to hospital.	Women with a history of gestational diabetes showed a relative risk of pancreatic cancer of 7.1. Studies showed that gestational diabetes mellitus could be one of the important risk factors for pancreatic cancer.
3	Peng et al., 2019 [31]	Cohort Study	Phenomenon increases with maternal age, obesity issues and decreases with daily physical activity	-	-	Women with GDM had a higher risk of developing PC in comparison with women who did not suffer from GDM, but the overall association was still low.
4	Wang Y, 2020 [32]	Systematic review and Meta-analysis	PCOS, maternal obesity or overweight, family history of type 2 diabetes mellitus (T2DM), prediabetes, previous history of fetal death and increased maternal age	-	Mixed identification methods for GDM from studies retrieved. Either self-reported, OGTT or glucose challenge test.	Two cohort studies found a significant positive association between GDM and pancreatic cancer risk, whereas another cohort study did not. Evidence of severe heterogeneity.
5	Quaresima P, 2021 [33]	Case report and Literature review	-	Obesity, heavy smoking, alcohol intake, history of diabetes, chronic pancreatitis, chronic cirrhosis, previous cholecystectomy and genetic predisposition, with approximately 5–10% of patients diagnosed with a pancreatic cancer having a family history of the disease. Presented with HELLP syndrome.	-	GDM shows a 7-fold increase in the risk of pancreatic cancer over the course of their lives.

Table 3. *Cont.*

#	Authors	Type of Study	Risk Factor for GDM	Risk Factor for PC	Identification of GDM	Association between PC and GDM
6	Simon J, 2021 [7]	Cohort study	-	Risk of PC increases by 80% in case of type 2 diabetes.	Before 2010, GDM screening was based on a two-step procedure for all women: the first test was on venous blood glucose 1 h after ingestion of 50 g of glucose, and in the event of a positive result, the second screening test was performed for oral glucose tolerance. Since 2010, recommended screening for these women is fasting blood glucose at the first prenatal consultation, and if it is not performed, an oral glucose tolerance test in the second trimester.	Over the eight years of follow-up, GDM was significantly associated with a higher risk of hospitalization with PC in the first and second Cox regression models adjusted for age and subsequent type 2 diabetes.
7	Choudhury AA, 2021 [34]	Literature Review	Insulin resistance, decreased chemerin levels, hereditary, reduced pancreatic insulin production similar to T2DM, obesity	-	Increased levels of glucose and C-reactive protein, lower levels of sex hormone-binding globulin and an increased chance of hyperinsulinemia when compared to pregnant women who do not have GDM.	It is reported that patients who have been diagnosed with DM are more likely to develop cancers such as pancreatic, colon, liver, kidney, bladder or BC. High linkage of GDM and development of cancer.
8	Slouha E, 2024 [35]	Systematic Review	Age, gestation, obesity and PCOS	-	Afamine, 1,5-anhydroglucitol and adiponectin markers.	Women with GDM have higher chances of developing breast, ovarian, cervical and uterine cancer and cancer in non-reproductive organs, like thyroid and pancreas.

2.3. Methodological Quality Assessment

Moreover, a quality assessment was performed to examine and evaluate the accuracy and quality of each article. The Newcastle Ottawa Scale (NOS) was used to evaluate the quality of cohort studies—with the lowest score being 0 and the highest being 8. The NIH quality assessment tool was used for the evaluation of case reports—0 being the lowest and the highest being 9. Lastly, the Cochrane quality assessment tool was used for systematic reviews and meta-analysis articles—with scores of 0 being the lowest and 7 the highest (Tables 4–6).

Table 4. Assessment of methodological quality of cohort studies, according to the adapted Newcastle Ottawa Scale (NOS).

References	Selection				Comparability		Outcome		Total Quality Score
	Representativeness of Exposed Cohort	Sample Size	Ascertainment of Exposure	Non-Respondents	Adjust for the Most Important Risk Factors	Adjust for Other Risk Factors	Assessment of Outcome	Statistical Test	
Peng et al., 2019 [31]	1	1	1	1	1	1	1	0	7
Simon J, 2021 [7]	1	1	1	1	1	1	0	1	7

Methodological quality classification based on total score: <5: low quality; 5–7: moderate quality; >7 high quality.

Table 5. Assessment of methodological quality of case reports, according to the adapted NIH quality assessment tool.

Reference	NIH Quality Assessment Tool-Criteria									
	Q'1	Q'2	Q'3	Q'4	Q'5	Q'6	Q'7	Q'8	Q'9	Total Quality Score
Quaresima P, 2021 [33]	1	1	1	1	0	0	0	0	0	4
Shi AW, 2018 [30]	1	1	0	1	0	1	1	0	0	5

Question 1: Research question clearly stated. Question 2: Study population clearly defined. Question 3: Participation rate of eligible persons at least 50%. Question 4: Uniform eligibility criteria across all participants. Question 5: Sample size justification. Question 6: Evaluating different levels of exposure. Question 7: Independent variables clearly defined and implemented consistently. Question 8: Statistical methods were well-described and confounding variables considered. Question 9: Outcome measures were clearly defined and results well-described. Methodological quality classification based on total score: Good: 7–9 criteria; Fair: 4–6 criteria; Poor: 0–3 criteria.

Table 6. Reporting the quality/risk of bias with Cochrane risk bias tool.

Author and Year	Random Sequence Generation	Allocation Conceal-ment	Participant and Personnel Blinding	Outcome Assessment Blinding	Incomplete Outcome Data and Biased Reporting	Further Biased Sources	Total Score
Tong, G.-X., 2014 [29]	+	+	+	+	+	+	6
Wang Y., 2020 [32]	+	-	?	?	+	-	2
Slouha E., 2024 [35]	+	+	?	+	+	+	5

Low risk of bias (+); High risk of bias (-); Unclear risk of bias (?).

3. Results

3.1. PRISMA Flow Diagram

Firstly, the total number of articles found without applying the criteria was recorded for all three databases. The total number of articles found was 1128, with 17 being from PubMed, 18 from Scopus and 1093 from ScienceDirect. After the criteria were applied—10-year publication window, review articles (literature, systematic and meta-analyses) and case reports, open access and published in the English language—997 articles were excluded as ineligible by the automation tools. Thus, 131 articles were recorded and screened. Moving on, 3 articles were excluded as they were duplicates, and 128 were evaluated. From those, a total of 121 articles were excluded for the following reasons—83 articles were excluded due to low relevance based on their titles, 30 from the content of their abstracts and 8 from the content of their main text. The articles were evaluated using the process of double-blind assessment—being evaluated by two different reviewers independently to eliminate bias of decision. One article was included from citations and a total of eight articles were included.

A table [Table 2] was then prepared to summarize the finding of those eight articles with the following categories: authors, risk factors of development of GDM, risk factors of development of PC, identification of GDM and, lastly, association between GDM and PC.

3.2. Methodological Quality Assessment

Additionally, three different quality assessments were prepared including the Newcastle Ottawa Scale (NOS), the NIH quality assessment criteria tool and the Cochrane risk bias tool.

3.2.1. Newcastle Ottawa Scale (NOS)

Firstly, the NOS is used to assess the quality and validity of non-randomized studies (case control and cohort studies). For this systematic review, two cohort studies—Peng et al. [31] and Simon J. [7]—were examined using the scale of 0 to 7 (0 being the lowest quality and 7 the highest). For the Selection category, both studies clearly stated the goal of their study and included an adequate sample size to support the research they wanted to conduct. Regarding the comparability, both studies included a control group for accurate comparison with the study group. Moreover, both groups included possible risk factors that might interfere or be a complication of GDM. However, for the Peng et al. [31] study, no statistical test was provided in comparison with the Simon J. [7] study, and Simon J.'s [7] study did not provide sufficient information on the outcome regarding the correlation between GDM and PC. Both studies received a score of 7 out of 8, suggesting that the quality and validity of their study accurate (Table 4).

3.2.2. NIH Quality Assessment Tool

The NIH quality assessment tool was used for the evaluation and methodological assessment of case reports. The score range is from 0 to 9; a score of 0 to 3 is classified as "poor", 4 to 6 as "fair" and 7 to 9 as "good". In this systematic review, two case reports were examined, including the studies of Quaresma P. and Shi A.W. [30,33]. In both studies, the research question was clearly stated, and the population sample was clearly defined. In the study of Quaresma P. [33], the participation rate was considered eligible as more than 50% of the population remained until the end of the study, and there was a uniform eligibility across all participants. The study received a total score of 4, entering the "fair" category. The Shi A.W. [30] study included a uniform eligibility criterion for all participants and evaluated the different levels of exposure among the population. The independent variables clearly defined and implemented consistently and thus the study received a total score of 5, again falling into the "fair" category. The studies overall received a moderate score (Table 5).

3.2.3. Cochrane Risk Bias Tool

For the Cochrane risk bias tool, three systematic reviews and meta-analysis studies were included: Tong G.-X., Wang Y. and Slouha E [29,32,35]. Six domains were used to classify and rate the context of each study with the following information, random sequence generation, allocation concealment, participant and personnel blinding, outcome assessment blinding, incomplete outcome data and biased reporting and further biased sources. The bias was assessed using the following criteria: high, low and unclear. The study of Tong G.-X [29] received the highest score of the three, which was 6, as it included all relevant information. The study of Slouha E. [35] received a score of 5, and the study of Wang Y. [32] received the lowest score of 2 (Table 6).

4. Discussion

Based on the systematic research conducted, data collected using the PRISMA guidelines and PICO model, the following results can be stated from the information summarized in Table 3.

4.1. Risk Factors for the Development of Gestational Diabetes Mellitus

Firstly, three out of the eight studies, namely Slouha E, Peng et al. and Wang Y, [31,32,35], concluded that increased maternal age increases the risk of development of GDM, and four out of eight studies, namely Slouha E, Peng et al., Quaresima, Wang Y and Tong G.-X., [29,31,33,35], stated that higher maternal weight and obesity are contributors to higher risks in the development of GDM. Based on the studies retrieved, it can be stated that the reason for this correlation might be due to higher nutrient intake, greater circulating adipokine and greater oxidative stress among pregnant women in advanced maternal stage [36]. The studies of Wang Y. and Slouha E. [32,35], stated that except for obesity and increased maternal age, PCOS as well as family history of T2DM, prediabetes and previous history of fetal death can also play an important role in the development of GDM [32].

4.2. Risk Factors for the Development of Pancreatic Cancer

Moreover, the study of Shi A.W. [30] states that the risk factors for PC are GDM, HELLP syndrome hemolysis, elevated liver enzymes and low platelets, a complication considered as a variant of pre-eclampsia [37], pulmonary hypertension and disseminated intravascular coagulation (DIC) in late pregnancy. Furthermore, the study of Quaresima P. [33] stated that obesity, heavy smoking, alcohol intake, history of diabetes, chronic pancreatitis, chronic cirrhosis, history of cholecystectomy and genetic predisposition for PC have an estimated rate of 5–10% of patients being diagnosed with PC. Additionally, HELLP syndrome was again identified as a risk factor. The study of Simon J. [7] states that the risk of PC increases by 80% in the case of type 2 diabetes.

4.3. Association of Gestational Diabetes Mellitus and Development of Pancreatic Cancer

When it comes to the association of GDM and the development of PC, the study of Tong, G.-X. [29] states that in the same manner that DM is related to PC, GDM can have the same impact. The study mentions five new pancreatic cancer cases being found in women with history of GDM and 49 without a GDM history, thus estimating the hazard ratio of GDM history being 7.1. The study of Shi A.W. [30] notes the same risk association showing that GDM can an important risk factor for the development of PC. Additionally, the study of Peng et al. [31] states that women with GDM had a higher risk of developing PC in comparison with women who did not suffer from GDM. However, the overall association was still low. Furthermore, the study of Wang Y. [32] showed that two cohort studies found a significant a positive association between GDM and risk of PC, whereas another cohort study did not. In the study by Quaresima P. [33], GDM showed a 7-fold increase in the risk of PC over the course of the women's lives. Moreover, the study of Simon J. [7] concluded that over the eight years of follow-up, women with GDM were significantly associated with a higher risk of hospitalization with PC. Moving on, the study of Choudhury AA [34] reports that patients who have been diagnosed with DM are more likely to develop cancers such as pancreatic, colon, liver, kidney and bladder cancer, and a high linkage of GDM and development of cancer can be observed. Lastly, the study of Slouha E [35] states that women with GDM have higher chances of developing breast, ovarian, cervical and uterine cancer, as well as cancer in non-reproductive organs, like the thyroid and pancreas.

5. Conclusions

Thus, based on the data examined, it can be concluded that GDM has an association with the development of PC and can be considered as a risk factor. A major set-back to this study was the limited data found, as this topic is not widely examined. However, based on the data collected and the quality assessments performed, the studies found are credible and valid enough to support the correlation and linkage between GDM and the development of PC.

Author Contributions: Conceptualization, S.T. and S.K.; methodology, S.T.; software, S.T.; validation, S.T., K.P. and D.K.; formal analysis, S.T. and M.-N.G.; investigation, S.T. and I.K.; resources, S.T. and I.K.; data curation, S.T., M.-N.G. and A.K. writing—original draft preparation, S.T.; writing—review and editing, S.T., I.K., S.K., T.P. and A.S.; visualization, S.T.; supervision, S.K.; project administration, S.K. All authors have read and agreed to the published version of the manuscript.

Funding: This research received no external funding.

Conflicts of Interest: The authors declare no conflicts of interest.

References

1. Harris, S. Europe Is Facing a Pancreatic Cancer Emergency. *Medscape*, 25 January 2024.
2. Perrin, M.; Terry, M.; Kleinhaus, K.; Deutsch, L.; Yanetz, R.; Tiram, E.; Calderon, R.; Friedlander, Y.; Paltiel, O.; Harlap, S Gestational diabetes as a risk factor for pancreatic cancer: A prospective cohort study. *BMC Med.* **2007**, *5*, 25. [CrossRef]
3. Stoffel, E.M.; Brand, R.E.; Goggins, M. Pancreatic Cancer: Changing Epidemiology and New Approaches to Risk Assessment Early Detection, and Prevention. *Gastroenterology* **2023**, *164*, 752–765. [CrossRef]
4. Gagliardi, J. *Mortality Rate of Pancreatic Cancer in Europe in 2022, by Country and Gender*; Health Pharma Medtech: Washington, DC USA, 2024.
5. *Cancer Stat Facts: Pancreatic Cancer*; NIH, National Cancer Institute: Bethesda, MD, USA, 2024.
6. Sarantis, P.; Koustas, E.; Papadimitropoulou, A.; Papavassiliou, A.G.; Karamouzis, M.V. Pancreatic ductal adenocarcinoma Treatment hurdles, tumor microenvironment and immunotherapy. *World J. Gastrointest. Oncol.* **2020**, *12*, 173–181. [CrossRef [PubMed]
7. Simon, J.; Goueslard, K.; Arveux, P.; Bechraoui-Quantin, S.; Petit, J.-M.; Quantin, C. Increased Risk of Hospitalization for Pancreatic Cancer in the First 8 Years after a Gestational Diabetes Mellitus regardless of Subsequent Type 2 Diabetes: A Nationwide Population-Based Study. *Cancers* **2021**, *13*, 308. [CrossRef]
8. McGuigan, A.; Kelly, P.; Turkington, R.C.; Jones, C.; Coleman, H.G.; McCain, R.S. Pancreatic cancer: A review of clinical diagnosis epidemiology, treatment, and outcomes. *World J. Gastroenterol.* **2018**, *24*, 4846–4861. [CrossRef] [PubMed]
9. Zhao, Z.; Liu, W. Pancreatic Cancer: A Review of Risk Factors, Diagnosis, and Treatment. *Technol. Cancer Res. Treat.* **2020**, *19* 1533033820962117. [CrossRef]
10. Roy, A.; Sahoo, J.; Kamalanathan, S.; Naik, D.; Mohan, P.; Kalayarasan, R. Diabetes and pancreatic cancer: Exploring the two-way traffic. *World J. Gastroenterol.* **2021**, *27*, 4939–4962. [CrossRef] [PubMed]
11. BioRender n.d. Available online: https://app.biorender.com/illustrations/65ff040d4603630b1370a481 (accessed on 25 March 2024).
12. Sapra, A.; Bhandari, P. Diabetes. In *StatPearls*; StatPearls Publishing: St. Petersburg, FL, USA, 2023.
13. Kerner, W.; Brückel, J. Definition, Classification and Diagnosis of Diabetes Mellitus. *Exp. Clin. Endocrinol. Diabetes* **2014**, *122* 384–386. [CrossRef]
14. *Types of Diabetes*; Diabetes UK: London, UK, 2019.
15. Lucier, J.; Weinstock, R.S. Type 1 Diabetes. In *StatPearls*; StatPearls Publishing: St. Petersburg, FL, USA, 2023.
16. Goyal, R.; Singhal, M.; Jialal, I. Type 2 Diabetes. In *StatPearls*; StatPearls Publishing: St. Petersburg, FL, USA, 2023.
17. Blogger, G. *Keeping Mom and Child Healthy after Gestational Diabetes Mellitus*; American Diabetes Association: Arlington, VA, USA 2024.
18. *IDF Diabetes Atlas*, 10th ed.; n.d.; Available online: https://idf.org/about-diabetes/diabetes-facts-figures/ (accessed on 7 May 2024).
19. Rph, C.L.I.; Tinong, R.T. The Incidence and Management of Type 2 Diabetes Mellitus after Gestational Diabetes Mellitus. *Cureus* **2023**, *15*, e44468. [CrossRef]
20. Alfadhli, E.M. Gestational diabetes mellitus. *Saudi Med. J.* **2015**, *36*, 399–406. [CrossRef]
21. Reece, E.A.; Leguizamón, G.; Wiznitzer, A. Gestational diabetes: The need for a common ground. *Lancet* **2009**, *373*, 1789–1797 [CrossRef] [PubMed]
22. Buchanan, T.A.; Xiang, A.H.; Page, K.A. Gestational diabetes mellitus: Risks and management during and after pregnancy. *Nat Rev. Endocrinol.* **2012**, *8*, 639–649. [CrossRef] [PubMed]
23. Mumtaz, M. Gestational Diabetes Mellitus. *Malays. J. Med. Sci.* **2000**, *7*, 4–9. [PubMed]
24. Naik, R.R.; Pednekar, G.; Cacodcar, J. Incidence and risk factors of gestational diabetes mellitus in antenatal mothers in Goa India. *Int. J. Reprod. Contracept. Obstet. Gynecol.* **2019**, *8*, 586. [CrossRef]
25. By Mayo Clinic Staff. *Fetal Macrosomia*; Mayo Clinic: Rochester, MN, USA, 2022.
26. By Mayo Clinic Staff. *Gestational Diabetes*; Mayo Clinic: Rochester, MN, USA, 2022.
27. Senat, M.-V.; Deruelle, P. Le diabète gestationnel. *Gynecol. Obstet. Fertil.* **2016**, *44*, 244–247. [CrossRef] [PubMed]

28. Preferred Reporting Items for Systematic Reviews and Meta-Analyses (PRISMA). 2024. Available online: https://www.prisma-statement.org/ (accessed on 7 May 2024).
29. Tong, G.-X.; Cheng, J.; Chai, J.; Geng, Q.-Q.; Chen, P.-L.; Shen, X.-R.; Liang, H.; Wang, D.-B. Association Between Gestational Diabetes Mellitus and Subsequent Risk of Cancer: A Systematic Review of Epidemiological Studies. *Asian Pac. J. Cancer Prev.* **2014**, *15*, 4265–4269. [CrossRef] [PubMed]
30. Shi, A.-W.; Shen, X.-F.; Ding, H.-J.; Liu, Y.-Q.; Meng, L.; Kalionis, B. Pancreatic carcinoma underlying a complex presentation in late pregnancy: A case report. *J. Med. Case Rep.* **2018**, *12*, 369. [CrossRef] [PubMed]
31. Peng, Y.-S.; Lin, J.-R.; Cheng, B.-H.; Ho, C.; Lin, Y.-H.; Shen, C.-H.; Tsai, M.-H. Incidence and relative risk for developing cancers in women with gestational diabetes mellitus: A nationwide cohort study in Taiwan. *BMJ Open* **2019**, *9*, e024583. [CrossRef] [PubMed]
32. Wang, Y.; Yan, P.; Fu, T.; Yuan, J.; Yang, G.; Liu, Y.; Zhang, Z.-J. The association between gestational diabetes mellitus and cancer in women: A systematic review and meta-analysis of observational studies. *Diabetes Metab.* **2020**, *46*, 461–471. [CrossRef]
33. Quaresima, P.; Saccone, G.; Pellegrino, R.; Vaccarisi, S.; Taranto, L.; Mazzulla, R.; Bernardo, S.; Venturella, R.; Di Carlo, C.; Morelli, M. Incidental diagnosis of a pancreatic adenocarcinoma in a woman affected by gestational diabetes mellitus: Case report and literature review. *Am. J. Obstet. Gynecol. MFM* **2021**, *3*, 100471. [CrossRef]
34. Choudhury, A.A.; Devi Rajeswari, V. Gestational diabetes mellitus—A metabolic and reproductive disorder. *Biomed. Pharmacother.* **2021**, *143*, 112183. [CrossRef] [PubMed]
35. Slouha, E.; Gates, K.M.; Al-Geizi, H.; Baah, E.; Clunes, L.A.; Kollias, T.F. The Relationship Between Gestational Diabetes and the Risk of Cancer: A Systematic Review. *Cureus* **2024**, *16*, e53328. [CrossRef] [PubMed]
36. Sun, M.; Luo, M.; Wang, T.; Wei, J.; Zhang, S.; Shu, J.; Zhong, T.; Liu, Y.; Chen, Q.; Zhu, P.; et al. Effect of the interaction between advanced maternal age and pre-pregnancy BMI on pre-eclampsia and GDM in Central China. *BMJ Open Diabetes Res. Care* **2023**, *11*, e003324. [CrossRef] [PubMed]
37. Weinstein, L. What Is Hellp Syndrome? Pre-Eclampsia Foundation, 2023. Available online: https://www.preeclampsia.org/hellp-syndrome (accessed on 7 May 2024).

MDPI AG
Grosspeteranlage 5
4052 Basel
Switzerland
Tel.: +41 61 683 77 34

Cancers Editorial Office
E-mail: cancers@mdpi.com
www.mdpi.com/journal/cancers

www.ingramcontent.com/pod-product-compliance
Lightning Source LLC
Chambersburg PA
CBHW061554220926
51850CB00005B/336
* 9 7 8 3 7 2 5 8 6 0 6 9 2 *